# Practical Otorhinolaryngology - Head and Neck Surgery

Zhonglin Mu • Jugao Fang
Editors

# Practical Otorhinolaryngology - Head and Neck Surgery

## Diagnosis and Treatment

PMPH PEOPLE'S MEDICAL PUBLISHING HOUSE

Springer

*Editors*
Zhonglin Mu
Department of Otorhinolaryngology
Head and Neck Surgery
The First Affiliated Hospital of Hainan
Medical University
Haikou
China

Jugao Fang
Department of Otorhinolaryngology
Head and Neck Surgery
Beijing Tongren Hospital
Capital Medical University
Beijing
China

ISBN 978-981-13-7992-5 ISBN 978-981-13-7993-2 (eBook)
https://doi.org/10.1007/978-981-13-7993-2



This Springer imprint is published by the registered company Springer Nature Singapore Pte Ltd.
The registered company address is: 152 Beach Road, #21-01/04 Gateway East, Singapore 189721, Singapore

# Preface

As science grows, imageology, endoscopic technology, and new materials are widely used. The development of medical imageology, such as the more realistic 3D and HD imaging, simulates endoscopy, actual dynamic images, the 3D HD quality toward-anatomy imaging; as the molecular biology continues to deepen, the diagnosis and treatment of the hereditary deaf and other genetic diseases have made great progress. A variety of implantable artificial hearing aid devices are gradually been applied in the clinic now. The continuous development of new technologies which have reflected tissues and organs' functional and molecular information, and the bioinformatics are widely used, contributing an important role in the development of this subject's medical precision. These achievements mentioned above inspire us to edit this book with strong desire.

During the compilation of this book, we always obey the "five attributes" (ideological, scientific, advancement, enlightenment, and practicability) and "three bases" (basic theory, basic knowledge, and basic skills) principle. We try to expand and improve the basic skills of clinicians at a professional level. Therefore, we refer to the classic teaching materials and the literatures in the field of otorhinolaryngology head and neck surgery both in China and abroad and strive to make it a concise book, with a clear structure and illustrations (with more than 300 pictures and 12 operation videos) to reflect the characteristics of the current times. Also, we are working toward perfection with our professional knowledge, will greatly appreciate for cooperation specialists.

China — Zhonglin Mu
China — Jugao Fang
30 June 2020

# Acknowledgements

The book is translated and revised by experts with clinical, teaching and scientific research background. In particular, I would like to express my sincere gratitude to those scholars for their outstanding contributions in writing and translation: Arthur Clement; Chaowei Zhang; Dian Wang; Emmanuel Costantine Makale; Hao Ruan; Jie Song; Joseph Akparibila Azure; Jiayi Tang; Koranteng Collins Osei; Lei Zang; Liping Wang; Nambalirwa Mary; Shun Ding; Weiqun Hu; Xiaoyong Han; Xiaohua Cheng; Ying Zhao; Yilong Wang; Zhengyang Xu.

# Contents

# Editors and Contributors

## About the Editors

**Zhonglin Mu** is a chief physician, professor, and doctoral adviser. He is mainly engaged in basic and clinical aspects of otology and rhinology, established the Department of Otorhinolaryngology Head and Neck Surgery of Hainan Provincial Hospital. His innovations enabled people in Hainan Province to experience the best services of otorhinolaryngologist.

At 2010, he was awarded the State Council Special Prize for a key expert in Hainan for his outstanding contribution to Hainan Province. He was the third-term chairman of the Otorhinolaryngology Head and Neck Surgery Association in Hainan Province; he was the first chairman of Otorhinolaryngology Physicians Association of Hainan Province. In addition, he has made outstanding contributions to the development of 2012 Hainan high-tech technological industry.

He has participated in writing nine books: 7-year national senior medical clinical medicine's professional teaching material (Otorhinolaryngology Head and Surgery), 5-year medical teaching material (Otorhinolaryngology Head and Neck surgery). His several articles were published at American Acta and other authoritative journals.

**Jugao Fang** is a chief physician, professor, and doctoral adviser, director of the Department of Otorhinolaryngology Head and Neck Surgery, Beijing Tongren Hospital, Capital Medical University.

He studied at renowned international Sloan Kettering Cancer Center in New York and later at American Houston MD Anderson Cancer Center. Furthermore, clinical head and neck tumors are his main occupational field, endoscopic surgeries and functional operations on tumors at head, neck, nose, and skull base and thyroid surgeries are all where he masters. In addition, he was honored as one of the "Top 10 China Doctors" for head and neck surgery and thyroid surgery. Apart from these, over 100 articles were published by him, containing over 40 articles collected in SCI. He is also a chief editor for over 10 books and a contributor of two Senior Otorhinolaryngology Head and Neck Surgery teaching materials. He has obtained several provincial science progress awards. Several national topics funded by China National Science Foundation and other resources were published by him. He is the vice-chairman of China Otorhinolaryngology, Head and Neck Surgery Association of, vice-Chairman of China Medical Association, vice secretory-general of the China Anti-cancer Association Head and Neck Tumor Professional Council Standing Committee, councilor of the China Disability Restoration Association, secretary-general of the Anti-laryngeal Cancer Restoration Professional Council and the executive director of the China Medical Health Promotion Association. He is also an editorial board member of some magazines, including the Chinese National Otorhinolaryngology Head and Neck Surgery, the China Otorhinolaryngology, Head and Neck surgery, the International Surgery, and the International Otorhinolaryngology.

## Contributors

**Xun Bi** Department of Pediatric Surgery, The First Affiliated Hospital of Hainan Medical University, Haikou, China

**Saiming Chen** Department of Otorhinolaryngology Head and Neck Surgery, The First Affiliated Hospital of Hainan Medical University, Haikou, China

**Xiaohua Cheng** Beijing Institute of Otolaryngology, Beijing Tongren Hospital, Capital Medical University, Beijing, China

**Jugao Fang** Department of Otorhinolaryngology Head and Neck Surgery, Beijing Tongren Hospital, Capital Medical University, Beijing, China

**Bo Feng** Department of Otorhinolaryngology Head and Neck Surgery, Chinese People's Liberation Army (CPLA) General Hospital, Beijing, China

**Yong Feng** Department of Otorhinolaryngology Head and Neck Surgery, Xiangya Hospital, Central South University, Changsha, China

**Yongjun Feng** Department of Otorhinolaryngology Head and Neck Surgery, The Second Affiliated Hospital of Hainan Medical University, Haikou, China

**Qiyi He** Department of Otorhinolaryngology Head and Neck Surgery, The Second Affiliated Hospital of Hainan Medical University, Haikou, China

**Jiajun Huang** Department of Otorhinolaryngology Head and Neck Surgery, The First Affiliated Hospital of Hainan Medical University, Haikou, China

**Jihong Huang** Department of Otorhinolaryngology Head and Neck Surgery, The First Affiliated Hospital of Hainan Medical University, Haikou, China

**Lihui Huang** Beijing Institute of Otolaryngology, Beijing Tongren Hospital, Capital Medical University, Beijing, China

**Lu Jiang** Department of Otorhinolaryngology Head and Neck Surgery, Xiangya Hospital, Central South University, Changsha, China

**Zhiqun Li** Department of Medical Imaging, The First Affiliated Hospital of Hainan Medical University, Haikou, China

**Dasong Lu** Department of Otorhinolaryngology Head and Neck Surgery, The Second Affiliated Hospital of Hainan Medical University, Haikou, China

**Xiaohui Mi** Department of Otorhinolaryngology Head and Neck Surgery, Chinese People's Liberation Army 91458 Military Hospital, Sanya, China

**Zhonglin Mu** Department of Otorhinolaryngology Head and Neck Surgery, The First Affiliated Hospital of Hainan Medical University, Haikou, China

**Rong Tu** Department of Medical Imaging, The First Affiliated Hospital of Hainan Medical University, Haikou, China

**Jianghua Wan** Department of Medical Imaging, The First Affiliated Hospital of Hainan Medical University, Haikou, China

**Xiaofeng Wang** Department of Otorhinolaryngology Head and Neck Surgery, The First Affiliated Hospital of Hainan Medical University, Haikou, China

**Xin Wei** Department of Otorhinolaryngology Head and Neck Surgery, Hainan People's Hospital, Haikou, China

**Desheng Xian** Department of Otorhinolaryngology Head and Neck Surgery, The First Affiliated Hospital of Hainan Medical University, Haikou, China

**Xiaoguang You** Department of Medical Imaging, The First Affiliated Hospital of Hainan Medical University, Haikou, China

**Xuejun Zhou** Department of Otorhinolaryngology Head and Neck Surgery, The First Affiliated Hospital of Hainan Medical University, Haikou, China

# Part I

# Otorhinolaryngology Head and Neck Surgery Pandect

With advances in science and technology and wide application of endoscopy, new materials and multidisciplinary integration, Otorhinolaryngology has evolved into Otorhinolaryngology Head and Neck Surgery. As a second clinical medical discipline, it mainly deals with the study of researching anatomy, physiology and diseases at auditory, balance, olfactory and other sensory organs and respiratory, swallowing, phonation, language and other organs. This chapter will introduce the application of the commonly used examination equipments, the imaging examination, the commonly used drugs, the common therapeutic technology, the robotic surgery system and the video navigation technology in otorhinolaryngology skull base surgery.

# 1 Common ENT Examination Equipment

Bo Feng, Xiaohui Mi, Xun Bi and Zhonglin Mu

## 1.1 General Examination Equipment

Currently, basic Otorhinolaryngology equipments include: light source, frontal mirror (headlight), otoscope, tuning fork, anterior rhinoscope, posterior rhino-scope, indirect laryngoscope, gun-shaped forceps, geniculate forceps, cerumen hook, spatula (tongue depressor), spray bottle or watering can, etc.

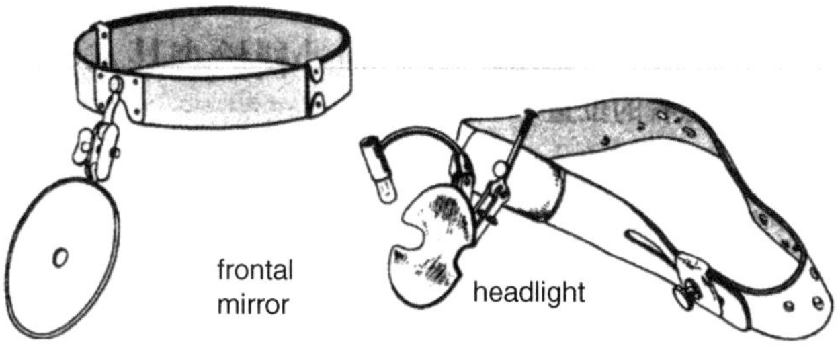


**Fig. 1.1** Frontal and headlamps

### 1.1.1 Frontal Mirror

Frontal mirror is a round concave condenser, it's generally 7.5 cm in diameter, 25–30 cm in focal length and about 1.25 cm in central peephole. It is used at bedside in operation. Its focusing is the main function for application (Fig. 1.1). The light source is projected onto the frontal mirror surface. After the light is reflected and focused on the inspection site, then inspectors observe the focused area through the mirror hole (Fig. 1.2).

Before wearing the glasses, firstly, adjust the tightness of the double-spherical joints appropriately to ensure the mirror flexible and not slippery to fall down. Secondly, wear the frontal mirror over the head and straighten the double spherical joints to ensure the mirror and the frontal plane parallel to

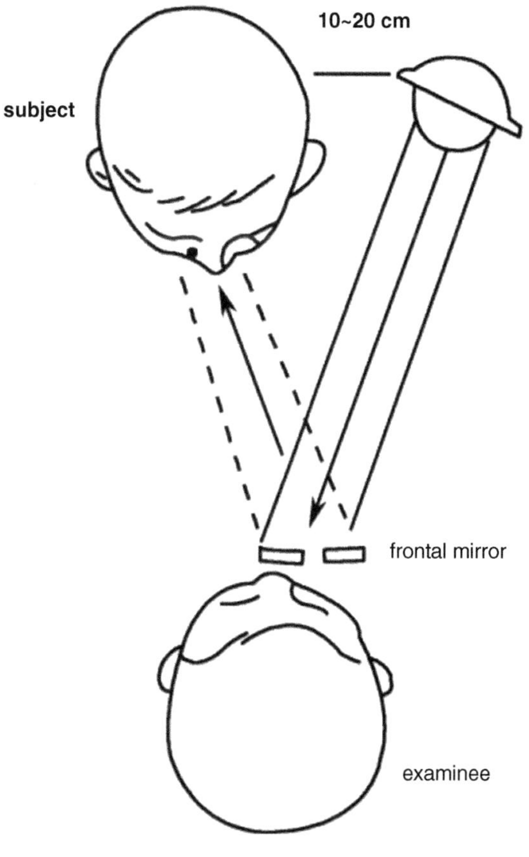


**Fig. 1.2** Light


B. Feng (✉)
Department of Otorhinolaryngology Head and Neck Surgery, Chinese People's Liberation Army (CPLA) General Hospital, Beijing, China

X. Mi
Department of Otorhinolaryngology Head and Neck Surgery, Chinese People's Liberation Army 91458 Military Hospital, Sanya, China

X. Bi
Department of Pediatric Surgery, The First Affiliated Hospital of Hainan Medical University, Haikou, China

Z. Mu
Department of Otorhinolaryngology Head and Neck Surgery, The First Affiliated Hospital of Hainan Medical University, Haikou, China




Z. Mu, J. Fang (eds.), *Practical Otorhinolaryngology - Head and Neck Surgery*, https://doi.org/10.1007/978-981-13-7993-2_1

the right eye or the left eye of the examiners. Thirdly, set the light source on the same side of the mirror, 10–20 cm above the ear of the examinee, to ensure that the light is projected onto the mirror surface. Finally, adjust the mirror to focus the reflected light on the examining site.

The examiner's sight line should be directly aiming at the reflected focal point for examination through the mirror hole.

To use it correctly, several points should be noticed:

1. Ensure the light focus, the sight line, the mirror hole in a line;
2. Suitable focal length, about 25 cm, adjust the projection of the light source and front mirror of the reflective angle, and adjust the patient's head position, so that the most accurate reflection of the light hits exactly where it's being examined;
3. Look up the binocular to establish the site;
4. Maintain a comfortable posture, do not twist the neck, bending waist, turn around to accommodate Light source and reflected light.

### 1.1.2 Other Commonly Used Examination Equipments

In clinical diagnosis and treatment, the commonly used examination equipments are: otoscope, tuning fork, the anterior rhinoscope, the posterior rhinoscope, the indirect laryngoscope, the gun-shaped forceps, the geniculate forceps, the cerumen hook, the spatula (the tongue depressor), the spray bottle or watering can, endoscopic (indirect nasopharyngoscopy), knee tweezers, cotton swabs, alcohol lamps, dirt basins, etc. (Fig. 1.3).

In recent years, lights and mirrors have been gradually replaced by headlights with better illumination and clearer

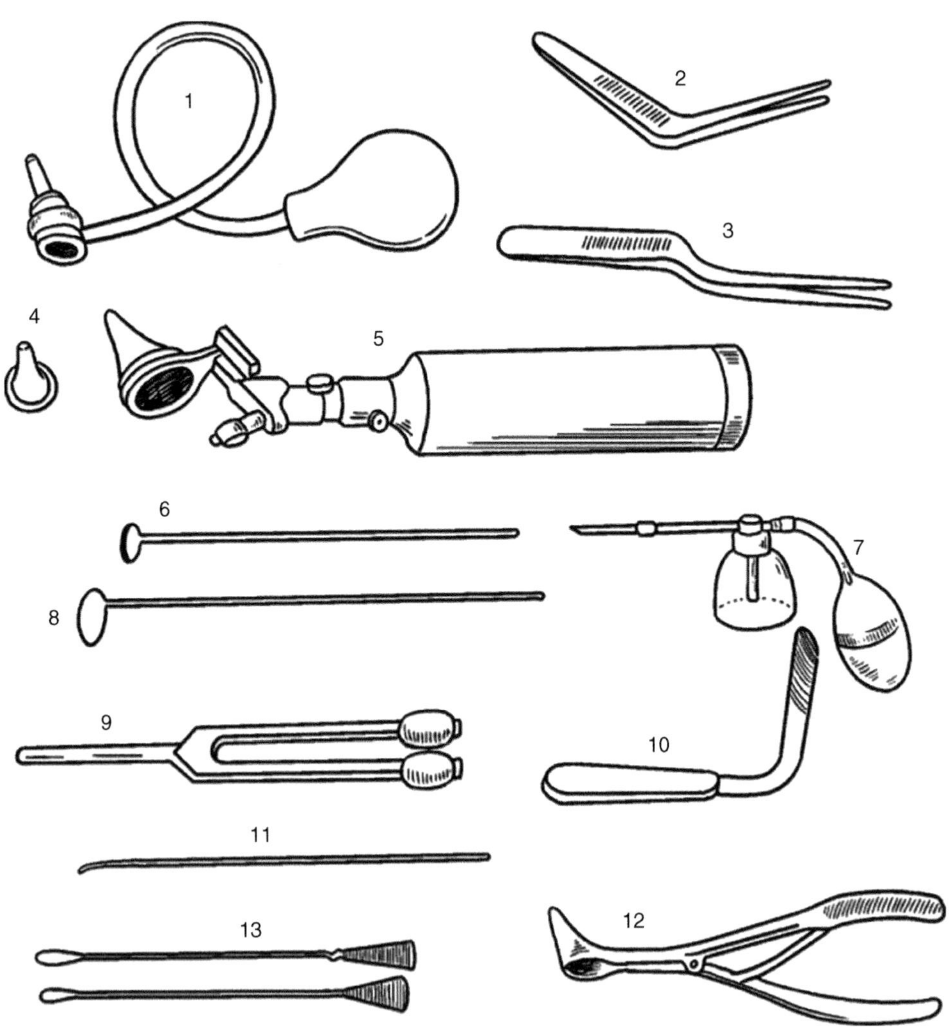


**Fig. 1.3** Otorhinolaryngology Head and Neck Surgery commonly used examination equipment: (1) Pneumatic otoscope, (2) Geniculate forceps, (3) Gun-shaped forceps, (4) Otoscope, (5) Electric otoscope, (6) Posterior rhinoscope, (7) Sprayer, (8) Indirect pharyngoscope, (9) Tuning fork, (10) Corner spatula, (11) Cerumen hook, (12) Anterior rhinoscope, (13) Cotton applicator

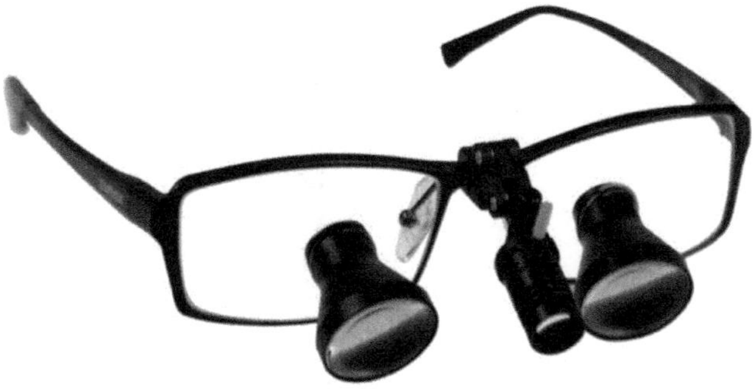

**Fig. 1.4** Frame LED magnifier

vision, such as cold light source lamp, LED headlight, LED magnifier (Fig. 1.4), electric otoscope, Electrosurgical stents and equipments with better lighting and higher definition.

## 1.2 ENT Comprehensive Diagnosis and Treatment Unit

Otorhinolaryngology Comprehensive treatment for examination and treatment designed with inspection chair, cold light source, set the spray, attractor, inflator, spotlight, self-induction heater, automatic sewage in one box, and some also optional reading light boxes, monitors, microscopes and image acquisition, endoscopic standard interface and other equipment, not only to the doctor's examination has brought great convenience, but also for routine treatment.

### 1.2.1 Basic Structure and Main Functions

The platform consists of the workbench, the electric inspection chair or the therapy chair. The introductions are as follow:

**Workbench**
Includes control panel, spotlight, spray gun, suction gun, cold light source, self-induction warmer, etc., and also can be equipped with reading lamp, monitor, etc. (Fig. 1.5). The main function:

1. Spray
   Can atomize the liquid medicine into tiny droplets and spray it on the body cavity or body surface. The advantage of the spray gun is that the atomized particles are small, evenly distributed, irritant and easy to operate.
2. Extract
   To attract negative pressure adjustable straw, used for ear, nose, pharynx, laryngeal secretions, pus extract.
3. Insufflation
   For the throat tube blowing and constant jet device to provide positive pressure air supply for the throat and external auditory canal purulent blood, secretions, foreign body cleaning and maxillary sinus rinse. It is characterized by adjustable pressure, flow changes with the pressure of the inflatable to meet the requirements.
4. Spotlight
   Overcome the short range of activities of vertical lighting, fever, light is not concentrated, scattered light interference, lack of brightness and can not be adjusted and other shortcomings, which is characterized by concentration, brightness adjustable, non-thermal radiation, light arm Large range of activities.
5. Self-Induction Heating
   For indirect laryngoscope warming pre-heating, when the mirror gets into the contact induction heating zone, the heater will automatically blow hot air, its advantage is easy to use, no fire hazards, and appropriate temperature.
6. Cold Light Source
   It provides light source to the endoscope, and its brightness is adjustable,
7. Automatic Sewage
   Automatic sewage will attract the process of storage in the dirt bottle automatically discharge dirt, automatic cleaning, which is characterized by automatic monitoring, automatic discharge, eliminating the need for manual cleaning liquid bottles caused by direct contact with infection.
8. Reading
   Can read X-ray, CT, MRI and other video film.

The workbench is also equipped with a conventional equipment article category placement area:

1. Instrument plate: placing cleaning equipment (tongue depressor, the anterior rhinoscope, the posterior rhinoscope, etc.);
2. Insertion tube: indirect laryngoscope, hooks, Tweezers, etc.;
3. Tank: placing cotton balls, gauze, Vaseline gauze, etc.;
4. Pollution equipment collection device: the used equipment will be placed in the classification within the collection box within the workbench;
5. Placement Area of drugs: 3% hydrogen peroxide solution, 1% ephedrine solution, 1–2% tetracaine solution.

**Fig. 1.5** Otolaryngology Head and Neck Surgery General Hospital equipment

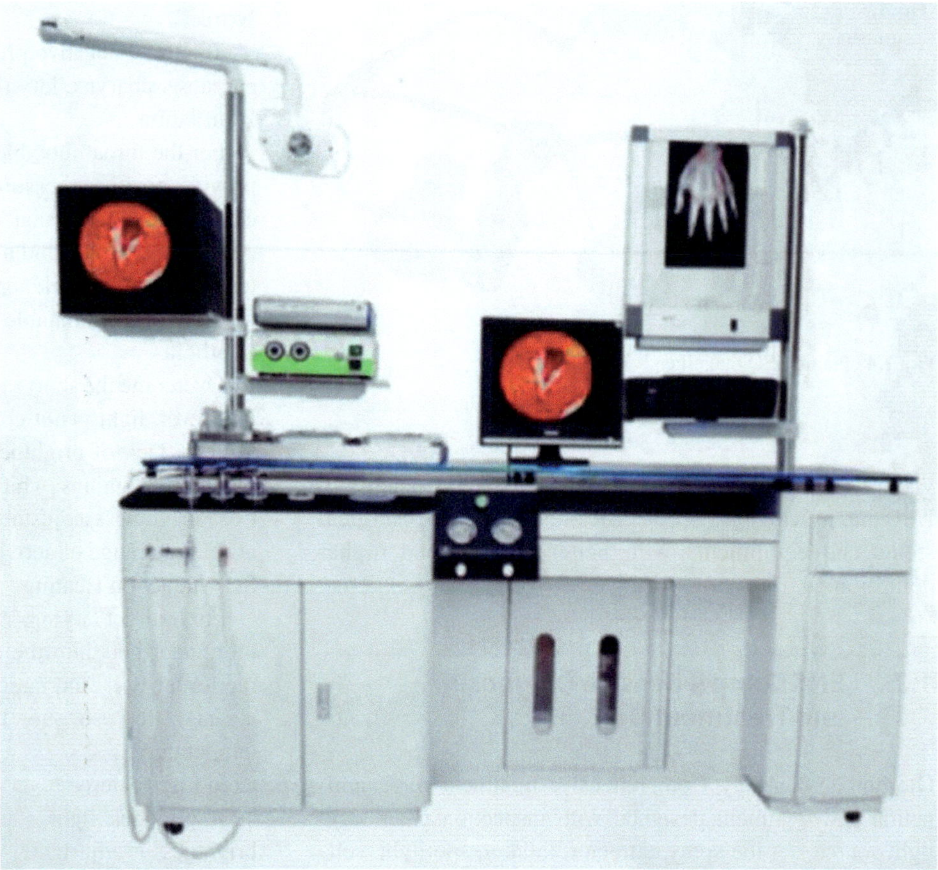

**The Electric Chair**
For the work of the main supporting facilities, which can be divided into two types: lifted and rotated inspection chair and therapy chair.

### 1.2.2 Classification

According to the station is divided into a single station and double station type. The single station workbench is only for one physician use. The double station workbench is designed for two physicians to work at both sides of the platform, also for the clinical teaching.

According to the style can be divided into writing desktop and screen style, the former is a combination of clinic and writing desk, set inspection, treatment, medical record writing and other work in one, for a relatively narrow place, such as a small room interval examination room or Treatment room; the latter is the combination of clinic and screen, can take full advantage of the limited space for clinicians to create a relatively independent working environment, suitable for more spacious places.

## 1.3 Endoscopy

The anatomic sites of the organs at the otolaryngology head and neck are concealed, so the traditional inspection cannot expose them. But the medical endoscope is a medical electrical device to provide the internal observation or imaging for the diagnosis and the treatment by inserting into the body. It constitutes cold light source, the objective lens, the image acquisition system and the eyepiece. It is divided into the rigid endoscopy and the flexible endoscopy.

### 1.3.1 Rigid Endoscope

Common endoscopes used in the otolaryngology head and neck surgery department include the rhinoendoscope, the optic endoscope, the esophagoscope and the bronchoscope. The angles of the rhinoendoscope view camera maybe at 0, 30, 70, 90, 120°and other degree angle and the scopic diameter may be 2.7–4.0 mm (Fig. 1.6). In recent years, there appears a variable perspective endoscope, which is more convenient to use. The rhinoendoscope is used to synchro-

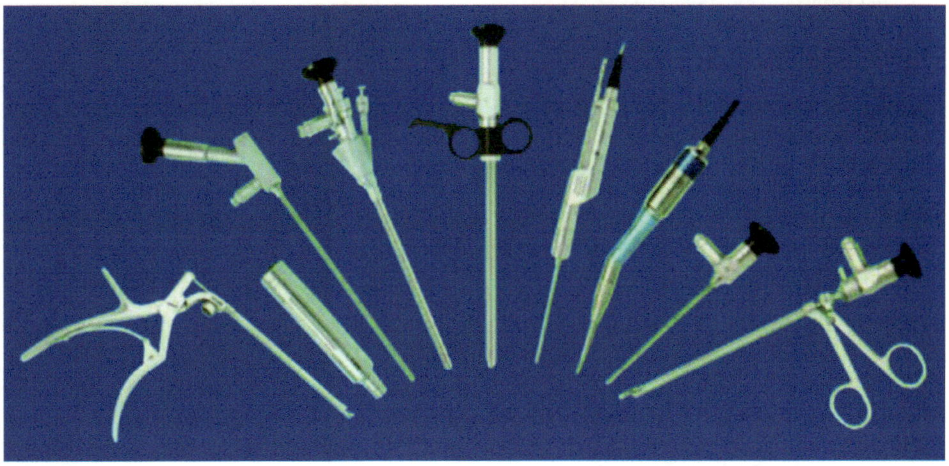

**Fig. 1.6** Endorhinoscopic instruments

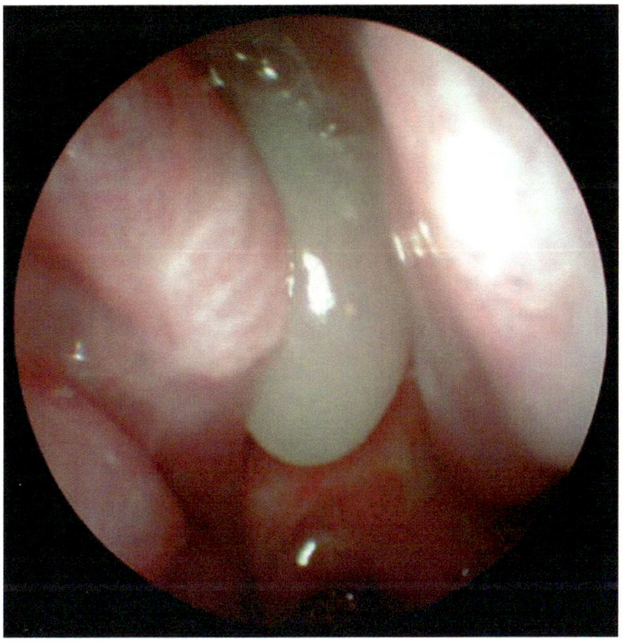

**Fig. 1.7** Endorhinoscopic rhinopolyp

nously observe the nose and the rhinal pharynx (Fig. 1.7) even the internal structure of the paransanal sinuses through the display monitor to make the vision clearer. The nasal and the Para nasal sinus disease' precision and accurate therapy could be made by the supporting surgical instruments.

Compared to the endoscopic size, the otoscopic diameter is smaller. It is mainly used to inspect the external auditory canal and the tympanic membrane. The tympanum could be observed through the tympanic membrane, which has great diagnostic value on the external and the middle ear diseases (Fig. 1.8). The otic operative vision is clear during operation (Fig. 1.9), so it is possible to observe the lesions hard to be perceived by the naked eyes, the residual cholesteatoma

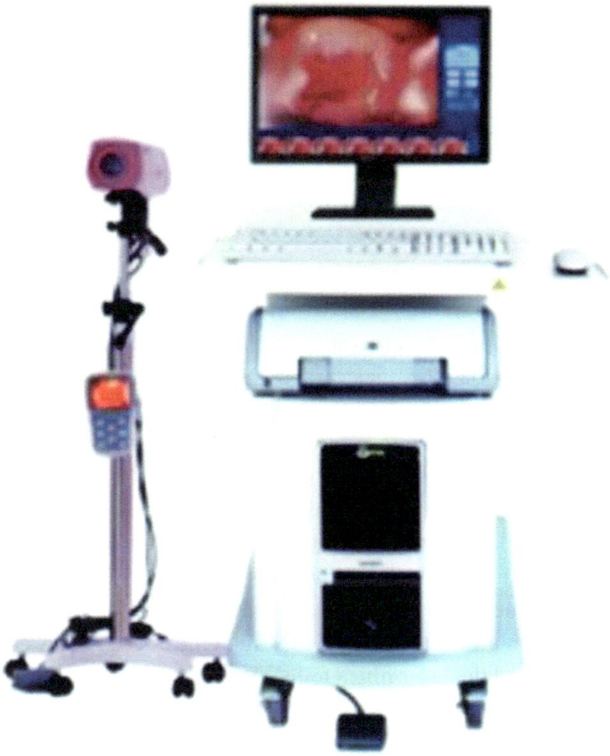

**Fig. 1.8** Otoendoscopic comprehensive imaging system

existing and so on, and it makes the middle ear surgery more precise, minimally invasive and safer. But both hands of the operators are inconvenient.

### 1.3.2 Soft Endoscope

Soft endoscope include fiber endoscope, electronic endoscope, etc. The fiber endoscope mainly includes the fiber

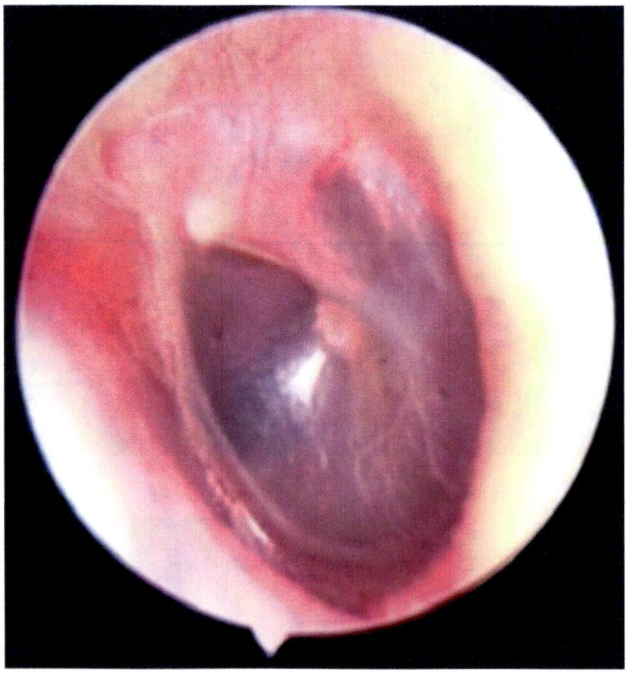

**Fig. 1.9** Clear endoscopic imagining of the tympanic membrane

rhinolaryngopharyngoscope, the Eustachian tube, and sometimes the fiber gastroscopy and the fiber bronchoscopy also can be applied. The fiber rhinolaryngopharyngoscope consists of three main parts, the cold light source, the endoscope and the imaging system (Fig. 1.10). Compared to the fiber endoscope, the electric endoscope replaces the fiber bundle with the electric micro image sensor, which is thinner and also displaying the imaging clearer (Fig. 1.11). Most of the widely used electric endoscopes at present are matched with the therapy pipes, which introduce the biopsy forceps and the laser fibers to facilitate the examination and therapy.

### 1.3.3 Narrow-Band Imaging

Narrow-banding imaging (NBI), being used in recent years, during which the light through special filters becomes 420 nm and 520 nm narrow-waves, and their composite wavelength corresponds to the spectrum of the hemoglobin absorption. The 420 nm length wave is easy to be absorbed by the mucosal fibrous tissues; and the 520 nm length wave effect on the sub-mucosa vessels, distinguishing the mucosal layer's lesions after digital processing and which an also highlight the mucosa-vascular distribution, contributing to detect the micro lesions early.

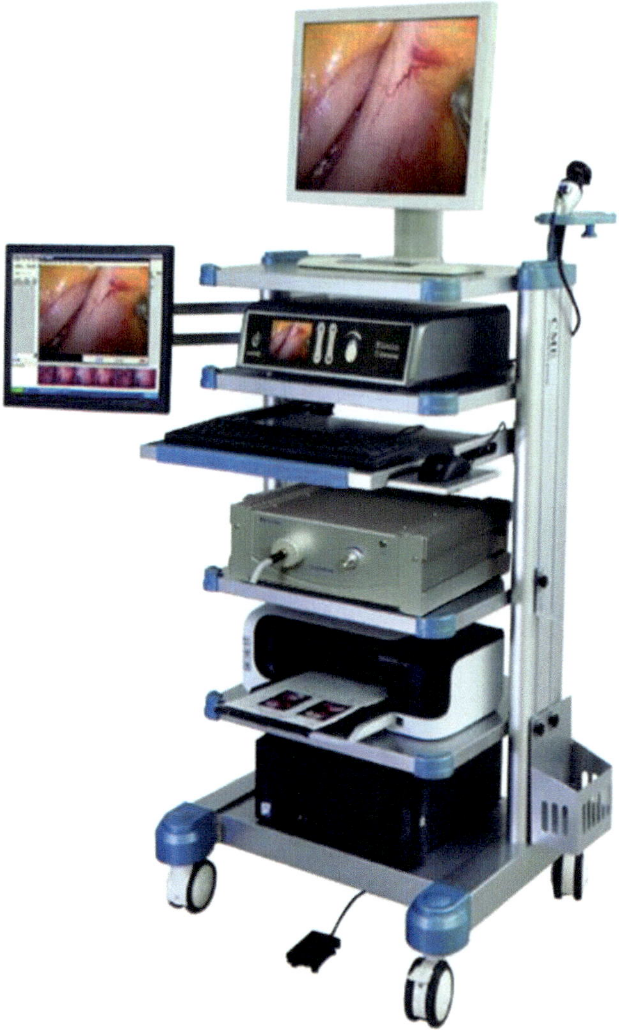

**Fig. 1.10** Fiber rhinolaryngopharyngoscope

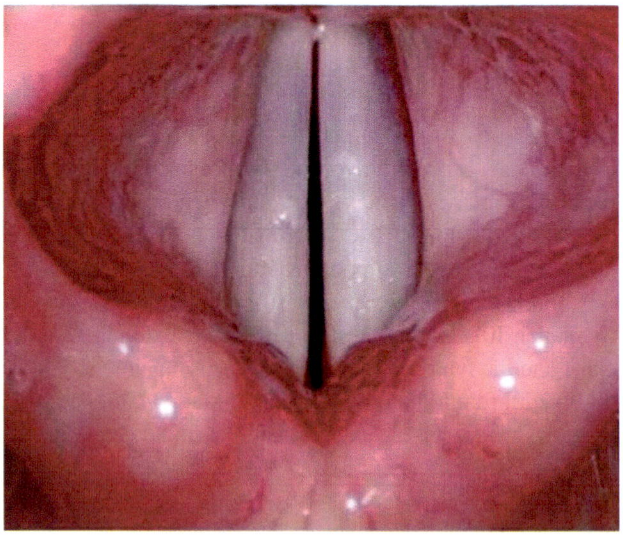

**Fig. 1.11** Electric rhinolaryngopharyngeal vocal cord inspection imaging

## 1.4 Other Special Examination Equipment

Otorhinolaryngology Head and Neck Surgery involves otorhinolaryngology, audiology, vestibular science, voice and other multi-branch disciplines, for more specialist examination equipment, see the relevant sections. This section will introduce the most commonly used pure-sound audiometer and the recent 3D-operation microscope and 3D-display system.

The pure-tone audiometer is equipment sending the pure tones, which are at different frequency and intensity and these are produced from the electronic oscillating and amplification circuit based on the electroacoustic principles, to the clients through headphones to respectively test each-frequency threshold-intensity (Fig. 1.12). Acoustic intensity would be indicated with 'dB'.

The recording curve of each frequency (hearing curve) is called the audiogram, and it could provide an accordance to the qualitative, quantitative and positional diagnosis.

Some hallmark of pure-tone acoustic curves have special significance on determining the causes of deafness (Fig. 1.13), such as at the bone-conduction audio threshold curve, the corresponding intensity at the 1000-Hz site is higher than that at the 4000-Hz site and at the 2000-Hz site has a sudden dropping, but both threshold extremities are at a normal range, which is a typical otosclerosis hearing curve; if the hearing loss is not severe but the corresponding intensity at the 4000-Hz and at the 3000-Hz hearings have evident loss, it is noise-induced-deafness's hearing curve.

Surgical microscope is the key and important equipment for ear microsurgery and otorhinolaryngology. In each of the two optical paths of some imported surgical microscopes, a

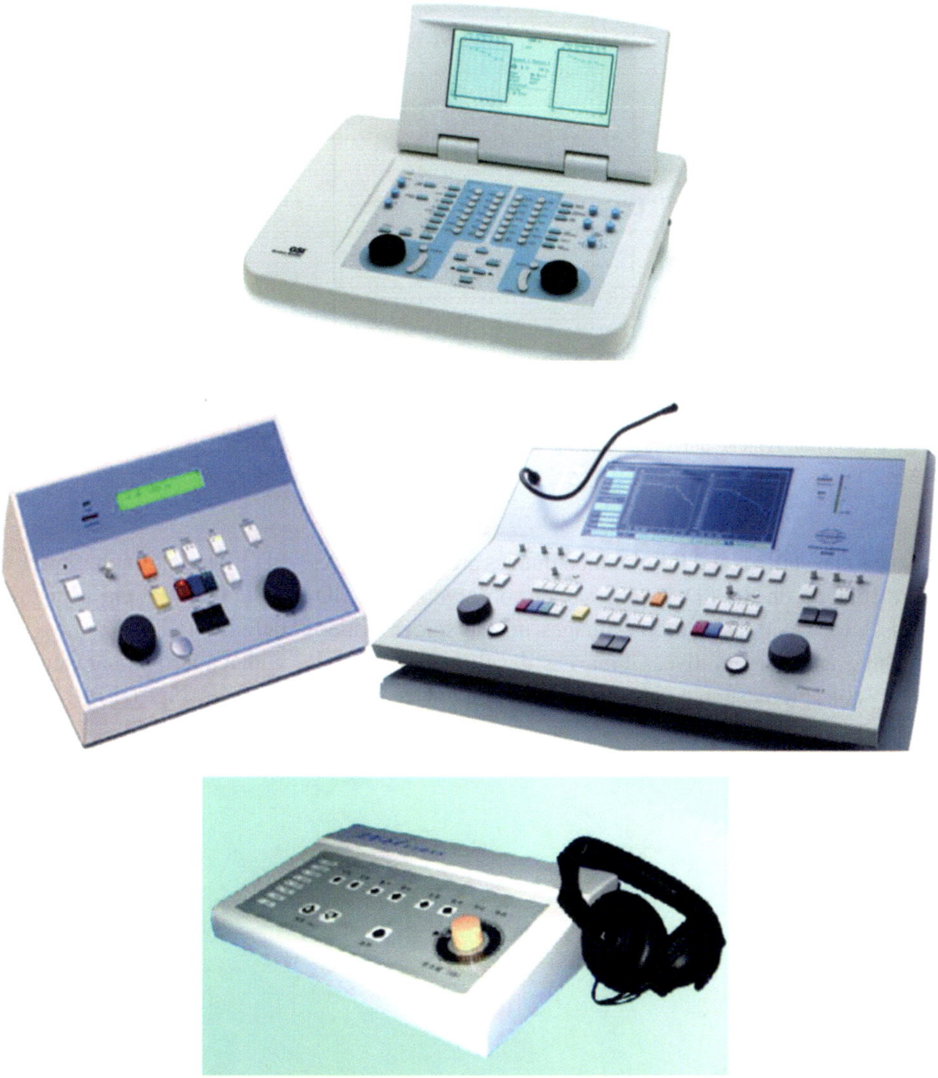

**Fig. 1.12** Pure sound audiometer

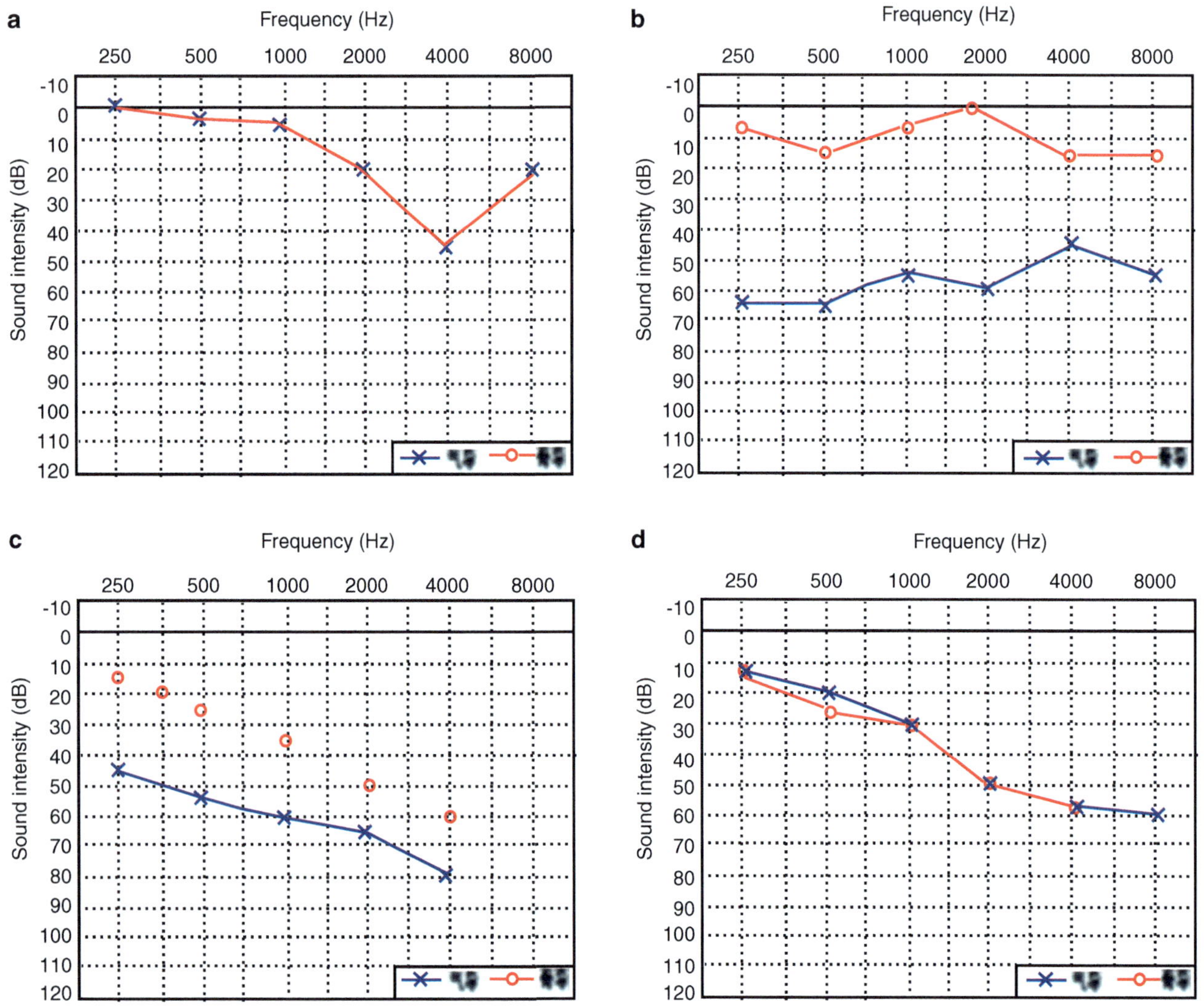


**Fig. 1.13** Four typical pure-tone hearing curves. (**a**) Noise-induced deafness, (**b**) conductive deafness, (**c**) mixed deafness, (**d**) sensorial deafness

camera is installed, and the obtained images are processed to be displayed on the 3D display screen, observers wear 3D glasses to watch stereoscopic images on the screen, video teaching and surgery live. China has developed a surgical microscope stereoscopic video demonstration device, by the 3D high-definition digital video camera, 3D high-definition LCD monitor and adjust the bracket, which has a 3D high-definition digital camera original lens modified and coupled with a micro-camera lens and focus light source Microphone Adapter (Fig. 1.14).

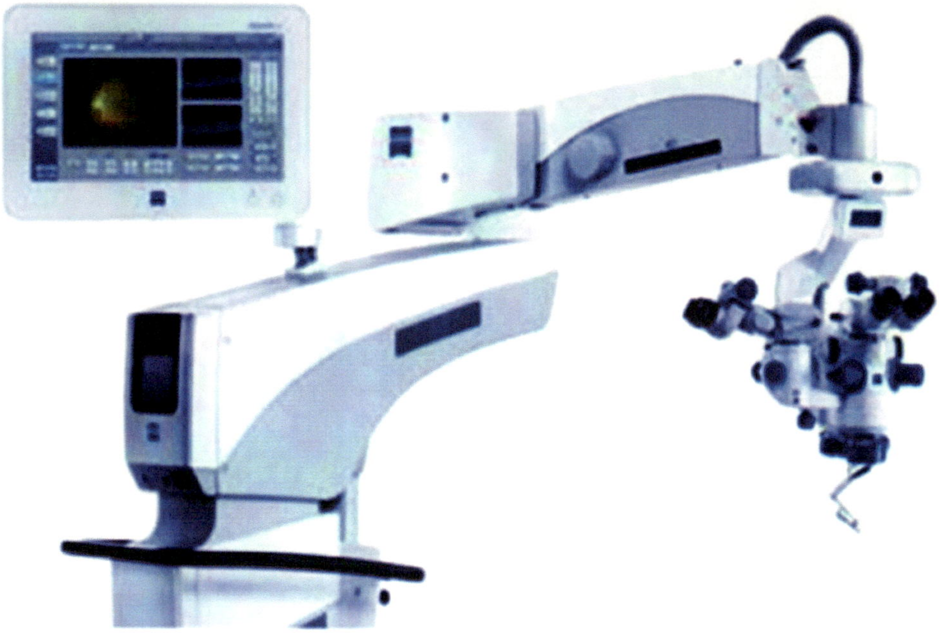

**Fig. 1.14** 3D operative microscope and display system

# Medical Imaging Examinations of Otorhinolaryngology Head and Neck Surgery

2

Zhiqun Li, Rong Tu, Xiaoguang You and Jianghua Wan

Medical imaging is the creation of technique and process for the visual representations of the interior of the body for clinical analysis and medical intervention, as well as the functions of certain organs or tissues (physiology). Medical Imaging is geared towards revealing hidden internal structures in the skin and bones, as well as to diagnose and treat diseases. Medical imaging experts also set up a database of normal anatomy and physiology to make it possible to identify abnormalities. Although imaging of excised organs and tissues can be performed for medical reasons, such procedures are generally considered to be part of pathology rather than medical imaging.

It mainly includes X-ray, CT, MRI and radionuclide imaging techniques, which have been developing rapidly in last two decades, and they are mainly characterized by clearer information of anatomy and pathological structures; more and more three-dimensional images, simulated endoscopic images and real-time dynamic images.

Some major MIE technologies used in ENT are briefly discussed as follows.

## 2.1 X-ray Examination

X-ray images are black and white images composed of different gray scales, reflecting a composite projection of differences in density and thickness of the tissue. Normal sinus and papillae are gas-filled, with a good density difference, suitable for X-ray examination. However, since X-ray images are overlapping images, radiographs often need to be performed from different perspectives to minimize overlap and display lesions.

For the soft-tissues organs and tissues, which lack density contrast, such as the pharynx, lead in high-density contrast medium can be introduced artificially to develop an imaging; it is called digital subtraction angiography (DSA).

Because X-ray images are overlapped images, positioning diagnosis is difficult. CT and MRI equipment and technology are developing rapidly. The images are clear and anatomical. The anatomic details are clear and the diagnosis value is high. Therefore, the application of X-ray film has been gradually reduced.

### 2.1.1 Oto-Temporal Site

At this site, the regular X-ray imaging includes the Schuller (or lateral-inclined) positioning and the Mayer (or axial) positioning, of which the former could display the tympanum, the tympanic tegmen, the mastoid cells and the sigmoid sinus ante theca, under which the mid-ear aditus, the external ear aditus and the tympanum super imposingly project at the inferior sub temporal maxillary junction to generate a round-translucency (Fig. 2.1), and the latter could clearly display the tympanum, the mastoid sinus and the mastoid sinus aditus (Fig. 2.2).

Ear X-ray film is currently clinically replaced by high-resolution CT imaging.

### 2.1.2 The Nose and Nasal Sinus

At these sites, regular X-ray radiograph mainly includes the rhinal sinus Waltz (or occiput mental) positioning and the Caldwell (or occiput frontal) positioning. The Waltz positioning imaging could display the rhinocavum, the anterior ethmoid sinus, the maxillary sinus, the eye orbit and the zygomatic arch, and the Caldwell positioning imaging could display the frontal sinus, the anterior ethnocide sinus and the eye orbit (Figs. 2.3 and 2.4).

Z. Li (✉) · R. Tu · X. You · J. Wan
Department of Medical Imaging, The First Affiliated Hospital of Hainan Medical University, Haikou, China


Z. Mu, J. Fang (eds.), *Practical Otorhinolaryngology - Head and Neck Surgery*, https://doi.org/10.1007/978-981-13-7993-2_2

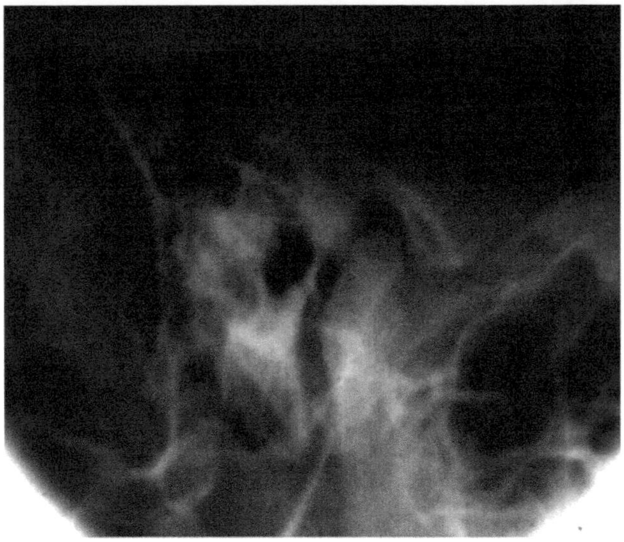

**Fig. 2.1** Mastoid Schuller positioning

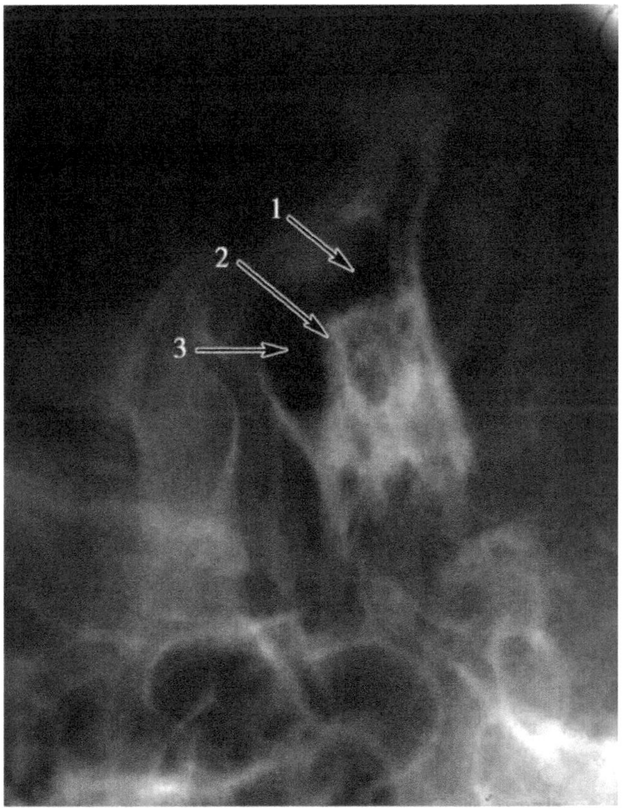


**Fig. 2.2** Mastoid Mayer positioning. (1) mastoid sinus. (2) bone bridge. (3) epitympanum

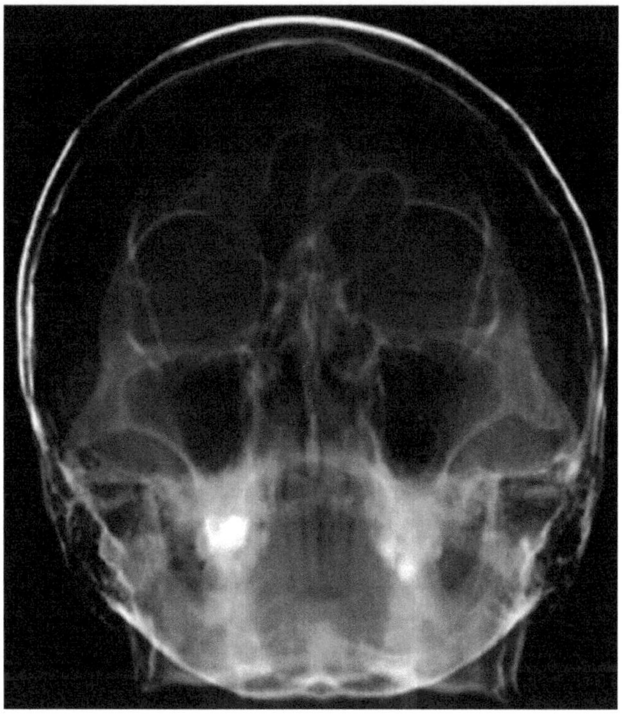

**Fig. 2.3** Waltz positioning

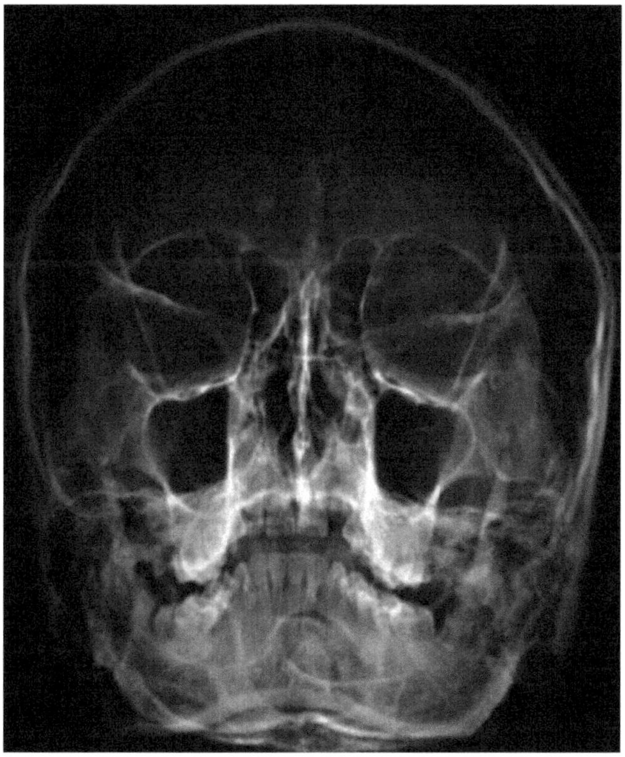

**Fig. 2.4** Caldwell positioning

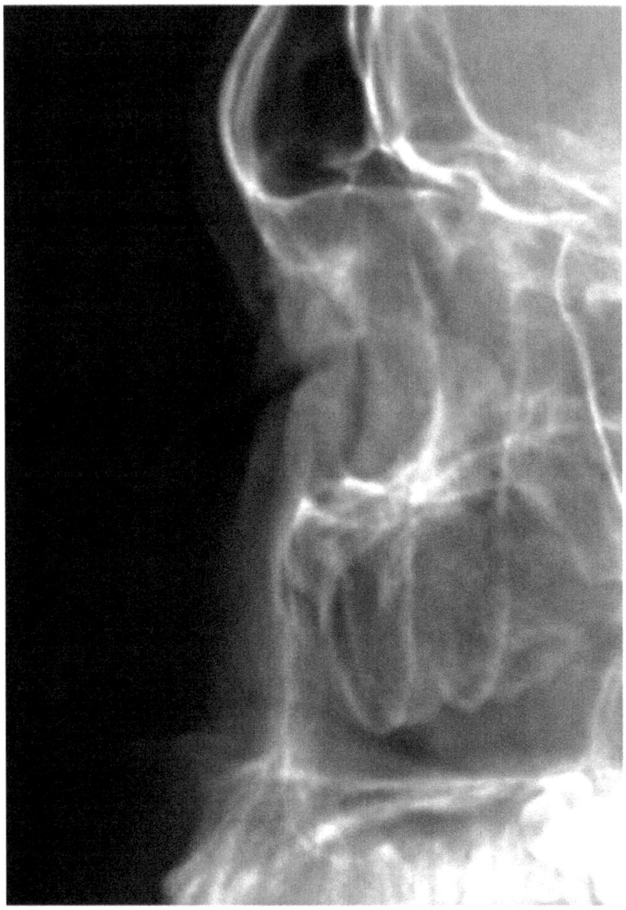

**Fig. 2.5** Lateral rhinal bone positioning of X-ray

At lateral rhinal bone-positioning imaging could display the rhinal bone and it could help master the bone fracture and unmatched the existing (Fig. 2.5)

### 2.1.3 Larynx and Pharynx

Laryngeal and pharyngeal X-ray imaging are mainly the lateral positioning imaging, displaying the structures, which includes the post-pharyngeal wall, the pre-cervical soft tissue, the pharyngocavum, the soft palatine, the lingual root, the epiglottis, the thyrocartilage, the laryngocavum, the vocal cords, the subglottic region, etc. Laryngopharyngeal structures are almost soft tissues and cartilages, so the X-ray imaging's value in clinic is limited. But the Barium imaging and the lipiodolography could display the deglutition and intracavum change, so they have certain value to some extent.

## 2.2 CT Examination

CT is the abbreviation of the x-ray computed tomography. CT images are a computer-reconstructed imaging, reflecting the X-ray absorption degree of certain-layer-thickness tissues. It is similar to the X-ray white-and-dark imaging, the higher the tissue density is, the more trending to whiter the images are, whereas, it would display a black-trending imaging.

Compared with the regular X-ray imaging, the CT images have characteristics as follows:

1. Cross-section Imaging

   It could reflect the tissues' and the organs' anatomic structures more stereoscopically and more accurately.
2. High-density-resolution

   Plain CT scan images could clearly display the organs constituted by soft tissues, such as the Brian, the eye orbit, the laryngopharynx, the acicular chin and etc. Enhanced scanning (re-scanning after injecting intravenous high-density contrast medium) images display the anatomic details of the blood vessels and micro-organs better.
3. Powerful Image Post-processing Function

   CT images are series of digital images constituted by pixels, so they can be post-processed with software, which include the 2D and the 3D reconstruction techniques and other analysis and displacement techniques. The 2D reconstruction technique mainly applies the coronary and the sagittal multiple (MPR) and curved (CPR) planar reformation, so it is helpful to display the anatomic relation between the lesion and the peristructures. The 3D reconstruction techniques contain the maximum intensity projection (MIP), the minimum intensity projection (minIP), the volume rendering technique (VRT), the surface shaded display (SSD), the CT virtual endoscopy (CT-VE) and so on. The 3D reconstruction techniques mainly help volume-reconstruction, so it has two advantages, strong three-dimensions and displaying clear anatomic relationship. and the CT-angiography (CTA) could straightly observe the tumor blood supply conditions. This technical application greatly expands the clinic CT application fields and improves the CT's diagnostic value.

### 2.2.1 Plain CT Scan

**Ototemporal Axis (Level), Coronary Position, Oblique Sagittal Position**

Ototemporal structures are fine; most of them are pneumatic bones and have relative-higher density contrast. In clinic, high-resolution CT (HRCT) imaging is often applied,

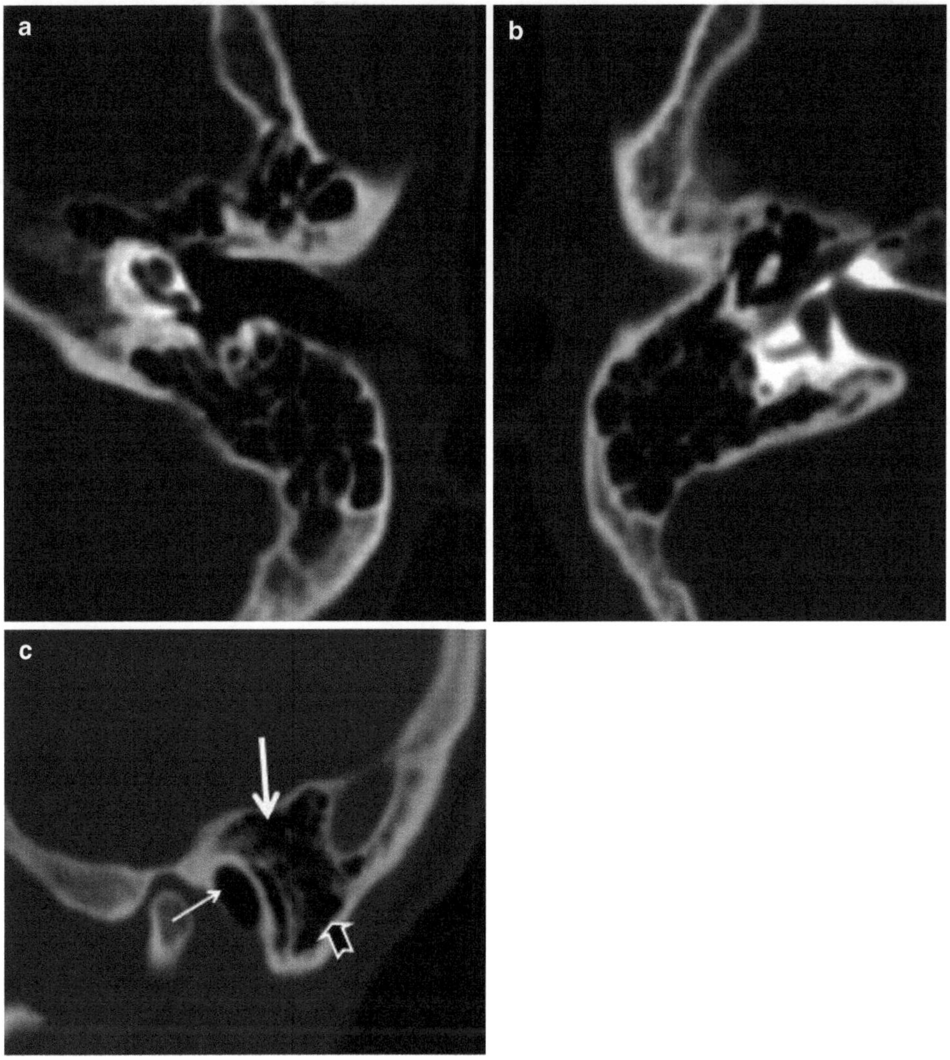


**Fig. 2.6** HRCT displays normal ototemporal structures. (**a**) Mainly display cochlea, tympanic cavum. (**b**) Mainly display ossicular chain (Malleus and incus junction), tympanic cavum, tympanic facial nerve segment, external semicircular canal and inner ear canal. (**c**) Temporal oblique sagittal reconstruction, which display the right tympanic cavum (tiny arrow), mastoid sinus (thick arrow) and mastoid cell (turning arrow)

because it could reconstruct random cross-section and display the ossicular chain, the tympanic cavum, the vagus, the mastoid sinus, even the facial nerve's, other structures and their micro lesions (Figs. 2.6 and 2.7).

Right lateral imaging mainly displays external ear canal, otosteon, semicircular canal and inner ear canal; left lateral imaging mainly displays tympanic cavum, otosteon and cochlea.

### Nose and Para Nasal Sinus

HRCT photography is the best rhinal and rhinosinuses examination and it could reconstruct their coronary images. The coronary images could display the osteomeatal complex structure (ethmoid infundibulum, the ethmoid bulb, the mid-turbinate, the uniform process, the meniscal tear, the midrhinomeatus, etc), and it has important reference value on clinic rhinal endoscopy operations (Fig. 2.8).

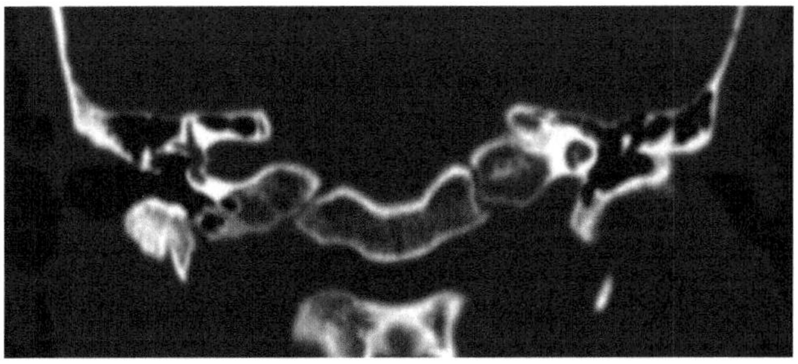

**Fig. 2.7** Ototemporal HRCT coronary reconstruction imaging

### Laryngopharynx

CT has relative-higher diagnostic value on pharyngolaryngeal lesion, because it could display the pharyngocavum, the laryngocavum, all the pharyngolaryngeal wall's

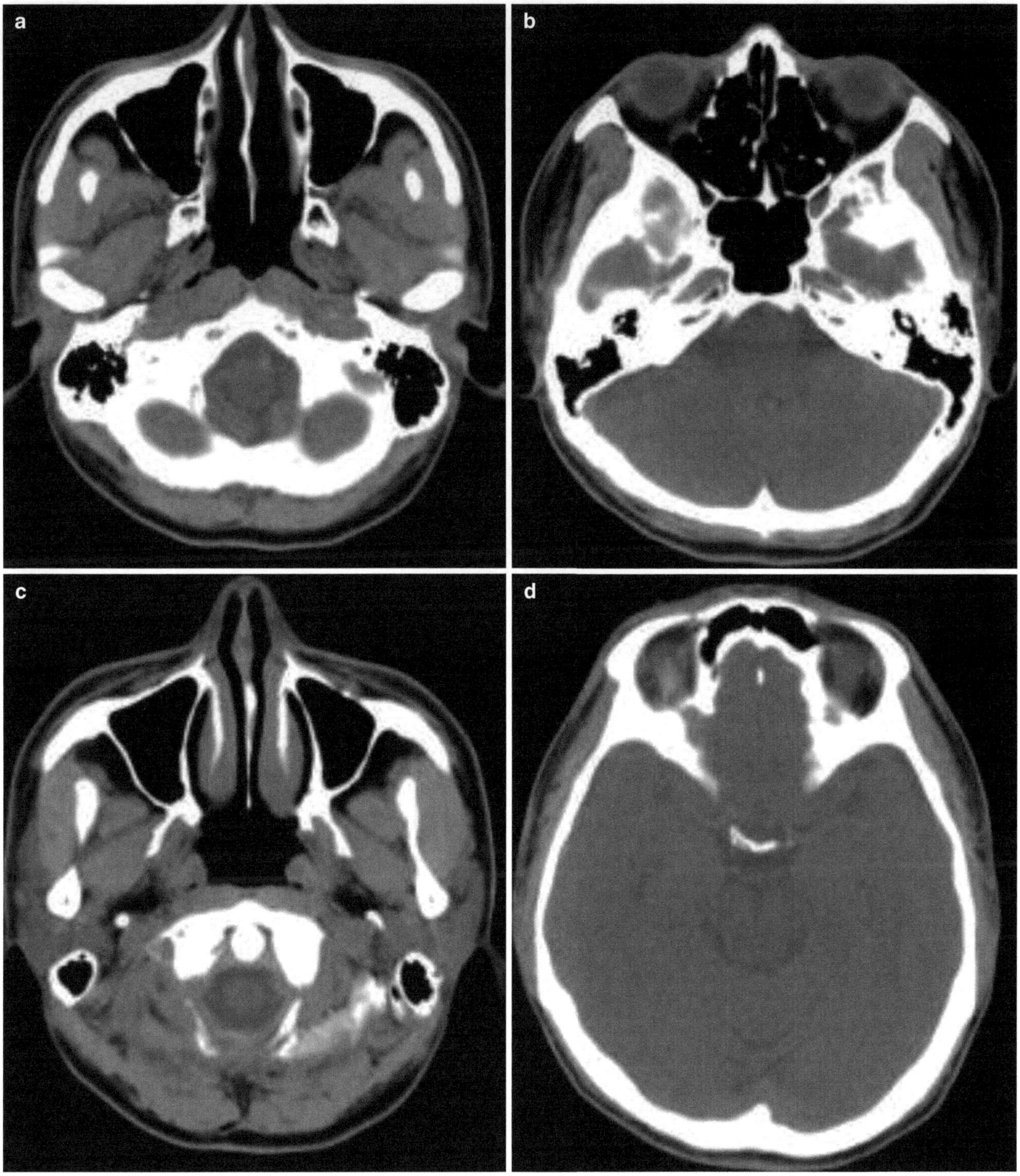


**Fig. 2.8** Axial rhinosinus CT. (**a**) It mainly displays bilateral rhinocavum, maxillary sinus, rhinal pharynx and mastoid. (**b**) From anterior back, it mainly displays bilateral ethmoid sinus, sphenoid sinus, petrous apex. (**c**) It mainly displays bilateral sub turbinate, maxillary sinus, rhinal pharynx, atlas and dentate. (**d**) It mainly displays frontal sinus and sellar region

layers' structures, the epiglottis, the aryepiglottic fold, the piriform recess, the vocal cords, the ventricular cords, the Parapharyngeal interval, the Parapharyngeal interval and their lesions, and it could also display the lymphatic metastasis (Fig. 2.9).

### 2.2.2 Enhanced CT Scan

It is mainly applied for the diagnosis and the differential diagnosis of the cervicocranial tumorous lesion, because it not only could display the tumor's range, boundaries, adjacent invasion

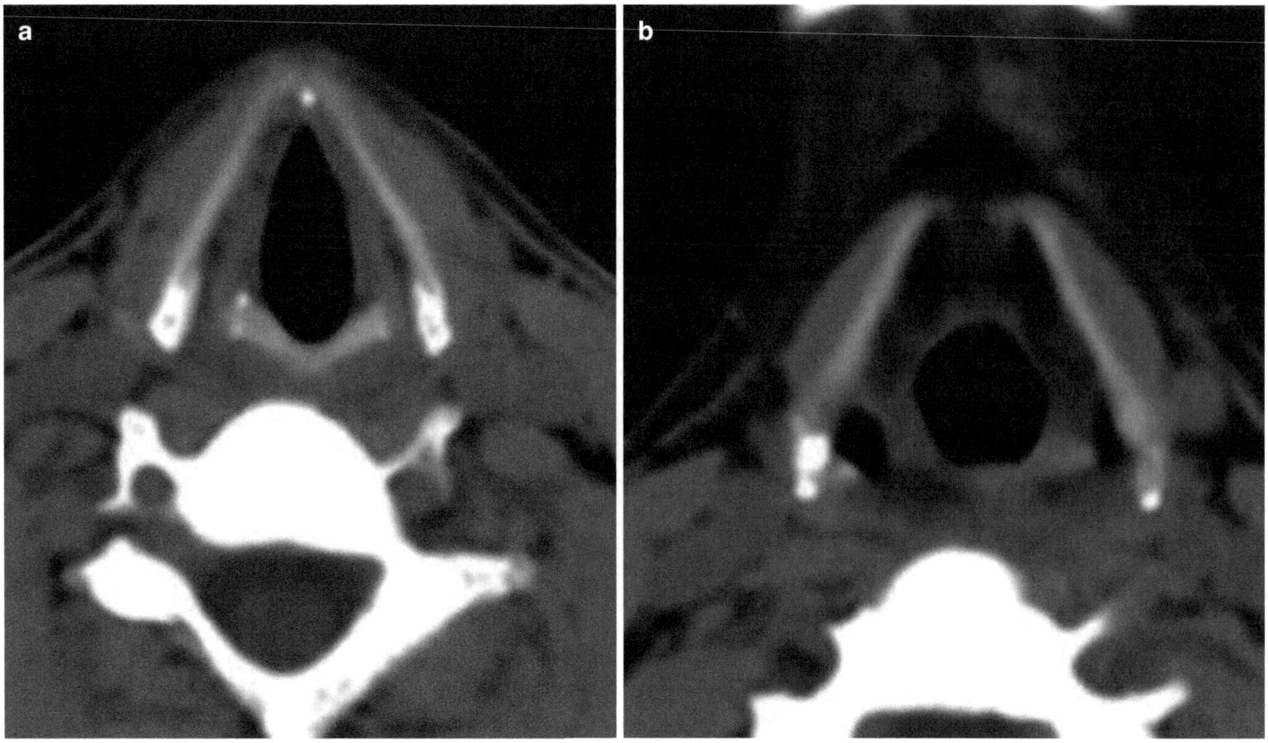


**Fig. 2.9** Laryngeal axial CT. (**a**) It displays laryngoventricular cavum, laryngoventricular wall, thyroid cartilage and arytenoid cartilage. (**b**) It displays oropharyngeal cavum, piriform recess, thyroid cartilage, etc

and lymphatic metastasis, but also display the tumor's blood supply and its relationship with the adjacent blood vessels.

### 2.2.3 CT 3D-Reconstruction

Craniocervical CT 3D-reconstruction mainly includes multiplanar reformation (MPR), maximum intensity projection (MIP), CT virtual endoscope (CTVE), curved planar reconstruction (CPR), volume rendering (VR) and so on. The MPR is used to display the ostiomeatal complex, the ossicular chain, the internal otovagus, the facial nerve, the laryngoventrium and so on.

The relationship between the tumor and its peripheral structures and the cervicocranial fracture as well (Fig. 2.10); the MIP could be used to display the relationship between the tumor and the adjacent blood vessels, the fracture at the nose and Para nasal sinus, the ototemporal site and the maxillofacial fracture; the CTVE is mainly used at larynx, its images are exactly like the fibrolaryngeal images but it could help observe the regions those hard to be observed under fibrolaryngoscope, such as the sub glottis region and so on; the cervicocranial CTA could be used to display the tumor blood supply vessels, the relationship between the tumor and the adjacent blood vessels, and the vascular lesion's range and its peripheral relations (Fig. 2.11); the VR could be used to display the rhinosteon fracture in a special way, because it could help differentiate the micro fracture and the normal pore channels (Fig. 2.12).

## 2.3 MRI Examination

Magnetic resonance imaging (MRI) is a digital imaging technique whose procedures are inputting the patient into a specific magnetic field to let the atomic nucleus (mainly hydrogen proton) in its body happen corresponding sagittal change, producing resonant phenomenon under the effect of the outside pulse signals and collecting and processing the information relieved from the atomic nucleus resonance by computer to produce a digital image. Because signals are generated from different tissues' and lesions' resonance, the imaging could be applied to help diagnose in clinic.

In the past 30 years, the MRI equipments' hardware has being developed gradually. The MRI imaging's producing rate and the imaging quality becomes higher. Its software functions become more powerful, not only display the tissues' anatomic structures, but also reflect the tissues' metabolism, functions and molecular characteristics. Its clinical application becomes wider and wider, because of which, the clinical diagnostic development has been greatly promoted.

The MRI imaging differs from the CT imaging, because it doesn't display the tissues' density. It represents the MRI signal intensity at tissues and the signal intensity is determined by several parameters; which mainly include the $T_1$ relaxation time, the $T_2$ relaxation time and other information. Besides, different tissues and lesions have their own proper $T_1$, $T_2$ and other parameters.

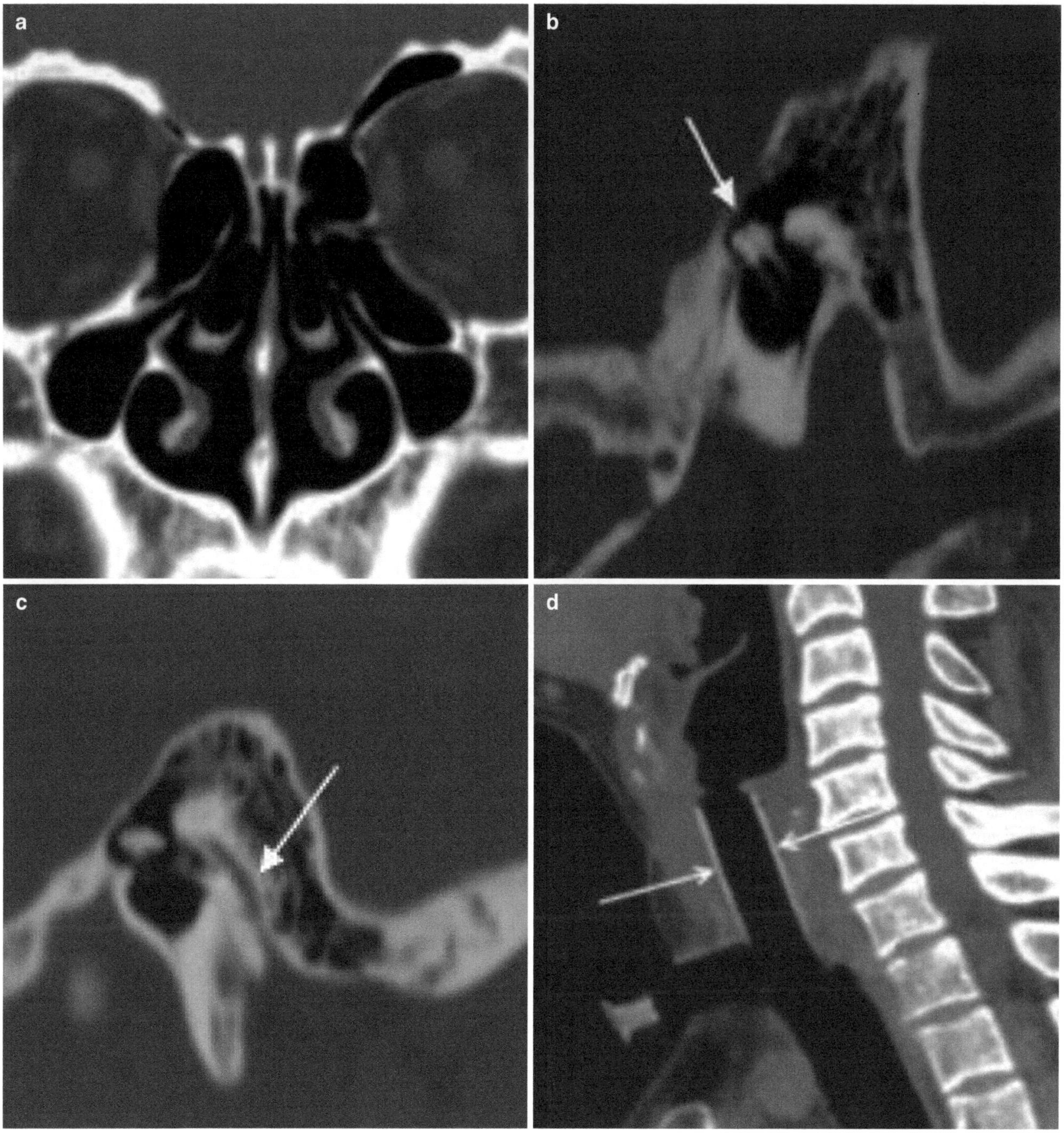


**Fig. 2.10** CT 3D-reconstruction images. (**a**) Coronary Para nasal sinus reconstruction imaging displays bilateral sinus-aditus-rhino meatus complex. (**b**) Temporal reconstruction imaging displays ossicular chain in the malleoli joint (arrow). (**c**) Facial nerve reconstruction imaging displays facial nerve mastoid segment (arrow). (**d**) Laryngo-reconstruction imaging displays laryngeal support (arrow)

MRI's high soft tissue resolution is evidently better than CT, the ultrasound and other imagings, this is also MRI's biggest advantage, and it is especially helpful at displaying the tumor, the inflammation, the congenital abnormality and other lesions.

MRI mainly has characteristics, including the multi-sequence imaging, the multi-azimuth imaging, the multiple functional imaging etc. Commonly, the MRI scanning technician or physician should choose the appropriate sequence or technique according to the clinic diagnostic requisition, so the clinic requisition should be as definite as possible to obtain the best diagnostic result.

The most commonly used sequences in clinic contain the $T_1$ weighted imaging ($T_1$WI) and the $T_2$ weighted imaging ($T_2$WI). Same tissue shot under different parameters weighted imaging has grey scale difference. The $T_1$WI mainly reflects the tissues' anatomy information and the $T_2$WI mainly reflects the lesion's information (Fig. 2.13).

Commonly used MRI section orientations contain the cross section (axial view), the coronary view and the sagittal

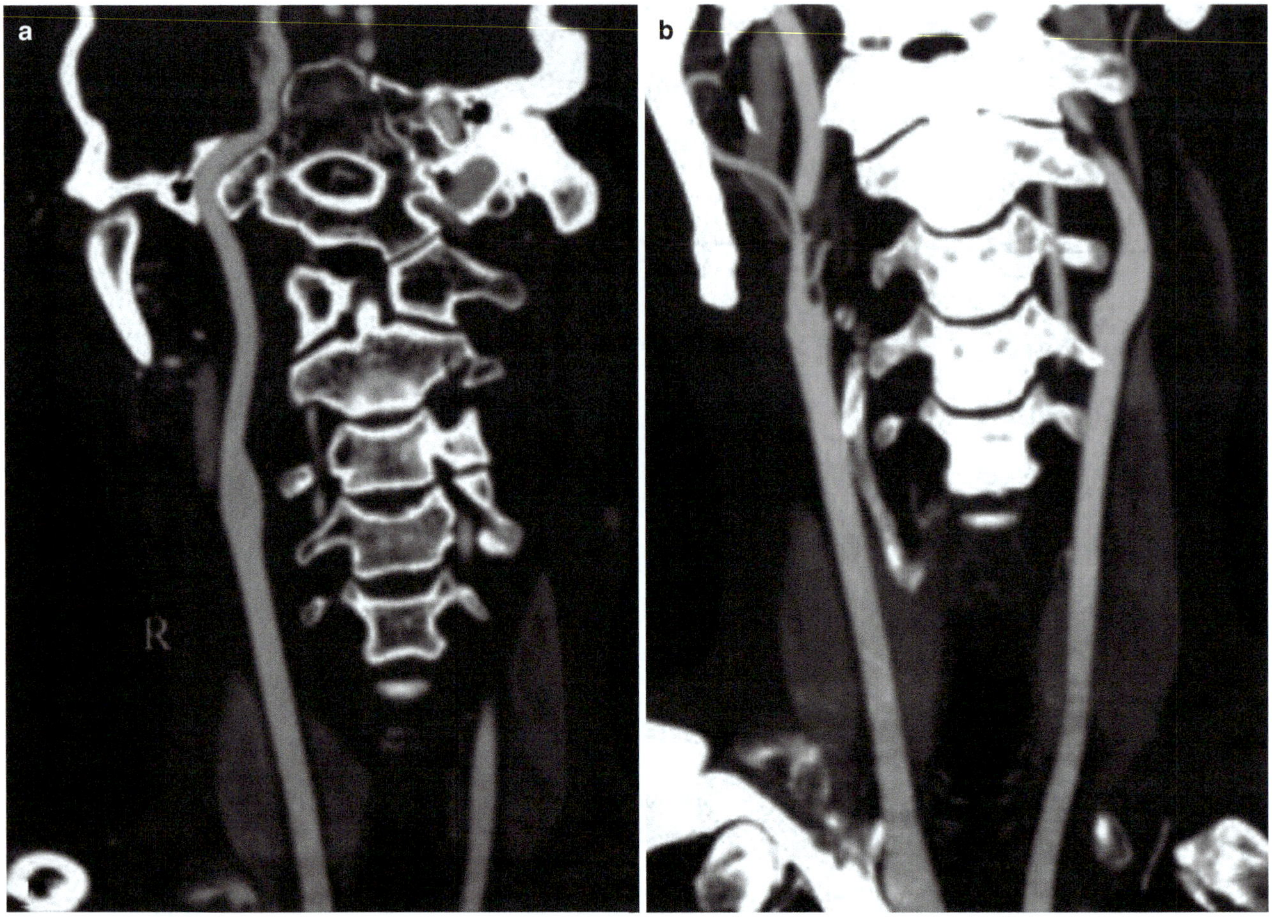


**Fig. 2.11** Cervical CTA imaging. (**a**) CPR imaging displays right lateral main cervical artery and intra-cervical artery. (**b**) MIP imaging displays bilateral main cervical artery, extra-cervical artery and intra-cervical artery

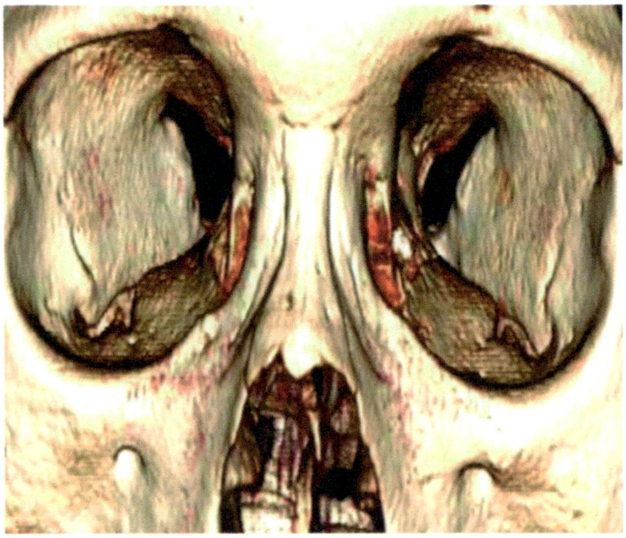

**Fig. 2.12** Common rhinal bone CTVR 3D imaging

view, the imaging could also be shot at random section based on the anatomic structural course characteristics to become the best tool to display the adjacent relationship between organs and tissues (Fig. 2.13).

Mostly-used specific cervicocranial MRI techniques include the angiography, the diffusion weighted imaging and the hydrography technique. The magnetic resonance angiography (MRA) could display any third or fourth degree vessel branches, especially the cerebral blood vessels, without the contrast medium. The MRA is non-traumatic and quality-reliable imaging examination; so it has become the efficient tools to examine the cervicocranial vascular diseases. The MRI diffusion weighted imaging (MRI-DWI) is a kind of functional imaging.

It could examine the water molecules diffusion motion in human tissues and accurately quantify the motion. Then speculate the lesion segments' pathologic ingredients through observing the microscopic diffusion motion state of the water

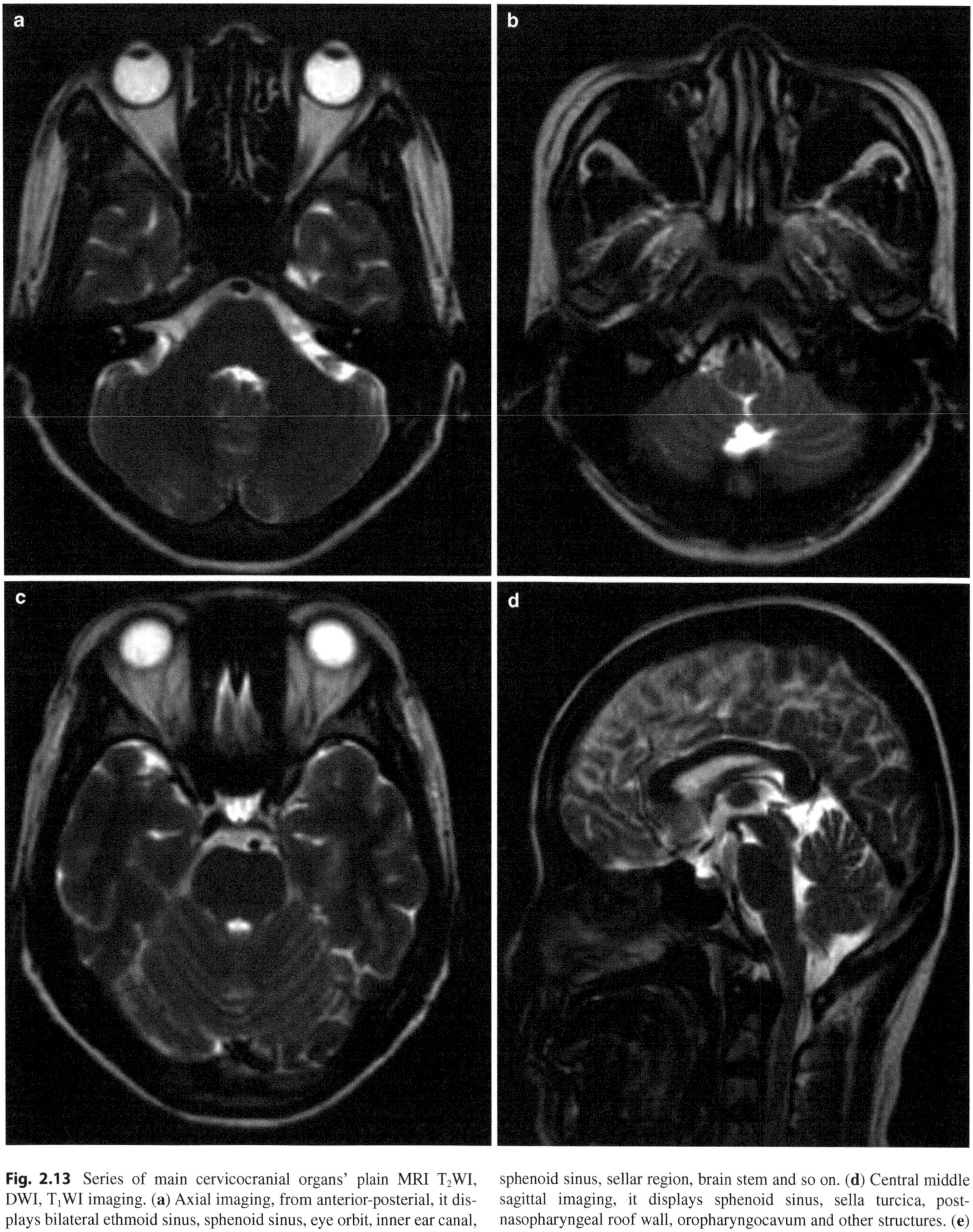


**Fig. 2.13** Series of main cervicocranial organs' plain MRI $T_2$WI, DWI, $T_1$WI imaging. (**a**) Axial imaging, from anterior-posterial, it displays bilateral ethmoid sinus, sphenoid sinus, eye orbit, inner ear canal, audio nerve, mastoid process and so on. (**b**) Axial imaging, it displays bilateral turbinate, maxillary sinus, nasopharyngeal region and their mucosa, etc. (**c**) Axial imaging, it displays bilateral ethmoid sinus, sphenoid sinus, sellar region, brain stem and so on. (**d**) Central middle sagittal imaging, it displays sphenoid sinus, sella turcica, post-nasopharyngeal roof wall, oropharyngocavum and other structures. (**e**) Axial DWI, rhinopharyngocavum represents no signals and mucosa displays linear high signal at rhinopharyngeal bedding imaging. (**f**) Axial $T_1$WI, it lies as image (**c**)

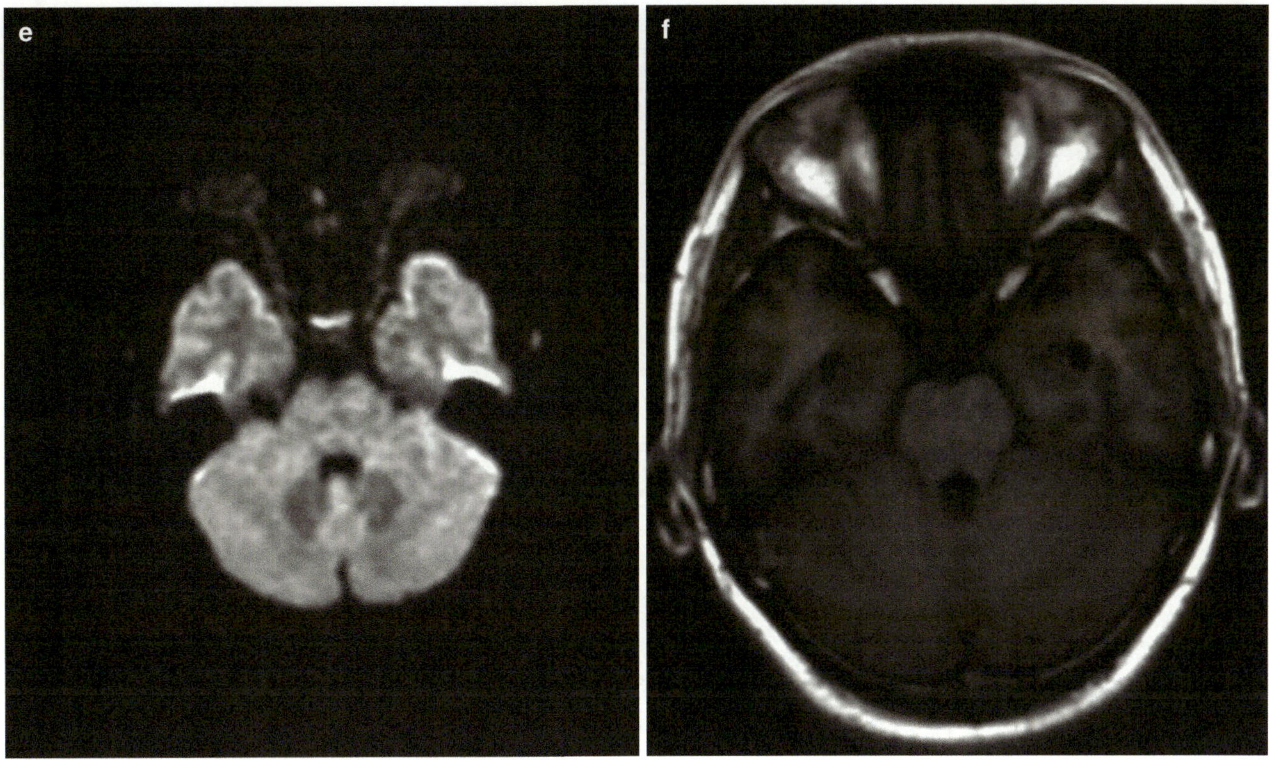


**Fig. 2.13** (continued)

molecules in tissues. The DWI technique could be used to differentiate diagnosis of the cystic lesions (cyst and abscess) and it has certain value at the etiologic diagnosis of the cervicocranial tumor and the lymph nodes swelling. Besides, the MRI hydrography could also be used at the ototemporal region to display the internal otic vagus structures and their lesions.

### 2.3.1 Plain MRI Scan

**Ototemporal Region**

Plain ototemporal MRI scanning's commonly used main sequences contain the $T_1$WI, the $T_2$WI and the steady free precession sequence (FIESTA at GE Company's device), they are mainly used to display the inner ear vagus, the audition nerve, the facial nerve and other structures, and the scanning orientation is commonly the cross section or the coronary section. Especially the hydrography technique (heavy $T_2$WI), the inner ear membranous labyrinth structure could be well displayed. MRI's value at displaying the facial audition nerve and the inner ear labyrinth has been gradually stressed in clinic, but its value at displaying the otosteon, the mastoid process, other pneumatic bone structures and their lesion is not good as CT (Fig. 2.14).

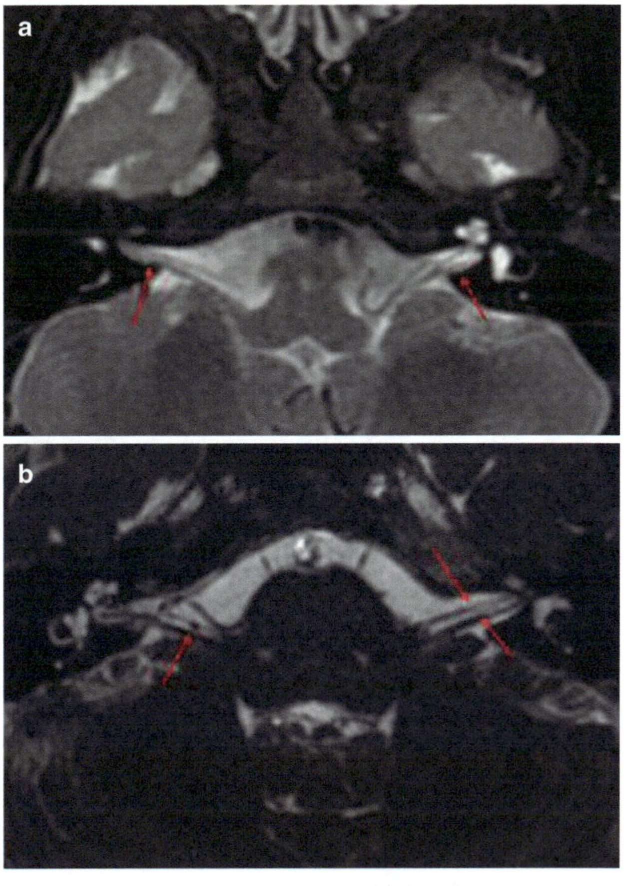


**Fig. 2.14** Mid-ear axial $T_2$WI (**a**) and FIESTA (**b**) sequence imaging, which displays bilateral inner ear canal, auditory nerve and inner ear structures

**Nose and Nasal Sinus**

MRI is an important addition to the CT examination. It commonly applies the $T_1$WI and the $T_2$WI sequence and the multi-azimuth scanning and it could help display the lesion

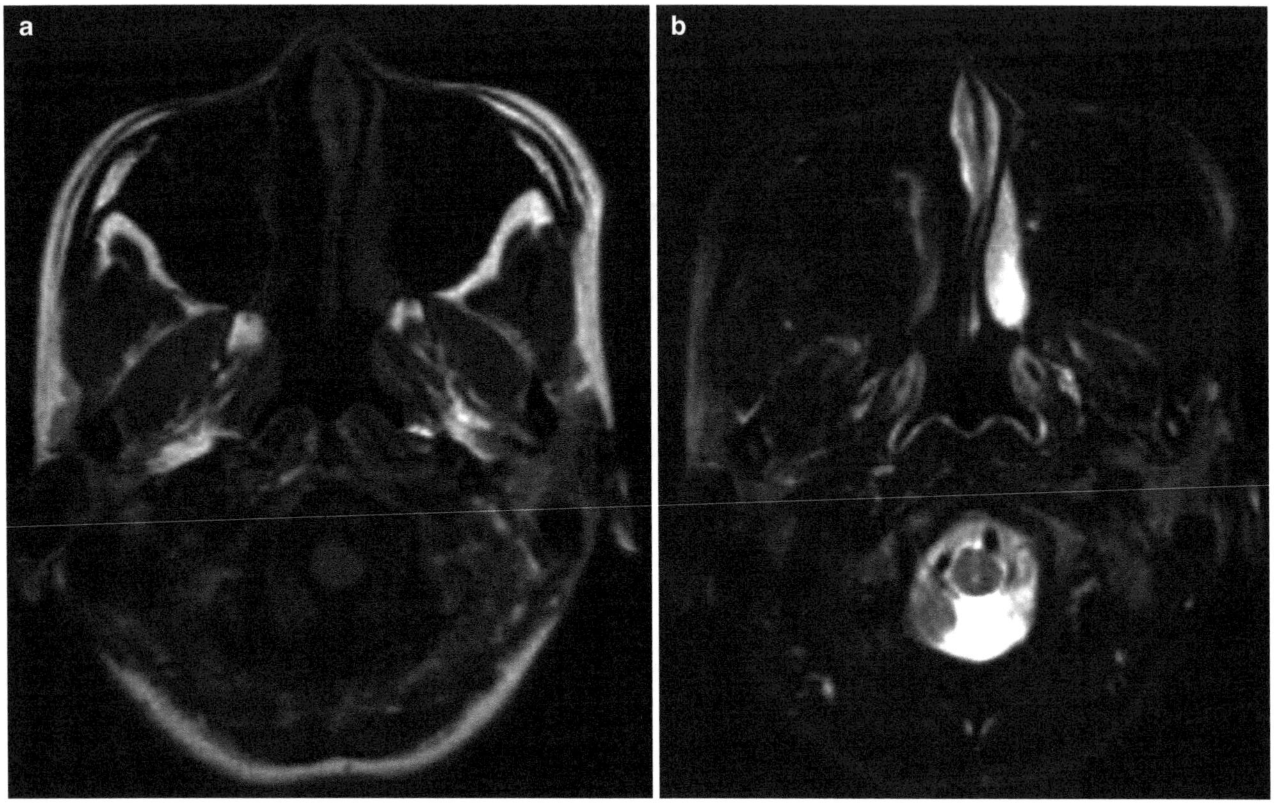


**Fig. 2.15** Nasal sinus MRI. (**a**) $T_1$WI, lateral maxillary sinus, rhinocavum, rhinopharynx, bilateral pharyngeal recess and their post-lateral muscle group. (**b**) $T_2$WI, displaying same structure as image A but clearly rhinopharyngeal mucosal layer

and its range to help differentiate the tumor from the inflammation, the mucosal cyst from the mucocele if combined it with the fat-inhibition technique (Fig. 2.15).

**Pharyngolarynx**

Laryngeal and pharyngeal lesion's MRI displacement and diagnosis value are evidently better than that of CT. Common sequences used at this region include the $T_1$WI, the $T_2$WI and the inversion recovery sequence (called STIR sequence at GE Company), the scanning slice thickness is 3-5 mm. If scanning combines with fat-inhibition technique and the enhance scanning if necessary, it could help clearly display the lesion, especially the tumor's boundaries, range, adjacent invasion and metastasis, to provide important foundations to clinic grading (Fig. 2.16).

### 2.3.2 Enhanced MRI Scan

Enhanced MRI scanning uses paramagnetic contrast medium, such as the G d-DTPA, after injecting which at cubital veins; apply sagittal, coronary and axial multi-orientational scanning. The enhanced scanning could improve the tissue contrast and evaluate the lesion tissues' blood supply condition and the relationship with their peripheral blood vessels, and it is mainly applied to the cervicocranial tumor localization, quantification, and orientation and differentiation diagnosis.

### 2.3.3 MRI Hydrography, Angiography, Neurography and Other Techniques

MR hydrography could display the inner ear labyrinth and its lesion, master the congenital abnormality existing as well. The MR neurography could display the relationship between the auditory nerve and the facial nerve and their adjacent nerves, especially helpful to diagnose the tinnitus and other diseases, which occur when, the vagal vessels oppressed the auditory nerves (Fig. 2.17). The MR angiography could display the relationship between the tumor and the blood vessels and the vascular lesion (Fig. 2.18).

## 2.4 Radionuclide Examination

Radionuclide imaging is an imaging technique visualizing human body by using radio-drugs. It mainly includes the single photon emission computerized tomography (SPECT) and the positron emission tomography-computed tomography (PET-CT). The SPECT's systemic bone scanning is a common method to examine the malignant tumor bony metastasis and it could help find the lesion six months earlier than the X-ray examination (Fig. 2.19), but it's short because its relative-worse-anatomic-resolution imaging and not-high specificity. The PET-CT are the imaging' which fuse the nuclear medical PET functional imaging and the anatomic

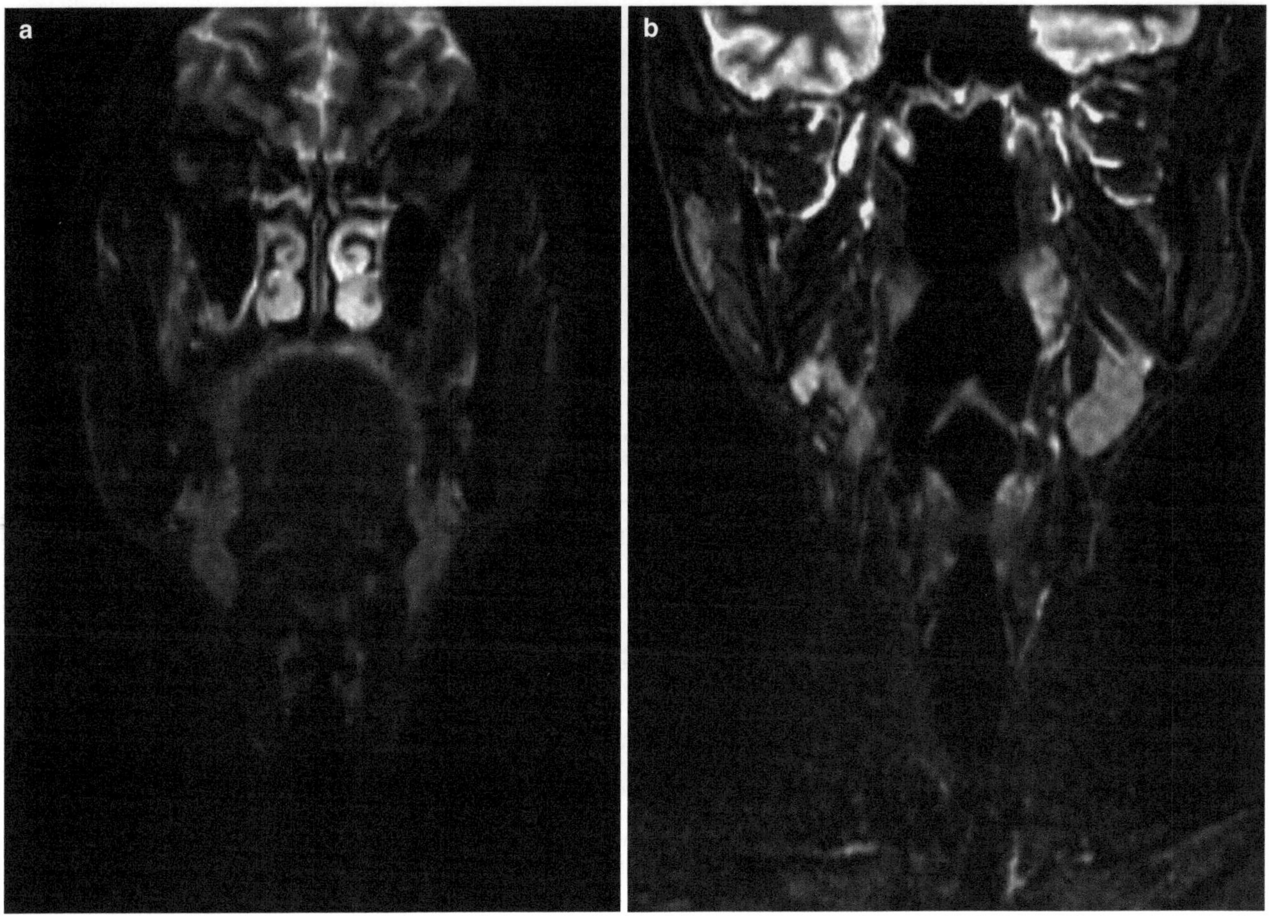


**Fig. 2.16** Cervicocranial coronary MRI $T_2$WI. (**a**) From upside down, it displays bilateral rhinocavum, maxillary sinus, laryngoventricular cavum and vocal cords. (**b**) From upside down, it displays superior nasopharyngeal wall, epiglottis, epiglottis vallecula, trachea and so on

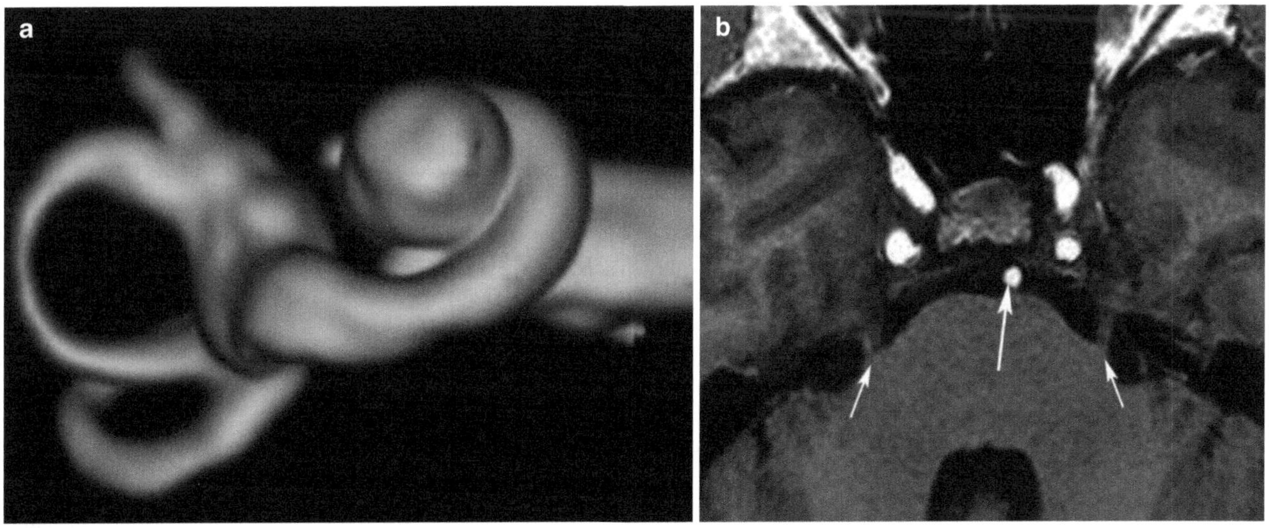


**Fig. 2.17** MRI hydrography, angiography and neurography. (**a**) MR 3D inner ear hydrography, which could display cochlea, vestibule and three semicircular canals. (**b**) Original MRA transverse section imaging, which could display basilar artery (long arrow) and trigeminal nerve (short arrow)

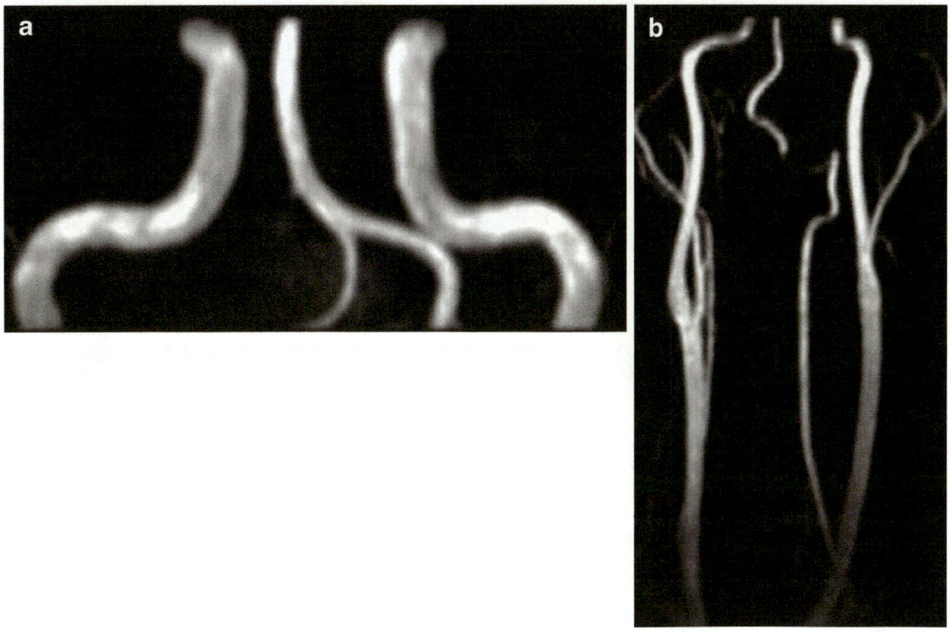


**Fig. 2.18** Cervicocranial MRA imaging. (**a**) 3D MRA, displaying sub cranial blood vessels. (**b**) 2D MRA, displaying bilateral cervical artery and vertebral artery system

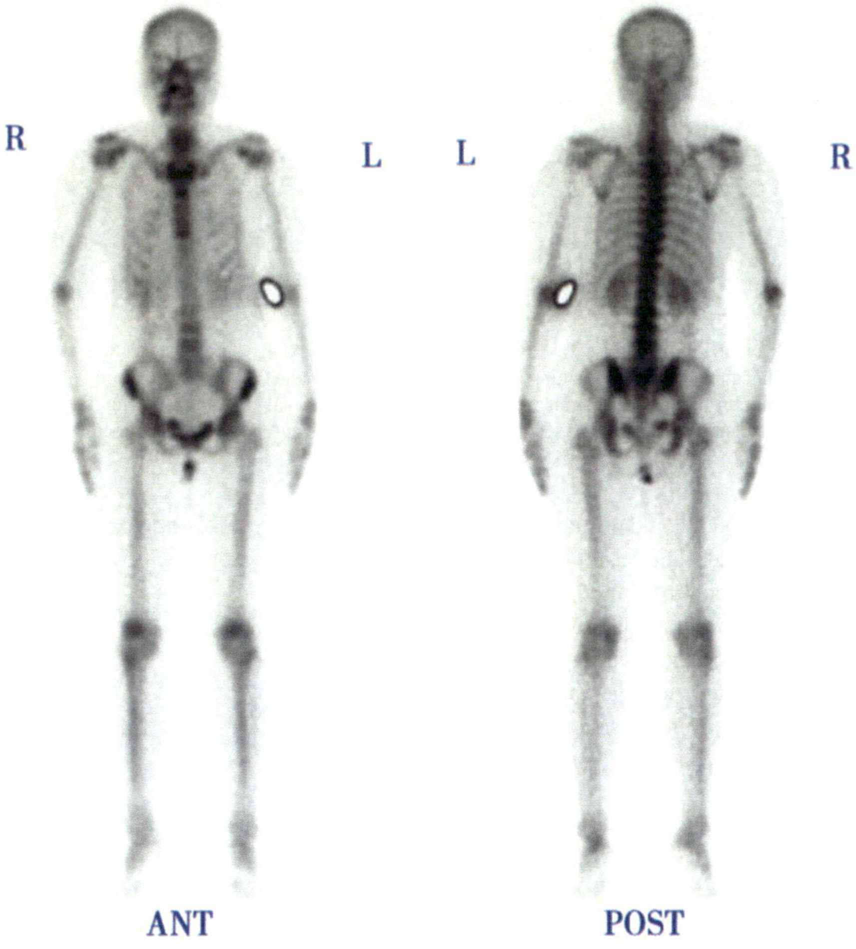


**Fig. 2.19** Systemic bone imaging, normal ante position imaging and post position imaging

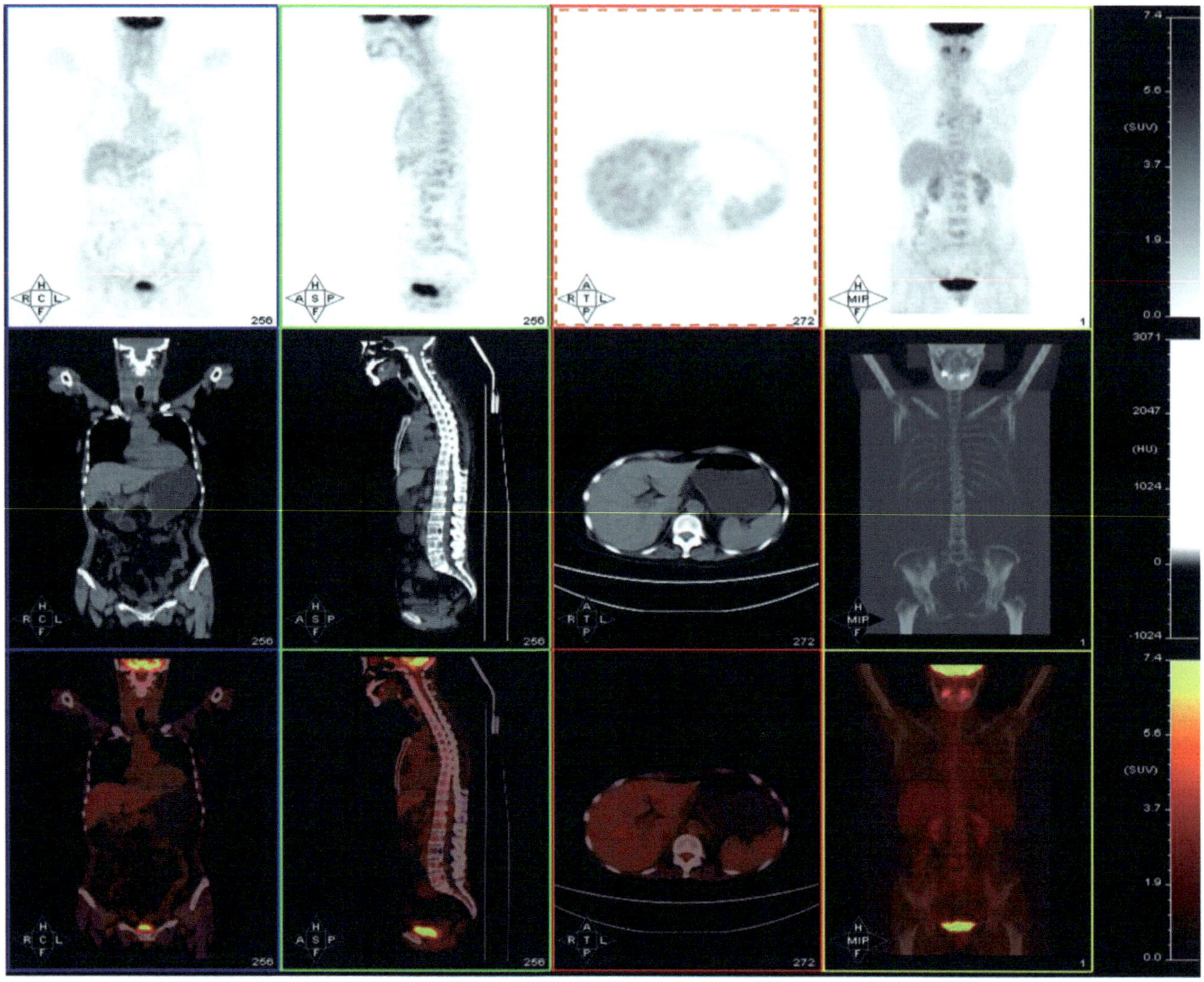


**Fig. 2.20** Normal PET-CT. First row: PET's coronary, sagittal, axial section imaging and normotopia imaging after injecting $^{18}$F-FDG radionuclide at trunk, except urinary bladder and brain, on which abnormal radial drug concentration isn't seen; second row: CT's coronary, sagittal, axial section imaging and maximum density osseous tissue 3D reconstruction imaging; 3th row: PET-CT fusion imaging (images are from Zhejiang University first affiliated hospital nuclear medicine department doctor Lili Lin)

CT imaging, and it could display the early lesion if the imaging could indicate fine anatomic information. The radionuclide imaging could be used to differentiate benign from malignant tumor, grade the malignant tumors, evaluate the efficacy, monitor the recurrence, evaluate the radio treatment's sensitivity and tolerance of the malignant tumors, seek the primary tumor lesion and so on [1] (Fig. 2.20).

## Reference

1. Zhang XL. Medical imaging. Beijing: High Education Publishing House; 2007. p. 84–103.

# Common Drugs Used in Otorhinolaryngology Head and Neck Surgery

# 3

Saiming Chen and Jihong Huang

## 3.1 Common Drugs of Ear

1. 3% Hydrogen Peroxide
   (a) Ingredients: 3% hydrogen peroxide.
   (b) Action: clearance and disinfection.
   (c) Application: acute and chronic suppurative otitis media, external otitis.
   (d) Usage: ear washing, three times daily.
2. 0.25–0.5% Chloramphenicol Cortisone Solution
   (a) Ingredients: 0.25–0.5% chloramphenicol and cortisone.
   (b) Action: disinfection, sterilization, swelling, and anti-allergy. The effect on the gram-positive bacilli is better.
   (c) Application: acute and chronic suppurative otitis media.
   (d) Usage: ear drops, three times daily.
3. 2.5% Chloramphenicol Glycerin
   (a) Ingredients: 2.5% chloramphenicol.
   (b) Action: the effect on the gram-negative bacteria is good
   (c) Application: acute and chronic suppurative otitis media.
   (d) Usage: ear drops, three times daily.
4. 1–3% Phenol glycerin Ear Drops
   (a) Ingredients: 1–3% phenol glycerin.
   (b) Action: sterilization, analgesia and DE tumescence.
   (c) Application: acute otitis media without tympanic membrane perforation and external auditory canal inflammation.
   (d) Usage: Ear drops, three times daily.
5. 4% Boric Acid Ethanol Ear Drop
   (a) Ingredients: 4% boric acid.
   (b) Action: disinfection and sterilization. Short ear tingling may occur, which explain to the patients.
   (c) Application: chronic suppurative otitis media and radical mastoidectomy (at unary operation cavity).
   (d) Usage: ear drops, three times daily.
6. 3–5% Sodium Bicarbonate Glycerin Ear Drops
   (a) Ingredients: 3–5% sodium bicarbonate.
   (b) Action: alkaline solution, dissoluble to soften cerumen.
   (c) Application: external auditory canal cerumen impaction.
   (d) Usage: ear drops, several times daily. After the cerumen softens, fetch it or wash with water.
7. Ketone (Fluorine) Alconazole Ear Drops
   (a) Ingredients: ketone (fluorine) conazole.
   (b) Action: ketoconazole is a broad-spectrum imidazole anti-fungal drug, which could strongly inhibit the candida, the yeast, and the skin fungi.
   (c) Application: combine with transdermal effect of the laurocapram (azone) to treat the fungal otitis, which is good at low dosage, short therapy course, good curative effect
   (d) Usage: eardrops.
8. 0.3% ofloxacin Eardrops
   (a) Ingredients: 0.3% ofloxacin.
   (b) Action: It is a fluoroquinolone and a broad-spectrum bactericidal sterilization drug, which mainly inhibit the bacterial DNA synthesis.
   (c) Application: bacterial otitis media, external otitis and myringitis.
   (d) Usage: For adults, six to ten drops/time, three times daily; for children, appropriately lessen the medication drops.

## 3.2 Common Drugs for Nose

1. Rhinal Mucosal Decongestant Drugs

   Apply them locally in the nose and combine them with the adrenergic receptor on the rhinomucosal vascular wall to reduce the rhinomucosal swelling. The common drugs

S. Chen · J. Huang (✉)
Department of Otorhinolaryngology Head and Neck Surgery, The First Affiliated Hospital of Hainan Medical University, Haikou, China



Z. Mu, J. Fang (eds.), *Practical Otorhinolaryngology - Head and Neck Surgery*, https://doi.org/10.1007/978-981-13-7993-2_3

include the 1% (0.5% for children) ephedrine and the xylometazoline (oxymetazoline nasal) spray.

(a) Ephedrine Rhinal Drops
 - Ingredients: 1% ephedrine hydrochloride.
 - Action: Reduce rhinomucosal edema and improve rhinal obstruction.
 - Application: it has an instant effect on remitting the rhinal obstruction, but it is an α- andβ-receptor stimulant, having relatively side effects on the heart and the nerve system, therefore, patients with hypertension, coronary atherosclerosis heart disease, the hyperthyroidism, glaucoma and prostatomegaly should be used carefully.
 - Usage: Rhinal drops while necessary.

(b) 0.05–0.1% Xylometazoline (Oxymetazoline) Spray
 - Ingredients: 0.05–0.1% xylometazoline (oxymetazoline).
 - Action: xylometazoline is an imidazoline derivatives, α-receptor agonist, which effect to contract the rhinomucosal vessels, reduce the congestion and improve the rhinal obstruction symptoms.
 - Application: acute and chronic rhinitis, rhinal sinusitis, allergic rhinitis, and hypertrophic rhinitis.
 - Contraindications: Patients with the atrophic rhinitis and the dry rhinal cavity and the patients who are receiving the single ammonia oxidase inhibitors (such as the isoniazid, etc.) are prohibited to use it.
 - Usage: adults and children older than 6-year-old: three sprays each side each time, once each morning and bedtime.

2. Mast Cell Stabilizing Agent

 2% sodium hyaluronate rhinal drops

 (a) Ingredients: 2% sodium hyaluronate.
 (b) Action: inhibit release of allergic substances.
 (c) Application: allergic rhinitis.
 (d) Usage: rhinal drops, three times daily.

3. Antihistamines Rhinal Spray

 (a) Levocabastine hydrochloride rhinospray
 - Ingredients: 0.05% levocabastine.
 - Action: antihistamine
 - Application: allergic rhinitis
 - Usage: rhinal spray, three times daily

 (b) Ketotifen Fumarate Aerosol
 - Ingredients: ketotifen fumarate
 - Action: antiallergic, antihistamine
 - Application: allergic rhinitis
 - Usage: rhinal spray, three times daily

 (c) Azelastine Hydrochloride rhinal spray
 - Ingredients: azelastine hydrochloride
 - Action: antiallergic, antihistamine
 - Use: allergic rhinitis.
 - Usage: rhinal spray, twice daily

4. Glucocorticoid rhinal spray

 (a) Beclometasone dipropionate aqueous rhinal spray
 - Ingredients: Beclomethasone.
 - Action: glucocorticoids, anti-inflammatory and anti allergic.
 - Application: allergic or vasomotor rhinitis
 - Usage: rhinal spray. For adults: totally four times daily two sprays per time, and for severe conditions, dosage could be increased but the daily intake should not be beyond 20 sprays; for children, two to four times daily one to two sprays every time.

 (b) Fluticasone Propionate rhinal spray
 - Ingredients: 0.05% fluticasone propionate.
 - Action: it has potent anti-inflammatory activity, but when it locally has an effect on the rhinomucosa, its systemic activity isn't detected.
 - Application: prevention and therapy of children and adults (not younger than 12) with seasonal allergic rhinitis and perennial allergic rhinitis.
 - Usage: Only rhinal inhalation: once daily, two sprays each nostril; the maintenance dose is once daily, one spray each nostril. The minimum dosage to effectively control the symptoms should be firstly applied, and only regular medication could help obtain the maximum efficacy.

 (c) Mometasone Furoate rhinal spray
 - Ingredients: 0.05% mometasone furoate.
 - Action: glucocorticoids, for local anti-inflammatory and anti-allergic.
 - Application: allergic rhinitis. Adults and children (not younger than 3).
 - Usage: rhinal spray. For adults: three times daily; for children not younger than 12 years, once each day, two sprays per rhinocavum; for children 3–11 year-old, once daily, one spray each rhinocavum [1].

 (d) Budesonide rhinal spray
 - Ingredients: Budesonide.
 - Action: glucocorticoids, for anti-inflammatory and anti allergy.
 - Application: Treatment of seasonal perennial allergic rhinitis and perennial non-allergic rhinitis, prevent rhinopolyps' regeneration after its resection and treat rhinopolyps symptomatically [2].
 - Usage: rhinal spray, one spray in the morning or evening respectively.

 (e) Triamcinolone Acetonide rhinal spray
 - Ingredients: triamcinolone acetonide

- Action: glucocorticoids, for local anti-inflammatory and anti allergy.
- Application: prevention and treatment of perennial and seasonal allergic rhinitis.
- Usage: rhinal spray. Fully shake it before using to make it even. For adults and children not younger than 12-year-old,once daily, two sprays each time each rhinocavum(220 μg/ daily); for children at 6~12-year-old, once daily, one spray each time each rhinocavum(110 μg/ daily). Regularly take medicines, and the maximum curative effect could be achieved after 1 week.

5. Spray Rhinal Allergen Blocking Drugs

   It is compounded by the chitosan hydrochloride and the polyethylene hydrogenated castor oil. After being sprayed into nose, it could prevent and adjuvant treats allergic rhinitis by reducing the allergen inhalation by the absorption effect. The patients allergic to chitosan should be cautioned to avoid its usage.
6. Rhinal Irrigation

   As a common post-endoscopic surgical therapy, rhinal irrigation could be applied to treat chronic paranasal sinusitis as well. Pathogenic substances and dirt accumulated in rhinal cavum could be dischargd by water flow so as to restore the normal physiological rhinocavum enviroment and the rhinocilia function and protect the rhinocavum [1]. Rhinal irrigation mainly contains isotonic saline, hypertonic saline and other natural sea salt. Basically, hypertonic saline over 3.5% is not suitable for rhinal irrigation; hypertonic saline 2%–2.3% and distilled seawater often be applied in clinic. Compared on the clinical effect, hypertonic saline is better than hypotonic saline, however, patients suffered dry rhinocavum should not be applied with hypertonic saline. As to brine, its temperature should be close to 37 °C (normal human body temperature) to reduce stimulation to the rhinomucosa and it should be applied twice daily due to personal needs (Fig. 3.1) [3].
7. Compound menthol camphor rhinal drops
   (a) Ingredients: totally 100 ml, including 1 g mint,1 g camphor and paraffm.
   (b) Action: lubricate rhinomucosal membrane, stimulate nerve endings, deodorization, promote rhinomucosal secretion.
   (c) Application: atrophic rhinitis, rhinitis sicca.
   (d) Usage: rhinal drops, three times daily.
8. Omalizumab for Injection

   As the world's first innovative targeted drug for asthma, omalizumab for Injection reduces inflammatory mediators and eosinophils by binding to circulating free lgE. It is suitable for patients with allergic rhinitis accompanied by asthma or nasal polyps [2, 3].

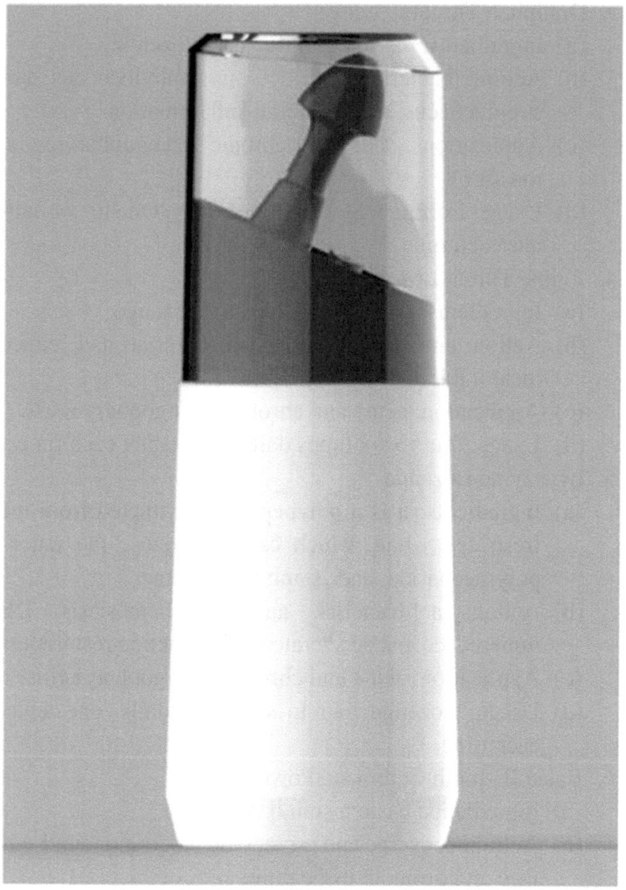

**Fig. 3.1** Nasal irrigator

## 3.3 Common Drugs of Throat

1. Compound Borax (Dobell) Solution
   (a) Ingredients: totally 100 ml, including 1.5 g borax, 1.5 g sodium bicarbonate, 0.3 ml phenol, 3.5 ml glycerol, and distilled water.
   (b) Action: alkaline solution, for antibacterial, antisepsis, disinfection and convergence.
   (c) Application: acute and chronic pharyngitis, tonsillitis and mouth wash.
   (d) Usage: diluted gargle, several three times daily.
2. Iodine Glycerol.
   (a) Ingredients: totally 100 ml, including 1.25 g iodine, 2.5 g potassium iodide, 0.5 ml peppermint oil, 25 ml distilled water, and glycerol.
   (b) Action: disinfection, lubrication and mild stimulation.
   (c) Application: chronic pharyngitis and atrophic pharyngitis, atrophic rhinitis as well.
   (d) Usage: apply on posterior pharyngeal wall and other lesion sites, three times daily.

3. Doniphan Throat Lozenge
   (a) Ingredients: 0.5 mg domifen each lozenge.
   (b) Action: bactericidal effect on staphylococcus and streptococcus, and local anti-inflammation
   (c) Applications: acute and chronic laryngopharyngitis, tonsillitis.
   (d) Usage: Lozenge. Several times daily. One to two tablets each time
4. Iodine Throat Lozenge
   (a) Ingredients: 0.0013 g iodine each lozenge.
   (b) Action: anti-inflammation, antibacterial, and reduce local inflammatory responses.
   (c) Application: acute and chronic laryngopharyngitis.
   (d) Usage: four to six times daily, One tablet each time.
5. Lysozyme Lozenge
   (a) Ingredients: it is a polypeptidase extracted from the fresh egg white, which can decompose the mucopolysaccharide, and 20 mg per lozenge.
   (b) Action: antibacterial, antivirus, hemostasis, DE tumescence and accelerate tissue function restoration
   (c) Application: acute and chronic laryngopharyngitis
   (d) Usage: Lozenge four to six times daily, one tablet each time.
6. Basic Bismuth Carbonate Powder
   (a) Ingredients: basic bismuth carbonate.
   (b) Action: converge and protect the mucosal wound surface and promote its healing.
   (c) Application: pharyngeal and esophageal mucosal damage, postoperative esophagoscopy.
   (d) Usage: Take it on tongue without water four to six times daily.
7. 1% Tetra Caine
   (a) Applications: Common mucosal superficial anesthetics. Apply it topically to anesthetize the mucosal surface during otorhinolaryngology operations, esophageal and tracheal inspection. It is a clinical error to apply it as an infiltration anesthesia drug.
   (b) Notice
      - Injection and surface anesthetic agents must be strictly reserved respectively, and marked with respective labels. The tetra Caine solution should be mixed with another color (such as eosin) so as to distinguish them.
      - Fresh preparation is the best, not suitable for long time.
      - Apply a small dose at first to observe whether the drug anaphylaxis existing or not, if it doesn't occur, an appropriate therapy dose could be applied, total of which commonly is not over 60 mg (6 ml) for adults.
      - While using the tetra Caine, adding a few epinephrine is necessary to contract the capillaries so as to slower the drug absorption and prolong the anesthesia time.
      - Enjoin the patients not to swallow the medicines (except for the esophageal inspection).
      - Children and pregnant women have low tolerance to this drug, so they should take it with great caution or not take it. During the medication period, the medical staff should pay close attention to their complexion, facial expression, pulse, respiration and so on.
   (c) poisoning symptoms: dizziness or vertigo, blurred vision, airisclose, panic terror, pallor, dry mouth, mydriasis or excitement, hallucination, delirium, talkative, wild laugh and weak pulse, reduced blood pressure, irregular and shallow respiratory and other symptoms. Once the poisoning is found, stop taking the medicine immediately, fetch the tetra Caine cotton piece in nose and perform the first aids. Intravenously inject the dexamethasone by 5 mg; to the excitement or the convulsions, give them the sedative (such as diazepam, 0.1–0.2 mg/kg, intravenous injection) or thiopental it is used to control the tic by a viable 2–2.5% by slow intravenous injection, and immediately stop injecting once the tic is under control but keep the needle incase the recurrent tic, but the total medicine is commonly not over 5 mg/kg. Simultaneously, set the patients in the supine positioning with head-down tilt, then quietly and closely observe their pulse, HR, respiration, Bp and consciousness till the poisoning symptoms are gone. The arterial respiration, endotracheal intubation, oxygen inhalation and other measurements could be applied if necessary.

## References

1. Bachert C, Zhang L, Gevaert P. Current and future treatment options for adult chronic rhinosinusitis: focus on nasal polyposis. J Allergy Clin Immunol. 2015;136(6):1431–40.
2. Chen Y, Chai X. Gist progress of monoclonal antibiotic therapy of chronic rhino-paranasal sinusitis accompanying with rhinopolyps. J Clin Otorhinolaryngol Head Neck Surg. 2018;32(10):789–93.
3. Heatley DG, McConnell KE, Kille TL, Leverson GE. Nasal irrigation for the alleviation of sinonasal symptoms. Otolaryngol Head Neck Surg. 2001;125(1):44–8.

# Common Treatment Technology in ENT

# 4

Qiyi He, Xun Bi and Yongjun Feng

## 4.1 Laser Treatment

### 4.1.1 Principle of Laser Therapy

Laser has five effects on organisms: thermal interaction, photochemical action, mechanical action, electromagnetic action and bio stimulation.

Medicine mainly uses its thermal interaction and photochemical action. Its therapeutic effects include physiotherapy, acupuncture and surgery.

1. Laser physiotherapy: weak laser directly irradiates the lesions could produce the anti-inflammatory analgesic effect and the vascular relaxation, promote the blood circulation and the metabolism and so on. It usually applies the He-Ne laser and the $CO_2$ laser;
2. Laser acupuncture: the laser acupuncture irradiation can approach the therapy purpose by penetrating skin without pain, asepsis;
3. Laser operation: the high-power laser-beam replaces the scalpel to operate, whose advantages are: less bleeding; high accuracy rate, light injury to target cell surroundings; relatively-lighter postoperative tissue swelling, less reaction; quicker wound healing, less infection, relatively-lighter scar.

During laser therapy, there should be strict secure measures, the medical personnel who contract the laser should wear the protective glasses, the patients' eyes should be pasted with unguents, the operation field surroundings should be under the saline gauze protection, especially while transferring oxygen through the airway, beware of breaking the air sac and cause a burning.

The laser has many advantages, such as its good directionality, high brightness, high monochromasis, good coherence; so it is widely used in medical field. The common otorhinolaryngological laser devices include the Nd: YAG optical maser, the $CO_2$ laser device, the argon-ion optical maser, and semiconductor laser device.

1. Nd:YAG Optical Maser

   It is a solid laser device, its laser wavelength is 1.06 pm, whose laser is the near infrared invisible light, its beam type is the pulse or the continuous wave, its output power is 1–100 W, its tissue penetration depth is about 4 mm, it can complete the solidification, the cutting, the gasification and so on and it is transmitted by the 300~700-μm quartz optical fiber. It could operate or treat in the deep intra cavum sites through various shapes of rigid tubes or endoscopes.
2. $CO_2$ Laser Device

   It is a gas laser device; it belongs to the non-contact laser. Its laser wavelength is 10.6 μm, the nearly infrared invisible light, its tissue penetration depth is about 0.23 mm, its beam types include the pulse, ultra-pulse and continuous wave, which are transmitted through the light-guide articulating arm and connected with the operative microscope and various endoscope through the adapters. Its general output power is 2~30 W, which could accomplish the burning, solidification, cutting, gasification and so on. Especially the folding light-guide arm and the microscopic sighting device passing through multiple joints, both of them make the focal spot smaller and the operation more accurate.
3. Argon-Ion Optical Maser

   It is a gas laser, its laser medium is the strongly ionized low-pressure argon, it's in the visible blue light spectrum, its wavelength is 488~515 nm and it is transmitted by the quartz optical fibers. Its beam type is the continuous

Q. He (✉) · Y. Feng
Department of Otorhinolaryngology Head and Neck Surgery, The Second Affiliated Hospital of Hainan Medical University, Haikou, China

X. Bi
Department of Pediatric Surgery, The First Affiliated Hospital of Hainan Medical University, Haikou, China



Z. Mu, J. Fang (eds.), *Practical Otorhinolaryngology - Head and Neck Surgery*, https://doi.org/10.1007/978-981-13-7993-2_4

wave, whose laser efficiency is 0.1%, output power is 1~10 W and tissue penetration depth is 0.84 mm, it has special affinity with the hemoglobin, and It is suitable for the therapy of the hemorrhagic diseases and the hemangioma.

4. GaAIAs Semiconductor Laser Device

   It is a relatively-new type laser device, its laser wavelength is 810 nm ± 25 nm, its tissue exposure mode contains the continuous, the single and the repeated pulses; it could be passed through the flexible optical fiber transmission, its output power is 0.5~20 W, It could operate the non-blood cutting, the gasification, the solidification.

### 4.1.2 Laser Therapy for Ear Diseases

1. Otic Diseases' Laser Therapy
   (a) Laser operation could be applied to the external otic surgeries, such as the pseudo auricular cyst, the mole, the wart and the otic benign tumor on the auricular, the external auditory canal, the lateral mastoid skin; the sebaceous cyst, the pre auricular fistula, the accessory auricles, the auricular and the periauricular skin micro lesion squamous carcinoma or the basaloma; the mid-ear surgeries, such as the tympanic laser boring, the tympanoplasty, the strapes laser fenestration surgeries and so on.
   (b) Local irradiation therapy could be applied to the acute external otitis, the external otitis furunculosa, the herpes zoster, the auricular eczema, the dermatitis, the anterior auricular fistula infection, the sebaceous cyst infection, the acute and the chronic secretory otitis media, the suppurative otitis media, the operation incision infection, the irradiation therapy reaction and so on. Joining the acupuncture irradiation as the adjuvant therapy could help treat the severe tinnitus Meniere's disease, etc.
   (c) Dos and Don'ts
      - Strict aseptic blanket should be applied during the auricular and the external ear canal laser operation to avoid the complicate postoperative auricular cartilage suppurative infection;
      - The intra-extra-ear canal laser operation is better in the operative microscope;
      - The local auricular irradiation therapy could be under an accurate laser dosage to avoid the auricular cartilage injury.
2. Rhinal Diseases' Laser Therapy

   The auricular and the rhinovestibular diseases should be applied to the low-power $CO_2$ laser irradiation therapy, and the YAC laser irradiation operation therapy could be applied to the chronic rhinitis, the chronic nasal sinusitis, the rhinopolyps and the epistaxis.
   (a) The laser operation could be applied to the external nose, the rhinovestibuler cutaneous nevus and thymion, the angioma, the anterior rhinoaditus atresia, the rhinal cavum adhesion, the rhinal septum capillary hemangioma and papilloma, the middle turbinate polyposis, the inferior turbinate hypertrophy, the rhinopolyps.
   (b) The local irradiation operation could be applied to the allergic rhinitis, the rhinal vestibular inflammation and furuncle, the middle septum anapetia and mucosal erosion, the intractable epistasis and the olfactory disorder as well.
   (c) Dos and Don'ts

      While the laser operation is applied to the external rhinal sites adjacent to the eyes, protect the eyes as much as we can by wearing the laser-protection glasses or covering the eyeball with the gauzes soaked by normal saline; it is suitable to operate under the endoscopic surveillance, the light beam should be focused as much as possible, the irradiation time should not be too long, and pay attention to injure the lamina cribiosa and the orbital contents while applying the laser operation on the rhinocavum topical and extratopical wall.
3. Laryngopharyngeal Diseases
   (a) Pharyngeal operation and therapies, such as tonsillectomy, adenoidectomy, benign pharyngotumorectomy, chronic pharyngitis, lymphatic follicular hyperplasia or hypertrophy, the lateral pharyngeal band gasification and local irradiation, the early nasopharyngeal cancer or the irradiation therapy residual focus gasification and carbonization.
   (b) The laser application in pharyngeal operation benefits from laser micro manipulation device invented in the 1970s, which couples $CO_2$ laser and binocular microscope through special adapters, solving the transmission problem of the laser beam directly entering laryngocavum and ensuring laser therapy accuracy.

      In recent years, laser fibrescope's invention has made it easier for manipulating laser to clear the lesion remotely, and it has many advantages, including clear operative vision, no hemorrhage, rapid postoperative recovery and good laryngal function remittance. To protect the vocal cords and the normal peripheral tissues better, certain pulse power (4~6 W) laser should be applied, and to avoid the repeated irradiation at one site, the skipping cutting mode should be applied.

      Laser could be applied to treat the vocal nodules, the vocal polyps, the laryngoscar stenosis, the benign laryngotumor, the arytenoid cartilage resection, the

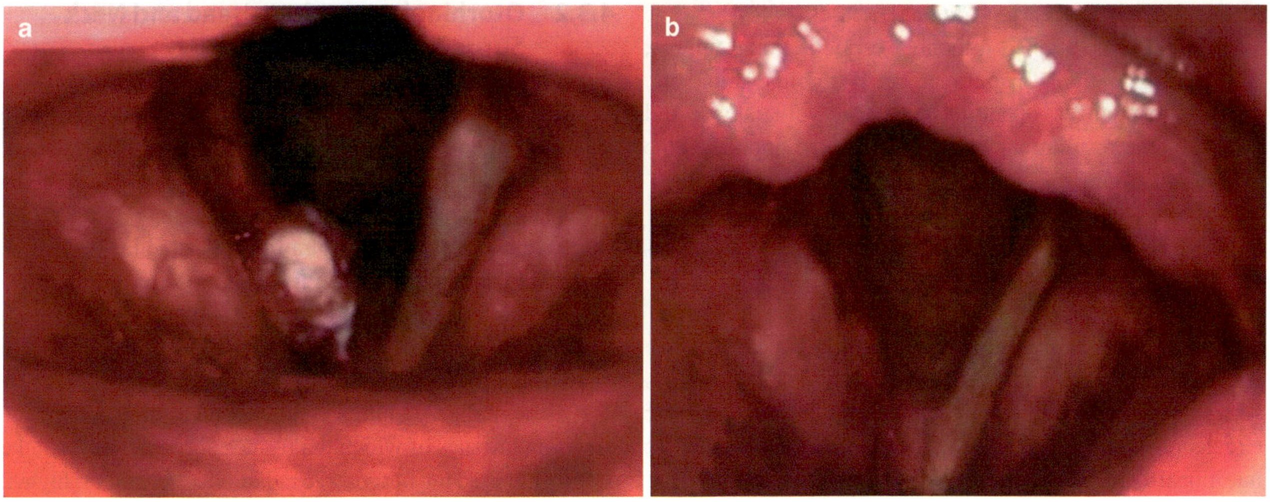


**Fig. 4.1** laryngocancer (glottic type) laser operation effect: (**a**) Pre-operation (**b**) 1 year postoperation

T1 stage laryngocancer, especially at the T1~2 stage glottic laryngocancer, the laser therapy has been the first choice (Fig. 4.1).

(c) Dos and Don'ts.

The area dealt every time should be limited as far as possible to avoid the possible laryngeal edema caused by too-large scope. If it is vital to apply the laser operation to the relatively bigger scope lesion, the pre-operative tracheotomy should be performed. Before performing the laser therapy, cautiously inspect the lesion's peripheral vascular channel to avoid accidentally injuring the laryngopharyngeal great vessels.

## 4.2 Cryotherapy

### 4.2.1 Principles of Cryotherapy

Cryotherapy is a therapeutic method, which utilizes the below 0 °C temperature, which could freeze and destroy the tissues, to freeze the lesion to treat. It could cause less tissue defections, deformation, dysfunction and other complications and thinner and shallower scar. But the cryopreservation would also reduce the molecular motion rate of some substances or in organisms or kill the biological cells.

1. Cryotherapeutic Mechanism
   (a) The refrigeration could induce the intracellular and the extra-cellular ice to cause cellular damage.
   (b) The refrigeration could cause the protein denaturation.
   (c) During the rapid cooling, all the intracellular components would cause the cell rupture because the uneven contraction-distention ratio.
   (d) The refrigeration could also cause the local blood circulation disorders.

   Common clinical freezing mediums are the Freon and the liquid nitrogen. The common coolers are the phase-change freezer (liquid nitrogen), the throttling expansion freezer (freon) and the thermal freezer, among which, the liquid-nitrogen phase-change freezer is a common one at otorhinolaryngology apartment.
2. Cryotherapeutic Method
   (a) Contract Method: directly contract the cryo-pencil with the lesion; most common method.
   (b) Spray Method: straightly spray the freezing medium onto the affected part.
   (c) Penetration Method: penetrate the cold scalpel bit into the affected tissue to destroy the lesion.
   (d) Tilt-pouring Method: pour the freezing medium onto the affected part.

### 4.2.2 Otorhinolaryngology Head and Neck Cryotherapy

1. Auricular Pseudocyst Liquid-Nitrogen Low-Temperature Cryotherapy

   Firstly, puncture to fetch all the cyst fluid, secondly, set the contract cryo-pencil on the cyst and count the therapeutic times, about 30 s, from −30 °C to −85 °C. One to three days after operation, the evident local swelling and infiltration could be observed, then they would scab and gradually cure 7~10 days later.
2. Chronic Rhinitis Cryotherapy

   Set the cryo-pencil on the inferior rhino-concha which will be frozen after performing the mucosal surface anesthesia, start recording time at −30 °C and accomplish the therapy after 30~45 s, remove the cryo-pencil when it warms up, and after the mucosal restoration (normally 1~1.5 min) completes, repeat the cryotherapy once again.

3. Cryotherapy of Cervico-Cranial Diseases

   It could be applied to benign cervico-cranial tumors, including angioma, papilloma, small fibroids, keloid etc. The post-cancer operation cavum cryotherapy could reduce the restoration and it could also be applied to the malignant tumors' palliative therapy.

## 4.3 Radiotherapy

The microwave's therapeutic effect mainly depends on the endogenous thermal and the thermal effect. The endogenous heat could enhance the local blood circulation, the lymphatic circulation, and the irradiated tissues' metabolism, improve nutritional status, accelerate tissue repair and regeneration process, and improve the tissues' immunity response ability. The mechanism of the thermal effect is unclear, but it is very effective on acute inflammation and endocrine gland diseases.

### 4.3.1 Mechanism

1. The clinical electromagnetic wave frequency is generally 500~2500 MHz, and it could help our body produce the bio microwave thermal effect.
2. While the low-power microwave irradiate on the affected area, it produce little heat but enough to dilate the capillaries and the arterioles, finally improve the local tissues' blood circulation and enhance tissue metabolism.
3. The microwave could increase local leucocyte nucleus antibody and enhance local immunity ability; therefore, inflammation development is under control. This mechanism could apply on the microwave irradiation therapy.
4. When the microwave carries too much energy; heat production would be high, which could promote protein denaturation, tissue coagulation, necrosis and eventual defluvium. During the therapy, the microwave help solidify the tissues. If there isn't any hemorrhage the microwave dosage output would be effected by the tissue coagulation. It's characterized by its even heating with uniform depth, its non-heating process, its limited action range, its clear boundary, its non-coke, its non-hemorrhage, its less-smoke production and its clear operation vision. This mechanism could be applied on the microwave operation therapy. Recently, the microwave material work-station has been developed, which could be Figured with various heating methods.

### 4.3.2 Otorhinolaryngology Head and Neck Surgery Microwave Therapy

1. Hypertrophic Rhinitis and Allergic Rhinitis Microwave Coagulation Therapy

   Through the tissue endogenous thermal effect occurrence, it helps locally instantaneous high temperature coagulation, tissue denaturation and vascular occlusion, so as to effectively reduce turbinate volume and improve rhino-cavum ventilation.
2. Cervico-Cranial Recurrent Malignant Tumor Microwave Irradiation Therapy

   The malignant tumor's water content differs from the normal tissues of which the former one is higher than the latter one, so the microwave radiation absorption is higher. The characteristic of the radiation makes it possible to efficiently kill the tumor cells and protect the normal cells to the hilt. Applying the interstitial microwave radiation combing with the radiotherapy and the chemotherapy, is very effective on the cervico-cranial recurrent cancer.

## 4.4 Low-Temperature-Plasma Radio-Frequency Ablation Therapy (LTPRFAT)

### 4.4.1 LTPRFAT Principle

It decomposes the lesion intra tissue cells at 100-kHz radiofrequency, then cut and ablate them at relatively-low temperature (40~70 °C). Its principle is to form a plasma film between the electrode and the tissues, in which the free electrophorus particles are accelerated to obtain the kinetic energy, the electric field and disrupt the intracellular molecular bonding to disintegrate in addition, so that the hyperplastic lesion tissues would be reduced or eliminated. So the LTPRFAT can be applied to treat chronic rhinitis, rhinopolyps, epistaxis, chronic pharyngitis, epiglottic cyst etc.

### 4.4.2 Otorhinolaryngology Head and Neck Surgery LTPRFAT

1. Rhinal Diseases LTPRFAT

   It includes treatment of rhinal active hemorrhage and rhinal easily bleeding benign tumors, such as the nasal hemangioma. After treating the peripheral lesion, treat the hemorrhagic spot. Its processes are: press the spot with cotton piece, then instantly remove the piece and contract the spot with the cryopencil immediately to accomplish the hemostasis. The rhinitis's therapy mainly focuses on rhinal agger, middle concha, middle meatus's lateral mucosa and the inferior concha's mucosa. While performing the inferior chonca's therapy of the chronic rhinitis, the cyberknife could draw a line from inferior to anterior, or singly fire at 4~5 spots. If the watery secretion is too much while treating the rhinal cavity diseases, the therapy could be affected, so wipe them with cotton swabs before treating. Recently, combing the cyberknife with the endoscope could help perform the intra-rhinocavum LTPRFAT.

2. Laryngeal and Lingual Root Diseases' LTPRFAT

   To treat the glandular pharyngitis, muffle the tongue with gauzes and choose the evidently-swelling follicles with the bending cryopencils with the spatula or under the indirect laryngoscope and treat 4~5 of them each time. The chronic amygdalitis LTPRDAT (Fig. 4.2) dissection, during which insert the cryopencil into the tonsillar lacuna till its peripheral skin becomes pale, five to six spots laterally each time. Some laryngopharyngeal tumors and cysts can also be dissected with the LTPRFAT (Fig. 4.3).

3. Otic Diseases' LTPRFAT

   It is mainly applied to eliminate the accessory auricles, the small external ear canal neoplasms.

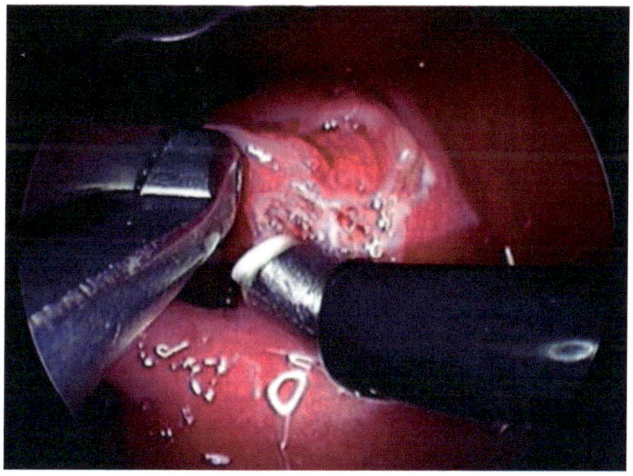

**Fig. 4.2** LTPRFAT tonsillar dissection

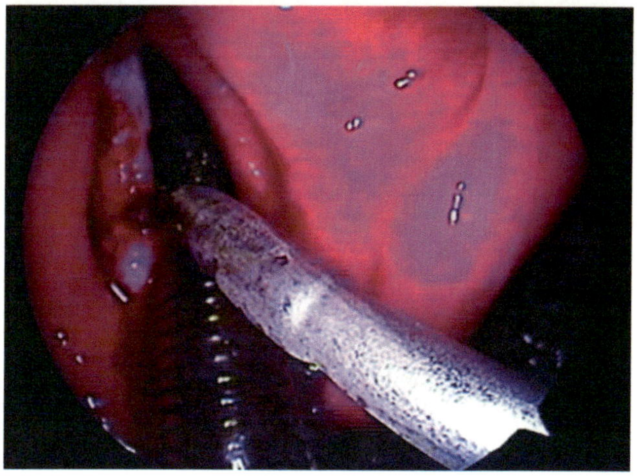

**Fig. 4.3** LTPRFAT glottic laryngocancer therapy

With recent new technology, low-temperature plasma radio-frequency operation devices cause the low-temperature plasma radio-frequency's energy to eliminate the lesion tissues at a relatively-low temperature. The low-temperature ablation technology can form a highly-aggregated plasma bodies region around the electrode through the electrolyte. The low-temperature plasma radio-frequency has many advantages: indirectly damage tissues which causes less peripheral tissue damage; the electric current doesn't flow through the tissues so the tissue thermal energy is less making the therapeutic temperature low; tissues then ablate at fixed sites, benefiting from the intra molecular interval.

The low-temperature plasma system has been widely applied to treat the obstructive sleep apnea hypopnea syndrome (OSAHS), chronic rhinitis, allergic rhinitis, chronic amygdalitis, tonsillar hypertrophy, and adenoid hypertrophy; all of which has obtained great curative effect [1].

## Reference

1. Du Y, Wang D, Zhang L. Diagnosis key points and treatment method fascicle. 2013.

# Application of Robotic Surgery System and Imaging Navigation Technology at Otorhinolaryngology Skull Base Surgery

5

Zhonglin Mu, Jugao Fang and Xiaohui Mi

## 5.1 Brief Introduction

As science and technology develop, especially the electronic information technology and the robotic surgery technology, integration of the imaging, the radio-surgery and the Horsley-Clarke technique, the robotics derives a variety of new treatment measures. The wide application of the rhinal endoscopic surgery takes some change on the skull-base surgical methods, such as at the endoscopic of pituitary adenoma resection surgery, the cerebrospinal rhinorrhea repair surgery, the optic nerve decompression via sphenoid sinus [1]; of which the operative access is easy, the trauma is small, the vision is clear and the complications are less, and it also widens the application of navigation system. The robotic surgical system is a kind of advanced robot platform, which is a kind of finer micro-invasive operation mode to perform complex surgeries.

Imaging navigator technology is also called frameless stereotaxic or computer—aided surgery (CAS). Random point at patients' head could be pointed on the 3D model corresponded by X- Y - Z coordinates, signed by a cross in preoperative imaging instructions to help obtain imaging information (by CT or MRI) of patients before operation and recorded in computer.

**Electronic Supplementary Material** The online version of this chapter (https://doi.org/10.1007/978-981-13-7993-2_5) contains supplementary material, which is available to authorized users.

Z. Mu (✉)
Department of Otorhinolaryngology Head and Neck Surgery, The First Affiliated Hospital of Hainan Medical University, Haikou, China

J. Fang
Department of Otorhinolaryngology Head and Neck Surgery, Beijing Tongren Hospital, Capital Medical University, Beijing, China

X. Mi
Department of Otorhinolaryngology Head and Neck Surgery, Chinese People's Liberation Army 91458 Military Hospital, Sanya, China

After anesthesia, registration would be performed to establish the corresponding relationship between patients' actual position and imaging, the sites where the surgical instruments' ending is and the actual surgical path during operation. On the basis of design thought above, otorhinolaryngology imaging system consists of three parts: imaging processing systems for recording and processing images data, coordinating digitizer system and professional computer software. On the basis of different coordinate positioning technologies, current imaging navigation system contains four categories.

### 5.1.1 Acoustic Conductive Imaging Navigation System

Set pinger on surgical instruments, then computer determines the location of surgical instruments by measuring the time required to transmit the sound waves from sonic emitter to microphone.

### 5.1.2 Mechanical-Arm Type Imaging Navigation System

Connect surgical instruments at the further end of mechanical arm and place position sensors inside the mechanical arm, then computer could measure the precise location of the end of the surgical instruments connected to the mechanical arm by the built-in sensor to obtain the mechanical arm's movement.

### 5.1.3 Electromagnetic Inductive Type Imaging Navigation System

Place magnetic field above the operation-related area and connect electromagnetic sensor to surgical instrument, then



Z. Mu, J. Fang (eds.), *Practical Otorhinolaryngology - Head and Neck Surgery*, https://doi.org/10.1007/978-981-13-7993-2_5

computer could accurately measure the position of the surgical instrument by detecting the position of the electromagnetic sensors in the magnetic field.

### 5.1.4 Optical Sensing Type Imaging Navigation System

According to the difference between luminescent mark and luminescence principle, it has two categories: active type (AOSINS) and passive type (POSINS).

AOSINS's positioning method: set the infrared light-emitting diode (led) on a probe or a surgical instrument, then the computer can pinpoint the probe or the surgical instruments by detecting the position of led; and on the other part, place the infrared led on the head frame connected to patient's head, then the head's movement can be watched on the computer.

POSINS's positioning method: install the reflector on the surgical instrument or the probe, and then the probe can be positioned by detecting the light reflected from the reflector.

As we can see above, AOSINS and POSINS differs from the light source, that the former needs a wire to connect led to the power source, nor is the latter one.

As a tool, the navigation system plays an important role on improving security level during otolaryngology skull-base surgeries. It provides precise positioning, and makes the operation more perfect after being combined with the endoscope; the robotic surgery system could perform a complex surgery accurately with less trauma and fewer surgical personnel.

## 5.2 Da Vinci Robotic Surgical System

**Definition**

Da Vinci robotic system (Fig. 5.1) is the second generation robotic surgery system and an advanced robotic platform. Otorhinolaryngology surgeons have already started to apply it in clinic, such as during trans-oral robotic surgery (TORS), because it could give a good feedback for oro-pharyngeal cancer, its advantages like no scar left at face and neck and smaller trauma, it costs shorter operative and postoperative healing time and shorter hospitalization time, it causes less bleeding, etc. It is mainly applied to parapharyngeal interval tumor, which is with an intact membrane of the capsule, at the anterior lateral internal carotid artery also bit distant from the internal carotid artery, in neck and thyroid masses or tonsils, oro-pharyngeal and ear parts as well, and it is also widely used in general surgery, gynecology, cardio thoracic surgery and urology [2] (Fig. 5.2).

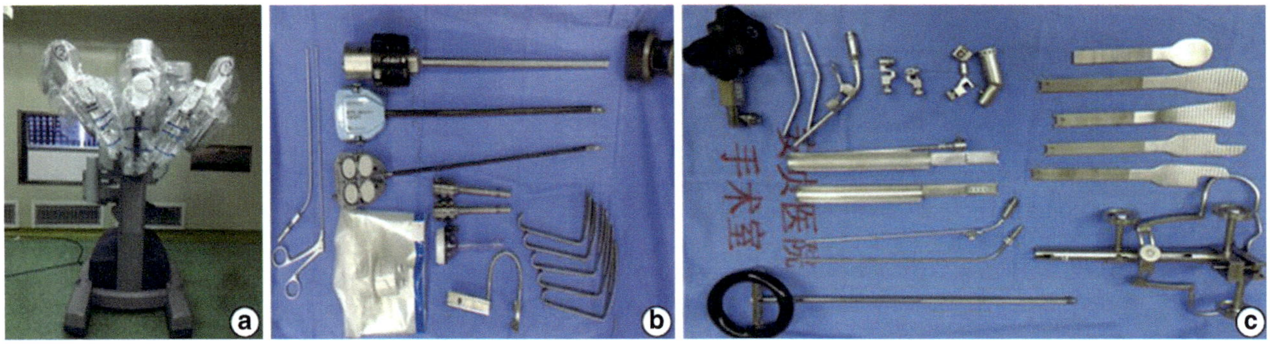

**Fig. 5.1** (**a**) Third generation Da Vinci robotic surgical system. (**b**) Operative equipments, including endoscope. Endo Wrist appliance and Da Vinci spreader. (**c**) Feyh-Kastenbauer spreader

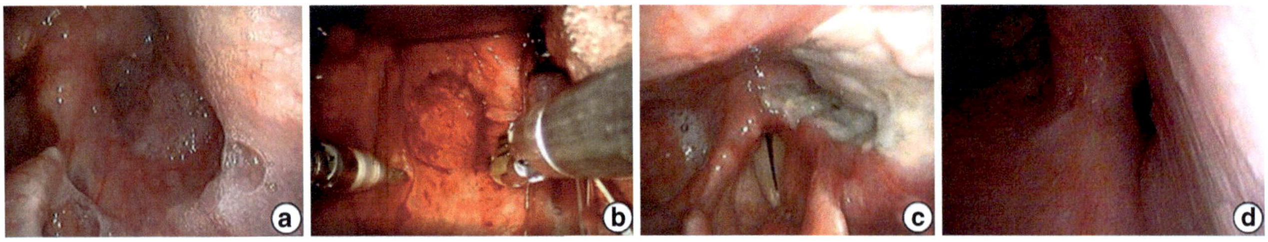

**Fig. 5.2** Da Vinci robotic surgical system transpolar hypo-pharyngeal tumor resection. (**a**) Preoperative laryngoscopy, displaying left lateral cauliflower shaped neoplasm in piriform recess, uninvolved at vocal cords. (**b**) Operative procedure, resecting left lateral piriform recess. (**c**) 1 week postoperative laryngoscopy, displaying abundant pseudomembrane at wound surface. (**d**) 13-month postoperative laryngoscopy, displaying no tumor recurrence

### Current Situation and Future in China

It costs much though it's huge and lacking of touching response caused. Its short operative experience and limited application spreading is another reason why it is not commonly applied in China.

As technology develops, many companies home and abroad have been reduced by R&D, which finally patronize a decreased price of Da Vinci robotic surgical system, Moreover, the related operations under the combined navigation of CT or B-mode ultrasound have made considerable progress. But with higher accuracy and more excellent functions. Simultaneously with Chinese development, it will be applied in Chinese medical center, TORS will be more common and represent a bright future.

## References

1. Ge WT, Han DM, Zhou B. Application and progression of imaging navigation system at otorhinolaryngology head and neck surgery. Chin J Otorhinolaryngol Head Neck Surg. 2001;36(4):305–6.
2. Meng L, Fang J, Wang J, Yuan X, Yang F, Rao Y, Feng Y, Wei Y. Primary experience of applying Da Vinci robotic surgical system on transoral laryngeal and hypopharyngeal tumor resection. J Clin Otorhinolaryngol Head Neck Surg. 2018;32(14):1065–70.

# Part II

# Otology

As an important peripheral organ for hearing and balance, ears play an important role in language communication and balance maintenance. Studying otology and oto-neuro surgery contributes to define the pathogenesis, the diagnosis and the treatment of otic diseases. This part will start from the otic applied anatomy and physiology, then mainly emphasis the otic semiology, clinical examination methods and the key points on diagnosing and treating the common otic diseases.

# 6 Applied Anatomy and Physiology of Ear

Zhonglin Mu and Xiaofeng Wang

## 6.1 Applied Anatomy of Ear

According to anatomical sites, ear contains the external, the middle and the inner ear, among which, the external ear includes the auricle and the external auditory canal, the middle ear contains the tympanic chambers, the tympanic sinus, the mastoid and the eustachian tube and the inner ear consists the osseous labyrinth and the membranous labyrinth. The membranous labyrinth hides in the osseous labyrinth and it contains the cochlea, the vestibule and the semicircular canals. The middle ear and the inner ear both locate in the temporal bone, and their physical structure is like what the profile maps of the external, middle and inner ear show.

### 6.1.1 External Ear

The external ear includes the auricle and the external auditory canal. The external auditory canal originates from the first branchial ditch, whose ectoderm epithelium extends into deep sites to develop the original external auditory canal. The posterior margin of the first branchial arch and the anterior border of the second branchial arch enclose the external ear aditus, and these two branchial arches produce the auricle.

**Auricles**

The Auricles of human beings is smaller than some low-grade-mammals' and most of them are inactive, but they still collect acoustic waves. Coordination of bilateral auricles can also help distinguish the sound's source orientation. Its surface is uneven and horn-shaped, so it has its own filtering characteristics, which can change the characteristics of sound waves by changing the incidence angle.

The auricle except for the lobule is made with the elastic cartilage, it is shell-like and often symmetrical bilaterally (Fig. 6.1). The auricle attaches to the head's flank generally at about 30° by the ligaments, the muscles, the cartilage and the skin. Auricle's rolling-outwards free margin is called the helix, which is developing from the helix crus above the external ear aditus. There is a roughly parallel arched ridge at the front of the helix, it is called the anthelix and its upper

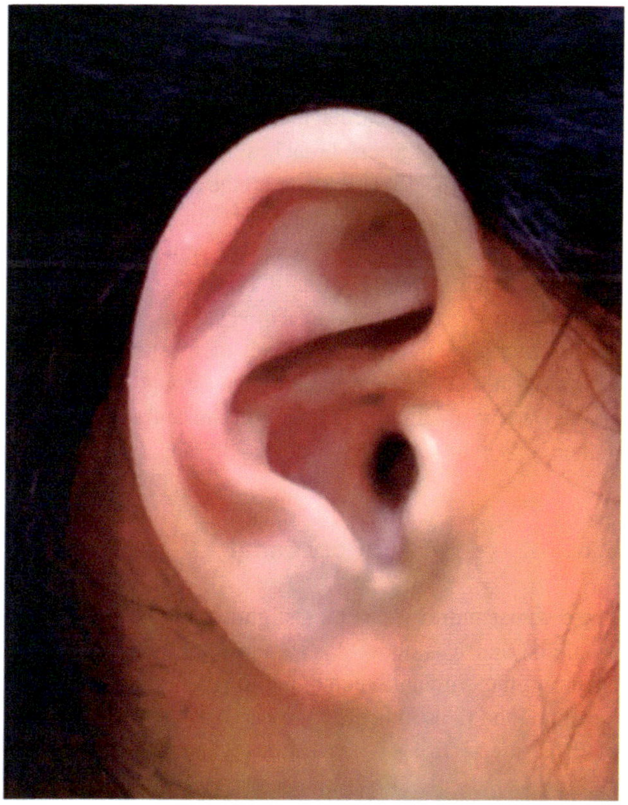

**Fig. 6.1** Auricle shape

Z. Mu (✉) · X. Wang
Department of Otorhinolaryngology Head and Neck Surgery, The First Affiliated Hospital of Hainan Medical University, Haikou, China



Z. Mu, J. Fang (eds.), *Practical Otorhinolaryngology - Head and Neck Surgery*, https://doi.org/10.1007/978-981-13-7993-2_6

ends divide into the anthelix crus. There is a narrow and curved chase between the helix and the anthelix, it is called the navicula or scapha. The deeply big fossa at the front of the anthelix is called the auricle concha, which could be divided into two parts by helix crus: the upper concha cymba and the lower concha cavum, and the concha cavum accesses into the external ear aditus. While wearing a hearing aid, these two parts are where the ear mold inserts, especially when the mold cannot be embedded into the concha cymba, the sound can leak out to cause the howl round. The protuberance at the front of the external ear aditus is called the tragus. The other tragus opposite to the tragus at antra-inferior anthelix is called the antitragus. The sunken between the tragus and the antitragus is called the intertragic notch. The none-cartilage part at inferior antitragus is the lobule.

The auricle's domination nerves are complex; They are the trigeminal nerve, the facial nerve, the branches of the glossopharyngeal nerve and the vagus, and the branches of the great auricular nerve and the minor occipital nerves from the cervical plexus. Among them, the great auricular nerve is the main nerve governing the auricle, so it should be possibly kept while performing the auricle fixation surgery, the rhytidectomy and the parotidectomy.

The auricular blood supply is abundant, which is from the branch of the external carotid artery. The anterior auricle is mainly supplied by the superficial temporal artery branch, and the posterior by the branch of the posterior auricular artery. The posterior auricle artery has small branches passed through the auricular cartilage and anastomosed with the superficial temporal artery branches at front of the auricle. The auricular vein accompanied with the auricular artery and flows back to the superficial temporal vein and the posterior auricular vein. The superficial temporal vein branches to the posterior auricular vein and finally affluxes into the internal jugular vein. The posterior auricular venous branches into the external jugular vein; sometimes the posterior auricular vein interlinks with the sigmoid sinus through the mastoid process, so the external ear's infection can cause the intracranial complications, which are extremely rare.

### 6.1.2 External Auditory Canal

The external auditory canal is a slightly curved lumen closed at an end and it is about 25–35 mm long from the concha cavum to the tympanic membrane. Its outer 1/3 is the cartilage part, and the rest is the bone part and the narrowest part of their intersections is the isthmus. The infants' external auditory canal only consists the cartilage part, but the bone part will gradually develop as they grow up.

The external auditory canal has related-thinner skin and it is related-tightly bonded to the perichondrium and the periosteum, so the pain is related-severer when the external auditory canal swells because of the inflammation. In the cartilage part's skin, the ceruminous glands, which have similar construction to the sweat glands, could secrete the cerumen and there are abundant hair follicles and sebaceous glands.

If the first and second bronchial arch dysplasia occur at embryonic stage, the auricle will deform, which may manifest as the incomplete auricle, the accessory auricle, the microtia, the macrotia, the preauricular fistula, etc. The bronchial cleft cyst or fistula can occur when the first bronchial cleft is not closed. The inner fistula adituses locate at the inferior isthmus wall, minority of whom can interlink into the middle ear, and its external adituses locate at the mandibular plane of the anterior sternocleidomastoid margin.

The superficial temporal artery, the posterior auricular artery and the deep branch of the maxillary artery supply blood to the external auditory canal. The superficial temporal artery locates at front of the ant-helix, and if open the skin, it would be easy to be found.

Sensory nerves of the auricle distribute abundantly, which include the branches of the trigeminal nerve, the vagus, the facial nerve and the glossopharyngeal nerve, and the great auricular nerve and the minor occipital nerve from the cervical plexus.

The Lymph of the external ear drains to the peripheral auricular lymph nodes. The anterior auricular lymph flows into the preauricular lymph nodes and the parotid lymph nodes, the post auricle lymph flows into the post auricular lymph nodes. Lymph of the sub auricle and the inferior wall of the external auditory canal flow into the sub auricular lymph nodes the superficial cervical lymph nodes and the deep cervical lymph node co group.

**Middle Ear**

Middle ear locates between the external ear and the inner ear. It contains the tympanum, the Eustachian tube, the tympanic antrum and the mastoid process. It is the main section of the sound wave conduction, through with a tiny shape, but it plays a vital role.

1. Tympanum

   Tympanum is a hexahedron-like gas 1–2 mL cavity in the temporal bone. It locates between the tympanic membrane and the external profile wall of the inner ear, it opens to the rhinopharynx by the Eustachian tube forwards and the tympanic antrum and the mastoid cells via the tympanic antrum aditus. It could be divided into three parts. The attic is the site above the superior margin of the dense tympanic membrane; the mesotympanum is the site between the superior and the inferior margin of the dense tympanic membrane; the hypotympanum is the site under the inferior margin of dense tympanic membrane. Its superior diameter is about 14 mm, its anteroposterior diameter is about 11 mm, its medial-lateral diameter is 2–6 mm and the smallest diameter appears at the tympanic promontory and the tympanic membrane.

The tympanum consists of the auditory ossicle, the muscles, the ligaments, the nerves and the blood vessels. Its mucosa is thin but there is abundant blood supply, covering the tympanic bony wall, the tympanic inner surface, and the surface of these contents mentioned above, and on its mucosa, many plica and small crypts is formed and the crypts' aditus opens towards the tympanum.

Ossicular chain consist of the malleus, the incus and the stapes (Fig. 6.2) Muscles here include the tympanic tensor muscle and the stapes muscle. Nerves here contain the tympanic plexus, the facial nerve and the tympanic chorda nerve. Artery blood here is mainly from the external carotid artery; vein here flows into the pterygoid venous plexus and superior petrous sinus.

2. Eustachian Tube

The Eustachian tube is a 31–38 mm long (average 36 mm) channel for communicating the tympanic cavum and the rhino pharynx, and it consists of the bone (external 1/3) segment and the cartilage (internal 2/3) segment (Fig. 6.3).

The opening nearby the tympanum of the Eustachian tube is called the tympanal opening, which is located above anterior wall of tympanum and under semicanalis tensoris tympani. The opening near nasopharyngeal is called the pharynx opening, locating at profile nasopharyngeal wall, 1 cm posterior to inferior nasal concha. The thickest part of eustachian tube is at pharynx and it becomes thinner gradually to external direction till isthmus, the narrowest position, and then expands gradually till drum opening. Eustachian tube of children is shorter but wider cavity, almost level of long axis to cause that the inflammation of the nasopharyngeal can invade tympanum, causing acute otitis media induced by this tube.

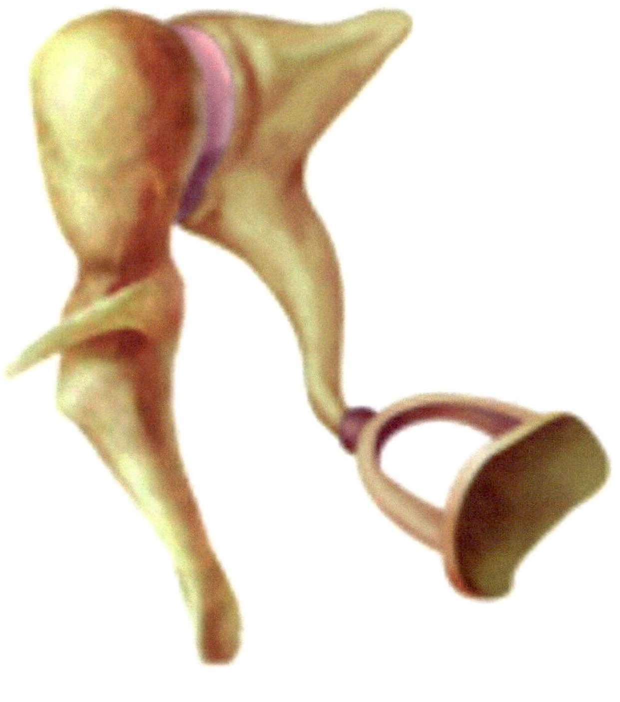

**Fig. 6.2** Ossicular chain: malleus, anvil and stapes

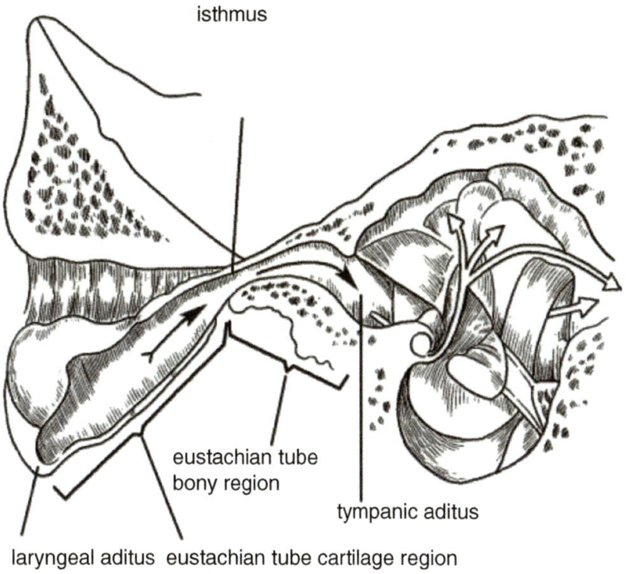


**Fig. 6.3** Eustachian tube

Normally at resting state, the Eustachian tube closes due to the passive elastic cartilage and the surrounding tissues pressure, and while swallowing and yawning, the Eustachian tube cartilage region opens because of the adjacent muscles' contraction. The muscles related to the Eustachian tube function are the palatine tensor, the palatine levator, the supra-pharyngal constrictor and the salpingo pharyngeus.

3. Tympanum Antrum

It is a pneumatic cavity at the supra posterior tympanum and a pivot connecting the tympanum and the mastoid cells. It is inborn but also varies much, so it's an important sign at the mastoid operation. The newborn's location is shallow but high because of the underdeveloped mastoid, at the supra-external auditory canal and only 2–4 mm to the bone cortex. But to the adults, it locates 10–15 mm to the mastoid cribrosa, its size and shape vary according to the mastoid gasification degree, but some adults may not have the tympanic antrum due to its under development or young-age inflammation, to which attention should be paired. There is a 6 mm round aditus between the tympanum antrum and the supra tympanum, which is called the tympanum antrum aditus.

4. Mastoid

It's located at the posterior-inferior temporal bone. It consists of many air cells, which have important clinical significance. The tympanum antrum exists in newborn but the mastoid does not. The mastoid, which is like a spongy cartilage, begins to take shape at the age of one. The mastoid's gasification usually begins at the late embryonic stage and continues growing at the infants and childhood.

Most of the mastoid air cells result from the tympanum antrum's gasification and few of them are the result of the infra-tympanum antrum in words gasification, which approaches to the mastoid region through the facial nerve vertical bone tube, so that sometimes cracking may occur at the facial nerve vertical bone tube. There are varieties of the cellular cells in the adults' normal mastoid, and the cells' size and quantity vary; The superior and the anterior mastoid region may be relatively big and the inferior mastoid region may be small.

The posterior mastoid cell boundary is adjacent to the sigmoid sinus and the cerebellum, and the supra-mastoid cells are adjacent to the temporal brain lobe via the tympanic roof. According to the mastoid gasification conditions, the mastoid could be divided into four types (Fig. 6.4).

**Diploetic Type**

Air cells here are small but plenty, similar to the cranial barrier and with relatively thicker bony cortex.

**Well-Pneumastised or Cellular Type**

Mastoid is entirely gasified with developed air cells, which are made up of the intercommunicating air cells and those air cells communicating with the tympanum antrum. The air cells here are relatively big, the bony walls between the cells are relatively thin and the mastoid is big too. The mastoid bone cortex here is relatively thin, the bone cortex would be easier to damage because of the inflammation then perforated to evoke the supramastoid sub periosteal abscess, which is more seen at infants.

**Sclerotic or Acellular Type**

Air cells here are undeveloped, so the mastoid is made up by dense bone cortex. The tympanum antrum exists but usually small. This type occupies 9.71% and bilateral ossification occupies 3.88% as the survey says.

**Mixed Type**

Two or three of three types above present.

### 6.1.3 Inner Ear

It is also called labyrinth. It is covered with a bony shell, so it is also known as the osseous labyrinth, located at the temporal petrous bone. The osseous labyrinth contains the membranous labyrinth, in which the lymph exists, and the space between the membranous labyrinth and the osseous labyrinth is called the perilymphatic interval, containing the outer lymph.

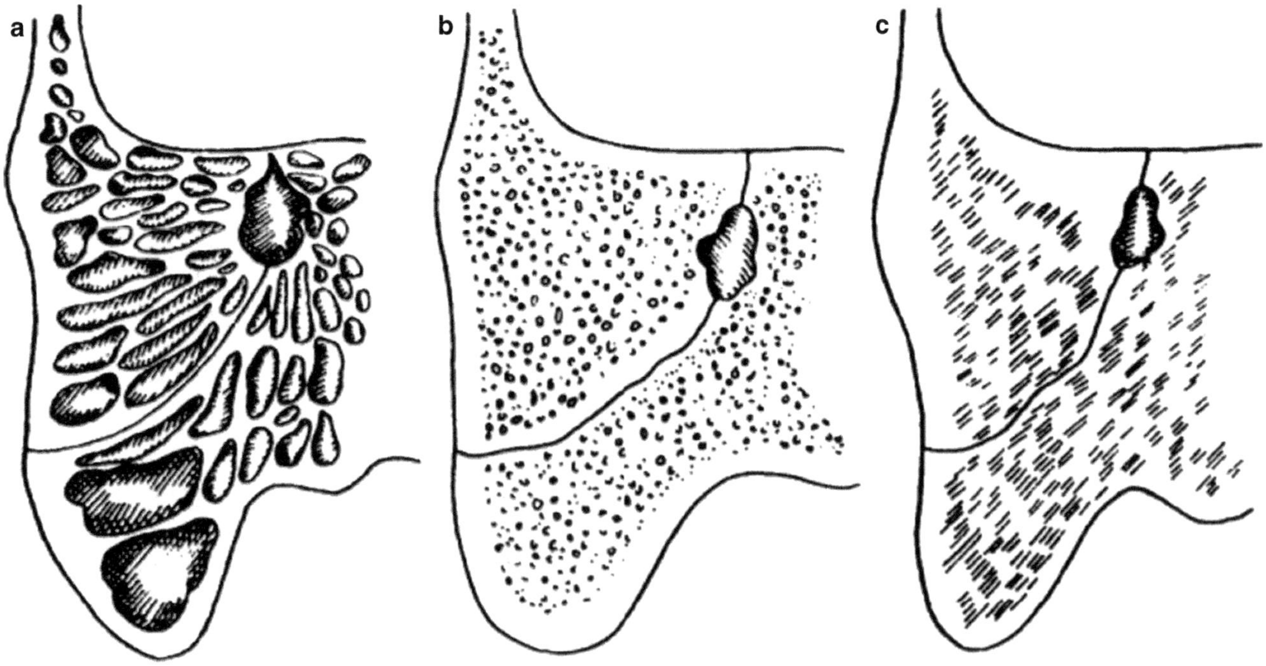


**Fig. 6.4** Mastoid types: (**a**) Well-pneumastised or cellular type. (**b**) Diploetic type. (**c**) Sclerotic or acellular type

1. Osseous Labyrinth

It is contributed by the dense sclerotic, which could be divided into the vestibule, the osseous semicircular canals and the cochlea.

(a) Vestibule

It is located between the cochlea and the osseous semicircular canals. It is an irregular 4 mm in diameter oval cavity, containing the auricle and the saccule inside. Its anterior-inferior site is narrow and communicates with the cochlear vestibular scale. Its post-superior site is wide, within five osseous semicircular canal aditus. Its outer wall is the intra tympanic wall, within the vestibular fenestra and the cochlear fenestra. Its superior wall is also where the facial nerve's labyrinth segment passes through. Its internal wall is the inner ear canal base, of which at the anterior, the oblique vestibular crest exists, and the spherical recess exists at the intra-inferior crest, the elliptical recess exists at the posterior. At the both recesses' wall's anterior site and the sub crest site, varieties of ostioles exist, where the fibrous nerve passes. At the posterior media crest, the vestibular intra-aqueduct aditus exists, which is also called the internal lymphatic aditus.

(b) Osseous Semicircular Canal

It locates at the intra-posterior vestibule. There are three almost 2/3 annulared small bone tubes at each side, which are respectively called external (horizontal), anterior (superior) and posterior (vertical) osseous semicircular canal and all of which are perpendicular to each other. All the osseous semicircular are both end at the vestibule, one of which is the osseous ampulla who is slightly-enlarged and the other are the general bone crus who is the combination of the anterior and the posterior osseous semicircular the other ending and the single bony crus who is the external osseous semicircular the other ending. Therefore, these three osseous semicircular canals has five aditus communicating to the vestibule.

(c) Cochlea

It locates at the front of the vestibule with a snail-shell-like shape. Its sharper ending trends intra-outwardly to the eustachian tube and its base trends posterior-inwardly, both of which contribute the inner ear canal base and there are several ostioles in the base, through which the cochlear nerves enter the cochlea. The cochlea is contributed with a central cone-like modiolus and an about two rolling osseous tube surrounding the modiolus. The modiolus could be divided into the superior vestibular scale and the inferior tympanic scale by the osseous spiral lamina, which embeds into the osseous cochlear duct and the cochlear duct separates both scales and they communicate at the modiolus apex by the helicotrema. The tympanic scale communicates with the tympanum through the cochlear fenestration and the cochlear penetration membrane could close the communication. The vestibular scale communicates with the tympanum through the vestibular fenestration and the stapes baseman plate and the annular ligament could close the communication. The cochlear inletting aditus exists adjacently to the cochlear fenestration, and through the aditus, the external lymph communicates with the subarachnoid space. The cochlear duct is about 30 mm.

2. Membranous Labyrinth

It is composed of the membranous tube and the membranous sac. It is fixed in the osseous labyrinth by the fiber bundles and suspends in the epilymph. It is filled with the endolymph. It could be divided into the utricle, the saccule, the membranous semicircular canal and the membranous cochlear duct, all of which communicates with each other (Fig. 6.5).

(a) Utricle

It is densely linked to the bone wall by the connective tissue, the micro vessels and the vestibular nerve. There are five aditus communicating with the membranous semicircular canal in its posterior wall and the utricle-saccule tubule communicating with the saccule. There is also the thickened sensory epithelium region on its intra-external basement, which is called the utricle macula, mainly censoring the head's static speed and linear acceleration on sagittal plane and affecting the tension of all the four extensors and flexors.

(b) Saccule

It is located in the saccula fossae at the intra-anterior -inferior vestibule. In its intra-anterior wall, the vestibular nervous terminal organs exists, which is called macula (acoustic macula), and the posterior macula region communicates with the cochlear duct through the sacculocochlear canal.

(c) Membranous Semicircular Canal

Three membranous semicircular canals located in their corresponding osseous semicircular canals and they occupy about 1/4 osseous semicircular canal's lumen cavity. They have three membranous ampullae, one single membranous crus and one general membranous crus, and all the five aditus are communicating with the utricle. In each membranous ampulla, there is a transverse sickle-like upheaving called ampulla crest, which is a balance sensor.

The membranous cochlear canal is a membranous canal in the cochlea. Its cross section is a triangle. Its extra lateral wall is a relatively-thicker spiral ligament, attaching on the extra lateral spiral canal wall between the vestibular nerve crest and the basal membrane crest, and it is covered with the pseudo strati-

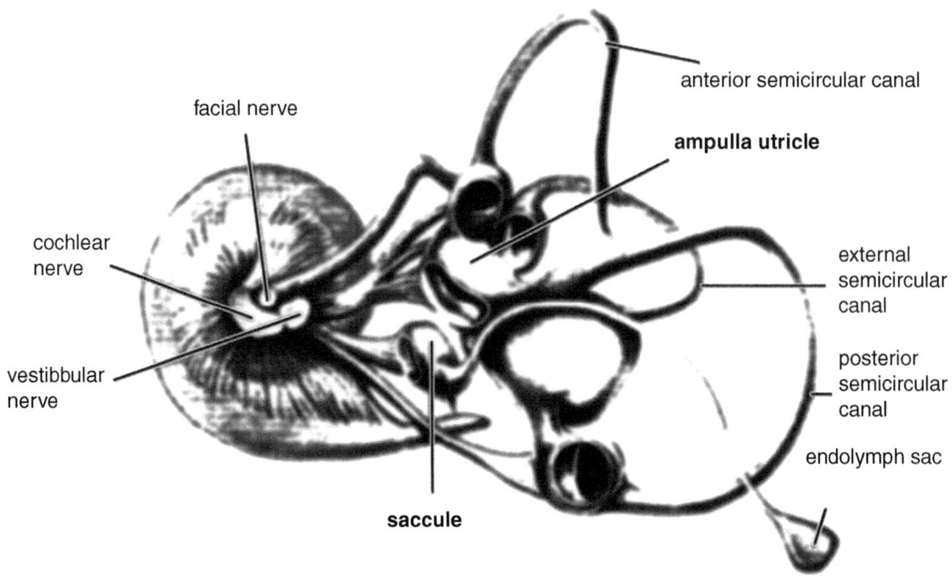


**Fig. 6.5** Membranous Labyrinth

fied epithelium who has abundant blood vessels, which called vascular stria. The cochlear bony canal could be divided into the superior vestibular scale and the inferior tympanic scale, both of which are filled with lymph. There is a thin film near the bony spiral plate base called vestibular membrane, and the vestibular membrane; the basal membrane and part of the spiral ligament form the membranous cochlear canal, which is filled with endolymph [1].

## 6.2 Physiology

Otic physiological functions contain the auditory and the equilibrium. To human, the ears are the only organ to accomplish the auditory. On the equilibrium sense, the eyes and the proprioception can also join to accomplish it except for the important role of ears. The reason why human beings could feel the beautiful sound with their hearts and make effect on their emotions and behaviors is the auditory development procedures, firstly the ear receives, conducts and senses the sound, transforms it into nerve signals, then the signals approach the auditory Center and they are sensed and finally the audition is developed.

### 6.2.1 Auditory Physiology

Sound has physical and physiological properties. It means sound waves in physiology and it refers to the subjective sensations caused by sound wave effect on the auditory organs. Its intensity is the objective sound energy, and the sensation to recognize the sound intensity when a certain-intensity sound wave effect on the human ears is called loudness, which is subjective.

The auditory physiology is the science searching and explaining various physiological phenomena and mechanisms during the auditory process. The process could be briefly expressed as: sound wave reaches the tympanum through air, then approaches the inner ear through the otostoen, the cochlea transforms the sound's vibration signals into biological signals and preliminarily analyses and synthesizes, and the signals would be ascended to all levels of the centers through the auditory nerve then perceived by the cortex.

Sound can be transmitted into ears by two routes: the air conduction through auricle, external ear, tympanic membrane and ossicular chain; the bone conduction through skull.

The auricle helps orientate the sound, especially the external auditory canal, a one-end-closed lumen, could resonant best with the four-times -wavelength sound wave due to physical principle, and the external auditory canal's resonance frequency is 3400 Hz, so the sound pressure at 3400 Hz range could increase 10~12 dB, what is called pressurization.

The middle ear's main functions are: impedance matching, resonance, staples reflection and Eustachian tube hydroelectricity. Among all of them, the impedance matching function is mainly related to three factors: area ratio of tympanic membrane and stapes base plate, length ratio of manubrium mallei and longer incus crus and the conical tympanic membranous buckle-like movement.

The inner ear and the auditory nerve have several mechanisms involved encoding the sound frequency and intensity. The cochlea converts the sound signals incoming ears into the audible biological signals and duly preliminarily analy-

ses and synthesizes the sound frequency and intensity. The sound's physiological process in the inner ear is the stapes vibration evokes the basal membranous displacement wave, then the wave ascends from the cochlea to top, based on the "traveling wave theory" that was found in 1960 by Bekesy, and the theory is the classic theory related to the cochlear passive mechanisms. However, the cochlea has a more subtle tuning function in physiological status, what is the 'cochlear active mechanism theory' raised at modern times.

The cochlear spiral organs communicate with the afferent neuro-fibers except for the efferent neuro-fibers, and they are under the auditory efferent system's domination. The efferent nerve which are dominating the spiral organs are the neurons adjacent to the superior olivary nuclei, and they are also called olivary cochlear bundle, dominating the outer hair cells.

In recent years, the olivary cochlear bundle's function is considered as inhibiting the efferent nerve electric potentials produced from the low and high intensity sound stimulation to enhance the auditory system's recognition ability to the relatively high intensity sound information.

### 6.2.2 Equilibrium Physiology

Human keeps balance by the coordination function of the balance-triad, which is constituted with the vestibular sense, the vision sense and the proprioception. If one system of the balance triad malfunctions, other two systems could still maintain balance after the compensation occurrence. But if two systems of the triad malfunction, the human equilibrium can't be maintained.

The vestibule system mainly dominates the equilibrium, and it is essential at maintaining balance. The semicircular canal's ampulla senses the head's rotation motion, meaning the head angular acceleration movement stimulation, and the otolith organs could sense the head linear acceleration movement stimulation. The gravity is also a linear acceleration movement, and when the head inclines, the otolith could sense the head's change relative to the gravity direction. Therefore, all the external force that could affect the human beings and evoke the vestibular equilibrium reaction could be divided into two categories, the angular and the linear acceleration movement.

Besides, the vestibule system also dominates the signals' integration, having the function similar to consciousness sensation and memory. On the other hand, it also has the function similar to the extra-pyramidal system, so it could adjust the body posture and the eye orientation and administrate the relatively meticulous movement. Its specific ability to maintain the body posture and the eyeball orientation equilibrium could ensure safety accurate orientation and clear vision especially the clear vision during movements counts on the vestibular effect. Therefore the vestibular regulating function could help human maintain a clear foreground while moving their bodies or heads to ensure a safe movements.

In brief, there are plenty of communications between the vestibular system and other nerve systems and the vestibular feedback system involves multiple systems, which may help explain why the dizziness or the vertigo symptom is common. The vestibule system has many close association with other nerve systems, especially the inter reaction effect between it and the autonomic nerves system which not only could effect on the kinetosis but also the 'vestibule-autonomic nerve system' diseases' pathogenesis and the researches on the vestibular feedback mechanism, the vestibular blood supply, the labyrinth fluids circulation rules, the related biological and immunity effect and so on play a vital role on the prophylaxis of therapy of the aerospace medicine and the clinic vertigo.

Recent studies show that the inner ear could receive the antigen stimulation then produce the immunity response. The response could protect the inner ear, but if it is too severe, the inner ear damage will be caused then the autoimmunity inner ear diseases be evoked.

## Reference

1. Peng YW, Wang HJ. Local anatomy. 5th ed. Beijing: People's Medical Publishing House; 2001.

# Common Signs and Symptoms and Examination Methods of Ear Diseases

7

Zhonglin Mu, Zhiqun Li and Jianghua Wan

## 7.1 Common Symptom of Ear Disease

### 7.1.1 Otalgia

It is a common symptom. It usually contains the throbbing pain, the oppressive pain, the stabbing pain, the knife-like pain, the tearing pain, the dragging pain, etc. The pain can be paroxysmal, intermittent or persistent. According to the etiology, it's categorized as follows.

1. Primary Otalgia
   (a) External Ear Otalgia
      Otic perichondrites, auricular frostbite, foreign bodies in external ear canal, external ear furuncle, trauma, acute diffusion external otitis, necrotic external otitis, etc.
   (b) Middle Ear Otalgia
      Tympanic membranous trauma, bullous myringitis, acute suppurative otitis media, barotraumatic otitis media, and middle ear cancer etc.
2. Secondary Otalgia
   (a) Periotic Lymphadenitis, Cervical Metastasis and Others
      They could cause otalgia by stimulating the great auricular nerve and the less occipital nerve
   (b) Temporal Mandibular Joint and Its Adjacent Tissue Disease
      It includes the tempura mandibular arthritis, the parotitis and others, which could cause the otalgia via the auriculotemporal nerve.
   (c) Oral and Rhinal Disease
      It includes the naso-rhinosinusitis, maxillary sinus tumor, dental carries, periodontitis, 2/3-anterior tongue ulcer and tumor, mouth floor cancer, etc, which can cause reflective otalgia via trigeminal ototemporal branch.
   (d) Pharyngeal Diseases
      It includes laryngeal nerve involvement at the post-tonsillectomy, the pharyngeal cancer, the pharyngeal abscess, the pharyngoulceration and so on, which could be transmitted into the Jacobson's plexus to cause the reflective otalgia
   (e) Laryngeal Disease
      It includes the laryngophthisis, the laryngeal cancer, the laryngo perichondritis and so on, which could cause the reflective otalgia via the outer-branch of the supralaryngeal nerve and the labyrinth nerve.
3. Neuropathic Otalgia
   It's more common. One is the ear herpes zoster evoked by the virus, another is the virus neuritis, during which the involved nerves' orientation sites pain occurs, and the glossopharyngoneuralgia is also accompanied with the otalgia.

### 7.1.2 Tinnitus

Tinnitus refers to the subjective auditory sensation in the patients' ears and head, but it doesn't have the corresponding sound source in the vital environment, and it's just a common symptom caused by the auditory function chaos, which is the human subjective otic sound without any external sound and (or) electricity stimulation. Its main mechanism at the auditory center is the auditory fiber nerves and all levels of the central neurons spontaneous electric dysrhythmias.

Z. Mu (✉)
Department of Otorhinolaryngology Head and Neck Surgery, The First Affiliated Hospital of Hainan Medical University, Haikou, China

Z. Li · J. Wan
Department of Medical Imaging, The First Affiliated Hospital of Hainan Medical University, Haikou, China



Z. Mu, J. Fang (eds.), *Practical Otorhinolaryngology - Head and Neck Surgery*, https://doi.org/10.1007/978-981-13-7993-2_7

For a long time, tinnitus is often divided into the subjective and the objective tinnitus. Sound of subjective tinnitus could only be heared by patients themselves, but sound of objective tinnitus could be heared by both patients of examiners, especially at myogenic tinnitus, tinnitus would occur corresponding with muscle contraction. To be precise, the tinnitus is a patients' subjective symptom and depends on the patient's physiopathological condition, so the categories above have its usage limit in clinic. According to the lesion sites, tinnitus could be divided into the otogenic tinnitus and the un-otogenic tinnitus, the former of which is caused by the lesion in the auditory system and the latter is the result of the diseases outside the auditory system, such as the anemia, the hypertension and so on. Based on its etiology, the tinnitus contains the physiological tinnitus and the pathological tinnitus, the former of which is the pulse sound, the respiration sound, the Eustachian tube opening sound and other sound produced at quiet environment when the arteries are under pressure while the internal body organs and viscera maintain their normal action state and when the blood flows and the latter is caused by the external mechanical, infectious and noise or drug induced.

### 7.1.3 Otorrhea

It is also called ear discharge, which is the abnormal liquid accumulation or outflow from the external ear canal, and it is an ear diseases' common symptom. Analyzing by the otorrhea's properties color and luster, odor, chemical result and so on could make differentiated diagnosis. The otorrhea's properties differ between diseases, and it could also converse at one disease' different stages.

1. *Serous Otorrhea*: It includes the external ear canal eczema, the allergic otitis media and other serous inflammatory exudation.
2. *Mucous Otorrhea*: When the secretory otitis media occurs, the mucous glands are hyperactive and its mucus exudation components increase, which contain the mucin, so the exudation fluid could be drawn into filaments.
3. *Purulent Otorrhea*: It is the otorrhea occurs at the otic furuncle, the diffusion external otitis, the suppurative parotitis outwards diabrosis and acute stage of purulent otitis media.
4. Watery Otorrhea: It is almost the cerebrospinal fluid otorrhea or from the vestibular outra-lymph. The congenital defection, the cochlear fenestration rupture or the vestibular fenestration rupture and the skull base fracture could also cause it.
5. Lipoid Otorrhea: Greasy skin is a normal physiological phenomenon caused by the excessive external ear canal' skin ceremonious glands secretion, but if the secretion is a white stinky-tofu-like mass, it is the cholesteatoma.
6. Bloody: Otorrhea it mainly occurs at the tympanic trauma, the temporal bone fracture, the bullous myringitis, the jungular glomerulus, the middle ear cancer and so on.

### 7.1.4 Deafness (Epicophosis)

Generally, hearing loss is collectively known as deafness. Its etiology and clinic features are extremely complex. It may be a special disease; it also can be the manifestation, reflection or symptoms of some external, middle or inner ear diseases and their adjacent organs' or the systemic diseases in auditory system.

According to the lesion property, it has three categories, the organic deafness, the functional deafness and the feigned deafness. Due to the diseases' on setting time characteristics, it has three kinds, the sudden deafness, the progressive deafness and the fluctuating deafness. Usually it is divided into the conductive deafness, the sensorineural deafness and the mixed deafness due to the lesion sites.

1. Conductive Deafness

   Hearing loss caused by acoustic malfunction at external ear canal and middle ear is called conductive deafness, so patients with conductive deafness have normal bone conductive audition range, but there would be autophonia.
2. Sensorineural Deafness

   If its lesion is at the organ of Corti's hair cells, auditory nerve or all levels auditory centers, the sound sensation and the nervous impulse conduction would dysfunction, and because of which the sensorineural deafness would occur, with the recruitment phenomenon. If the lesion is at the auditory nerve and its conductive accesses, it is called nervous deafness (post-conchlear deafness); and if the lesion is at the cerebral cortex auditory center, it is called central deafness.
3. Mixed Deafness

   It occurs when the acoustic system and the sensorineural system both damages. According to the lesion sites' difference and the invasion degrees' difference, it could manifest as acoustic-as-priority or sensory-as-priority mixed deafness. The mixed deafness occurs when the patients with both the conductive deafness and the sensorineural deafness caused by the external and (or) the middle ear lesion as well as the hair cells of organ of Corti or auditory nerve lesion, such as the patients with long-term chronic suppurative otitis media

not only have the conductive deafness evoked by the tympanic perforation and the ossicular destruction but also have the sensorineural deafness caused by the long-term toxin absorption and injury to the cochlear hair cells.

4. Feigned Deafness

   It is also called cheating deafness. It refers to the condition where patients without any auditory system diseases claim that they lose their hearing and pretend no response to sound, or that the patients' hearing is only with slight loss but they exaggerate the performance degree. The feigned deafness motives are complex and their performances vary. The objective audiometry, such as the acoustic immittance, the auditory evoked potentials, and oto-acoustic emission can accurately identify the feigned deafness, but it is still necessary to differentiate the diagnosis from the functional deafness.

5. Functional Deafness

   It is also known as mental deafness or hysteria deafness, which is non-organic deafness. The patients with functional deafness are often with the mental psychic trauma history and manifestation as unilateral or bilateral sudden severe hearing loss, with or without tinnitus or vertigo, and the functional deafness could recover occasionally or rapidly by suggest-ionization therapy.

### 7.1.5 Ataxia

It refers to the condition that the patients can't maintain their postures and balance because of the motor coordination disorder under a normal muscle tension, which means that the random motor range and coordination disorder occur. While examining, the ataxia caused by the muscular paralysis and the visual accommodation disorder should be firstly excluded. The examinations include the Romberg test, the rotation test, the finger-to-nose test, the treadmill test, the eyes-closed walking test and so on. Some common tests used in clinic are as following:

1. Sensory Ataxia

   It refers to the condition that the central afferent nerves can't reflect the somatic sites because of the deep sensory disorder at body and (or) all fours. Its characteristics is that the symptom is obvious when the eyes are open and it would aggravate in darkness or with closed eyes, so are the lower limb symptoms. The sensory ataxia's etiology may be perineurial degeneration, posterior root lesion, posterior bundle lesion, brainstem lesion, cerebrovascular lesion, and parietal lobe lesion.

2. Vestibular Ataxia

   It refers to the ataxia caused by the vestibular disorder. Patients with vestibular ataxia would manifest as the unstable standing, the vertigo, the nystagmus and the balance loss but none limb movement disorders. Its injury may be in the inner ear labyrinth, the vestibular nucleus or the central nerve system.

3. Cerebellar Ataxia

   It refers to the condition that the balance disorder, the unstable standing and (or) tread, the limbs in-coordination, the dysmetria, the adiadochocinesia, the motion starting and ending delay, the continuous motor disorder and the cerebellar nystagmus caused by the injured various cerebellar afferent and efferent nerves.

4. Hybrid Ataxia

   It refers to the coexistent ataxia evoked by several causes.

### 7.1.6 Vertigo

It is a motor or orientation illusion, it refers to the condition that the patients sense by themselves or their outside environment quiet views plane-rotate along with a certain orientation, swing or float. It is a spatial orientation sensory disorder, which mainly occur when the peripheral or the central vestibular lesion suddenly onsets and it is one of the most common clinical symptoms. Based on the onsetting sites the vertigo could be divided into several types.

1. Central Vertigo

   It has slow onset. Its most illusion is the rightwards-or-leftwards swings and the upwards-or-downwards floats, it is progressive, it last a relative-longer time, which could be over 10 days. Its onsetting has no relationship with the head position change, it's often without the tinnitus or the hearing loss, it often accompanies with various types' nystagmus and other central nervous system damage symptoms; it include the acoustic neuroma, and cerebellar tumor.

2. Otogenic Vertigo

   It often onsets suddenly; Patients with otogenic vertigo would sense that themselves and their surrounding views rotate or swing, and the sensation would aggravate when the head position changes; it only lasts for short time, several minutes or several hours; it often accompanies with tinnitus, hearing loss, it is mostly with horizontal nystagmus, accompanying with nausea, vomiting and other automatic nervous symptoms, and it has the spontaneous remission and the recurrence tendency; it include the Meniere's disease, the labyrinthitis, and the otic toxic drug poisoning.

3. Systemic Disease Vertigo

   Its manifestations vary; one of which is floating sensation, another is numbness sensation or sensing the inclination and the linear waggle. It may occur during hypertension, severe anemia, heart diseases, cerebrotraumatic sequelae, hypoglycemia, the neurosis, cervicovertigo, and otovertigo.

## 7.2 Examination Method of Ear

### 7.2.1 Common Examination Method

1. Inspections
   (a) Observe the auricular shape, size, location, and pay attention to the congenital deformities existing, such as the accessory auricle, the protruding ears, the microtia, and the auricular defection existing.
   (b) Observe the congenital preauricular fistula, which often locates at the anterior helix crus and whose orifice could be seen; the congenital first branchial fistula is often similar to the preauricular fistula, but the other fistula orifice could often be found at auricle or posterior ear, in external ear canal, at cervix or other sites.
   (c) Observe the auricular inflammation existing: the auricular swelling often suggests the inflammation or the frostbite; observe the existing of the unlimited thickening, the herpes clusters, and anabiosis.
   (d) Observe the auricular scar existing, such as the sarcoma; observe the metastasis existing, such as the posterior auricular abscess pushes the auricle forwards.
   (e) Observe the auricular hypertrophic neoplasm, pigment ulceration and others existing, such as the base cell carcinoma and so on.
   (f) Observe the posterior auricular sulcus change, existing and so on, such as the postauricular subperiosteum abscess.
   (g) Observe the external ear canal meatus change: atresia and stenosis existing; neoplasm, cerumen, and cholesteatoma dander occurrence; swelling, blisters, erosions and others existing; hair follicles furuncle existing; secretion existing, based on whose properties the external ear canal or the middle ear diseases could be briefly concluded, such as the external ear canal carcinoma, the middle ear cancer and others whose secretion is bloody, and the cerebrospinal fluid otorrhea whose secretion is watery.
2. Palpation

   Touch unilateral auricle with single thumb or index finger to sense the existing of the thickening, the fluctuation, the sclerosis, etc. The limited thickening fluctuation sense but without swelling could suggest the serous perichondritis, which is called auricular pseudocyst; the swelling accompanies with the fluctuation sense and the tenderness pain suggests the abscess;

   Press bilateral mastoid surface with single or both thumbs to observe the existing of the tenderness pain, the subcutaneous masses, etc: the tenderness pain may suggest the mastoiditis; the mastoid subcutaneous lymphatic swelling may suggest the external otitis and the otitis media; the enlargement, the tenderness pain and the fluctuation sensation suggest the posterior auricular subperiosteal abscess; the retro-inferior to subcutaneous auricular masses suggest the parotid tumor; if it hurts while opening mouth while pressing the anterior tragus, the temporomandibular arthritis could be suspected.

### 7.2.2 Radiology

1. X-ray Examination
   (a) Temporal lateral radiograph: Schuller's position or Lentz's position;
   (b) Axial temporal radiograph: Mayer's position;
   (c) Inner-ear-canal orbit-access position;
   (d) Other projection positions: temporal post-anterior oblique position (Stenver's position), temporal fronto-occipital position (Towne's position).
2. CT Examination
   (a) Regular high-resolution plains scan;
   (b) Combine CT scan with coronary or sagittal reconstruction [multi-planer reconstruction (MPR)] when necessary is the most common clinical technique;
   (c) Others: 3D reconstruction technique, such as ossicular chain or petrous bone maximum intensity projection (MIP) and surface shadow display (SSD) and other techniques, could enlarge the otic bony structure to more easily observe the subtle lesion change and stereopsis.
3. MRI Examination

   2D or 3D angiography, for displaying the positional relationship between the aberrant vessels and the auditory nerves; inner ear 3D hydrography technique, for clearly displaying 3D structure of nerves, vestibular cochlear membranous labyrinth and semicircular canal.

### 7.2.3 Endoscopy

1. Electric Otoscope

   It is an amplifier otoscope with own light source. Turn on the light, set it in the external ear canal, and then the subtle tympanic membranous lesion could be observed. The otoscopic lens set in the external ear canal could adjust the ear canal size, and it include the disposable type and the repetitive type, of which the latter need disinfection before a second use to prevent the bacteria and the virus spread. The electric otoscope is convenient to take, and it doesn't need any other light source, so it especially fit the bedridden patients, infants, etc, and the external ear canal cerumen should be cleaned up before using it. The electric otoscope equipped with otic blown balloon could also be applied to observe the tympanic motor condition.

2. Otoscope

   It includes the rigid tube type and the fibrous type. It consists of a camera lens, a lens body and a light source interface, The rigid oto-endoscopic camera lens has three viewing angles, 0°, 30° and 70°; it can be equipped with the camera system and the imaging system, which could not only observe the subtle external ear canal and tympanic morphologic change but also shoot the photographic documents, so as to perform the operation of external ear canal, the tympanic membranous and the tympanic cavum lesion. The fibrous otoscope has a relative-big advantage in observing the tympanic concealed sites and the intra-cochlear fine structures.

3. Eustachian Tube Scope

   Pass the 30° angle rigid or fibrous otoscope through the tympanic tresses sites and enter it into the tympanic cavum to observe the eustachian tube's tympanic aditus area and its surroundings. The eustachian tube cartilage segment is relatively hard to be observed, so it is also practical to observe the eustachian tube's pharyngeal aditus conditions from the nasopharyngeal sites, then the fibrous otoscope could cross through the eustachian tube pharyngeal aditus and enter the eustachian tube to observe, coordinating the eustachian tube's internal air-blowing to observe the cartilage segment's mucosal change conditions.

### 7.2.4 Vestibular Functional Examination

It manly provides the vestibular functional status by observing the spontaneous or the induced body signs, and it could provide the basis for the diseases' localization diagnosis and occupational deviation. The vestibular system has extensive communications with the eyes, the spinal cords, the cerebellum, the automatic nervous system and other systems, involving the multiple departments' diseases, so that it has great value on differentiating the diseases' diagnosis. The examination contents contain the spontaneous nystagmus, the gaze nystagmus, the tracking nystagmus, the optokinetic nystagmus, the positional nystagmus, the vestibular nystagmus and the balance ability evaluation.

1. Nystagmus Test

   The nystagmus is the most evident and important sign of the clinical vestibular responses. The nystagmus is an involuntary, unconscious and mostly rhythmic eyeball's back-and-forth concussion movement. The nystagmus contains the spontaneous type and the induced type. The eyes' concussion evoked by the pathological stimulation at vestibular. The nystagmus reaction evoked by the hot (and) or cold, rotating or other physiological stimulation at vestibular organs is called induced nystagmus.

   The nystagmus examination is often the naked-eye observation under natural light. The examiner finger ending should be 30–60 cm from the patients both eyes. First guide the patients to look straight, and then stare at the left, the right, the upper, the lower, the supra-left and the supra-right oblique angle. The staring angle should be <45°, because the staring angle >45° could evoke the oto-muscular extreme nystagmus (end-point nystagmus). The vestibular nystagmus fast phase tends to unilateral side; the pendular nystagmus without fast or slow phase mainly occurs at congenital otic disease; the cerebellar diseases' nystagmus could also be pendulum type, the horizontal type or the rotating type nystagmus. The oblique nystagmus, the vertical nystagmus and the separated type nystagmus which could cause the fast phase while staring to the right and(or) left are all central nystagmus.

   The nystagmus could also be observed through the Frenzel glasses or the infrared video patches (Fig. 7.1).

   The electro-nystagmography is to observe the nystagmus by the skin electrode method, where the cornea displays a positive potential relative to the retina, neither is the retina to the cornea, both of which constitute a potential difference axis, so while setting pairs of electrodes at the eyeballs' surrounding skin, the eye movement would record the peripheral electric field potential change, whose graph is the electro-nystagmogram.

2. Rotation Examination

   It is a physiological stimulation. It makes the semicircular canal sense the angular acceleration. The rotation stimulation is the comprehensive response after the bilateral labyrinth is stimulated, so it not only needs unilateral labyrinth assessment; besides, the test equipments are complex and expensive.

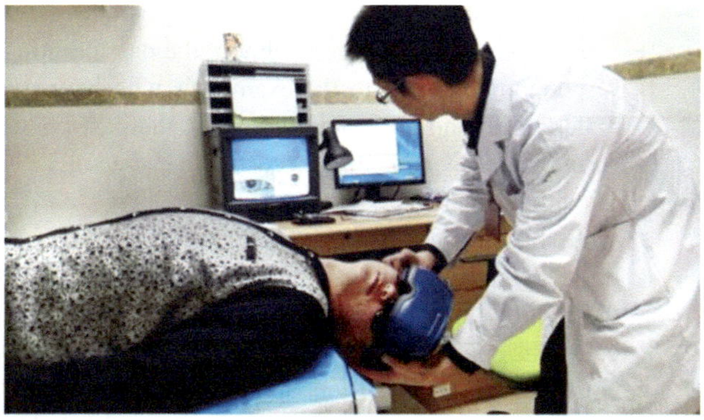

**Fig. 7.1** Infrared video patches

Its common stimulation methods include the angular acceleration rotation test and the sinusoidal harmonic acceleration test (SHAT). Its clinic significances are: the phenomenon that the nystagmus unilateral trends occur under angular acceleration rotation but it lessens or disappears when the angular acceleration increases is called vestibular revive; It mainly reflects the vestibular insufficient activity, suggesting the vestibular peripheral lesion; the vestibular damping is that the directional preponderance phenomenon only exists under the high intensity stimulation and it mainly occurs at the central lesions, such as the cerebrovascular lesion and the posterior skull-base tumor.

3. Balance Examination

   The vestibular main function is to maintain the human balance by maintaining its muscular tension, so the vestibular system's lesion would cause the posture and tread. The methods to examine the balance function are too many, including the static and the dynamic balance examination.

   (a) Static Balance

   - Romberg's Test

     Let the examinees stand up with their feet together, and their ten fingers tie at front of the chest and tighten towards two sides, then observe that whether the examinees' bodies' inclination existing or not while opening and closing their eyes. The normal persons are without any inclination during the test and their result is negative. The labyrinth or the cerebral lesion could prompt the examinees incline spontaneously.

   - Past-Pointing Test

     The examinee and the examiner sit face to face and the examiner's hands are at front with two index fingers extended. Please the examinee raises both hands, then ask the examinee try to respectively contract its own index fingers with the examiner's. Test several times respectively with both opened eyes and both closed eyes, then conclude. To the normal people, the eyes opening or closing won't make any sense on the accurate contraction between the four fingers without the past-pointing phenomenon, but to the examinees who have the labyrinth and the cerebral lesions, the past-pointing phenomenon could occur.

   (b) Dynamic Balance

   Its basic principle is: the vestibular neuro-system project the oto-muscular movement to the head through the internal longitudinal fasciculus and project to the caudal ending through the vestibular spinal cords to maintain the trunk and the lower limbs muscular excitability. When there is no vision information and ankle proprioception information, the vestibular feedback is the main postural modulation factor.

   - Tread Test

     Draw a concentric circle with two 0.5~1.0 m radius circles and equally divide the circle into 12 parts, one of which occupies 30°. The examinees stand up in the circular center with blindfolded eyes, and reach both arms forwards, then tread one hundred times by average 80~110 times/min speed, each of which should be with a right angle between the thigh and the calf. The examiners should observe the body rocking existing, the relative positional change existing between the head and the body, the both arms' positions going up or down or declination existing and the footsteps migration distance.

   - Walking Test

     Blindfold the examinees' eyes, and ask them to move backwards or forwards by 5~10 steps, during which the examiners observe the tread and calculate the error angle between the beginning and the ending point. If the angle is >90°, evidence of bilateral vestibular function difference is revealed.

4. Vestibular Functional Examination Results Evaluation

   There isn't any standard and unified evaluation method. As the clinical practice displays, various vestibular functional examination results vary greatly, so consideration of various factors' influence to the examination result, especially the patients' clinical manifestation, is vital while evaluating various vestibular functional examination results.

   The vestibular peripheral abnormality's vestibular functional examination characteristics are: the unilateral semicircular canal miopragia suggests the ipsilateral vestibular miopragia, or the contralateral vestibular functional enhancement caused by stimulation; if the directional preponderance suggests that the patients are at acute stage or some vestibular pathway sites are abnormal (non localizable); the fixation inhibition phenomenon may occur.

   The vestibular central abnormality's vestibular functional examination characteristics are: the open-eyes staring nystagmus, the reverse staring nystagmus, the downwards staring nystagmus may occur; the cog wheeling and the smooth pursuit abnormality and the optokinetic nystagmus abnormality would occur; the visual suppression would fail.

### 7.2.5 Hearing Examination

It contains two categories: the subjective audiometry and the objective audiometry. The former contains the stopwatch test, the tuning fork test, various pure-tone tests, speech audi-

ometry, etc. The latter includes the non conditional reflex and the reflex audiometry, the impedance audiometry, the electric response audiometry, the oto-acoustic emission audiometry, etc.

1. Tuning Fork Test

   It is one of the common methods to distinguish the deafness properties; the C-key octave tuning fork is the common tuning fork, and its vibration frequency contains 128, 256, 512, 1024 and 2048 Hz, among which the 256 Hz and the 512 Hz are the most common ones. The common examination methods include:

   (a) Rinne Test (RT)

   It is also called gas--bone-conductive contrast test, which is an examination method to contrast the ipsilateral examined otic gas conduction and bone conduction. Choose and vibrate the $C_{256}$ tuning fork, and set it at the examinees' otomastoid tympanic area to test its bone conductive audition, record the time till the sound can't be heard, and simultaneously transfer the tuning fork 1 cm from the external ear canal's external aditus to test its gas conductive audition and record the time till the sound disappears.

   Result analysis: if $T_{AC} > T_{BC}$, it is the positive("+") RT, which is of the normal people or the sensorineural deafness; if $T_{BC} > T_{AC}$, it is the negative ("-") RT, or if $T_{BC} = T_{AC}$, it is the "±" RT, both of which are of the conductive deafness.

   (b) Weber's Test (WT)

   It is also called bone conductive deviation test, which is used to compare bilateral otic bone conductive audition strength. Choose and vibrate the $C_{256}$ or the $C_{512}$ tuning fork, set it at the anterior forehead or the central cranial top and ask the examinees to distinguish the side where they hear a relatively louder sound. Record with the"→" as the deviation side and the "=" as non-deviation sign.

   Result analysis: if both ears are at same audition, normal or same injury level, it is "WT=“; if the conductive deafness occurs, the affected lateral oto bone conduction is better, which is "WT→affected ear"; if the sensorineural deafness occurs, the normal otic audition is better, which is "WT→normal ear".

   (c) Schwabach's Test (ST)

   It is also called bone conduction contrast test, which is used to distinguish the examinee's bone conduction difference from the normal ones'. Set the vibrating $C_{256}$ tuning fork on the examiners and the examinee's mastoid tympanic sinus area simultaneously to test and compare their bone conductive time difference.

**Table 7.1** Tuning fork examination result comparison

| Examination method | Normal | Conductive deafness | Sensorineural deafness |
|---|---|---|---|
| RT | + | – or ± | + |
| WT | = | → affected ear | → normal ear |
| ST | ± | + | – |

   Result analysis: if the difference is 0, it is "ST±", which mean that the examinee is normal; if the examinee's time is longer, it is "ST+", which means that the examinee has the conductive deafness; if the examinee's time is shorter, it is "ST-", which means that the examinee has the sensorineural deafness. The tuning fork examination result comparison is as chart say (Table 7.1).

   (d) Gelle's Test (GT)

   It is method to test whether the examiners who are with complete tympanic membrane have the fixed stapes or not. Set the vibrating $C_{256}$ tuning fork on the examinees' tympanic sinus area, and simultaneously alternate the external ear canal compression and decompression with the blowing otoscope.

   Result Analysis: if the examinee could sense the sound intensity fluctuation, which means that the bone conductive sound reduces while compressing and restores while decompressing, it is GT+, which indicates that the stapes movement is normal; but if the sound doesn't change during the process, it is the GT-, which indicates that the stapes is fixed.

2. Pure-Tone Audiometry

   Pure tone is single frequency sound; its threshold refers to the over half times' minimum sound-pressure sound recognition at the specific sound condition test. It reflects each frequency minimum sound audition level, which the examinee could reach to at a peace environment through recognizing the sound from the earphone and the bone conductive vibrators. The pure-tone threshold could be recorded on the audition table to make an auditory chart, whose horizontal axis represents the "frequency", and vertical axis represents the "decibel (dB) loss". If the difference between the bone conduction and the gas conduction is >10 dB and the bone conduction is at the normal range, it is the conductive hearing loss; if the difference is zero or <10 dB and both of the two conduction are normal range, it is the sensorineural hearing loss; and if the difference is >10 dB and the bone conduction is at normal range, it is the mixed hearing loss.

   Sometimes the masking is required during the pure-tone audiometry, which is aimed to expel the other ear's participation to obtain the true threshold of the examining ear. The masking time should be according to the difference between the sound intensity and the intra-otic sound

attenuation value, whether, which is more than the unexamined otic bone conductive threshold. Commonly, the Hood platform method would be applied but be cautious to avoid that the masking voice intensity is too small to mask or too big to excessively mask (conduct to examining ear).

3. Speech Audiometry

It is an audiometry to test the examinees' speech auditory threshold and speech recognition ability by the auditory stimulation, speech signals. The examination contents include the speech auditory threshold and recognition ratio, of which the former contains the speech sensation and recognition threshold, between what the speech sensation threshold refers to the speech audition level which could sense 50% test materials and the speech recognition threshold refers to the speech audition level which could hear 50% test materials, and the latter refers to the correct hearing percentages of the speech signals in audiometry materials. If draw various speech levels' speech recognition rate into one curve, the nerve would be the speech audio graph. When the posterior cochlear (auditory nerve) lesion occurs, the pure tone audition is good but the speech recognition rate is relative-lower. Besides, about the audiometry materials, check appendix one, among which the audiometry material Mandarin developed by the CPLA general hospital otorhinolaryngology boffin is a favored one in China in clinic.

4. Acoustic Impedance Admittance Test

It is an objective method to test the middle ear audio conduction system and the brainstem auditory pathway functions, and it is called acoustic immittance on the international. Its basic examination contents are the tympanogram, the static compliance value and the staples acoustic reflex.

(a) Tympanogram

It is applied to test the tympanic membranous and the ossicular chain's compliance to the detection sound under the influence of the external ear canal's pressure change.

Method: probe the otobyon scopic head into the examining otic external ear canal, rapidly increase the pressure to +1.96 kPa(+200 mm $H_2O$), then the tympanum would be pressed inwards tightly and the acoustic compliance would decrease, after then, gradually reduce the external ear canal pressure, the tympanic membrane would recover and loose, the acoustic compliance would increase till the external ear canal's and the tympanic membranous internal pressure is equal, when the acoustic compliance is maximum. Since then, the external ear canal would be negative pressure, the tympanic membrane would be absorb tightly outwards and the acoustic compliance would reduce. The acoustic compliance's change following the external ear canal pressure's change presents a peak-shaped curve, which is also called tympanic immittance or tympanic function curve (Fig. 7.2)

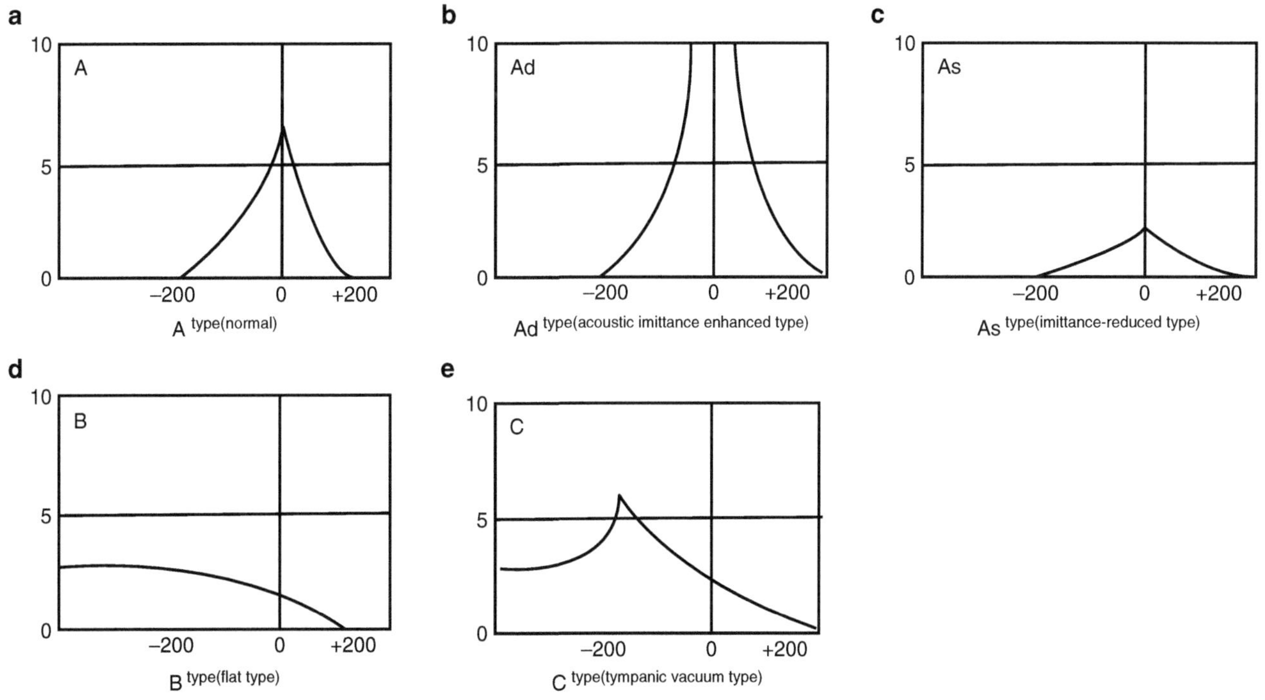


**Fig. 7.2** Tympanic immittance curve category

- Type A

  It is the normal type, whose pressure apex point is around 0 daPa in ±50 daPa range, but the −100 daPa is abnormal. The adults' normal acoustic immittance range is 0.3~1.65 mL and the children's is 0.35~1.4 mL. This type presents at examinees who have complete tympanic membrane and normal movement, suitable middle otic pneumatic cavity, and normal eustachian tube function.
- Type Ad

  It is an acoustic immittance enhanced type, and its amplitude is more than A type but its apex point is the same as A type. It mainly presents when the examinees are with loose tympanic membrane or tympanic healed perforation, ossicular chain disruption, combination of the loose tympanic membrane and the abnormally patulous Eustachian tube or other middle ear acoustic system hyperactivity.
- Type As

  It is an acoustic immittance reduced type, its tympanic activity is low, and its amplitude is lower than A type. It mainly presents at the examinees with otosclerosis, ossicular-chain-tympanum scar adhesion, ossicular fixation, evident tympanic thickening and other conditions when the middle ear acoustic system activity is limited.
- Type B

  It is an acoustic immittance no-change or flat type, where the tympanic membrane and the middle ear system don't move act and the acoustic stiffness evidently enhances and the internal tympanum is almost without or tiny pneumatic cavity when the external ear canal internal pressure changes. Its curve is flat without apexes. It mainly present at the examinees with tympanic effusion, adhesion, large swelling masses and internal granulation filling, evident middle ear adhesion, also tympanic membranous perforation, cerumen embolism and probe-external ear canal extra wall contract.
- Type C

  It is tympanic negative pressure type, whose apex point is below −100 daPa, it mainly present when the eustachian tube dysfunction and the tympanic vacuum occur.

(b) Static Acoustic Compliance

It is the maximum acoustic compliance when the external ear canal and the tympanic pressure are equal, which is the difference between the tympanic immittance graphic apex point and baseline. The normal static acoustic compliance's range is 0.30~1.60, and individual value varies too much, it could be effected by various middle ear diseases, so it's inaccurate to set it as a single diagnosis index.

(c) Stapes Acoustic Reflex

A certain intensity (70~100 dB over threshold) sound stimulation could evoke bilateral stapes reflective contraction to change the middle ear acoustic compliance by enhancing the ossicular chains and the tympanic stiffness. In clinic, it could be applied to differentiate various lesions on the reflex pathway, and the tympanic function condition's objective detection, the brainstem lesion localization, the auditory neuroma diagnosis, the non-organic deafness differentiation, the facial nerve paralysis localization diagnosis and prognosis evaluation, subjective auditory threshold estimation and so on. The Metz recruitment test and acoustic reflex attenuation test could be applied to differentiate the oto-cochlear deafness and the posterior cochlear deafness from each other. While adapting the hearing aids, the acoustic reflex threshold could be a reference to determine the reasonable gain and the saturation acoustic pressure level.

5. Electric Response Audiometry (ERA)

It is a method to record the auditory system potential change evoked by the acoustic stimulation by modern electronic techniques. It suits to test the acoustic threshold, differentiate the functional deafness and the organic deafness from each other, the cochlear and the posterior cochlear lesion from each other and localizable diagnose the auditory neuroma and some central lesion of the infants or the adults disable to cooperate with examination. The common ERA contains the electrocochleography and the auditory brainstem response (ABR).

(a) Electrocochleography

It is the method to record the near field potentials originating from the oto-cochlear and the auditory nerve after acoustic stimulation and the potential is at short latency evoked potential range. It could record three types' potentials.

- Active Potential

  It is sum of all the single neuron's active potentials, mainly consisting of a negative wave ($N_1$~$N_3$) group. If it is from the whole basement membranous active potentials also evoked by short sound, it is called whole nerve action potential; if it is the potential evoked by the stimulation sound with frequency characteristics, it is called compound active potential.
- Cochlear Micro Potential

  It is mainly produced from the outer hair cells at oto-cochlear basal gyrus.
- Summating Potential

  It is the sum of the intra-cochlear nonlinear multi-component potentials; it is produced because of the asymmetric basal membranous activity; so its amplitude is proportional to the basal membranous displacement (Fig. 7.3).

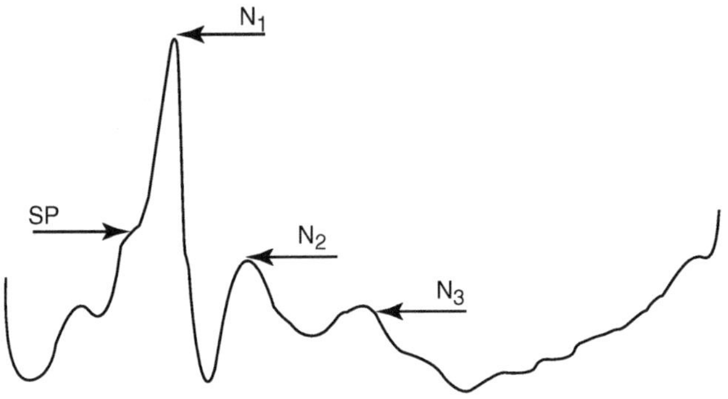


**Fig. 7.3** Electrocochleograph

The electrocochleograph is the only clinical audiometry, which could master the unilateral otic function; it needs not mask the other ear to avoid shadow hearing while localizating and qualitative diagnosis. However, almost examinees intolerant to accept the electro-probe, which causes the external ear canal tympanic electrode placement a bit difficult, but the electrode placement evidently impacts the recording results, therefore, it has a bit clinic application limits.

(b) ABR

It is at AEP rapid response range, which is to record the series of neurogenic electrical activities in the post sound-stimulation latency stage 10 ms. At the 1–10 ms latency stage, response wave I, II, III, IV, V, VI and VII would present, of which the wave I, III and V are the most evident ones. Commonly, wave I is of the auditory nerve, wave II is of the cochlear nucleus, wave III is of the supra-olivary complex, wave IV is of the extra-lateral lemniscus, wave V is of the subra-colliculus, wave VI is of the medial geniculate body and wave VII is of the thalamus.

Identification and analysis to response waveforms:

- Basic Waveform Knowledge

  Normal ABR would present Seven positive spikes in the post-stimulative 10 ms. During the auditory threshold detection, wave V identification is vital, but wave I, III, V are also important on the lesions' localization diagnosis, and the time interval between two normal adjacent waves is about 1 ms. As to the waveform, the wave V is the steadiest and its amplitude is the highest, and in normal ears, wave V could also be observed even with the sound 5~10 dB.

- Wave Latency Stage and Interphase

  The time range from the second the stimulating sound occurs to the second the wave presents is called wave latency stage, and the time interval between two random waves is called wave interphase. When the stimulation sound intensity reduces, the wave interphase extends, but the stimulating acoustic influence intensity at the early potentials is more obvious than the late potentials.

  The wave I~V interphase is also called brainstem conductive time or central conductive time. The wave I latency stage lengthen caused by stimulating acoustic intensity reduction is more obvious than other contents, so the wave I~III and the wave I~V interphase contraction isn't that evident. The wave latency stage and the wave interphase, especially of which the former, are important diameters to judge whether the ABR is normal or not.

- Inter-auricle Difference

  The bilateral otic wave latency stage's, interfacial and amplitude difference with the normal ones is another important parameter to judge the examinees' ABR, and if the former two is over 0.4 ms, the ABR is abnormal.

  The ABR usually applies the short sound stimulation, it mainly reflects the audition threshold at 3000~4000 Hz and it lacks frequency characteristics. Tone burst has a certain rise time and fall time, which would be several milliseconds or several decades millisecond, and it has relatively-better frequency specificity, therefore, the tone burst is a good sound stimulation signals to balance the neural synchronization response and the frequency specificity. The tone burst ABR evaluation is has characteristics such as its objection, its frequency specificity and its high accuracy, and it is mainly applied on the infants early hearing loss definite diagnosis, audition threshold evaluation, hearing aids fitting estimation, and feigned deafness identification.

(c) Acoustic Emission

Kemp detected the acoustic signals produced from the cochlea firstly in 1978, and defined it as a audio energy produced at cochlea and relieved into the external ear canal through the ossicular chain and the tympanic membrane, and it is called oto-acoustic emission (OAE). It reflects the active mechanical activity in cochlea. According to that the stimulation sound exists or not, it contains the spontaneous OAE (SOAE) and the echoed OAE (EOAE); according to the stimulation sound difference, the EOAE contains the transiently EOAE (TEOAE), the stimulus-frequency EOAE (SFEOAE) and the distortion production OAE (DPOAE). The SOAE is the single or multiple and narrow banding frequency spectrum and the static acoustic signal much similar to the pure tone recorded in the external ear canal without any outer acoustic stimulation, and 50~70%

normal people could be detected with the SOAE; the TEOAE refers to the OAE evoked by short tone, clicking sound or other short-job stimulation sound; the SFOAE refers to the oto-acoustic emission signals recorded in the external ear canal, which has same frequency as the stimulation sound's and is evoked by a single low-intensity continuous pure-tone stimulation; the DPOAE is the oto-acoustic emission signals evoked by two continuous pure sounds which have different frequency but with a certain frequency ratio, and whose frequency and the stimulation acoustic frequency are different but there is mathematical expression relationship to describe their relationship. The oto-acoustic emission is nonlinear, phase locking, repeatable and steady. If it increases intensely, it could be linear; the phase locking property refers to that the oto-acoustic emission phase depends on the acoustic stimulation signals phase position and the phase changed is fixedly corresponding to the stimulation phase change. The oto-acoustic emission represents the intra-cochlear active energy-dissipative mechanical activities, and it is a phenomenon in the cochlear active mechanical process.

Because the EOAE detection is objective, non traumatic, simple and sensitive; recently in clinic, it is mainly applied to the infants' and the newborns' audition screening, the cochlear deafness's early quantitative diagnosis, the identification between the cochlear and posterior cochlear deafness.

# Common Ear Diseases

# 8

Zhonglin Mu, Bo Feng, Yong Feng, Lu Jiang, Lihui Huang
and Xiaohua Cheng

## 8.1 Congenital Malformation of Ear

Congenital ear malformations include auricular malformation, external ear canal atresia, middle ear malformation and inner ear malformation.

Congenital external ear malformation and congenital middle ear malformations are both common ear abnormalities. Unilateral ear malformation is more common, while 25–30% of the patients have bilateral malformation. Congenital external ear and middle malformation are usually divided into microtia/atresia and middle ear malformation. Patients with congenital external ear malformation usually have two physiological defects, i.e. facial defects and hearing impairment. Plastic surgery and hearing improvements are urgent wishes of the patients and their families.

### 8.1.1 Congenital Auricular Malformation

Congenital auricular malformation is caused by abnormal development of the first and the second branchial arch. Genetic factors are the main causes of this abnormal development. Half of the malformations in the ear, nose, and throat region affect the ear. Malformations of the external ear (pinna or auricle with external auditory canal [EAC]) are collectively termed microtia. Microtia is a congenital anomaly that ranges in severity from mild structural abnormalities to complete occuring absence of the external ear (anotia). Microtia occurs more frequently in males (2-3:1), is predominantly unilateral (70–90%), and more often involves the right ear. The reported prevalence varies from 0.83 to 17.4 per 10,000 births. Microtia may be genetic (with family history, spontaneous mutations) or acquired. Malformations of the external ear can also involve the middle ear and/or inner ear. Microtia may be an isolated birth defect, but associated anomalies or syndromes are described in 20–60% of cases, depending on the study design. These generally fit within the oculo-auriculo-vertebral spectrum; defects are located most frequently in the facial skeleton, facial soft tissues, heart, and vertebral column, or comprise a syndrome. Diagnostic audiological investigation of microtia includes clinical examination, audiologic testing, genetic analysis and, especially in higher grade malformations with EAC deformities, computed tomography (CT) or cone-beam CT for the planning of surgery and rehabilitation procedures, including implantation of hearing aids.

**Clinical Manifestation**

Auricular malformation includes anotia, protruding/prominent ear (also called Dumbo ears), monkey ear, accessory auricle, macrotia and microtia. Anotia and microtia are often accompanied with atresia, external ear canal stenosis or middle ear malformation.

A German doctor Max has proposed the following classification system:

**Electronic Supplementary Material** The online version of this chapter (https://doi.org/10.1007/978-981-13-7993-2_8) contains supplementary material, which is available to authorized users.

Z. Mu (✉)
Department of Otorhinolaryngology Head and Neck Surgery, The First Affiliated Hospital of Hainan Medical University, Haikou, China

B. Feng
Department of Otorhinolaryngology Head and Neck Surgery, Chinese People's Liberation Army (CPLA) General Hospital, Beijing, China

Y. Feng · L. Jiang
Department of Otorhinolaryngology Head and Neck Surgery, Xiangya Hospital, Central South University, Changsha, China

L. Huang · X. Cheng
Beijing Institute of Otolaryngology, Beijing Tongren Hospital, Capital Medical University, Beijing, China



Z. Mu, J. Fang (eds.), *Practical Otorhinolaryngology - Head and Neck Surgery*, https://doi.org/10.1007/978-981-13-7993-2_8

- Type I: Auricular malformation is slight, auricular size is slightly smaller than normal ear, and each part of auricular structure can be clearly distinguished;
- Type II: Auricular size is 1/2~1/3 of normal size, auricular structure is partially preserved;
- Type III: Severe malformation of auricle, usually like a peanut (Fig. 8.1).

**Diagnosis**
Inquire if there are similar cases in the family, the history of other diseases and drug history of mother during pregnancy. Although the diagnosis could be made according to physical examination, it is still necessary to make a comprehensive examination for accurate anatomical description of malformation of middle ear, inner ear and facial nerve. Examination of auditory function, ear X-ray and CT scan are helpful to identify the auditory function, ear canal, mastoid, ossicular chain and inner ear.

**Treatment**
When patients ask for auricular plastic surgery, the surgery can be performed according to their individual conditions. It is usually done at around six years old before accepting education. Some surgeons advise surgery after 10 years old because thoracic growth at that time is not influenced if limb cartilage is removed to reconstruct the auricle. Artificial materials, such as silicone stent and high-density porous polyethylene (Medpore) can be used to reconstruct auricle. It has been reported that the artificial auricle made with biological silicone by 3D printing technology is used to reconstruct the auricle. To improve hearing of patients with bilateral severe malformation of ear canal atresia, canalplasty and tympanoplasty should be performed before entering school. Bone-anchored hearing aid (BAHA) could be used after birth to improve hearing and speech development as early as possible, BAHA is available, and bone bridge implant is optional.

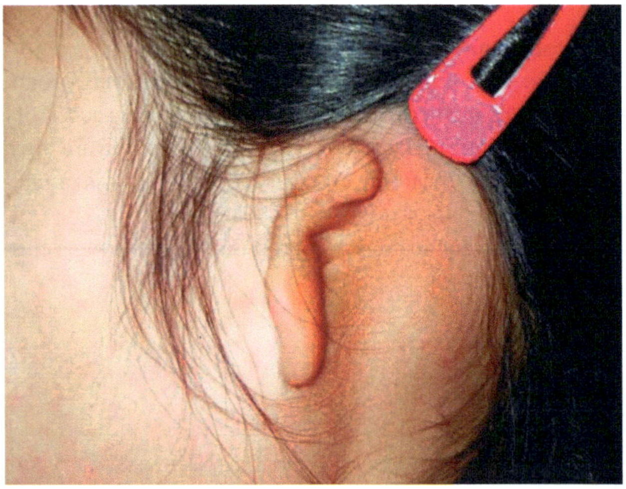

**Fig. 8.1** Congenital auricular malformation

### 8.1.2 Congenital Malformation of External and Middle Ear

#### 8.1.2.1 External Auditory Canal Malformation
It is classified as external ear canal stenosis and atresia including cartilaginous and bony atresia (Fig. 8.2).

#### 8.1.2.2 Middle Ear Malformation
It includes malformation of tympanic cavity, tympanum antrum, mastoid and Eustachian tube. The most common malformations are ossicular chain and facial nerve malformations.

**Ossicular Chain Malformation**
Ossicular chain is a lever structure which includes malleus, incus and stapes. Stapes transmits sound by direct connection with vestibular window, so almost all the auditory reconstruction surgeries focus on the stapes.

Classification of ossicular chain malformation by Okano in 2003 is as follows:

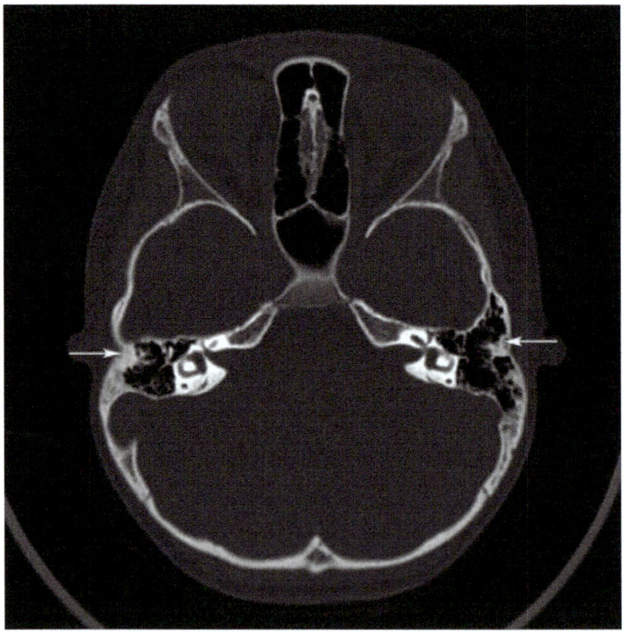

**Fig. 8.2** Bilateral atresia of external ear canal (arrow) CT scan

- Type I: discontinuity between the incus and the stapes with mobile stapes;
- Type II: congenital fixation of the stapes with ossicular deformity;
- Type III: congenital fixation of the malleus and deformity of the incus with mobile stapes.

Okano classification is a relatively simple and practical one.

#### Facial Nerve Malformation

The proportion of facial nerve malformation in ear malformation is high and correlates with severity of ear malformation. At 1994, Tongjia Leng analysed 250 cases with congenital external and middle ear malformation of which 26.7% were facial nerve malformation and 59.2% were chordal tympanic nerve malformation. The most common malformation of facial nerve is; bony defect of Eustachian tube and cover of vestibular window by Eustachian tube. The most common malformation of chorda tympani is absence of nerve. Care must be taken on bony defect of Eustachian tube. Though bony defect of Fallopian tube in middle ear may not be showed on CT scan, it can be judged by some indirect signs such as Eustachian tube abnormalities at geniculate ganglion, defect of vertical segment, defect of vestibular window and pyramidal process.

### 8.1.2.3 Diagnosis and Treatment

Diagnosis can be made based on physical examination of auricle and external ear canal, moderate and severe conductive hearing loss, and CT scan showing malformations of external ear and middle ear.

#### Classification of Ear Malformations

De la Cruz Ear Malformation Classification (Table 8.1)

Jahrsdoerfer Grading System (Only for Bony Atresia (Table 8.2)

Firstly, bone conduction threshold should be confirmed as normal by audiometry or ABR, and inner ear should be identified as normal by imaging examination.

Treatment Regimen

If inner ear development is well identified by auditory tests and CT scan, both feature and hearing can be improved by combination of pinnaplasty, canalplasty and tympanoplasty. Such surgery is challenging because of high incidence of facial nerve malformation, temporal bone abnormality, hypoplasia of tympanum and mastoid in patients with external and middle ear malformation. If a doctor chooses patients with wrong indications or does not know well about the anatomy of temporal bone of patient with ear malformation; facial paralysis, sensorineural hearing loss and other severe complications can occur. Therefore, appropriate preoperative evaluation is essential.

Preoperative evaluation of patients with bony atresia is usually based on Jahrsdoerfer grading system (Table 8.3). Generally, patients with 6 scores or more are indicated for surgery, patients with 8 scores or more may regain good hearing following canalplasty and tympanoplasty (air-bone gap <25 dB). In patients with 5 scores or less, surgical risk may outweigh the benefit.

Patient with a score of 4 or more can be treated with vibrant soundbridge (VSB), and those with a score of 3 or less are not indicated to take surgeries. VSB is a device implanted in the middle ear, which is applied for mixed hearing loss, conductive hearing loss and sensorineural hearing loss. Kiefer

**Table 8.1** De La Cruz ear malformation classification

| Minor malformation | Severe malformation |
|---|---|
| Normal pneumatization of mastoid | Poor pneumatization of mastoid |
| Normal oval window and footplate of stapes | Defect or malformation of oval window and footplate of stapes |
| Good relationship between facial nerve and footplate of stapes | Abnormal facial nerve course |
| Normal inner ear | Abnormal inner ear |

**Table 8.2** Jahrsdoerfer grading system

| Parameters | Scores |
|---|---|
| Stapes present | 2 |
| Oval window present | 1 |
| Middle ear space | 1 |
| Facial nerve position | 1 |
| Malleus-incus complex | 1 |
| Mastoid pneumatized | 1 |
| Incus-stapes connected | 1 |
| Round window present | 1 |
| Appearance external ear canal | 1 |
| Maximum total score | 10 |

**Table 8.3** Evaluation of patients with congenital middle ear malformation for reconstruction surgery by Jahrsdoerfer grading system [1]

| Scores | Operation indication |
|---|---|
| 10 | Excellent |
| 9 | Very good |
| 8 | Good |
| 7 | Fair |
| 6 | Marginal |
| <5 | Poor |

et al. reported that combined VSB implant and pinnaplasty could be applied for bilateral ear malformation. Although VSB has many advantages over tympanoplasty such as: reconstruction of the external ear canal is not needed, no postoperative complications like atresia and infection in external ear canal, no recurrent conductive deafness, small external volume and easier to bury in hair; it is an expensive implanted device for hearing loss. Nevertheless, VBS implantation cannot take place of classical tympanoplasty which is the best choice for patients with well-developed temporal bone.

Patients with 5 scores or less should implant Bone-anchored hearing aid (BAHA). Patients younger than 3 years old are suggested to wear soft band BAHA but not titanium-nail implantation which is indicated for patients older than 3 years old. The thickness of bone cortex for implant should be more than 4 mm. Titanium nail should be anchored as one-stage operation. Canalplasty is indicated for congenital external and middle ear malformation, especially for those with canal stenosis with a diameter of less than 2 mm. Poorly developed mastoid is not indicated for auditory reconstruction to avoid acquired cholesteatoma in the canal.

The results of hearing improvement following auditory reconstruction vary from patients. The poorer long-term result than short term result may be related to factors such as lateralization of tympanic membrane, repeated stenosis and infection of canal (18.3–31%), refixation of ossicular chain, sensorineural hearing loss etc.

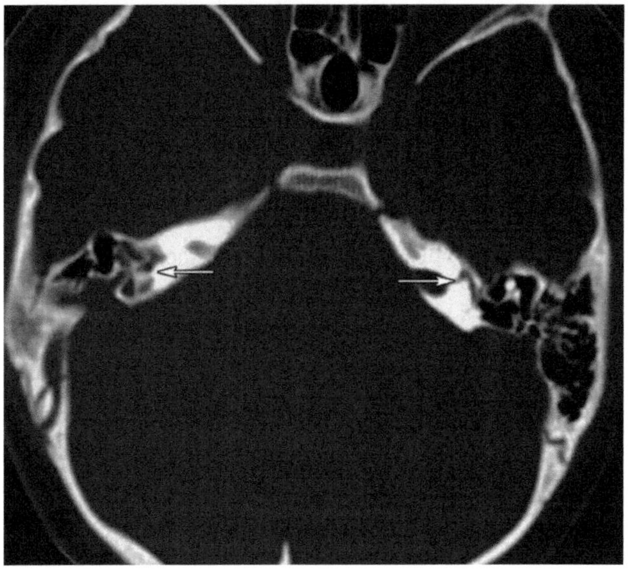

**Fig. 8.3** CT scan of Michel malformation of bilateral inner ear (arrow)

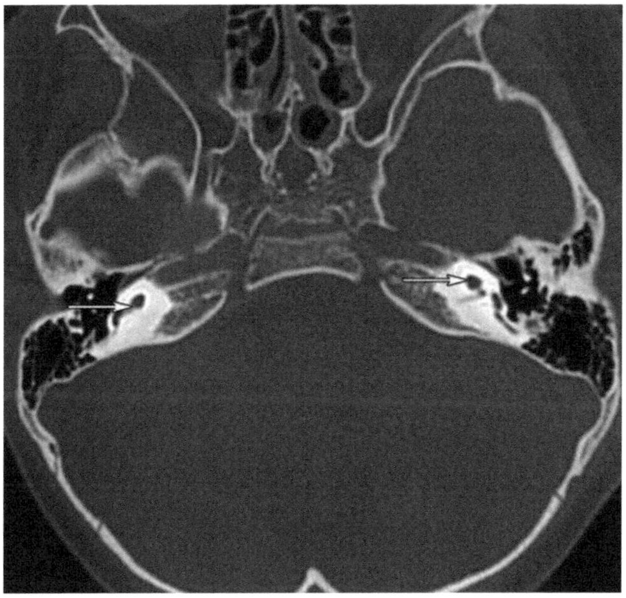

**Fig. 8.4** Mondini malformation of bilateral inner ear (arrow) CT scan

### 8.1.3 Congenital Inner Ear Malformations

Congenital inner ear malformation is a rare disease with an incidence of 1/2000–1/6000. It is subdivided according to the malformation sites into cochlear malformation, vestibular malformation, semicircular canal malformation, bony labyrinth malformation, internal auditory canal malformation, inner ear nerve malformation, blood vessel malformation etc. It includes malformations like hypoplasia, absence, deformation, translocation, stenosis etc. Common inner ear malformations are as follows.

1. Michel malformation

   Also known as Complete labyrinthine aplasia of inner ear. Complete absence of auditory and vestibular function (Fig. 8.3).
2. Mondini malformation

   Severe cochlear hypoplasia with a normal basal turn and a cystic fuse of middle and apical turn (Fig. 8.4).
3. Common Cavity malformation

   In common cavity malformation, developmental arrest occurs at the fourth week of gestation and is defined as a single cavity that represents the undifferentiated cochlea and vestibule (Fig. 8.5).
4. Enlarged vestibular aqueduct

   The width in the middle of the long axis of the aqueduct exceeds 1.5 mm. It may be related to SLC26A4 gene mutation (Fig. 8.6).

If the patients with external and middle ear malformation have severe inner ear malformation and thus profound sensorineural hearing loss, care must be taken to perform external and middle ear surgery except for auricular plastic surgery for patients' psychological and social need. Patients with indications choose to have cochlear implantation.

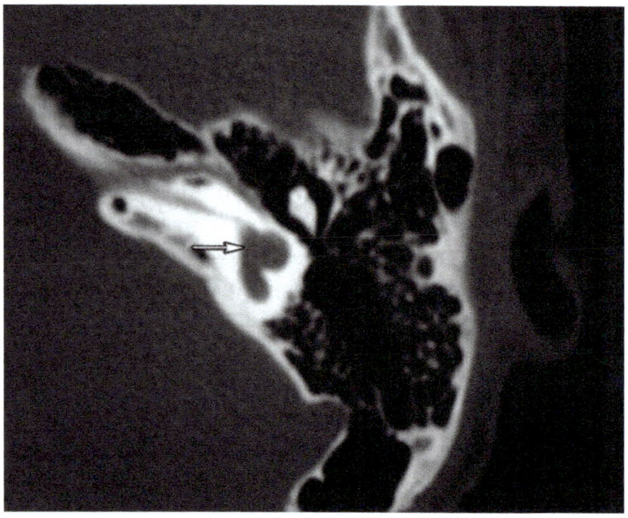

**Fig. 8.5** Common cavity malformation (arrow) CT scan

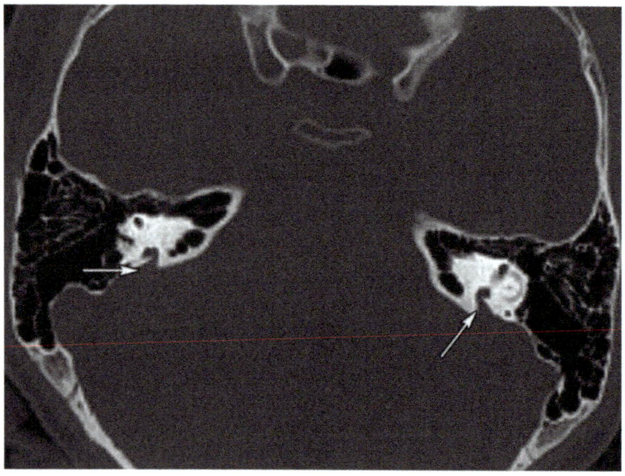

**Fig. 8.6** CT scan of bilateral aqueduct vestibule expansion (arrow)

### 8.1.4 Congenital Pre-auricular Fistula

Congenital pre-auricular fistula is a common otological disease, which occurs due to abnormal integration of hillock node at the first and second brachial arch or poor closure of the first brachial arch at embryonic stage.

**Clinical Manifestations**

1. Symptoms

   Usually asymptomatic, or local swelling, pain or festering following infection.
2. Signs

   Fistula is usually unilateral. Generally, the orificium fistula is located before helix crus, and the other end is blind. A little white sticky and caseous secretion may be extracted from the orificium while being pressed.

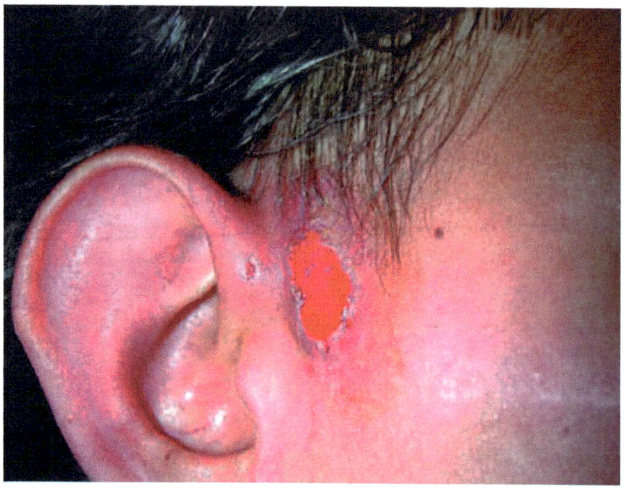

**Fig. 8.7** Congenital preauricular fistula

Repeated infection may lead to formation of cyst or abscess which may transform into purulent fistula or scar once it ruptures (Fig. 8.7).

**Therapy**

1. No treatment is needed if there is no infection. Systemic antibiotics for acute infection. If abscess forms, incision and drainage are needed followed by surgical resection once infection is controlled.
2. Surgical indications
   (a) A history of recurrent or persistent infection;
   (b) No previous infection, but local itch and exudation of secretion;
   (c) No symptoms, but surgery required by patient.

Injecting a little methylene blue solution into the fistula before operation and guiding with a probe during surgery is helpful to remove the fistula completely.

## 8.2 Trauma of Ear

### 8.2.1 Trauma of External Ear

**Clinical Manifestation**

1. Local symptom
   (a) Auricular hematoma

   It usually occurs after ear contusion. External force may break the blood vessel of auricle, and thus lead to blood deposit between cartilage and perichondrium. Soft semicircle and reddish subcutaneous mass may appear on auricle skin. Patient may have no obvious symptoms except local pain. Infection or gradual organization and calcification may occur if hematoma is not treated promptly.

(b) Hemorrhage

Anterior superficial temporal artery and posterior auricular artery are the main blood supply of auricle which forms a rich anastomosis. Injury to these arteries may result in severe bleeding which could be paused temporarily by direct pressure.

2. General symptoms

Patients may feel dizzy and usually don't have general symptoms following simple auricular trauma. Patients with trauma of other organs may have changes of vital signs such as blood pressure, pulse and respiration, and symptoms of corresponding organs.

**Examination**

Firstly, pay attention to the patient's vital signs. Secondly check the injured area and the surrounding areas. The patient's vital signs must be checked before the injured site and other organs are examined.

Examination and management may be performed at the same time for serious injuries. In unconscious patient or seriously injured patient; doctors have to make a primary diagnosis based on experience with careful examination of the patient (Fig. 8.8).

**Diagnosis**

Diagnosis can made based on the traumatic history and physical examination. Severity of injury must be assessed preliminarily, including depth and contamination of wound, vital signs, complications and so. Injury of middle ear and inner ear may result in hearing loss, tympanic membrane perforation, hemotympanum, vertigo, or facial paralysis. Temporal bone must be taken into consideration.

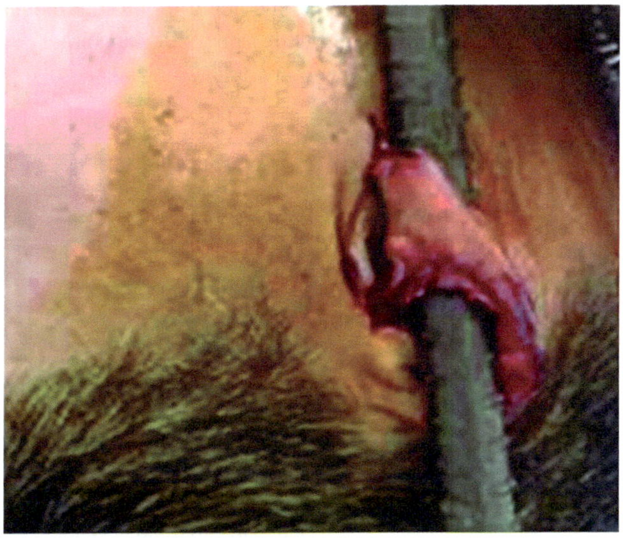

**Fig. 8.8** Auricular trauma

**Treatment**

1. The management of auricular hematoma

The auricular hematoma is not easy to be absorbed due to few subcutaneous tissue and poor blood supply of auricle. The accumulated blood can be extracted with a thick needle and dressed with pressure. If it does not heal following repeated operations, it can be incised parallel to the helix so that the hematoma can be exuded, or the blood clot can be removed. Pressure dressing and prevention from infection are essential.

2. Management of the external ear canal

Prevention from infection is the primary objective. The ear canal must be disinfected strictly and must not be irrigated with any liquid. The dust, cerumen and debris can be removed with suction, curettage and cotton swab. The ear canal should be kept as dry as possible. Nail purple oil is not recommended because it may disturb examining the wound. Sterilized antibiotic gauze or iodoform gauze can be used to pack the canal to prevent from infection and stenosis if necessary. If too much granulation tissue blocks the canal, it can be removed with curettage followed by canalplasty once the infection is under control.

3. General Management

**Systemic Management**

Adequate broad-spectrum antibiotics are recommended for prevention of infection. Tetanus immunoglobulin is required for deep wound.

### 8.2.2 Tympanic Trauma Tympanic Membrane Trauma

**Clinical Manifestations**

Sudden ear pain, immediate hearing loss accompanied by tinnitus, a small amount of bleeding in the external ear canal and vertigo. Occasionally, they may present with dizziness, nausea and mixed hearing impairment.

**Examination**

Tympanic membrane has many irregular shapes or fissure shaped perforation. There can be a little bloodstain within the external ear canal or blood scab. Small amount of blood can be found around the edge of the Tresses (Fig. 8.9). When there is plenty of bleeding or aqueous humor outflow, it suggests cerebrospinal fluid otorrhea caused by the fracture of the temporal bone or skull base. Conductive or mixed hearing damage can result from audition examination.

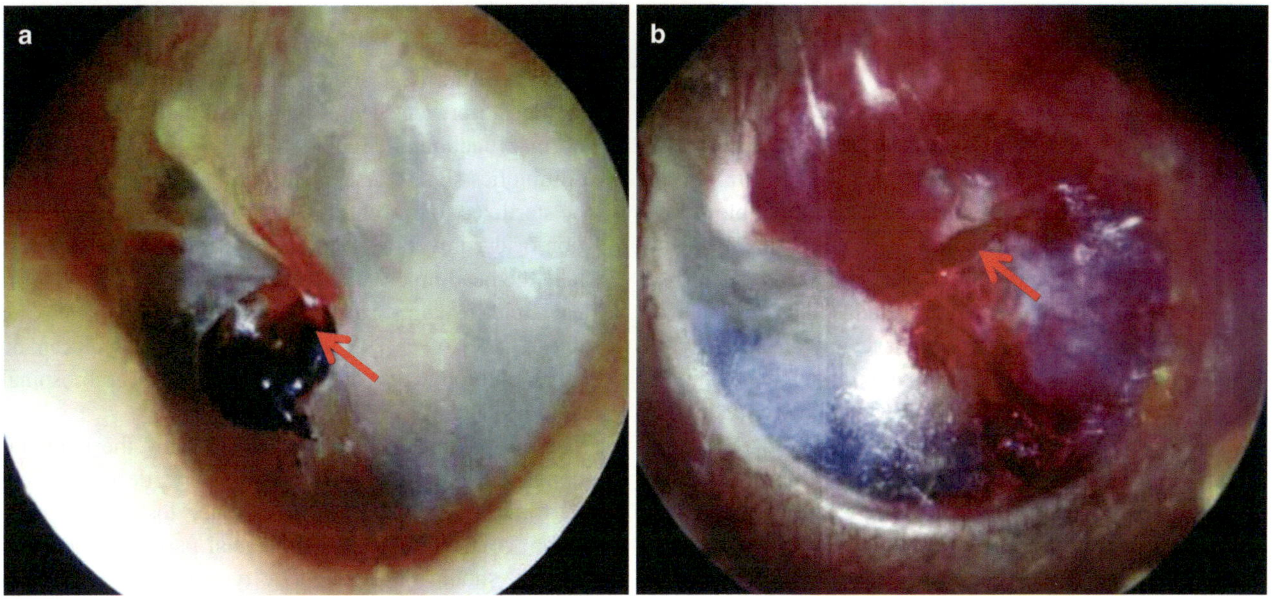


**Fig. 8.9** Tympana perforation. (**a**) Tympanum perforation, little bloodstain. (**b**) Tympanum fissure perforation

**Treatment**

1. Clear foreign matter in the external acoustic canal and block it with sterilized cotton ball.
2. Avoid catching a cold. Don't violently blow your nose.
3. Irrigating or dripping medicine to the external ear canal is forbidden. Most traumatic perforations can self-heal after about 3–4 weeks. If the perforation is too large to heal spontaneously myringoplasty should be considered.

### 8.2.3 Temporal Bone Fracture

**Classification**

1. Longitudinal fracture

   Longitudinal fractures comprise 80% of all temporal bone fractures. They are frequently caused by a lateral force over the mastoid or temporal squama, also usually produced by temporal or parietal blows. The fracture line parallels the long axis of the petrous pyramid. It starts in the pars squamosa (mastoid or external auditory canal), as seen in the image above (Fig. 8.10 the temporal bone transverse fracture), and extends through the posterosuperior bony external canal, continues across the roof of the middle ear space anterior to the labyrinth, and ends anteromedially in the middle cranial fossa in close proximity to the foramen lacerum and ovale. The most common course of the fracture is anterior and extralabyrinthine; however, although rare, intralabyrinthine extension is possible. Again, bilateral temporal bone fractures are present in 8–29% of all fractures, according to the medical literature.

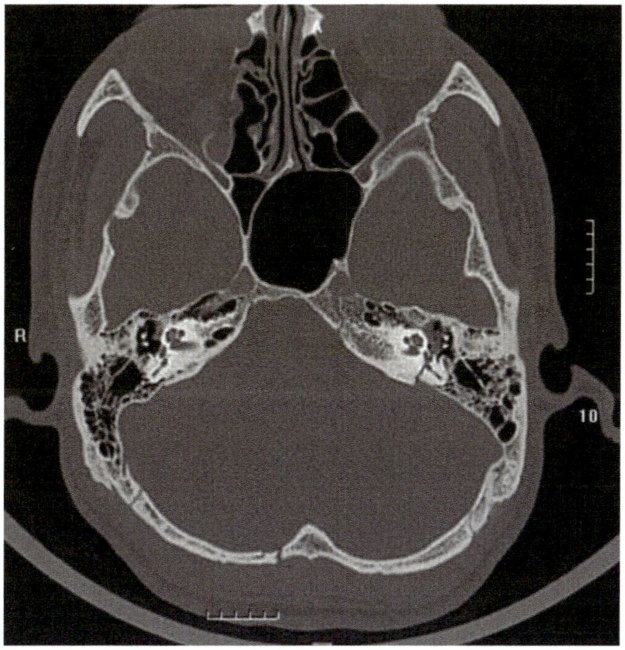


**Fig. 8.10** The left temporal bone transverse fracture CT scan

Signs and symptoms include bleeding into the ear canal from skin and tympanic membrane laceration, hemotympanum, external auditory canal fractures, ossicular chain disruption that produces conductive hearing loss, and facial nerve paralysis. Twenty percent of longitudinal fractures injure the facial nerve and cause paralysis. The injury site is usually the horizontal segment of the nerve distal to the geniculate ganglion. CSF otorhinorrhea is common but usually temporary. Sensorineural hearing loss may occur as a result of concussive damage. Vertigo occurs but is not related to the severity of the fracture.

2. Transverse fracture

   Transverse fractures comprise 20% of all temporal bone fractures. They are usually caused by a frontal or parietal blow but may result from an occipital blow. The fracture line runs at a right angle to the long axis of the petrous pyramid and starts in the middle cranial fossa (close to the foramen lacerum and spinosum). It then crosses the petrous pyramid transversely and ends at the foramen magnum. It may also extend through the internal auditory canal and injure the nerves directly. Cochlear and vestibular structures are usually destroyed, producing a profound sensorineural hearing loss and severe ablative vertigo. The intensity of the vertigo will decrease after 7–10 days and then continues to decrease steadily over the following 1–2 months, leaving only an unsteady feeling that lasts approximately 3–6 months, until compensation finally occurs. Intense nystagmus (third degree) is present since the initial fracture, with the fast component beating away from the fracture site. The nystagmus is easily seen by the naked eye. Nystagmus also decreases progressively in intensity (third degree, second degree, first degree) and then finally disappears.

   Rarely, a mixed hearing loss may occur. Facial nerve injury occurs in 50% of transverse fractures. The injury site is anywhere from the internal auditory canal to the horizontal segment distal to the geniculate ganglion. Pneumolabyrinth may be noted.

   Histopathology reveals hair cell loss, ganglion cell loss, and supporting cell loss. In rare cases, labyrinthitis ossificans occurs secondary to the trauma or subsequent infection. This must be kept in mind when cochlear implant is considered after a temporal bone fracture.

3. Mixed fracture

   These patterns, which extend both longitudinally and transversely, are common. According to some authors, these patterns occur more often than isolated transverse or longitudinal fractures. A range of 62–90% of temporal bone fractures were designed as a mixed pattern in medical literature.

4. Petrous apex fracture

   Rarely-seen. It can damage the second-sixth cranial nerves leading to corresponding eye symptoms and trigeminal neuralgia or facial sensation disorder. The petrous apex fractures can damage the internal carotid artery, leading to the fatal bleeding.

   The temporal bone fractures can be accompanied by cerebrospinal fluid leak. Cerebrospinal fluid leakage is light red in the early stage, gradually turns into crystal and the test result is sugary liquid (glycosuria test paper can be used).

**Treatment**

1. Keep airway clear and perform tracheotomy if necessary.
2. Control hemorrhage and infuses fluid or transfuses blood in time to prevent hemorrhagic shock and maintain the normal function of circulation.
3. Antibiotics should be applied in time and the ear should be sterilized to prevent infection of the encephalic infection or ear infection. If there is cerebrospinal fluid leak, take the head-up or half supine posture; most cerebrospinal fluid leakage can stop spontaneously. If leaking doesn't stop over 2–3 weeks, the dural defect can be repaired through the ear canal to control the cerebrospinal fluid leakage.
4. The peripheral facial paralysis caused by the temporal bone fracture should be operatively decompressed. Perforation of tympanic membrane, loss of acoustic chain, conduction deafness or facial paralysis and other malady should be repaired by tympanoplasty or facial nerve operation.

## 8.3 Disease of External Ear

### 8.3.1 Furuncle of External Auditory Canal

It is also called local otitis externa, mainly refers to acute suppurative lesions of the cartilaginous skin which occurs in the external ear canal as Fig. 8.11. Pathogenic bacterium is mainly the staphylococcus aureus and pseudomonas aeruginosa.

**Clinical Manifestation**

*Symptoms and Signs*

Patients have pain and drainage. Sometimes, a foul-smelling discharge and hearing loss occur if the canal becomes swollen or filled with purulent debris. Exquisite tenderness accompanies traction of the pinna or pressure over the tragus. Otoscopic examination is painful and difficult to conduct. It shows the ear canal to be red, swollen, and littered with moist, purulent debris and desquamated epithelium.

*Otomycosis* is more pruritic than painful, and patients also complain of aural fullness. Otomycosis caused by *A. niger* usually manifests with grayish black or yellow dots (fungal conidiophores) surrounded by a cottonlike material (fungal hyphae). Infection caused by *C. albicans* does not show any visible fungi but usually contains a thickened, creamy white exudate, which can be accompanied by spores that have a velvety appearance.

*Furuncles* cause severe pain and may drain sanguineous, purulent material. They appear as a focal, erythematous swelling (pimple) (Fig. 8.11).

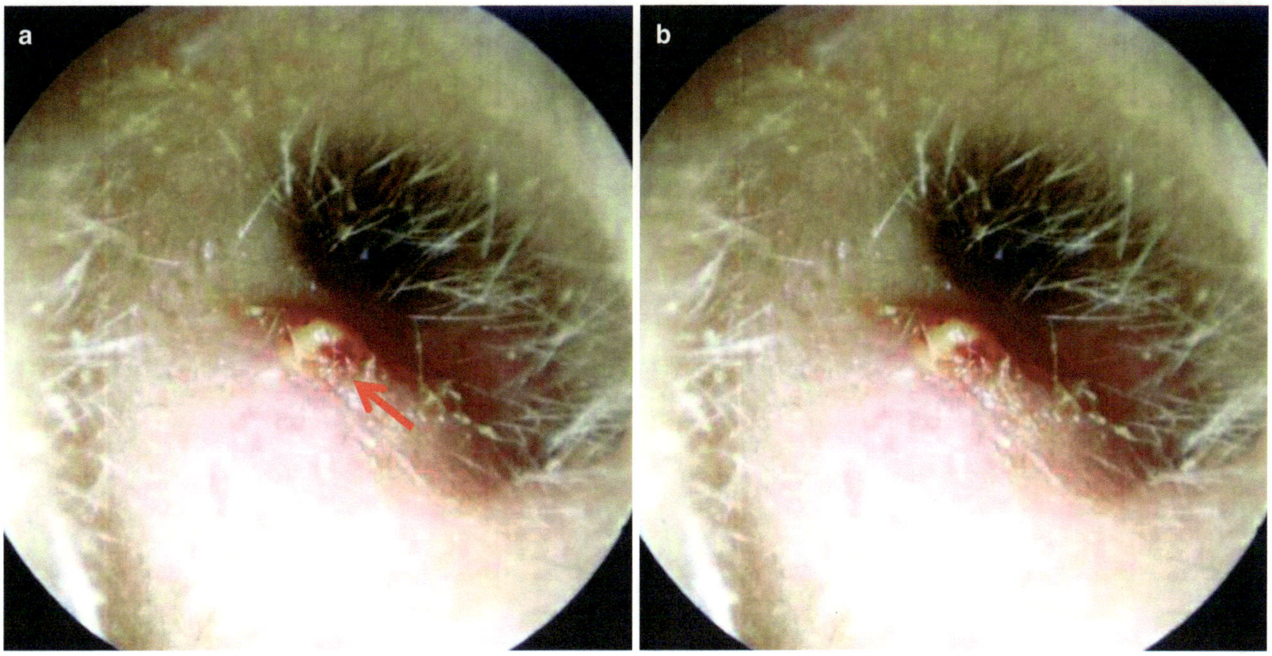


**Fig. 8.11** Furuncle of external auditory canal

**Treatment**

1. Local therapy

   When the furuncle is not mature, sterilize the area locally with ethanol, apply the detumescence gauze dipped with ichthammol on the furuncle, and use antibiotics when necessary. In the presence of purulent bolt, incise with sterile scalpel after ethanol disinfection, remove the abscess, apply the antibacterial gauze with erythromycin on and replace it every day until the lesion is involuted. When the abscess is fluctuated, incise along the external ear canal after the ethanol sterilization to drainage.
2. Systemic therapy

   Patients with fever or systemic disease may be treated with oral or intravenous antibiotics according to local or systemic antimicrobial susceptibility tests result and do analgesic therapy when there is severe pain.

### 8.3.2 External Ear Canal Cholesteatoma

**Clinical Manifestations**

Often occur in adults. Uninfected people have no symptoms. Patients with Severe cholesteatoma showed ear coagulation sensation; tinnitus and secondary infections have ear pain, headache and smelly secretion in the external ear canal.

**Specific Examination**

1. The deep section of the external ear canal is blocked with white or yellow cholesteatoma, and the canal surface is covered with multilayer flaky substance (Fig. 8.12).
2. After removing the related-bigger cholesteatoma, there could appear bone destruction and absorption at the external ear canal, obviously expanded bony part of the external ear canal.
3. Entire tympanum membrane can be congested and invaginated.

The big external ear canal cholesteatoma invades the mastoid to damage its sclerotin (Fig. 8.13), complicating with the cholesteatoma's type middle ear mastoitis, causing peripheral facial paralysis.

**Diagnosis**

Pathogenic exam result of cholesteatoma could confirm the diagnosis.

**Treatment**

1. In the absence of concurrent infection, cholesteatoma is easier to be taken out and removed like cerumen.
2. In the presence of infection, pay attention to control infection. Partially remove or all of cholesteatoma.

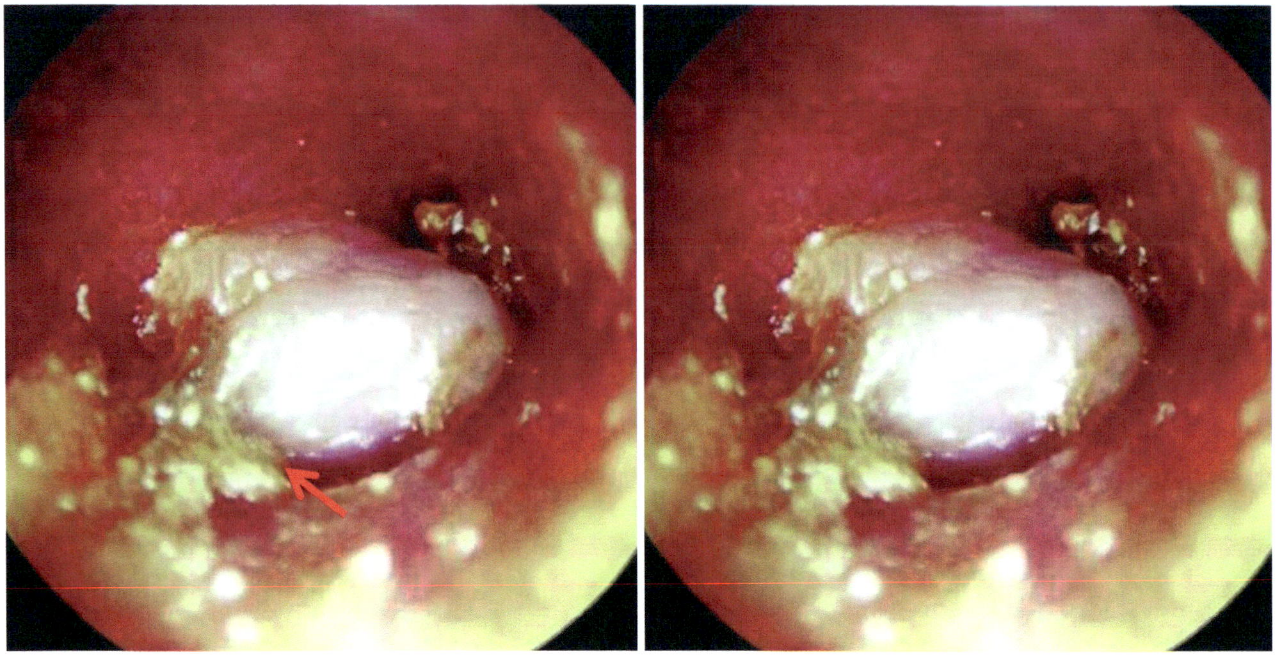

**Fig. 8.12** The external ear canal cholesteatoma

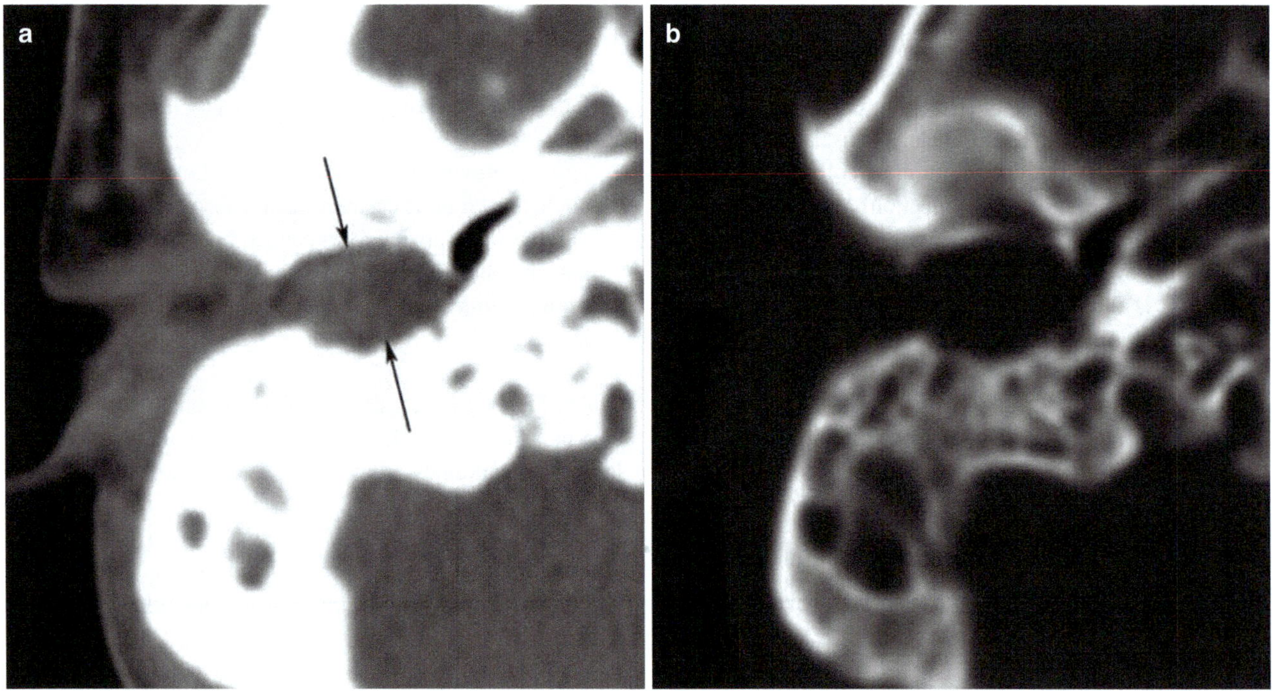


**Fig. 8.13** Axial CT scan: external ear canal cholesteatoma. (**a**) Soft tissue fenestra, manifesting soft tissue density shadow filled in right external ear canal (arrow). (**b**) Bone fenestra, manifesting bone destruction of the right external ear canal, harden bone edge and slightly enlarged external ear canal; unwell gasified mastoid and increased mastoid sinuses density

3. In patients with severe infection, the chlosteatoma is to be removed under general anesthesia and operating microscope. Control the infection by applying broad-spectrum antibiotics. Follow-up, observe and remove the residual or regenerative cholesteatoma after surgery.
4. Patients with the external auditory meatus cholesteatoma which has invaded the mastoid should be treated by radical mastectomy or modified mastectomy.

## 8.4 Diseases of Middle Ear

Middle ear disease is common in otorhinolaryngology, head and neck surgery, with symptoms such as ear discomfort, pain, swelling sensation, occlusion sensation, otorrhea, hearing loss, tinnitus, dizziness, etc. Trauma, infection or pressure change caused by obstruction of eustachian tube in the middle ear are most causes of the disease. Fever, malaise and other symptoms are associated with infective middle ear disease. Otitis media is the most common one among middle ear disease.

Classification criterion of otitis media in 2012 by the academy of otolaryngology of Chinese Medical Association is as follows.

1. Secretory otitis media (SOM)
2. Suppurative otitis media
   (a) Acute suppurative otitis media
   (b) Chronic suppurative otitis media: resting stage; active stage.
3. Middle ear cholesteatoma
4. Special otitis media
   (a) Tuberculous otitis media
   (b) HIV positive otitis media
   (c) Mesotoxic otitis media
   (d) Fungal otitis media
   (e) Necrotizing otitis media
   (f) Radioactive otitis media
   (g) Aero-otitis media [2]

### 8.4.1 Secretory Otitis Media

**Clinical manifestation**

1. Hearing loss

   Most of patients with acute secretory otitis media have the history of upper respiratory tract infection, with gradual hearing loss, and louder speech.
2. Otalgia

   Acute secretory otitis media may cause slight otalgia at the onset, and it develops while secondary infection to patients with chronic SOM.
3. Inner ear occlusion sensation

   Adult patients always complain of occlusion or distention sensation and can be relieved temporarily by pressing the tragus.
4. Tinnitus

   Not heavy generally, but there could be a "crackling" sound. While the head moves, yawning or blowing the nose, gurgling appears.
5. Acoustic immittance

   The acoustic immittance test has great value to diagnose. The flat type (type B) is the typical curve of the disease, sometimes-high vacuum type (type C). All the acoustic reflexes disappeared.

**Examination**

1. Tympanic membrane

   Acute SOM will cause hyperemia at pars flaccid or entire tympanic membrane, manifestation as shortened, deformed or disappeared cones light, shifted-to-posterior and obvious malleus's axillary process. The tympanic membrane is yellowish, orange-red glossy or amber when the tympanic effusion happens. For the chronic SOM, the color is grayish blue or milky white as shown in Fig. 8.14. There is hairy line on tympanic membrane, and when the head position changes, it's still parallel to the ground. The bubbles could be seen through the tympanum membrane and may increase while doing eustachian tube insufflation.

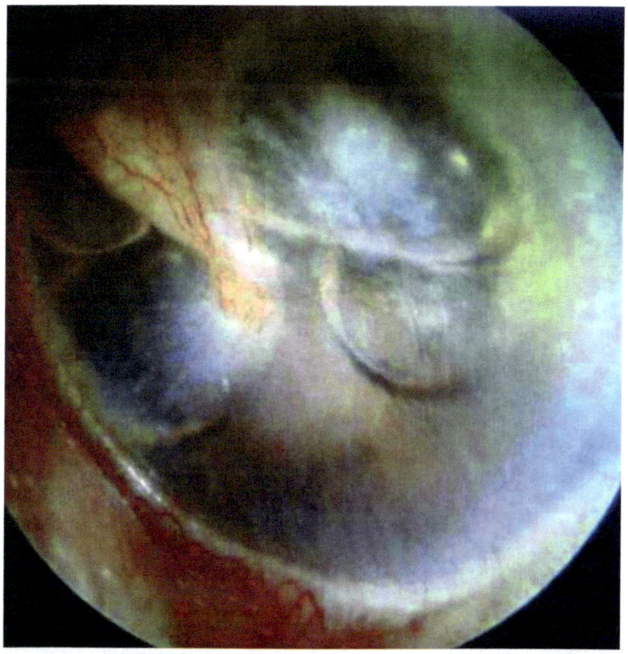

**Fig. 8.14** Secretory otitis media, manifesting fluid flat tympanum hydrous and inside bubbles

2. Pneumatic otoscope examination

   It manifests the tympanum membrane movement limitedly.
3. Audition test

   Tuning fork test and pure tone threshold test show conductive deafness. In severe cases, hearing loss of about 40 dBHL can be found, mostly low frequency, and could be improved after eliminating the effusion. Acoustic immittance figure is mostly flat type (Type B). Vacuum type (Type C) suspects the dysfunction of eustachian tube, including cavum tympanum hydrops appearing in part of them. Severe patients could reach 100 dBHL at ABR test and can't be used to diagnose nerve deafness.
4. Imaging diagnosis

   Ossa temporal CT scan: different degrees of hydrops occur in the pneumatic cavity of middle-ear system. Most of CT values are under 40 Hu.

   Mastoid MR Examination: the mastoid, mastoid cells without any signals, becomes hypersensitive and has high specificity diagnosis value (Figs. 8.15 and 8.16).

**Differentiate Diagnosis**

Tympanotomy could help make a definite diagnosis.

**Treatment**

The first choice for the patients is 3-month non-surgical therapy grasping the surgical indications strictly. Etiology therapy, improving the middle ear ventilation drainage and removing the tympanic effusion are the therapeutic principles of the disease.

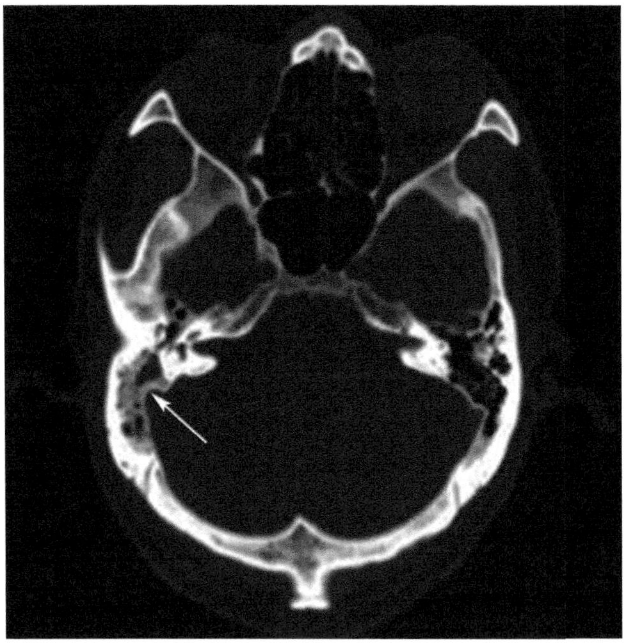

**Fig. 8.15** Bilateral mastoid plain CT scan (bone fenestra). Well-gasified left nidus Vespa, right mastoid nidus Vespa filled with slightly high-density fluid (arrow)

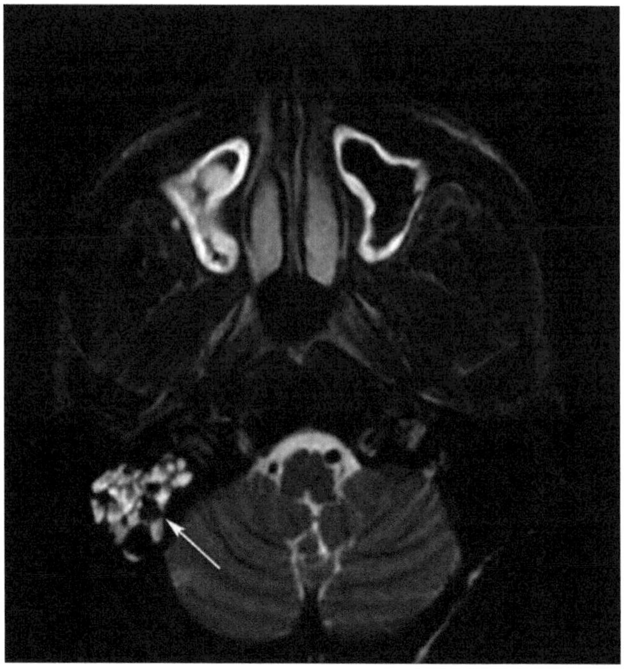

**Fig. 8.16** Bilateral mastoid plain MR scan ($T_2$WI). Well-gasified left nidus Vespa without signal manifestation, right mastoid nidus Vespa filled with $T_2$WI-high-signal fluid (arrow)

1. Non-surgical therapy
   (a) Antibiotics: select the appropriate antibiotics according to the severity of the lesion at acute phase.
   (b) Keep the nasal cavity and the eustachian tube unobstructed: inhale intranasal with 1% ephedrine solution and antibiotics contain hormones alternately, 3–4 times each day.
   (c) Promote cilium movement and excretion function: dilute mucin beneficial to ciliary excrete, lower superficial tension of eustachian tube mucosa and the opening pressure of the eustachian tube.
   (d) Takes glucocorticoid drug, dexamethasone, prednisone orally as adjuvant therapy.
2. Surgical therapy
   (a) Eustachian tube insufflation: Valsalva maneuver. Wave's ball method outraging method at chronic phase
   (b) Tympanic puncture and drainage: local anesthesia for adult patients and general anesthesia for infants.
   (c) Tympanotomy: Considered for patients with mucous effusion which cannot be cleaned by puncture. A radial or arc-shaped incision is made in the interior and lower quadrants of tympanic membrane with tympanic knife. Mucosa of tympanic wall should not be injured. After tympanic incision, fluid cavity should be absorbed.
   (d) Tympanoplasty: If the effusion is too viscous to be discharged and the eustachian tube function is difficult to return to normal in a short time after head radiotherapy, tympanoplasty can be considered (Fig. 8.17).

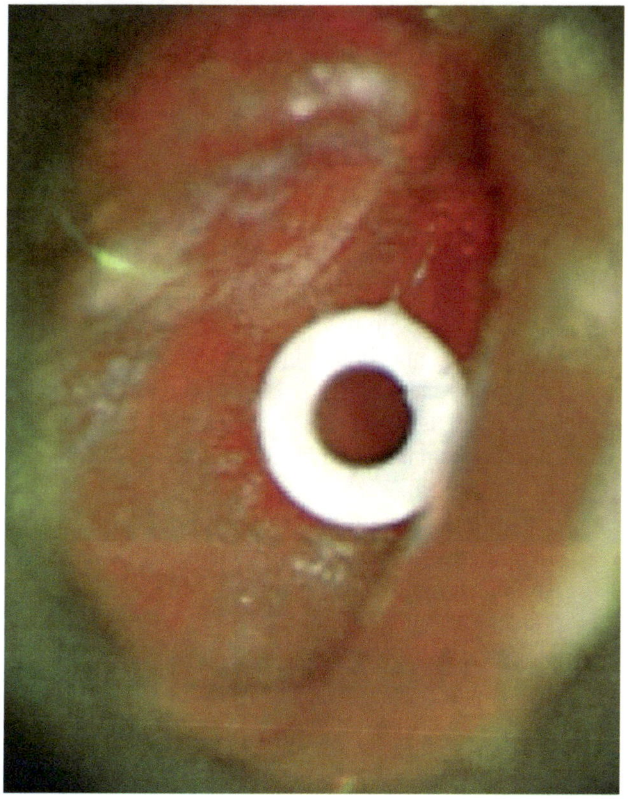

**Fig. 8.17** Tympanoplasty

(e) Long-term repeated attacks, suspecting granulation tissue formation or other irreversible lesion formed in the middle ear mastoid cavity or ossicular ossicles destruction, early simple mastoidectomy, epitympanotomy, upper tympanostomy or posterior tympanostomy should be performed to clear the lesion.
(f) Active treatment of nasopharyngeal or nasal diseases.
(g) Balloon angioplasty: In the early twenty-first century, Europeans developed a kind of balloon dilation catheter to treat sinusitis. Ockermanm (2010) and it was first applied to the eustachian tube by imputing the saccule at the Eustachian tube orifice to expand the tube under guidance of nasal endoscopy on a cadaveric head model. A slight crack at eustachian tube cartilage was found but no injury to the bone which confirms the feasibility and security of the balloon angioplasty. Subsequently, he applied it in the clinic, and found that the function of eustachian tube was significantly improved after surgery without any obvious complications. The results of 2-year follow-up showed that the balloon dilatation had a good long-term effect.

Secretory otitis media is closely related to dysfunction of eustachian tube, and dysfunction of eustachian tube may be related to dysfunction of tensor veli palatinis and decrease of surfactant in eustachian tube. Balloon dilatation of eustachian tube can cause small tear in the submucosa of eustachian tube, thinning the submucosa and enlarging the lumen. Moreover, the teared tissue is repaired by fresh scar tissue, i.e. collagen fibers are compressed and filled by fibroblasts, neovascularization and inflammatory cells, instead of collagen fibers, which are regenerated and repaired. Therefore, it is not easy to restenosis. After enlarging the eustachian tube lumen, it can improve drainage and restore ciliary function. It may also redistribute the active substances on the surface of eustachian tube mucosa and help to restore its function.

Surgical methods: After general anesthesia, the nasal cavity was contracted by 1% adrenaline for 5 min. The nasal cavity and nasopharynx were examined by 0 nasal endoscopy. The tip of 70 or 30 or 45 duct was placed at the nasopharyngeal orifice of the eustachian tube, and the guide wire was introduced into the eustachian Pump pressure, swell balloon, slowly add to 10 atmospheric pressure, maintain 2 min, pump decompression, suction to negative pressure, exit balloon and guide wire.

If the nasal cavity can not be inserted into both nasal endoscopy and balloon catheter implant due to anatomical reasons, nasal endoscopy can be inserted through oropharyngeal approach, and balloon catheter can be inserted through nasal cavity.

### 8.4.2 Acute Suppurative Otitis Media

**Clinical Manifestations**

1. Systemic symptoms are chills and fever. Children have severe systemic symptoms, such as high fever, convulsions, vomiting and diarrhea. Once the tympanic membrane is perforated, the body temperature gradually decreases and the symptoms of the whole body are obviously alleviated
2. Otalgia: deep ear throbbing pain or tingling, can radiate to the ipsilateral head or teeth, the pain is intense, causing restlessness, unable to sleep. Children cry endlessly, turn their head and neck, grasp their ears with their hands and refuse to eat. After tympanic membrane perforation and purulence, the earache is relieved.
3. Tinnitus: deafness, stuffy hearing, hearing loss gradually. When the earache is severe, deafness is often neglected, occasionally accompanied by vertigo, and deafness is alleviated after tympanic membrane perforation.
4. Otorrhea: After tympanic membrane perforation, there are mucopurulent efflux, which can be blood and water samples at first, and then become purulent.

**Examination**

1. Otoscopy

   Otoscope examines tympanic membrane congestion, which is at first congestion of the flabby malleolus stalk, then radial congestion of the tense part, and finally diffuse congestion and bulging outward. Finally, tympanic membrane perforation, because of small perforation, pus pulsatile overflow, visible flashing pulsatile light, known as "beacon sign", necrotic can see large tympanic membrane perforation (Fig. 8.18).
2. Ear palpation

   Mild tenderness appears at the tympanum antrum site of mastoid.
3. Audition examination

   Conductive deafness often.
4. Hemogram

   Quantity of WBC and neutrophils increases, and the hemogram gradually becomes normal after tympanum tresses.

**Treatment**

The principle is anti-infection, drainage and removing roots.

1. Systemic therapy
   - (a) Apply the antibiotics early at full dose:

     After doing tympanic membrane tresis, take the abscess for fine culture and drug sensitization. Choose the appropriate antibiotics due to the reference result, and stop the pills after keeping treating for couple days after the symptoms are gone.

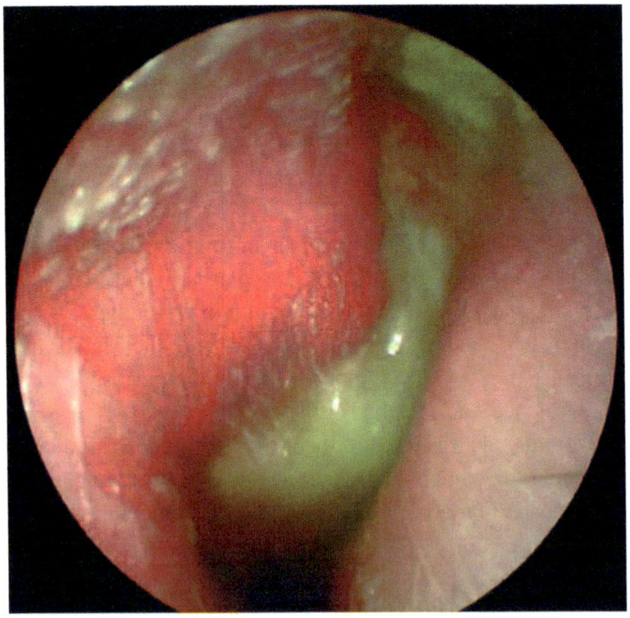

**Fig. 8.18** Acute suppurative otitis media under microscopy

   - (b) Rest enough, adjust the diet and keep bowels open. The severe patient should pay attention to the support therapy like applying the glucocorticoids, etc. Ask the pediatrician to cooperate while necessary.
2. Local therapy
   - (a) Ear inhalation

     Use 2% phenols to do ear inhalation before the tympanic membrane tresis; after perforating, use 3% peroxide to clear the external ear canal and inhalation antibiotics ear drops.
   - (b) Tympanic membrane incision therapies: accurate tympanic membrane dissection can be unobstructed drainage, is conducive to the rapid dissipation of inflammation, so that systemic and local symptoms are alleviated.
   - (c) Short-term uses of nasal congestion drugs: such as 1% ephedrine nasal drops, reduce the swelling of nasopharyngeal mucosa; help restore Eustachian tube function.
3. Etiology therapy

   Active therapy of chronic diseases of the nose and pharynx.

### 8.4.3 Chronic Suppurative Otitis Media

Chronic suppurative otitis media is chronic suppurative inflammation at middle ear mucosa, bone periosteum or bone cortex, its clinical features are long-term intra-auricular pus, tympanic membrane perforation, hearing loss, etc.

**Clinical Manifestation**

1. Intra-auricular discharge the overflow can be discontinuous or persistent. Secretions can be sticky or thin, sometimes with blood. Amount of secretions differ, and discharge would increase when water flows into ear.
2. Hearing loss: Hearing loss degrees differ.
3. Tinnitus: Some patients may be with paroxysmal or persistent tinnitus.

**Examination**

1. Tympanic membranous perforation

   It would locate in dense part, and size and shape of perforation usually differ, which can be manifested as central small perforation, kidney shaped perforation or large perforation, but there are residual edges in the tympanic membrane, and there is no destruction of the tympanic ring. Smooth tympanum antrum mucosa or slight tympanum antrum edema would be observed through proliferation (Fig. 8.19). Ossicular chain is usually complete or only partial malleus handle is necrotic.

2. Hearing test generally result manifest as mild conductive hearing loss.
3. Mastoid X-ray imaging or Temporal CT scan

   Mastoid may manifest as gasified type or barrier type, soft tissue shadow would be seen in middle ear. No cortex damage would be noticed (Fig. 8.20).

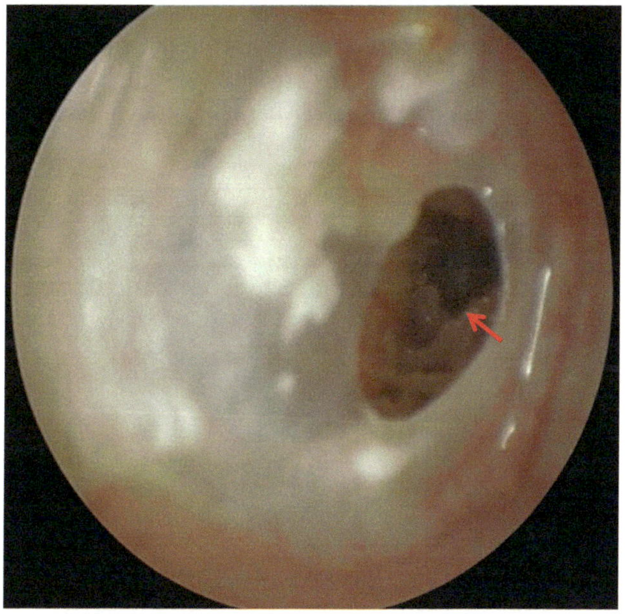

**Fig. 8.19** Tympanic membranous perforation

**Treatment**

If drainage is unblocked unblocked, local medication can be used, such as 0.3% ofloxacin ear drops, 2.5% chloramphenicol glycerin ear drops and 3% boric acid ear drops. 3% hydrogen peroxide solution can be used to wash ears before medication. The principle of treatment is to prevent recurrence and to restore hearing by tympanoplasty after inflammation control. In inflammatory stage, antibiotics should be selected reasonably according to the results of bacterial culture and susceptibility test. When the local purulent secretion is large, it should be cleaned with 3% hydrogen peroxide solution, cleaned or sucked up by an aspirator, and then dripped with antibiotic ear drops, such as 0.3% ofloxacin solution and 0.5% chlortetracycline solution. After inflammation control, tympanoplasty can be considered to reconstruct hearing.

### 8.4.4 Cholesteatoma of the Middle Ear

Cholesteatoma of the middle ear is a cystic structure located in the middle ear. It is composed of stratified squamous epithelium and contains cholesterol crystals, exfoliated skin cells, keratins and bacteria. It is not a true tumor. According to the pathogenesis, it is usually divided into acquired primary cholesteatoma and acquired lipoma. Cholesteatoma can be secondary to chronic suppurative otitis media. Chronic suppurative otitis media can also be secondary to bacterial infection of cholesteatoma. Therefore, this disease is called chronic otitis media with cholesteatoma.

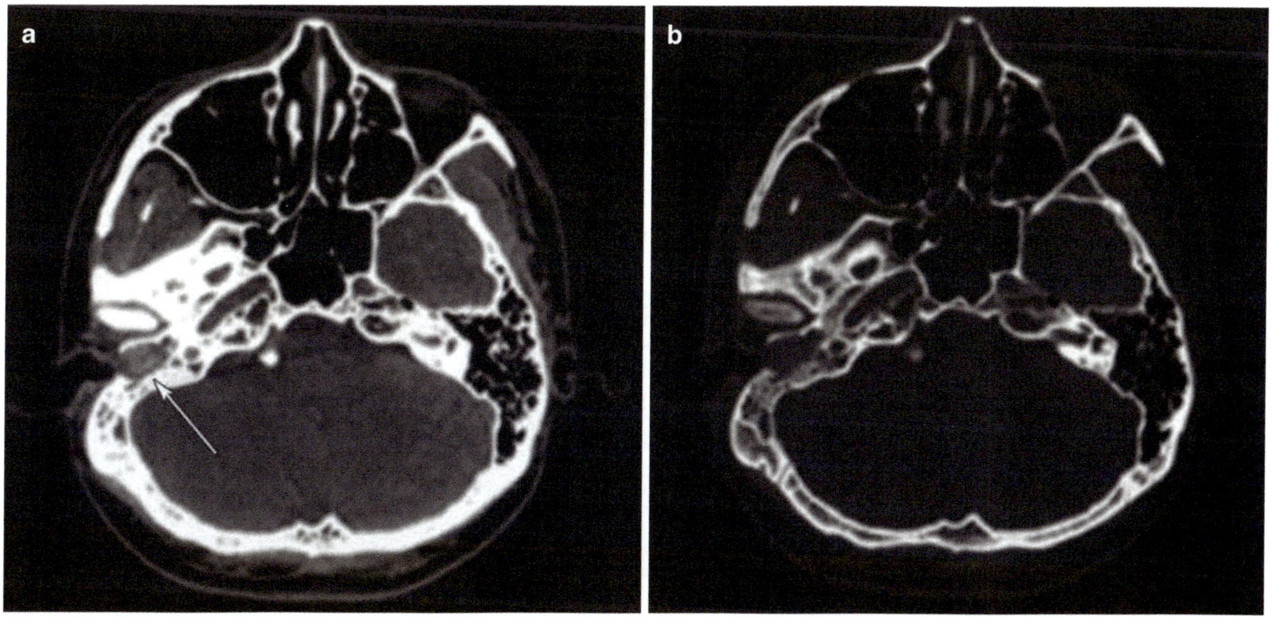


**Fig. 8.20** Temporal axial CT scan of right chronic middle ear mastoid otitis. (**a**) Soft tissue window CT plain scan; (**b**) bone window CT plain scan. Well-gasified left mastoid, no abnormality; small right mastoid nidus vespa, within high density shadow, middle ear cavity and mastoid sinus enlarges and little sclerotin damage within soft tissue density shadow stuff (arrow)

**Clinical Manifestation**

1. Acquired primary cholesteatoma is rare. No Otorrhea or tympanic membrane perforation can be found before infection. Acquired cholesteatoma is characterized by long-term otorrhea, pyotympanic membrane perforation and hearing loss
2. Long-term persistent or intermittent otorrhea. Stench exists.
3. Complication: Cholesteatoma of the middle ear may cause intracranial and extracranial complications, such as subperiosteal abscess, peripheral facial paralysis, labyrinthine inflammation, epidural abscess, thrombophlebitis of the sigmoid sinus, meningitis, brain abscess and even hernia, because of its strong bone destruction characteristics. Serious cases may cause death
4. There are marginal perforations in the relaxation or tension. From the perforation, there are grayish-white scaly or bean dregs-like substances in the tympanic chamber with strong odor (Fig. 8.21)

**Examination**

1. Audiological test

   It is usually a severe conductive hearing loss, such as lesions and the cochlea. Mixed hearing loss.
2. CT examination

   For patients with clinically suspected cholesteatoma high-resolution temporal bone CT scan, to accurately understand the cholesteatoma scope, ossicular's change. The destruction of the facial nerve canal, semicircular canal, tympanic cavity, etc. Which is typically characterized by soft tissue shadow in the middle ear, homogeneous density, dense and sharp border, and often accompanied by bone destruction (Figs. 8.22 and 8.23).

**Treatment**

Once the middle ear cholesteatoma is diagnosed, it should be operated as soon as possible. There are many kinds of surgical methods, mainly open and close (wall-closing) two types. Endoscopy can be used for wall-closure surgery to see areas that are difficult to be seen under the operating microscope, such as the upper tympanic chamber, tympanic sinus, eustachian tube and so on, which is expected to greatly reduce the incidence of residual lesions. After cholesteatoma is com-

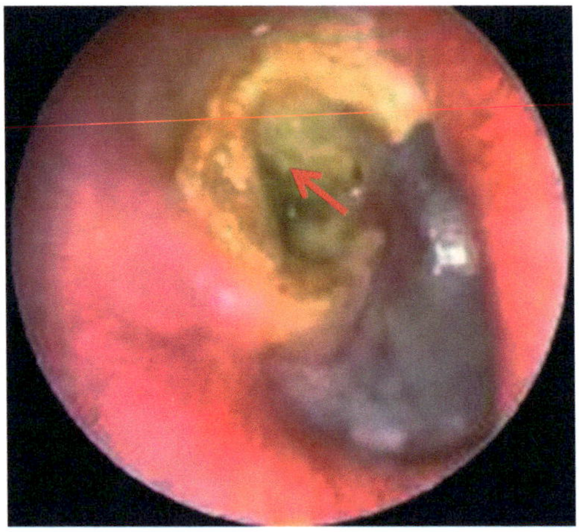

**Fig. 8.21** Middle ear cholesteatoma endoscopy

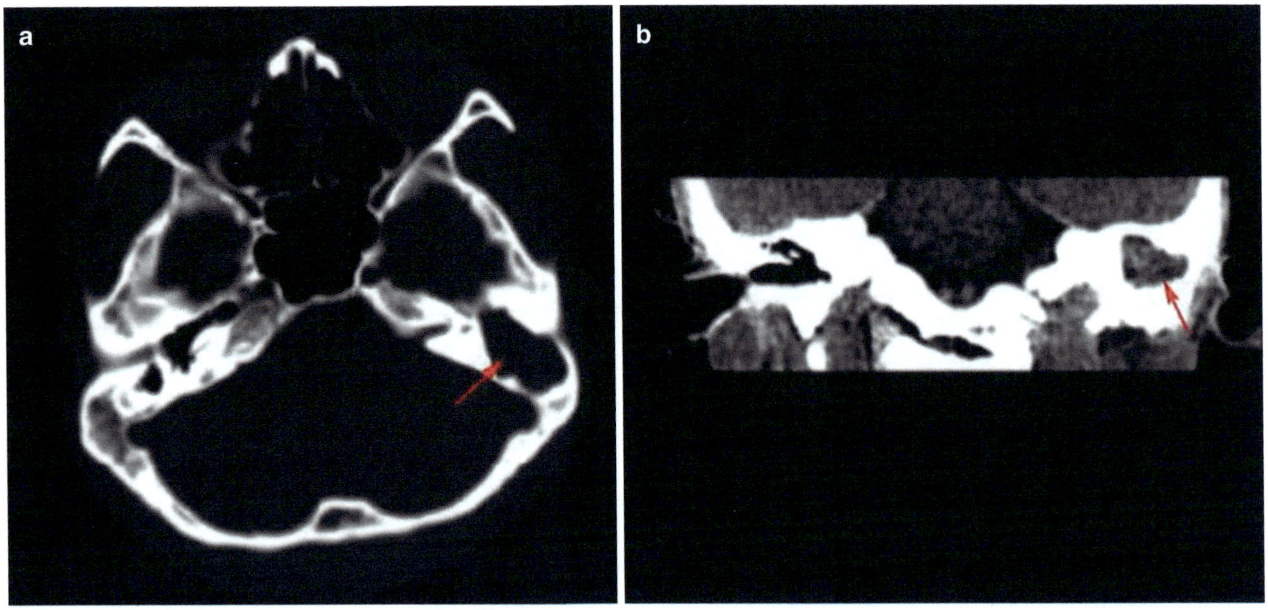


**Fig. 8.22** Left mastoid cholesteatoma's temporal CT scan manifestation. (**a**) Bone window axis. (**b**) Soft tissue window coronary reconstruction. Left mastoid is sclerosis type, where left mastoid sinus and aditus extend and large sclerotin damage zone could be seen, within soft tissue density shadow stuff (arrow) and its peripheral sclerotin has hyperplasia sclerosis

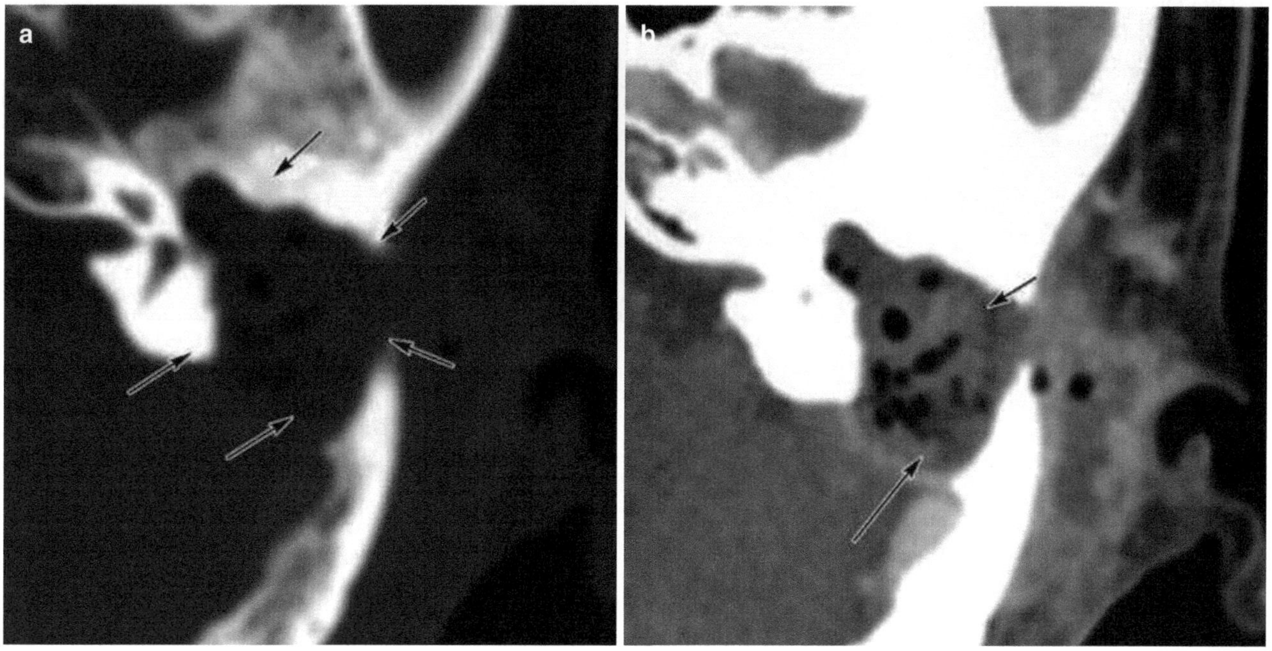


**Fig. 8.23** Temporal axis CT plain scan imaging manifest large cholesteatoma. (**a**) Bone window says left mastoid sinus enlarges, sinus wall sclerotin damage and sclerotin hyperplasia sclerosis (arrow); (**b**) enhanced scanning says non-enhance mastoid intra-sinus soft tissues, sinus cavity and its adjacent soft tissues communicate and constitute a sinus canal (short arrow),internal wall sclerotin damage and involved endo-cranium (long arrow)

pletely removed, ossicular chain reconstruction and tympanoplasty can be performed as appropriate to preserve or improve hearing.

### 8.4.5 Sequelae of Otitis Media

1. Atensive/Adhesive Otitis Media;
2. Tympanosclerosis;
3. Cholesterol granuloma of the middle ear;
4. Occult otitis media.

## 8.5 Otosclerosis

**Clinical Manifestation**

1. Hearing loss

   There is no cause for gradual hearing loss in both ears. Hearing loss is slow and gradually aggravated. Excessive fatigue, excessive tobacco and alcohol, and after pregnancy and childbirth can cause hearing loss significantly aggravated. Affect patients' social activities.
2. Tinnitus

   Tinnitus intermittent or persistent bass tinnitus. Most occur simultaneously with deafness.
3. Willis mishearing

   It is better for the patient to have a better hearing in the noisy environment than in the quiet environment. This phenomenon is called Willis's wrong listening or Willis's auditory perversion.
4. Vertigo

   A few patients experienced mild transient vertigo after head movement.

**Examination**

1. Signs

   The outer ear canal is more spacious, the tympanic membrane is normal, and the activity is good. Sometimes, at upper quadrant of tympanic membrane, a red area is seen, which is the manifestation of hyperemia of the promontory mucosa. This phenomenon is called Schwartz sign, which is one of the characteristics of clinical otosclerosis.
2. Audiometry
   (a) Tuning fork test RT 256 Hz negative, 512 Hz positive showed early hearing damage; 256 Hz and 512 Hz were negative, suggesting that hearing damage aggravated. Gelle test, a test of the mobility of the ossicles, is negative.
   (b) Pure tone audiometry Bone conduction hearing curve is V shape under 1000 Hz or 2000 Hz region decreased said Kaladze notch, suggesting that the stapes floor be fixed, will be eliminated after a successful operation.

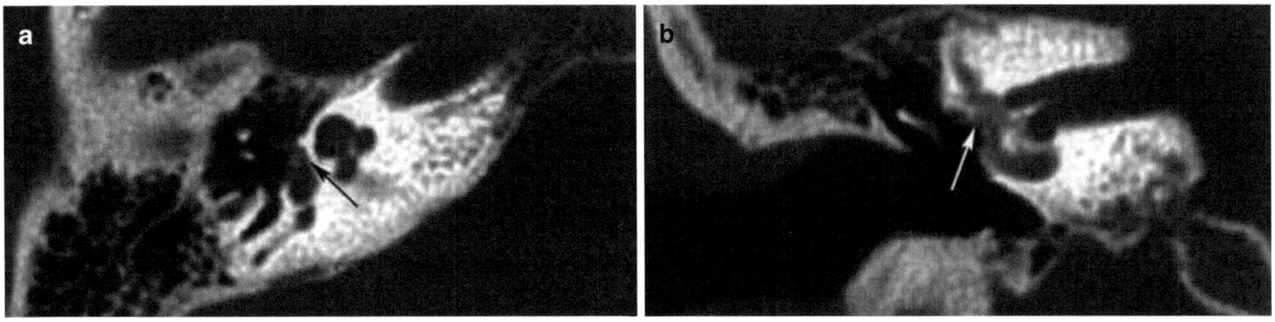


**Fig. 8.24** Otic sclerosis HRCT imaging. (**a**) Axis imaging, manifestation thickened stapes basal plate (arrow); (**b**) Coronary reconstruction imaging, manifesting bone labyrinth sclerotin absorption, density reduction and point calcified lesion (arrow)

(c) Acoustic impedance test: The tympanic curve showed A type, As type or biphasic curve, and the reflex threshold of stapes muscle increased or disappeared.
(d) Auditory brainstem response test: I wave and V wave latency prolongation or threshold increases.

3. Imaging examination

Temporal bone X-ray showed no lesions at middle ear and mastoid. High resolution spiral CT scanning of the temporal bone revealed thickened stapes floor, and sclerosis of the vestibular window, cochlear window, bony labyrinth and inner ear tract as Fig. 8.24.

**Treatment**

1. Surgical method: Stapes surgery and inner ear fenestration were selected according to the condition. Stapes surgery includes stapes swing and stapes resection. Fenestration of stapes floor and implantation of artificial auditory ossicles. Stapedectomy can use hand drill, drill and laser.
2. Medical therapy: Sodium fluoride therapy and chondroitin sulfate therapy.
3. Hearing aids can be selected for those who are not suitable for or unwilling to undergo surgery, and cochlear implants can be performed for those with severe bilateral deafness.

## 8.6 Disease of Facial Nerve

### 8.6.1 Facial Nerve Anatomy

1. Facial nerve composition

Facial nerve is composed of motor nerve, parasympathetic nerve, taste fiber and sensory nerve fiber.

(a) The motor nerve originates from the motor nucleus at the lower part of the pons, and innervates all facial expression muscles except the levator palpebrae superioris, buccal and stylohyoid muscles of stapes.
(b) Parasympathetic nerve originates from the superior salivary nucleus and distributes in lacrimal gland, submandibular gland and sublingual gland respectively through the sphenopalatine ganglion and the mandibular ganglion.
(c) The gustatory fibers mainly connect the anterior 2/3 gustatory receptors of the tongue and pass through the genicular ganglion to the nucleus tractus solitarius.
(d) The sensory fibers are mainly the skin sensation of the auricle and part of the external auditory canal.

2. The course of facial nerve

According to route of facial nerve motor nerve fibers, courses can be divided into the following sections.

(a) Superior nuclear segment: It originates from facial nerve center at cerebral cortex and descends towards facial nerve motor neuclei.
(b) Nuclear segment: It is course of facial nerve in pons.
(c) Cerebellopontine angle segment: It is the segment from subpons edge to inner ear aditus.
(d) Inner ear canal segments: It is the segment from inner ear aditus to inner ear canal basement.
(e) Labyrinthine segment: It is the segment from inner ear canal basement to geniculate ganglion.
(f) Tympanic segment: It is the course at tympanic inner membrane, from geniculate ganglion to pyramidal eminence. It divides into greater superior petrosal nerve which ends at lacrimal gland.
(g) Mastoid segment: It is the segment from pyramidal eminence to stylomastoid foramen, during which it divides stapes muscle and tympanic chord nerve.
(h) External temporal segment: It is the segment which ends at pathetic muscle through parotid gland after crossing stylomastoid foramen.

### 8.6.2 Diagnosis of Peripheral Facial Paralysis

Peripheral facial paralysis is caused by facial nerve nucleus or lesions below the nucleus.

**Clinical Manifestation**

The main manifestations are facial muscle disorders of voluntary movement, including the disappearance of frontal lines, inability to frown, raise eyebrows, incomplete closure of eyes, shallow nasolabial sulcus, droop and tilt to the opposite side, more obvious when speaking and showing teeth, leakage of breath when whistling, and easy outflow along the mouth corner when drinking water. There may be a loss of taste, tear or saliva secretion. The face is stiff and expressionless when facial paralysis is complete on both sides.

Etiological diagnosis:

1. The causes of peripheral facial paralysis can be preliminarily understood by detailed inquiry and medical history collection. These causes include congenital facial nerve deformities, bacterial and viral infections such as otitis media, herpes zoster, temporal bone fractures caused by trauma, and facial neuritis.
2. Physical examination

   Detailed physical examinations, including static and motor examinations, otolaryngology and nervous system examinations, and general examinations. Examination can provide valuable clues for diagnosis. House-Brackmann classification is usually used to assess the degree of facial paralysis (Table 8.4).
3. Imaging examination

   CT, MRI and ultrasonography.
4. Localization diagnosis
   (a) Lacrimal gland secretion test
   (b) Stapes reflex
   (c) Taste test
   (d) Saliva secretion test
5. Electrophysiological diagnosis
   (a) Electromyography
   (b) Nerve electrogram
   (c) Nerve excitability test

### 8.6.3 Common Peripheral Facial Paralyses

1. Bell's Palsy

   Bell's palsy is an acute peripheral facial paralysis of unknown origin, also known as idiopathic facial paralysis. It can occur at any age, but more people are 20–40 years old.

   The exact cause is unknown, but it may be related to ischemia caused by vasospasm, viral infectious immune response, heredity and other factors. The clinical manifestations were sudden and rapidly aggravated peripheral complete or incomplete facial paralysis. There may be a history of cold wind or viral infection. Early stage may be accompanied by side ear or subauricular pain, a small number of facial and tongue numbness, facial tactile abnormalities. The mastoid process may have tenderness, the posterior part of the tympanic membrane may have slight congestion, but it will disappear in a few days. To diagnose this disease, other diseases causing peripheral facial paralysis should be excluded.

   Treatment is divided into non-surgical treatment and surgical treatment. Non-surgical treatments include glucocorticoids, vasodilators, vitamins, physiotherapy, acupuncture and moxibustion, etc. Pay attention to cornea protection. Surgical treatment is mainly facial nerve decompression, but its indications, timing and scope of decompression are still controversial.
2. Auricular herpes zoster

   Herpes zoster virus infection of facial nerve induced peripheral facial paralysis, also known as Hunt syndrome, was reported by Ramsay hunt for the first time in 1910. The clinical feature is ear herpes accompanied by peripheral facial paralysis. First, common in the early stage of severe earache, the hyperemia, cluster appeared herpes conchae and around after herpes broken exudate (Fig. 8.25). Peripheral facial paralysis occurs later, can be incomplete facial paralysis, severe cases can be complete

**Table 8.4** House- Brakeman facial nerve functional recovery assessment criteria

| Damage degree | Level | Definition |
|---|---|---|
| Normal | I | Bilateral symmetry, normal function of each district |
| Mild facial paralysis (just perceptible) | II | Slight facial nerve movement inability, complete eye closure under slight force. Slight facial asymmetry while strongly smiling, slight synkinesis, no facial spasm |
| Moderate facial paralysis (significant difference) | III | Obvious inability of facial nerve movement, no facial appearance loss, possible eyebow raisement disability, complete eye closure while under force, powerful mouth movement while forcing but asymmetric, obvious synkinesis and spasm |
| Moderate and severe dysfunction | IV | Obviously inable facial muscle movement, appearance loss, eyebow raisement disability, unable to completely close eyes even while under force, asymmetric mouth movement, obvious synkinesis and spasm |
| Severe facial paralysis | V | Slight facial movement, palpebral closure disability, only slight quarrel movement at mouth corner, synkinesis and spasm disappeared |
| Complete facial paralysis | VI | Facial muscle movement disability, tension loss, no synkinesis, no spasm |

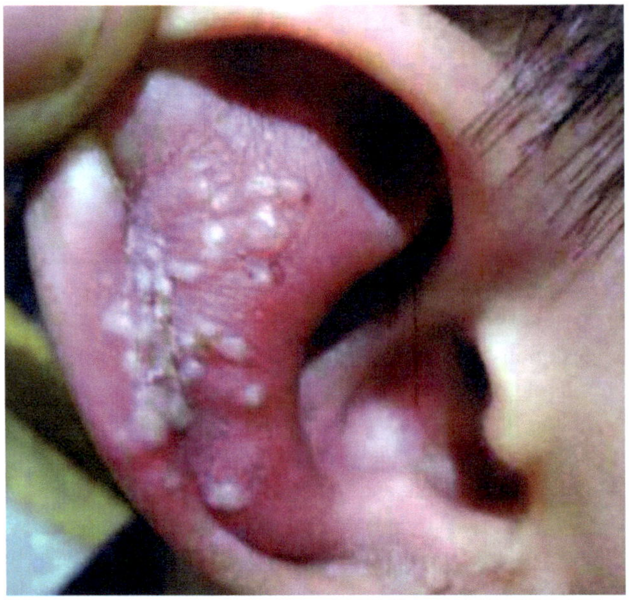

Fig. 8.25 Auricular herps zoster

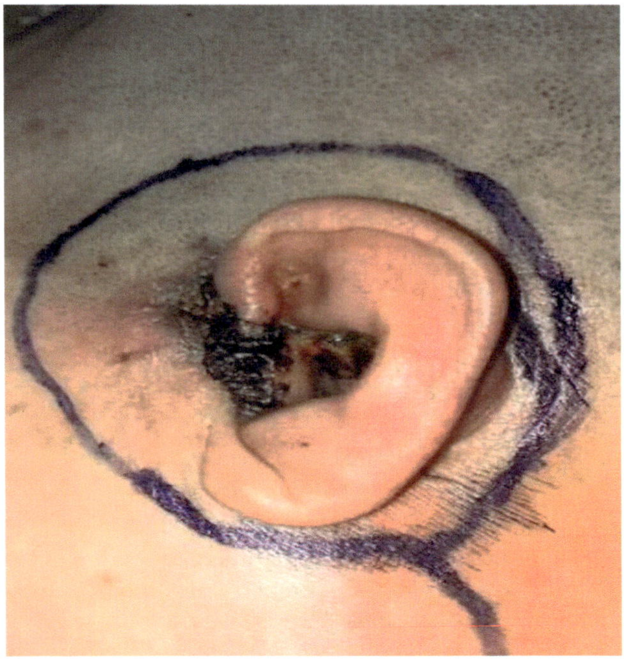

Fig. 8.26 Basal cell carcinoma of external ear

facial paralysis. If the virus invaded the cochlear nerve, vestibular nerve, trigeminal nerve, can appear ear, deafness, tinnitus, vertigo, facial pain. Other patients may have other neurological symptoms and signs. The therapy principle is similar to Bell facial paralysis.

## 8.7 Malignant Tumor of Temporal Bone

**Temporal Bone Malignant Tumors**

It accounts for 1/5000–1/20,000 of otological cases, and squamous cell carcinoma (SCC) is the most common. Squamous cell carcinoma accounted for 60–80% of the external auditory canal, middle ear and mastoid process, followed by adenocarcinoma, cystadenocarcinoma and basal cell carcinoma (Fig. 8.26), and melanoma was rare (Moffat et al.) summarized six histological types of squamous cell carcinoma: highly differentiated, moderately differentiated, poorly differentiated, clear cell morphology, spindle and verrucous squamous cell carcinoma. The incidence of squamous cell carcinoma of the temporal bone is 1/1,000,000,000–6/1,000,000,000, of which 60–70% occur in the auricle, 20–30% in the external auditory canal, and 10% in the middle ear and mastoid process. Age is more than 50–60 years old, there is no gender difference. The vast majority of auricles are basal cell carcinomas. The following is limited to squamous cell carcinoma of the temporal bone.

**Etiology**

The main cause is exposure to ultraviolet or excessive radiation, such as radiotherapy for nasopharyngeal carcinoma, especially in people with delicate skin. In 18 cases of temporal bone tumors, 39% (7/18) were radiation-related tumors (after radiotherapy for nasopharyngeal carcinoma): 5 squamous cell carcinomas and 2 sarcomas. For uncovered sites, such as squamous cell carcinoma of the external auditory canal, it may be related to genes. In addition, the correlation between chemical agents, such as chlorine-containing disinfectants, has also been reported. Chronic suppurative otitis media mentioned in previous literature is a significant pathogenic factor, which has not been confirmed yet. Most middle ear cancers with chronic otitis media are infected by human papillomavirus (HPV). About 50% of patients had a long history of otorrhea before using antibiotics.

**Clinical Manifestations**

The first symptoms are mostly otorrhea, and intraauricular hemorrhage or hemorrhagic secretions are more common. Hearing loss is conductive in the early stage. Tumors can invadc along bone walls or existing vascular and nerve pathways, and cochlear damage can lead to sensorineural deafness. With the growth of tumors, there are earache, dizziness and facial paralysis. Diffusion from the external auditory canal to the temporomandibular joint, parotid gland or directly through the weak external auditory canal bone wall, petrous scales bone suture or cartilage notch of the external auditory canal invaded the infratemporal fossa, causing difficulty in opening the mouth, external auditory canal, preauricular mass, etc. (Fig. 8.27); invasion of the fifth, sixth, fifth, eighth, nineteenth, eighth, eighth, eighth, eighth, fifth, fifth, fifth, fifth and fifth cranial nerves could cause corresponding

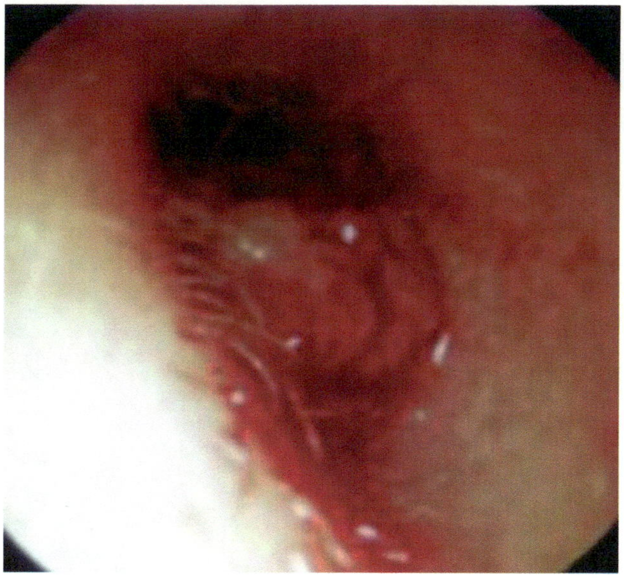

**Fig. 8.27** Soft tissue mass with slight enhancement in the left external auditory canal

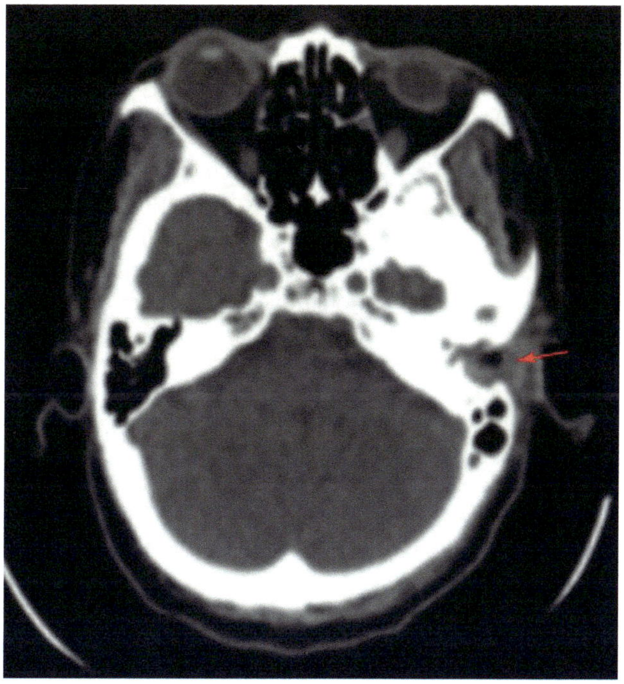

**Fig. 8.28** Axis CT of temporal bone demonstrates carcinoma of the left auditory meatus (arrow), with slight bone destruction of the external auditory

symptoms; invasion of the jugular foramen, causing internal Jugular Artery massive hemorrhage of the internal carotid artery; attacks the tympanic cap, dura mater and temporal lobe upwards, causing headache and meningitis. Late stage may have cervical lymph node enlargement and distant metastasis (Fig. 8.28).

**Surgery and Reconstruction**

1. Surgical methods for temporal bone cancer are limited T1 stage of external auditory canal, especially for the posterior wall of external auditory canal, which can be resected sleeve-like. Previously, the tumors were resected completely together with the skin of external auditory canal, but now they are only between simple tumor resection and extended partial temporal bone resection (LTBR).
   (a) Lesions confined to the external auditory canal: Most skull base surgeons advocate LTBR for patients with stage T1 and T2 who refuse or cannot be enlarged for medical reasons: removal of cartilage and bone of the external auditory canal, tympanic membrane and malleolus, incus, and other adjacent tissues. Surgical procedure: The external auditory canal was closed into a dead space and mastoidectomy was performed to enlarge the facial nerve recess. The upper tympanic cavity was enlarged as far as possible. The tympanic bone was ground down to the tympanic ring. The temporomandibular joint was dissected from the Tragus Cartilage and the anterior external auditory canal bone. The anvil-stapes joint was separated and the whole cylindrical tissue was removed. The operation can enlarge the superficial parotid gland, temporomandibular joint and condyle. LTBR is more conducive to complete resection of tumors than conventional mastoidectomy. Many studies have shown that the survival rate of routine mastoidectomy plus post-operative radiotherapy is similar to that of LTBR (Fig. 8.29).
2. Tumors beyond the external auditory canal: tumors originating from the middle ear and mastoid process, regardless of their size, belong to stage T3 or T4. They should be treated as follows: (1) small patch resection; (2) subtotal temporal bone resection (STBR); (3) total temporal bone resection (TTBR), also known as extended temporal bone resection.

1. *TTBR procedure:*

   These involve a complete removal of external auditory meatus, auricle and surrounding skin. Parotid gland, facial nerve, ascending ramus of mandible, zygomatic arch, temporomandibular joint, pterygoid muscle and foramen ovale were resected to protect trigeminal nerve. The internal carotid artery and the external carotid artery were separated in the upper neck. The internal carotid artery was completely resected with the cerebral nerves (IX, X, XI) and the medial jugular vein. The posterior vertebral artery was separated from the communicating branch of the neck 1 and the deep side of the carotid muscle to remove the stylomastoid foramen and expose the carotid artery into the cranial orifice. The middle cranial

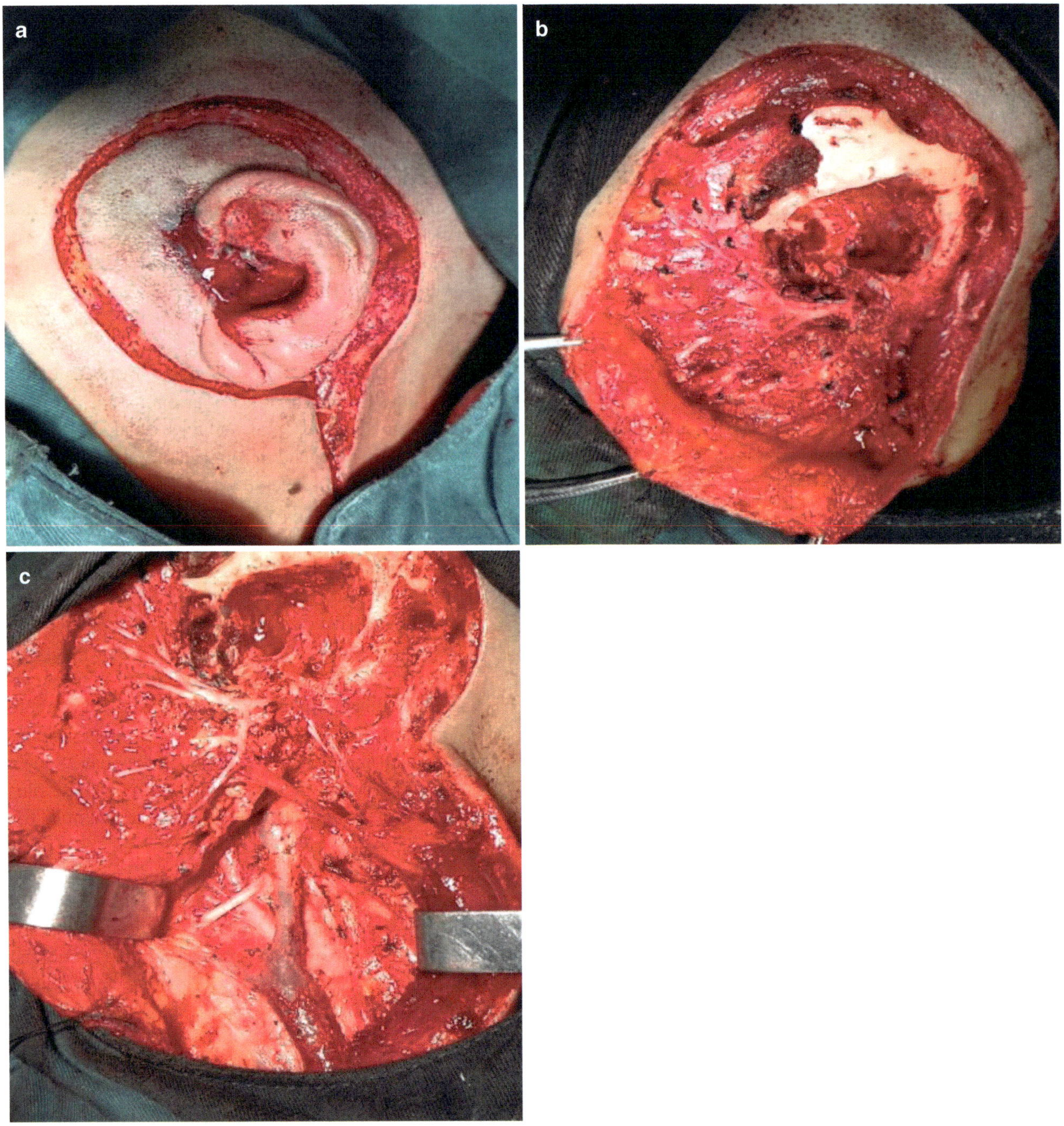

**Fig. 8.29** (**a**) Total auriculectomy. (**b**) Superfical parotidectomy and Lateral temporal bone resection. (**c**) Neck dissection

fossa was resected to expose the trigeminal nerve and the carotid artery in the petrous region. The dura mater of the middle cranial fossa and the transverse sinus were ligated behind the sigmoid sinus. The clival bone adjacent to the petrous apex and the carotid artery canal was resected forward. Carotid artery was excised and transplanted. Suboccipital incision was performed to direct the jugular bulb and foramen magnum. The dura mater was resected backward to sigmoid sinus, through communicating sinus to tentorium cerebellum, and forward to superior petrosal sinus. In the sacrificial group, 6 cranial nerves were removed to release the temporal bone. If the extent of resection is large, it must be carefully separated and resected layer by layer, especially in occipital condyle, clivus, carotid artery or cavernous sinus. Note that basal venous plexus hemorrhage is more frequent.

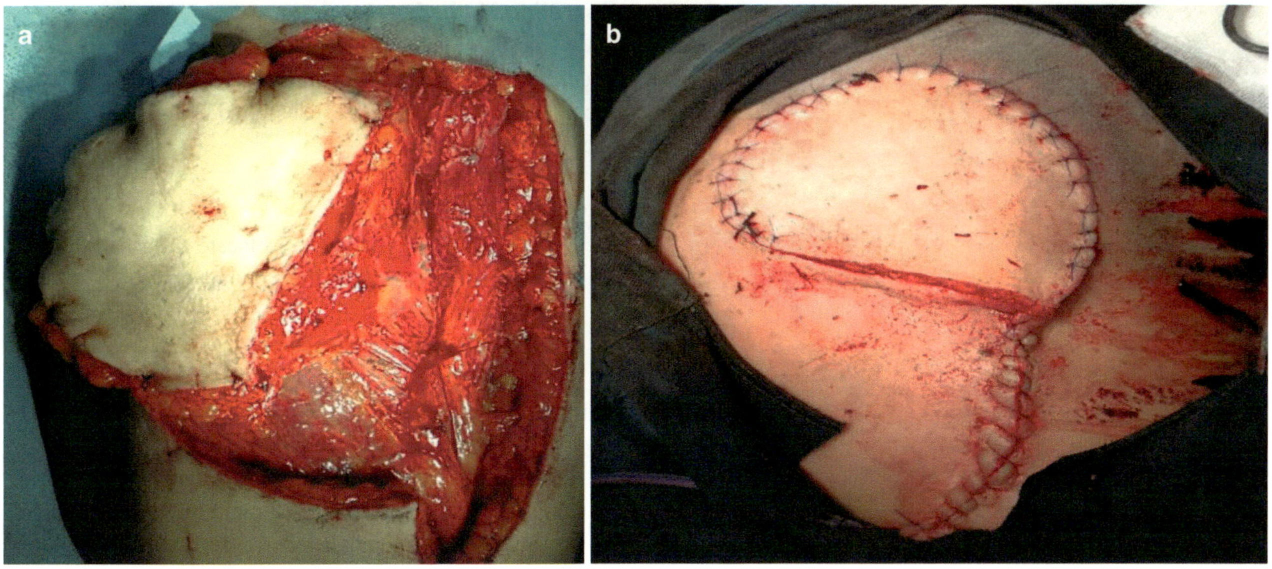


**Fig. 8.30** (**a**) Anterolateral thigh (ALT) flap. (**b**) Defect following reconstruction with an anterolateral thigh (ALT) flap

2. *Reconstruction*

   Mostly local musculocutaneous flaps, such as temporalis, trapezius, pectoralis or platysma cervicalis, were mostly used for reconstruction, and the surface was covered with skin or subcutaneous mucosal grafts. Temporal myocutaneous flaps are the most commonly used. It is believed that microvascular flaps can repair large meningeal defects or carotid artery exposure. The dura mater can be repaired with artificial meninges or fascia lata. Nerve transplantation can reconstruct facial nerve or other brain nerves, such as nerve pairs IX and IX. Some scholars believe that hypoglossal nerve should not be used to repair facial nerve, because the loss of hypoglossal nerve function will aggravate the loss of glossopharyngeal nerve and vagus nerve symptoms (Fig. 8.30).

## 8.8 Implantable Artificial Hearing Device

With the rapid development of a multidisciplinary clinical audiology, ear microsurgery technology, bio electronic technology and biomedical engineering technology, a variety of artificial implantable hearing device constantly available, has been widely used in clinical therapy for hearing loss, different types and different degrees of loss of patients. Implantable artificial hearing device comprises a semi implantable bone anchored hearing aid (BAHA), vibrant implantable Sound bridge (VSB), cochlear implant (CI), bone bridge, auditory brainstem implant (ABI) and auditory midbrain implant system implant (AMI), etc.

### 8.8.1 Bone Anchored Hearing Aids

Bone anchored hearing aid (BAHA) is a semi-implantable hearing device through bone conduction mode, which is constituted with the fixture, the titanium abutment and sound processor, among which the sound processor receives and amplifies the sound and converted to sound vibration the base and the titanium implant, and the bone conduction sound vibration directly to the cochlea, the inner ear and the auditory nerve auditory stimuli produced (Figs. 8.31 and 8.32). For patients with unilateral sensorineural hearing loss, BAHA is used to transfer the sound from the affected side to the contralateral cochlea, which can reduce the negative effect of the head shadow effect. It can expand the sound field and improve the speech recognition and comprehension ability of the patients in the noisy environment.

**Indications**

Patients with unilateral or bilateral conductive or mixed hearing loss due to various causes have partial hearing loss, expect to improve language communication ability, unable or unwilling to choose hearing reconstruction surgery, and unwilling or unable to wear ear canal hearing aids. Patients with unilateral sensorineural hearing loss due to various reasons are unwilling or unable to wear ear canal hearing aids. Children should be about 3 years old and have sufficient thickness of the skull to implant titanium screws, young people can wear BAHA soft band (BAHA soft land) first.

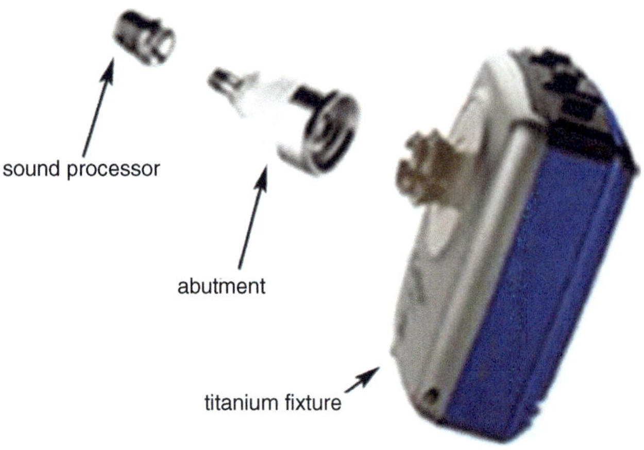


**Fig. 8.31** BAHA structural diagram

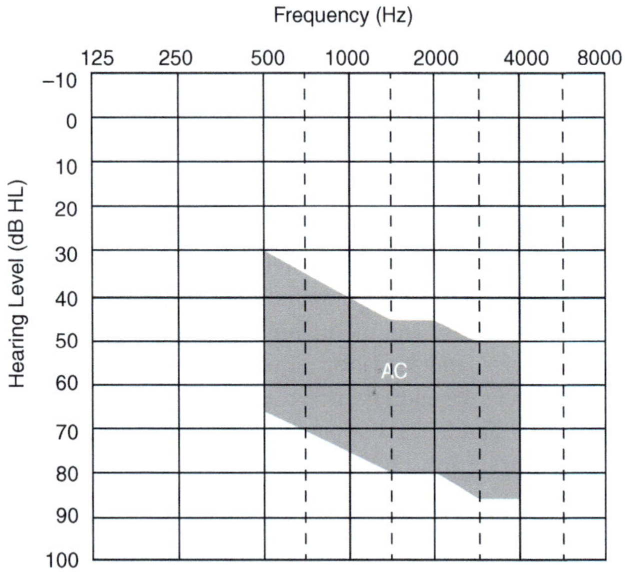


**Fig. 8.32** VSB implant sensorineural deafness gas-conductive threshold range

**Contraindication**

1. Skull thickness is not enough or the bone soft, prone to implant instability.
2. Patients with posterior cochlear lesions.
3. Persons with severe mental retardation.
4. Patients with severe mental illness.
5. Poor overall condition, cannot tolerate surgery.

The relative contraindications of BAHA implantation include osteogenesis imperfecta, Paget's disease, severe osteoporosis, etc.

**Operation Methods**

BAHA implantation can be performed under local anesthesia or general anesthesia, with simple operation and high safety. It can be completed in two phases, and can be completed in one phase.

1. One-stage operation
   (a) the BAHA model is use to locate the insertion point behind the ear, from the mastoid bone region at the midpoint of the external ear canal 5.0~5.5 cm. A U shaped flap with a diameter of about 2.5 cm is placed in front of the pedicle to expose the mastoid periosteum.
   (b) drill a deep 3~4 mm round hole and screw in the titanium screw.
   (c) reposition the flap and suture the incision.
   (d) after 3~4 months (about 6 months), titanium screws and bone tissue achieved good osseointegration and undergo the next stage operation.
2. Two-stage operation
   (a) Place the flap along the original incision and remove the subcutaneous tissue around the screw
   (b) drill a round hole on the top of the screw with a disposable drill.
   (c) the base is fixed to the screw by this hole.
   (d) reduction flap.
   (e) The patients were followed up for 6 weeks. After the local healing, the sound processor was installed on the base.

**Complication**

The most common complications are skin and soft tissue infections. Patients with diabetes, immune suppression or long-term immunosuppressive drugs often require a longer bone fusion time, and the incidence of wound infection is relatively high.

### 8.8.2 Vibriant Acoustic Bridge

The Vibrant Sound Bridge (VSB) is a kind of artificial semi implantable middle ear hearing device developed according to the principle of electromagnetic induction. It was manufactured by MED-EL company in Austria. It won the European CE, American FDA and China food and Drug Administration certification respectively. At present used in many hospitals to carry out surgical implantation of VSB. Its biggest advantage that it does not destroy the normal anatomic structure of the middle ear, and retain the integrity of ossicular chain. VSB consists of two parts: audio processor (AP) and vibrant ossicular reconstructive prosthesis (VORP). Floating MS transducer (FMT) can be surgically fixed to the ossicular chain, cochlear window or vestibular window.

**Indication**

1. In patients with moderate or severe sensorineural hearing loss, the threshold of air conduction is within the shadow range at Fig. 8.32. The effect of traditional hearing aid is not satisfied or unwilling to wear hearing aids, and the whole frequency hearing loss is higher than that of low frequency.
2. Mild, moderate or severe conductive deafness or mixed hearing loss in adults, including the etiology of otosclerosis, chronic suppurative otitis media (including middle ear cholesteatoma), congenital external ear atresia, congenital middle ear deformity and other bone conduction threshold in the shadow range at Fig. 8.33.
3. Air bone gap less than 10 dB, some scholars' think that can be less than 15 dB.
4. Speech recognition rate is above 50%.
5. The past 2 years the hearing fluctuation is less than or equal to 15 dB.
6. There is no abnormality in the skin of the implant site.
7. Normal developments, normal brain function, the correct expectations.

**Contraindication**

1. Posterior cochlear deafness or central hearing loss.
2. Active period of middle ear infection.
3. Chronic effusion of the middle ear.
4. Perforation of tympanic membrane with repeated infection of middle ear and high expectation value.

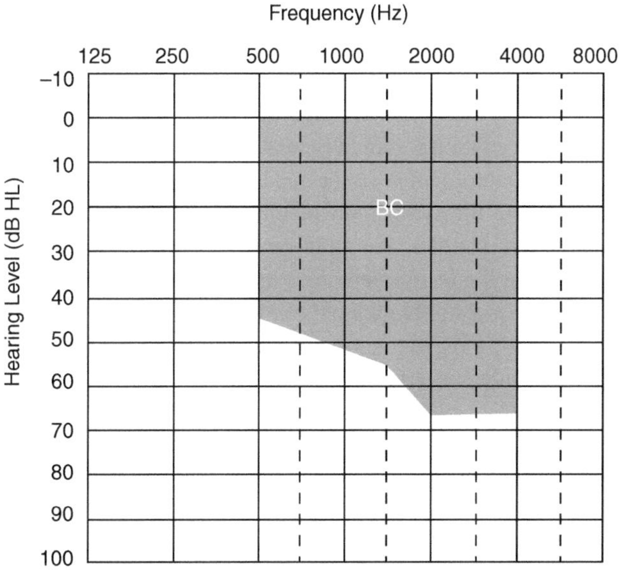


**Fig. 8.33** VSB implant conductive or mixed deafness bone-conductive threshold range

**Surgical Method**

The surgical approach using postauricular incision, can use S or C shaped incision for mastoidectomy, the facial recess opened in the ear tympanic, skull surface implant bed receiving coil and the modem, and then by the facial recess into the wire and MT in the middle ear cavity through small titanium clips on FMT FMT will be fixed in the long process of incus, or directly to the package of FMT fascia placed vertically in the round window membrane in vitro auditory processor in the ear and the corresponding position of the receiving coil. The posterior ear incision can also be applied for VSB implantation through the external ear canal approach.

**Complication**

VSB implantation may occur under the scalp hematoma, wound healing, facial nerve, chorda tympani nerve, ossicular chain (long limb of incus necrosis) or inner ear damage, cause taste changes, facial paralysis, hearing loss was not significantly improved or aggravated, tinnitus, vertigo, labyrinthitis, very small due to device failure again operation. SB implantation is not recommended for MRI examination at present.

### 8.8.3 Cochlear Implant

Cochlear implant (CI) is a biomedical device that helps hearing impaired people engineering their hearing and speech communication skills. This Engineering device has been used in clinic since 1970, and has a history of more than 40 years. With the development of related science and technology, products are constantly updated and replaced. The number of electrodes ranges from single-conductor to 24-conductor. The types of electrodes are straight, curved, soft and ultra-soft. Speech processing technology is constantly upgrading. At present, hundreds of thousands of people around the world have received CI implantation and benefited from it. In 2003, China first formulated the Guidelines for Cochlear Implantation. In 2006 and 2013, the Guidelines were revised comprehensively to provide guidance for clinicians, hearing and speech rehabilitation workers, and to further standardize cochlear implantation in China and improve overall treatment.

**Indication**

Patient selection criteria: cochlear implants are mainly used for the therapy of severe or profound sensorineural hearing loss.

1. Selection criteria for patients with pre-lingual deafness
   (a) implantation age is usually 12 months ~6 years old. The younger the implantation age, the better the effect.

(b) If 3-6 months wearing of hearing aids does not effect, Children with severe or profound hearingloss at both ears should be considered to take direct cochlear implantation.
(c) No operative contraindication.
(d) The guardians and (or) implanted patients have the correct understanding and proper expectation of cochlear implantation.
(e) they have the condition of hearing and speech rehabilitation education.

2. Selection criteria for patients with postlingual deafness
   (a) Postlingual deafness patients of all ages.
   (b) Biaural severe or profound sensorineural hearing loss, relying on hearing aids can not carry out normal auditory and speech communication.
   (c) No operative contraindication.
   (d) The implanter himself and/or his guardian have a correct understanding of cochlear implantation and appropriate expectations.
   [Contraindication]
   - Absolute contraindication
     Severe deformities of the inner ear, such as Michel deformity cochlear deformity, absence or interruption of the auditory nerve, acute suppurative inflammation of the middle ear and mastoid.
   - Relative contraindication
     Frequent seizures can not be controlled; severe mental, intellectual, behavioral and psychological disorders, can not match the hearing and speech training.

Guidelines for the clinical practice of cochlear implantation in special conditions.

1. White matter lesions
   If white matter lesions is shown on MRI, intelligence, neurological signs and MRI should be reviewed. If there is no setback of mental and motor development, no deformity of outer hearing and speech system, no positive pyramidal signs or signs of change at neurological examination, but only high signal lesion at cerebral white matter on MRI (like DWI), observe inspections above with the interval of 6 months. If the high signal lesion does not expand on MRI, cochlear implantation could be considered.
2. Auditory neuropathy (auditory neuropathy spectrum disorder)
   It is a kind of special sensorineural hearing loss, which is caused by the dysfunction of inner hair cells, auditory nerve synapses and (or) auditory nerve itself. Audiology has its typical characteristics, manifestations of otoacoustic emission (OAE) and (or) cochlear micro phonics (CM) and normal auditory brain response (ABR) thousands of missing or severely abnormal. At present, cochlear implant is effective for most patients with auditory neuropathy, but it may be ineffective or ineffective for some patients, and the patient and/or guardian risk must be informed before the operation.
3. Bilateral cochlear implantation
   Bilateral implantation can improve the acoustic source localization, speech understanding under quiet and background noise, and help to obtain more natural sound perception, and promote the development of hearing, speech and music appreciation ability. Bilateral simultaneous implantation or sequential implantation can be selected, and two times of sequential implantation, the shorter the operation interval, and the more conducive to postoperative speech rehabilitation.
4. Cochlear implantation for residual hearing
   Patients with residual hearing loss, especially those with high frequency hearing loss, are suitable for electrode implantation with residual hearing preservation. Postoperative acoustic and electrical stimulation mode can be selected, but the risk of loss or loss of residual hearing in patients and/or guardians should be told before the operation.
5. Artificial cochlea implantation in the abnormal-inner-ear-structure
   Abnormal inner ear structure related to artificial cochlea implanting includes common cavity deformity, undeveloped cochlea, ossified cochlea, cochlea stenosis, etc. The artificial cochlea could be applied to most of the patients with any symptoms above. Organize the preoperative case discussion, handle cautiously during surgery and it is suggested to monitor facial nerve. There will be difference at personal effect after surgery.
6. Artificial cochlea implantation in the chronic-otitis-media accompanying with tympanic membrane tresses.
   If the inflammation is under control, the patients should be offered one-stage or phased operation. One-stage operation is radically treating the lesion (or mastoid cavity autologous tissue padding or the ankylotia), repairing the tympanum membrane and implanting the artificial cochlea simultaneously; phased operation is clearing the lesion, repairing the cavum tympanic membrane tresses or blocking the external ear canal firstly and implanting the artificial cochlea about 3–6 months after the former surgery.

**Pre-operation Evaluation**

1. Medical history taking
   Knowing the etiologic agents by asking the medical history. The point of ear medical history should be on the etiology and process of hearing loss, which could be concluded from the history of the audition, titinus and dizziness, the ototoxicity drug exposure, noise exposure,

systemic acute and chronic inflammation, past otology medicine, family hearing loss, wearing hearing aid, development factors (systemic or local developmental deformity, intelligence development, etc) and other pathogenesis (epilepsy, mental condition, etc.) and to the hearing-loss infants, there should also be the history of the maternal fetation, the parturition, the infant growth, and speech growth. Besides, to all the patients, the doctors should ask about the speech-language ability (lamprophonia, understanding ability, presentation ability, etc) and desire to improve communicating.

2. Systemic or ear examinations

   It includes systemic examination, the examination of the auricular, the external ear canal, the cavum tympanumic membrane, etc.

3. Audition and vestibular function examination

   (a) exam items

   - Pure tone audiometry

     It includes the threshold value of the air and bone conduction. The infants under 6 years old could be applied the behavioral audiometry, including observing, visual reinforcement audiometry and play audiometry.

   - Acoustic immittance

     It includes the cavum tympanum imaging and the stapes muscle reflex.

   - Auditory evoked potential:

     It includes the ABR, 40 Hz, audition event related potential or auditory steady-state response (ASSR) and cochlear micro phonics exam.

   - oto acoustic emission (OAE)

     Do oto acoustic emission or temporary evoked oto acoustic emission (TEOAE) to the deformity.

   - Speech audiometry

     It can be divided into speech recognition rate test and speech recognition threshold test. Choose the accurate speech test material, open and (or) closed type (Appendix A).

   - Aided effect evaluation

     Aided audition threshold test and (or) speech recognition test after optimization match.

   - Auricular function exam (patients with the dizziness history and able to cooperate)
   - Bone promontory stimulation test (if necessary)

   (b) audition inclusion criteria

   - The pre-lingually deafened

     It's needed to do both the subjective and objective comprehensive audition evaluation.

     – objective auditory assess: click ABR reaction threshold >90 dB nHL, 40 Hz audition event-related potential reaction threshold (under 1000 Hz) > 100 dB HL. Audition steady-state response threshold (not less than 2000 Hz frequency) > 90 dB nHL; f ailed at oto acoustic emission of both ears (except for the neurotic)

     – subjective auditory assess: average threshold of single ear's behavioral audiometry>80 dB HL, aided audition threshold (over 2000 Hz frequency) > 50 dB HL; aided speech recognition rate (closed type disyllable) ≤70%, conclude that the patients can't cooperate can't get benefit from the hearing aid.

   - the post-lingually deafened

     Patients with average auditory threshold of ears' pure tone air conduction over 80 dB HL has profound hearing loss; patients have severe hearing loss if the open-phrase recognition rate of its good-hearing ear is less than 70%.

     Remnant audition: patients with good audition to the low frequency, whose audition threshold over 2000 Hz >80 dB HL and communication hearing-aid cannot help, could be implanted the artificial cochlea; To the patients whose remnant audition cannot be detected, it should be informed of to the patients themselves or their guardians that the bad hearing restoration risk after surgery.

4. Imaging evaluation

   As regular, CT scan the thin layer of the temporal, do the inner ear MRI and the skull MRI, 3-dimensionally reconstruct cochlea if necessary.

**Operation-Related Request**

1. Request to the physicians

   The physicians should have abundant middle-ear-mastoid microsurgery experience, been professionally and systemically trained at artificial cochlea operation and done 20 artificial cochlea implantation cases personally under guidance of experienced physicians at least.

2. Request to the operation room and basic equipment

   The room should be in good asepsis condition and contain the operating microscope, otology drill and relevant device.

3. Pre operative preparation

   Preoperative conversation should be done by the operation doctor and the audiologist, letting the patients or their guardians know about all the risk and complications possibly occur during the surgery, know the benefit and risk the patients could get from implanting the artificial cochlea and sign their name on the informed consent (Appendix B).

4. Operation procedure and methods

   As regular, operate through the mastoid crypt entrance access cochlea fenestra or cochlea fenestra entrance access at post auricle incision. The detail should be according to the relevant request of all types of the artificial cochlea implanting device.

5. Interoperation monitoring

   Do the electrode immittance test and electricity-evoked nerve reaction test due to the artificial cochlea device to know the integrity of electrode and auditory nerve reaction to electric stimulation.
6. Disposal after operation

   Take imaging (skull X-ray imaging) after operation to eliminate the electrode's location and the rest exams are is like other common oto operation.
7. Surgery complications

   Common complications include the cavum tympanic membrane tresses, the external ear canal injury, abnormal smelling sense, dizziness, titinus, facial muscle tics and pain, infection, scalp hematoma, cerebrospinal fluid leakage, facial nerve paralysis, meningitis, intracranial hematoma, shifting and exposure of the implantation service, electrode prolapsed, split or necrotic flap, etc. The complications should be dealt due to the relevant conditions.
8. Switching-on and debugging

   Turn the device on about 1–4 weeks after surgery usually, debug 1–2 times during the following 1-month and arrange the time due to the patients' condition. Lengthen the debugging interval properly after the audition stabilizes and finally debug the device once a year. Switching-on and debugging methods should be done according to the technical requirements. If the contralateral ear benefits from the hearing aid, it is advised to fit hearing aids.

**Audition Speech Restoration After Implanting**

The patients who implant the artificial cochlea have to be trained by scientific audition speech restoration training to promote their development of the diagnosis, expression and speech application ability. The guardians or patriarchs of infant patients implanted the artificial cochlea should master vital audio speech restoration information and skills under professional guidance at qualified rehabilitation institution, practice actively, try to be supporters, guides and accompanists of all the hearing-impairment children restoration education process to maximum the restoration effect. Adult with artificial cochlea implant should accept the guidelines of the audition adaption training and speech recognition training due to suggestions of doctors.

Restoration evaluation at the artificial cochlear implant includes the assessment of the implantation sound field, speech audition ability and language ability. The 'flying love, a Chinese audiometry software and the International simplest Chinese speech test set for adults with cochlear implantation developed by Xin Xi's group (from China), containing the most latently developed Chinese AzBio sentences, Chinese CNC mono-syllabary and Chinese BKB-SIN test, reflect the mandarin recognition assessment system for adult cochlear implant initially develops, which is enough to filtrate cases before operation and finish post-operation long-term restoration assessment. To this infant cochlear implant whose speech language ability can't finish the audition, language and speech test above, investigators should interview the teachers of patriarchs close to the infants to finish the evaluation paper. Suggested papers are meaningful auditory integration scale (MAIS), infant-toddler MAIS (IE-MAIS), patriarchs/parents evaluate ability of communication hearing (PEACH), teacher EACH (TEACH), meaningful using speech scale (MUSS) and Mandarin context development of infants (MCDI). To the long-term efficacy of big samples, investigators should evaluate the audition sense with result of the categories of audition performance (CAP) and speech expression ability with result of speech intelligible response (SIR). To evaluate the life quality of pre- and post-implanting artificial cochlea, Nijmegen cochlear implant questionnaire (NCIQ) is suggested.

### 8.8.4 Bone Bridge

Bone Bridge is the latest active cross-flap bone conductive audition implant device applied in clinic, including an implant and a head-mounted audition processor. The implant is made with receiving coil, a modem and a bone conductive floating mass transducer (Fig. 8.34). The implant has MRI compatibility and is able to do the 1.5 T MRI. Compared to the BAHA, there is no implant exposed to obviously decrease the wound infection incidence and no need to do follow-up skin care, what makes it a trend for the bone bridge to replace the BAHA. Bone bridge has been applied in clinic over 5 years, but it just breaks the ice in China.

**Clinical Indications**

It includes the conductive, the mixed and the unilateral sensory deafness of adults and infants over 5 years old caused by multiple reasons. It also contains the ankylotia, ineffective tymossiculoplasty (weak bone conduction of gas >30 dB HL), otosclerosis, tympanosclerosis, abrupt deafness and acoustic neuroma.

**Operation Method**

According to the preoperative CT scan result and position of patients, arranging proper bone bed and insert the implant after placing the implant behind the mastoid cavity or sigmoid sinus, fix the implant with two bone cortical screw (should we replace a professional word of 'bone cortical') and place the receiving coil on the skull. Switch on and debug when the operation area heals and the flap detumescence.

**Complications**

The bone cortical screw loosening occurs only in clinic aboard. There are few reports because at the beginning stage the bone bridges are used in China.

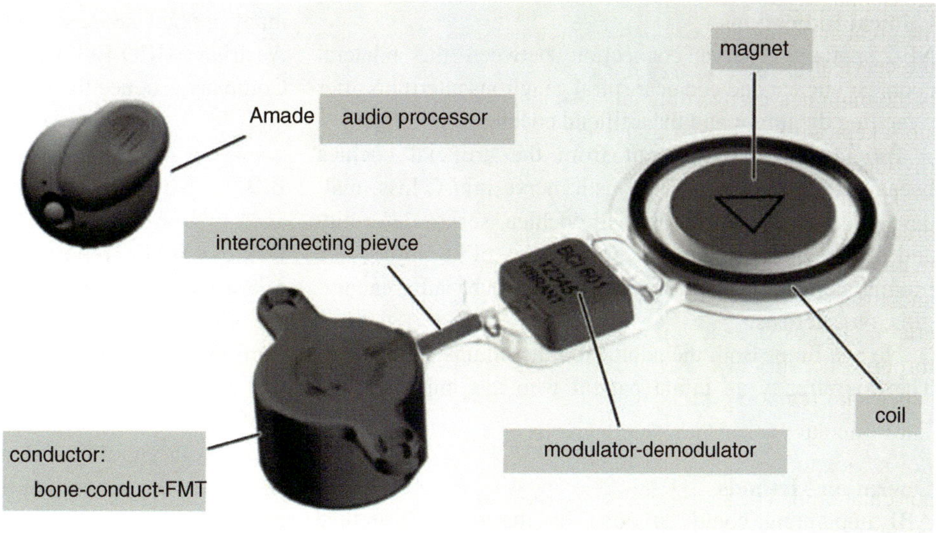


**Fig. 8.34** Contents of bone bridge

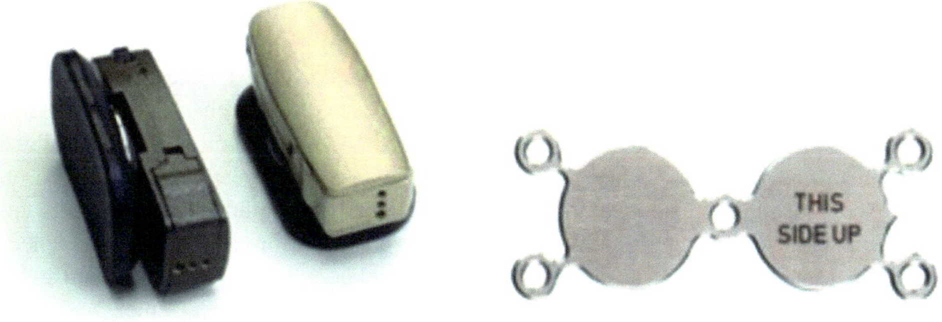


**Fig. 8.35** Sound processing and implant of implant bone conductive hearing-aid system

### 8.8.5 Implant Bone Conductive Hearing-Aid System

The latest China-made bone conductive hearing-aid system consists the sound processing and the implant (Fig. 8.35). The implant is packed with titanium enclosure and is the thinnest (only 2.6 mm) and smallest in size compared to other same-type productions. The implant is fixed with 5 titanium screws on subcutaneous mastoid, absorbing magnetically with the sound processing outside the skin to achieve transmitting the sound. The production has advantages like easy to operate, causing little injury, without exposure in vitro and others. Difference between topic system and Bone Bridge is that the energy converter in topic system is in the sound processing in vitro.

**Clinic Indications**

1. Conductive or mixed hearing loss but still can benefit from the amplified sound.

   The pure acoustic bone conductive threshold of the affected ear tested under 0.5 kHz, 1 kHz, 2 kHz and 4 kHz isn't more than 45 dB HL.
2. Bilateral symmetrical conductive or mixed hearing loss.

   Difference between the pure acoustic bone conductive threshold of both ears under 0.5 kHz, 1 kHz, 2 kHz and 4 kHz isn't more than 10 dB HL or average threshold at every frequency is not more than 15 dB HL.
3. Deep unilateral sensorineural hearing loss and cannot apply the air conductive contralateral routing signals hearing aid. The pure acoustic air conductive threshold of health ear at 0.5 kHz, 1 kHz, 2 kHz and 4 kHz isn't more than 20 dB HL.

### 8.8.6 Auditory Brainstem Implant

Auditory brainstem implant (BMI) has similar form as the artificial cochlea. The electrode array is inserted into crypt outwards the fourth encephalcoele by surgery and straightly stimulate the auditory neurons in the brainstem cochlear nuclear complex cross the cochlea and auditory nerve to produce audition. There are already over 1000 patients implanted. ABI is mainly produced by the Australian Cochlear Company and Austrian MED-EL Company.

**Clinical Indications**

NF-2 patients' nerve connection between the bilateral cochlear nuclear and cochlear spiral ganglions interrupts after removing the tumor and the artificial cochlea don't effect.

Patients can't get benefit from the artificial cochlea because of the cochlea or acoustic nerve injury, loss, mal-development, dysneuria, ossified cochlea, severe deformity and other symptoms, caused by varieties of etiologies like trauma, congenital deformity, auditory, neuropathy, meningitis, otosclerosis.

No age limit. Both the adults and the infants could be in. There is already an infant patient who has implanted the BMI.

**Operation Methods**

ABI implanting could be done by the translabyrinthine approach, retro-sigmiod approach or retro-sigmoid-inner ear canal approach and other operation methods. The translabyrinth approach is the most common one. An ideal method should entirely remove the tumor and also completely expose and accurately locate the implanting field to avoid from damage to the important blood vessels, nerve and functional zone.

**Complications**

Severe complications include death, cerebellar injury, persistent facial paralysis, meningitis, cranial nerve injury, cranial hydrops, pseudo-meningocele etc. Less severe complications contain the cerebrospinal fluid leak, temporary cranial hydrops, traumatic hematoma, slight infection, disequilibrium, perilous-implant infection, flap infections, temporary facial paralysis, temporary phonation or swollen difficulties, headache, flat problems, and non auditory response.

**Post Implanting Debugging and Effect**

The ABI implant switches on and debugs mostly six weeks after operation. First switching-on should be done under electrocardiogram monitoring to prevent the vital signs' change evoked by stimulating brainstem formation. Do regular postoperative debugging to fit personal requirements of patients. Debugging includes ensuring the threshold, the maximum comfort threshold, non auditory sensation response intensity of each electrode, tone-sensation grading evaluation, ordering the electrode pairs due to the tone, programing ABI language processor and eliminating speech manifestations.

All in all general effect of ABI is worse than the artificial cochlea according to data present.

### 8.8.7 Auditory Midbrain Implant

Auditory midbrain implant (AMI) has similar formation as the ABI. Place the electrode into the inferior colliculus or its central core to stimulate to produce the audition. There aren't many applied cases, so we need do further relevant research. Austrian MED-EL Company and Australian Cochlear Company produce the implant.

## 8.9 Sudden Deafness

Dekleyn firstly reports it at 1944. Most of the scholars relate its pathogenesis to the blood circulation disorder, the virus infection, the labyrinth fenestrated membrane rupture, the trauma, the poisoning, etc. Those whose etiology isn't explicit could be called the idiopathic abrupt deafness. It is defined by the Chinese Medical Association Otorhinolaryngology Head and Neck Surgery branch (2015) as the sensorineural hearing loss abruptly occurs inward 72 h with unclear pathogenesis, during which audition loses not less than 20 dB HL between two adjacent frequencies. Definition from the U.S. guideline in 2012 is the sensorineural deafness rapidly develops without clear pathogenesis inward 72 h, whose hearing loss at three successive frequencies isn't less than 30 dB. As research result from the Chinese Abrupt Deafness Research Center shows that the median onset age is 41-year-old, there is no obvious imbalance gender ratio, the left deafness onsets more than the right. The bilateral abrupt deafness incidence is low, about 1.7–4.9% of all cases, which is only 2.3% at researches of Chinese Research Center.

**Clinical Manifestation**

1. Suddenly happened hearing loss
2. Tinnitus (about 90%)
3. Ear stuffy-fullness feeling (about 50%)
4. Dizziness or giddiness (about 30%)
5. Paracusia acris or weak hearing
6. Periodic paraesthesia (common in anakusis)
7. Some patients develop mental disorders like anxiety, somnipathy and influence the living quality.

**Diagnosis**

Diagnosis gists from Chinese Medical Association Otorhinolaryngology Head and Neck Surgery branch at 2015:

1. The sensorineural hearing loss abruptly occurs inward 72 h with, during whom audition loses not less than 20 dB HL between two adjacent frequency, most of whom is unilateral and minority of whom is bilateral occurred or occurs at both ears by step.
2. Unclear pathogenesis (including the systemic or local factors)
3. May be accompanying with the tinnitus, the ear stuffy-fullness sensation, and the periodic paraesthesia etc.

4. May be accompanying with the dizziness, vomiting and nausea.

In 2012, the U.S. Guideline recommended diagnosing despite other neurologic diseases, examine the auditory, despite the retro-cochlear lesions and intensely deprecate the CT scan and other Regular lab examinations.

**Treatment**

Because the pathogenesis is unknown, there is no unified pattern to treat. Most of the therapy methods are experience-depend. Main measurements include the drug therapy, including the vasodilator dextran-40, calcium antagonist nimodipine, antihistamine methionine betahistine, glucocorticoid (oral or intra-tympanic injection), anticoagulation batroxobin, heparin, etc., and other methods like hyperbaric oxygen (HBO).

- Therapy guidelines In 2015 Chinese Medical Association Otorhinolaryngology Head and Neck Surgery branch point out that typing the abrupt deafness according to the auditory curve could guide the therapy and prognosis, the improving-inner-ear-microcirculation drug and the glucocorticoid effect on all types of abrupt deafness, proper combined drugs are more effective than the single drug, the effect order at all types should be low frequency decline type (best) > flat decline type (better) > high frequency decline type and anacusia type (worst).

1. Basic treatment advice
   (a) Abrupt deafness acute onset stage (inwards 3 weeks):
   Main change is the inner ear vasculopathy. Suggest applying the glucocortocid plus hemarheology therapy (including the hemo-dilution, improving the flow and decreasing the viscosity or fibrinogen, which is done by drugs like the ginkgol biloba extract (GBE), batroxobin, etc.
   (b) Application of glucocorticoid:
   Oral: prednisone 1 mg/kg per day (top 60 mg), taken at a drought in the morning, thrice daily, stay on it for 2 more days if it effects, no need to back-titrate. Withdrawal straightly if no response. The hormone could also be administrated by vein. Reckoning analysis due to the prednisone dosage, it should contain methylprednisolone 40 mg or dexamethasone 10 mg, same courses as oral hormone. The hormone therapy is priorly suggested to systemic injection. The local injection is for the rescue therapy, including the intra-tympanic or retro-auricle injection. The intra-tympanic injection should apply the dexamethasone 5 mg or methylprednisolone 20 mg, quaque omni die (QOD), 4–5 times. Retro-auricle injection should apply the methylprednisolone 20–40 mg or dexamethasone 5–10 mg, qod, 4–5 times. If the patients difficult in subsequent visiting, it could be applied the diprospan 2 mg (1 ml), retro auricle injection once. About these patients have hypertension history, diabetes history and other medical histories, the glucocorticoid or local administration due to the condition under close attention to blood pressure and blood glucose monitoring could be used to them with their permission.
   (c) Abrupt deafness could make secondary nerve injury, which can be cured by taking the nutritive psychotropic drugs (such as the mecobalamine, nerve nutrition factors, etc.) and antioxidants (such as the lipoid acid, the ginkgo biloba extract, etc.) at and after acute staging.
   (d) Same type drugs aren't suggested to be combined utilized.
   (e) It is still debatable about the hyperbaric oxygenation response, so the hyperbaric oxygenation isn't the best therapeutic regime. If the regular treat response isn't good, the rescuing measure should be considered.
   (f) The drug withdrawal could be advanced if audition restoration rates isn't good during the courses and delayed due to the condition. To these patients who don't get good efficacy, the hearing aid, the artificial cochlea or other auditory assistance devices could be applied according to the hearing loss degree.
2. Recommended grading therapy proposal
   The anacusia type, the high frequency decline type and the flat decline type have low curing rate, so the patients with any of them should be active treated as soon as possible.
   (a) Low-frequency decline type
      - It may be caused by the membranous labyrinth hydrops, so there should be salt-restriction. The patients should not be transfused too much transfusion and better no saline solution;
      - patients with average hearing loss <30 dB have high self-curing rate, could orally take drugs, including the glucocorticoid, the methionine betahistine, the improving venous-return drug (such as the aescuven forte) etc. and could also be considered to intra-tympanic or retro-auricular administration of the glucocorticoid (such as the methyprednisolone, the dexamathesone, the diprospan, etc.); patients with average hearing loss ≥30 dB could be venously injected the ginkgol biloba extract (GBE) + the glucocorticoid; minority of patients, getting no efficacy with regimen but exacerbating the ear stuffy-fullness sensation, can be treated with lowering-fibrinogen drug (such as the batroxobin) and other improving-venous-reflux drugs.

(b) High-frequency decline type
- improving microcirculation drugs (such as the ginkgol biloba extract (GBE)) + glucocorticoid;
- the ion channel blockers (such as the lidocaine) have good efficacy to decrease the high-tone tinnitus;
- the nutrition neurotic drugs could be considered (such as the mechobalamine, etc)

(c) All-frequency hearing loss (including the flat decline type and the anacuria type)
- decreasing-fibrinogen drug (such as the betroxobin);
- the glucocorticoid;
- the improving-inner-ear-microcirculation drugs (such as the ginkgol biloba extract (GBE).

The combined medication therapy is suggested.

The U.S. Guideline recommends that the intratympanic injection should be the rescuing therapy when other therapies failed and the initial hormone therapy (including the oral and intratympanic injection) and the hyperbaric therapies could be applied appropriately. No commendation to other drug therapy regimens.

Recommended efficacy grading by the Chinese Medical Association Otolaryngology Head and Neck surgery branch (2015):

1. *Recovery* The damaged frequency audition threshold reinstated to the normal, the health-ear level or the quality premorbid.
2. *High-efficacy* Average audition at the damaged frequency increases over 30 dB.
3. *Efficient* Average audition at the damaged frequency increases 15–30 dB.
4. *Inefficient* Average audition at the damaged frequency increases less than 15 dB [3].

## 8.10 Benign Paroxysmal Positional Vertigo

The benign paroxysmal positional vertigo (BPPV) is the temporary dizziness concomitant with nystagmus evoked when head moved to a specific location. Because most of the BPPV is self-limited diseases, curing after several days or months, it is 'benign'. It was firstly reported by Barany. BPPV is the most common peripheral vertigo disease, occupying 1/4 of vertigo diseases and whose morbidity is 10.7/100,000–64/100,000.

**Etiology**

The etiology of the BPPV isn't ensured. It can be idiopathic and also secondary to factors following:

1. When the age-related change or anaplasis occurred red in the labyrinth, the maculae utriculi degenerate, the otolith detaches and drops into the semi buccal tube (often in the posterior, occasionally in the lateral and the anterior).
2. Trauma

   Slight head trauma or head accelerating novation like the whiplash injury. The otolith dropping into the semi buccal tube can also occur after the stapes surgery?
3. Ear disease

   The mid-ear mastoid inflammation like the various labyrinthitis, the chronic suppurative otitis media, the Ménière disease catalase, the perilymphatic fistula, etc.
4. insufficient blood supply to inner ear

   It is caused by the arteriosclerosis and the hypertension, the capsule colloid membrane pinch outs and the otolith drops into the semibuccal tube.

**Pathogenesis**

There are many theories about the BPPV's pathogenesis, whose trendency is the cupulolithiasis theory and the canalithiasis theory (Fig. 8.36)

1. Cupulolithiasis theory

   It is reported by Schukne in 1969, the basophil granules after the utriculus otolith degeneration drop into the semi buccal tube (mainly the posterior canal) edge crest, what evokes the concentration difference between the endolymph and the edge crest to cause the ratio change and finally changes the ridge crest gravity and the linear acceleration into sensitivity (Fig. 8.36). But theory, if only the semi buccal cal tube keeps vertical to the ground, the gravity-sensitive ridge crest skewing should also be still and cause continuous vertigo and nystagmus. But the dizziness or the nystagmus in this disease could only last temporarily in few seconds, short time, so it's not enough to explain the short-term and the fatiguability of the nystagmus. Motility found that there are only 28% of the ridge crest otolith drops at the posterior canal, 21% at the lateral and 13% at the anterior in the normal ossa temporal which defends the cupulolithiasis theory.
2. Canalithiasis theory

   As research results show, the degenerated otolith crushing isn't attached to the ampullae edge crest but floating in the endolymph of the semi buccal tube. When the head moves to the stimulating area, the tube is vertical to the ground and the otolith moves by the opposite osit-smpullae direction and drops in the lowest sites of the semi buccal tube, what guide the endolymph to move the ampullae edge crest to opposite-utriculus direction, finally stimulate the ampullae edage sensory hair cells and evoke vertigo and nystagmus.

   In fact, a main difference between the cupulolithiasis theory the canalithiasis theory is that the otolith sedimentation attach is attached to the edge crest or floating in the smi buccal tube. If there are plenty of the otolith granules, there could be both simultaneously.

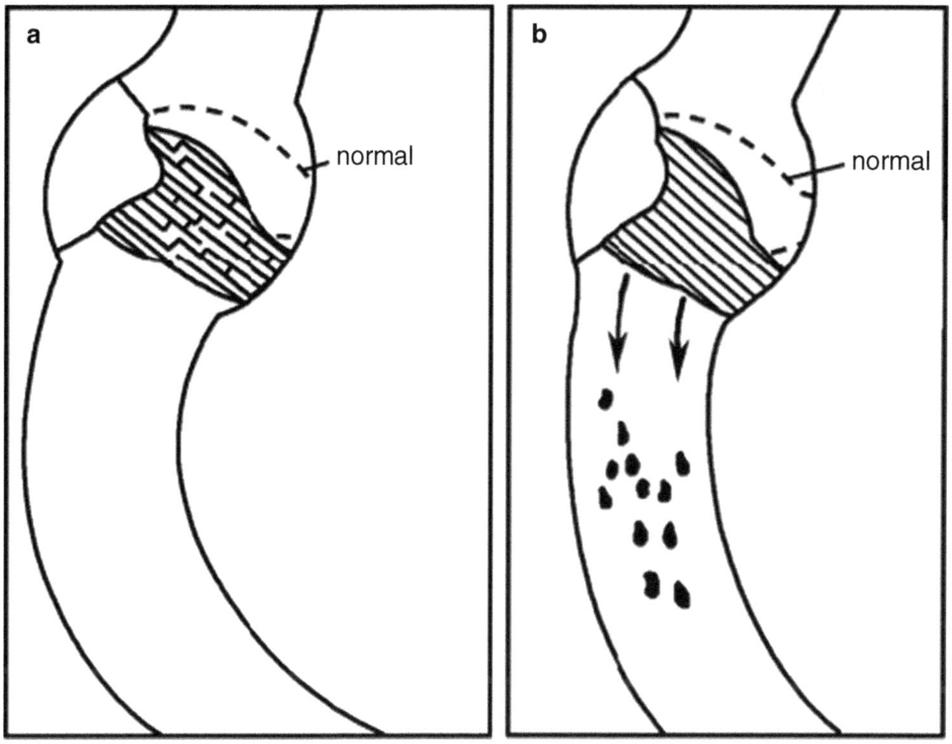


**Fig. 8.36** Pathogenesis pattern graph of the cupulolithiasis theory and the canalithiasis theory

**Pathology and Pathophysiology**
The views differs at that the substance existing on the semi buccal tube and the ridge crest is the otolith or the others. Welling (1997), Pames (1992) and others find that those granules floating in the semi buccal tube is basophilia, considering it as the translocating otolith. Motility (1992) found that there is basophil existing on 22% of the ridge crest in 566-ossae temporal, often being seen at the lateral and anterior sites. He considered it common that sedimentation occurs in the semi buccal after death, and the sedimentation maybe not the otolith, but also can be the cell debris like the macrophage, the WBC and possibly the crushing developed from the labyrinth micro hemorrhage. Besides, because of the trauma, the mid-ear surgery and the inflammation, there could be WBC and endo-membrane debris in the endolymph aggregating in the semi buccal tube to cause same reaction as the otolith translocation and finally evokes the BPPV.

**Clinical Manifestation**
Typical onset manifestation is that the severe rotational vertigo occurs while heading up or turning over but disappears soon, repeat action could invoke the vertigo again but accompanying with the tinnitus and no hearing loss. According to the locations the change occurs, the manifestations are different.

1. Posterior canal BPPV (PC-BPPV)

   Happen abruptly and often be evoked while the sudden prone, head moves toward one profile or stretching the neck, sudden acceleration or deceleration while in vehicles and crouching 3–6 s (incubation period) after suddenly moving head or stimulating the site, the patients sense the temporary rotating nystagmus and fatiguable. Accompanying with the vertigo, there is the top heavy sensation or floating sense, unsteadily. The period could last for several hours, couple days even over 1 year at the long-term. There is also vomiting and nausea sensation while being attacked, but without any hearing disorders, tinnitus etc. and none central nerve manifestations and signs. Comfortable during the incubation stage.
2. Horizontal canal BPPV (HC-BPPV)

   Vertigo happens in short time too, and often occurs while turning over. While the patients turn over to the affected side, the vertigo or the nystagmus is severe, but when the head moves vertically like raising-head-up or erection after stooping, there isn't any uncomforted. It is a short-term manifestation, lasting several days or about 1 month. Compared to the PCBPPV, the incubation stage is short as 2–3 s but the lasting may be longer. The fatigue feeling may be occurring or may not.
3. Anterior canal BPPV (Slo EC-BPPV)

   With low morbidity and may be ensured due to the vertical substance's direction at rotational vertigo.

**Examination**
1. Dix-Hallpike positioning nystagmus test

   The most common test method is at the post-canal and the anterior canal. The procedures are ensured by the nystagmus direction: (1) Sitting position, the investigator

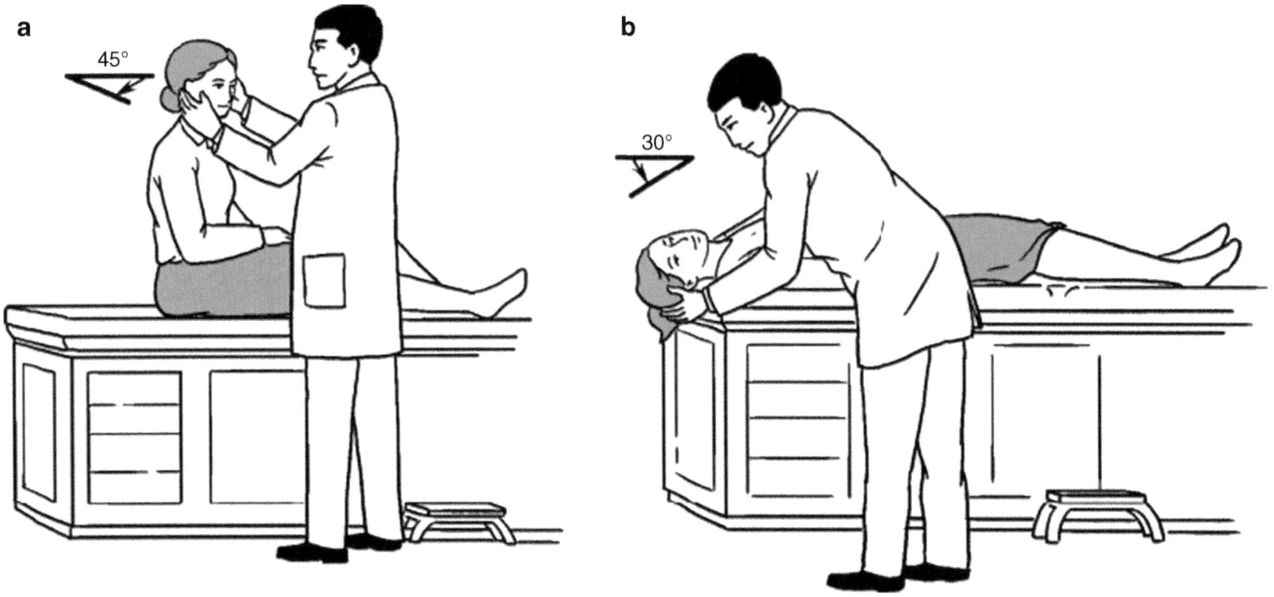


**Fig. 8.37** Dix-Hallpike test. (**a**) Sitting positioning detroverse the head by 45°; (**b**) The investigator support and move the head to the supine suspension position, 30° to the horizontal plane

support and dextroverse the patients' heads by 45°with both hands, (2) the investigators support, rapidly move the head to the supine suspension position with both hands, whose angle of the horizontal plane is 30° and 45° to the vertical plane, stay for 30 s and resume into the sitting position after investigation the vertigo and nystagmus conditions (Fig. 8.37). Investigate the other side by the same way. Typical PC-BPPVs always causes temporary vertigo and vertical rotatively nystagmus after 5–15 s' incubation and it lasts for less than 30 s, with fatiguability.

2. Roll test

   Horizontal position. The investigators support and rapidly detroverse the head to left or right by 90° by both hands and investigate the vertigo and nystagmus conditions (Fig. 8.38). The typical HC-BPPV rapidly causes severe rotative vertigo and toward-earth nystagmus after several seconds' incubation and it lasts for over 30 s, without fatiguability.

3. Audiometry

   There is usually no abnormal audiological manifestation, except for that the canalithiasis is secondary to other inner-ear disease.

4. Nystagmus electro-graph examination

   Most of the results are normal. If the BPPV is secondary to the some inner-ear disease, the relative vestibular function could change.

5. Imaging examination

   The neck X-ray imaging or MRI, the temporal CT scan and others could help differentiate diagnosis.

**Diagnosis and Differential Diagnosis**

1. Diagnosis gist
   (a) The temporary vertigo history when the head moves to a specific position.
   (b) Positioning nystagmus test could appear dame nystagmus characteristics and has incubation stage (<30 s).
   (c) Ascertain the BPPV type due to the history and Examination result (Table 8.1) [4].
2. Differentiate diagnosis

   The BPPV should be differentially diagnosed from the central vertigo, the vestibular neuritis, the Ménière disease, the cerebrovascular diseases and other dazzling diseases (Table 8.2).

**Treatment**

1. General therapy

   Escape position could evoke vertigo and rest in bed while vertigo occurs, avoiding the head novation, rapid retroversion, etc. Pay attention to the psycho-therapy, eliminating the psycho-burden.
2. Medical therapy
   (a) Drug therapy: choose the antidinic drugs due to the condition to inhibit the vestibular nerve excitement, alleviating the vertigo, controlling the nauseating, vomiting and other autonomic manifestations.
   (b) Positioning therapy: The Brandt-Daroff positioning therapy method. Close the eyes stand and twist toward one side till the occipital touches the Examination table. Keep the position till the vertigo

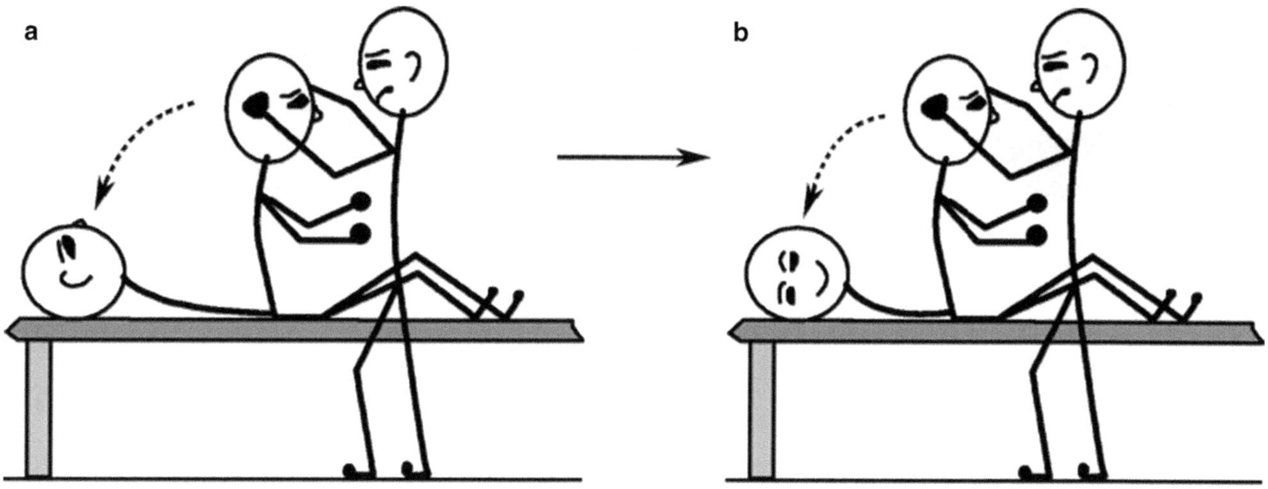


**Fig. 8.38** Roll test. (**a**) At the supine positioning and keep the head in middle. (**b**) The head rapidly detroverse to right or left by 90°

**Table 8.1** Differential diagnosis of positioning vertigo

| | Central vertigo | BPPV | Alcoholic vertigo | Cervical vertigo |
|---|---|---|---|---|
| Vertigo | | | | |
| Incubation | No | 2–20 s | No | Yes |
| Lasting time | Continuous | 2–40 s | Lasting while staying still | Short-term |
| Nystagmus | | | | |
| Direction | Unsteady | Towards inferior ear | | Steady |
| Occurring position | Plenty | One | Plenty | One |
| Fatigued | × | √ | × | √ |
| Property | Vertical or oblique | Rotating or horizontal | Rotation or horizontal | Horizontal |

**Table 8.2** Differentiate points on BPPV

| Differentiate points | PC-BPPV | HC-BPPV | SC-BPPV |
|---|---|---|---|
| Evoking test | Dix-Hallpike test | Roll test | Dix-Hallpike test |
| Lasting time | <30s | >30s | <30s |
| Incubation stage | 5–15 s | <3 s | 5–15 s |
| Fatiguability | √ | × | √ |

goes and sit up. Twist to another side after 30 s. Repeat as above till the vertigo symptoms disappear.

(c) Otolith repositioning maneuvers: choose different positional maneuvers according to the different BPPV types.
   - The PC-BPPV: Epley or Semont repositioning maneuvers (Fig. 8.39)

     Surgical therapy: to intractable BPPV, the patients should do the ampullae neurectomy, the vestibular neurotomy, the semi buccal occlusion, etc. if it influences the living quality of patients even after inefficient traditional therapy [5].

**Prognosis**

BPPV has high self-healing nature. The PC-BPPV can be self-healed after about 39–47 days, and the HC-BPPV's is 16–19 days. Symptoms of 30% of the patients last over 1 year. The recurrence rate after 2 years is about 20%, and 55% after 8 years. The recurrent patients could do the repositioning maneuvers again.

## 8.11 Ménière Disease

Ménière disease is a kind of inner ear disease with specific endolymphatic hydrops, manifesting as recurrent rotating vertigo, fluctuant sensory hearing loss, tinnitus and (or) aural fullness sensation. Its pathogenic change is endolymphatic hydrops (Fig. 8.40).

**Clinical Manifestation**

1. Clinic symptoms:

   The pathological base of the meniere disease is the hydro labyrinth. Its main clinical manifestations are shown in the following:

   (a) Recurrent rotating vertigo, lasting for 20 min even several hours, occurs twice at least;often accompanying with the nausea, the vomiting balance disorder but no consciousness loss; may accompanying with the horizontal or horizontally rotating nystagmus.
   (b) At least once sensory neuro deafness at pure tone test.
   (c) Indirect or persisting tinnitus, the ear stuffy-fullness sense
   (d) Despite other diseases could cause vertigo.
2. Clinic staging

   The clinic staging is according to average audition threshold under the pure-tone test investigation and the speech recognition rate (Table 8.3):

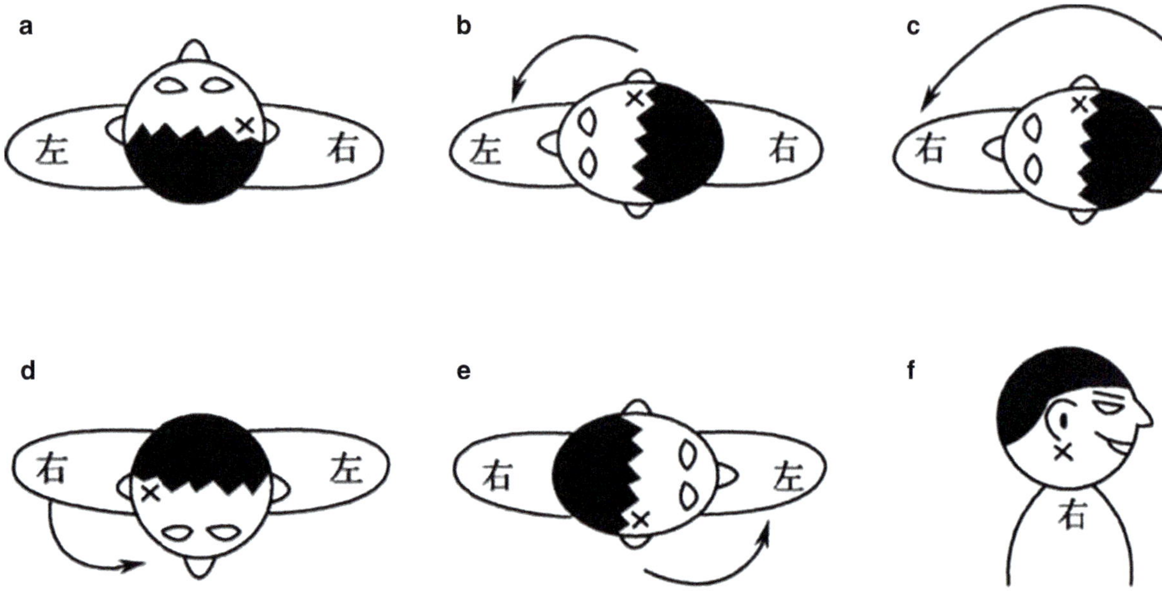


**Fig. 8.39** HC-BPPV positioning maneuvers

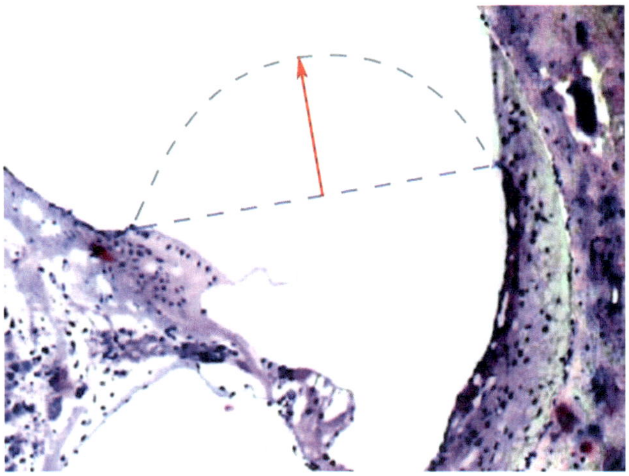

**Fig. 8.40** Diagram of endolymphatic hydrops in guinea pig cochlea

**Table 8.3** The meniere's clinic staging

| Stages | Average threshold of pure-tone (dB) | Speech-recognition rate (%) |
|---|---|---|
| I | ≤25 | ≥70 |
| II | 26–40 | ≥50 |
| III | 41–70 | ≥50 |
| IV | >70 | <50 |

The prophase: indirect normal audition or slight low-frequency hearing loss.

The mid-phase: indirect low frequency and high-frequency hearing loss.

The late stage: over moderate-severe all-frequency hearing loss, no audition undulation.

The pure-tone threshold applies the average value of threshold at the 250 Hz, 500 Hz, 1000 Hz and 2000 Hz, and it is the worst auditory range before therapy.

**Examination**

1. Enquire the medical history and the vertigo recurrence history
2. Examination
   (a) Otoscopy
   Normal tympanic membrane
   (b) Vestibular function Examination
   While the vertigo occurs, the nystagmus and the balance disorder appear. The indirect idiopathic and evoked vestibular function examinations are often normal. The evoked vestibular function examination at the effected side declines or completely disappears.
   (c) Audition
   Sensory deafness. Upward-sloping audition curve at the early stage, flat or decline curve at the later stage. The audition has the undulation and the recruitment phenomenon.
   (d) Glycerinum test
   After taking the 50% glycerinum by 2.4–3 ml/kg, the 250–1000 Hz auditions improved to positive, ≥15 dB.
   (e) Imaging examination
   The inner ear and the cerebellopontine angle CT scan or MRI Examination help differentiate diagnosis the Ménière disease. The temporal CT scan occasionally manifests the badly gasified peripheral aqueduct vestibuli, with short and straight lumen. Some

patients manifest the straightened and slimmed aqueduct vestibuli under membranous labyrinth MRI. The intra tympanic injection of the gutamide dilution through the auripuncture is recently applied to prepare the three dimensional fluid attenuated inversion recovery MRI (3D-FLAIR MRI) 24 h later, which is used to distinguish the intra-, the peri-lymph gap boundary, manifest the hydro labyrinth condition and is possible to offer accurate proof to differentiate diagnose the Ménière disease.

**Diagnosis Gist**

1. Paroxysmal vertigo occurs not less than 2 times, lasting 20 min to several hours and often accompanies with the automatic nerve system dysfunction and the disequilibrium, without consciousness loss.
2. Undulating hearing loss that the low-frequency audition loses at the early period and gradually the audition loss worsen along with the disease processing. At least do one sensory neurologic hearing loss at pure-tone test. There could be the recruitment phenomenon.
3. often accompanying with the tinnitus and (or) the ear fullness feeling.
4. Automatic nystagmus may happen.
5. Despite the vertigo caused by other diseases, such as the benign paroxysmal positioning vertigo, the labyrinthitis, the vestibular neuritis, the drug toxic vertigo, the paroxysmal deafness, vertebrobasilar artery insufficiency and the intracranial space-occupying lesion.
6. The suspicious diagnosis (unconfirmed the Ménière disease): (1) only for once vertigo occurs, the pure-tone test result is the sensory neurologic hearing loss, often accompanying with the tinnitus and the ear fullness feeling; (2) not for less than twice vertigo occurs, lasting 20 min to several hours. Normal audition, without tinnitus and the ear fullness feeling; (3) undulating low-frequency sensory neuro-hearing loss, accompanying with the recruitment phenomenon, no obvious vertigo occurrence. Diagnosis fit any one of three above is a suspicious diagnosis.

**Treatment**

1. Drug therapy

   Drugs act at controlling the acute onset treatment and long-term dealing especially the undulating stage therapy of vertigo. The ideal criteria of the drug therapy is to achieve aims following: (1) eliminating the vertigo; (2) build a new sensory equilibrium function with rapid and complete vestibular compensation; (3) alleviating the nausea, vomiting and other symptoms at automatic neurodysfunction. Treat as regular emergency therapy while onset to alleviate the vertigo, nausea and the vomiting.

   (a) Benzodiazepines

      Diazepam

      Is the mostly common used in the benzodiazepine which has a better vestibular sedation function and is helpful to treat the vertigo, vomiting and could against the anxiety simultaneously.

   (b) Antiemetic drugs

      They have the sedation, the anti-cholinergic and the antiemetic function, including the dimenhydrinate, the metoclopramide, the phenergan, the anisodamine, the scopolamine, the atropine, etc.

   (c) Vasodilator

      Such as the betahistine, the radix salvia miltiorrhiza, the niacin, etc.

   (d) Diuretics

      Such as the hydrochlorothiazide, the chlorealidone and the chlorobenzene pteridine. Supply potassium while taking the thiazide.

   (e) Ca2+ antagonists: intermittent period available flunarizine and nimodipine.

   (f) The middle ear administration: Cochlear window film has a semi permeable effect of intratympanic injection of drugs through the penetration into the inner ear and therapeutic effects of antagonists: intermittent period available flunarizine and nimodipine currently used gentamicin or steroids to intra tympanic injection therapy [6]. The injection of gentamicin in the tympanum can destroy the secretory function of the vestibule dark cells to alleviate the membrane labyrinth and water accumulation. But because gentamicin has the risk of hearing loss, it is more suitable for patients with severe hearing loss. Steroid injection into tympanic cavity not only increases cochlear blood flow, but also inhibits immune mediated inflammatory response, and avoids the influence of amino glycoside drugs on hearing. Commonly used drugs with dexamethasone and methylprednisolone.

2. Surgical therapy

   It is suitable for frequent seizures, heavy symptoms, longer course of disease, ineffective drug therapy, and a significant impact on work and life. It is divided into destructive surgery and non-destructive surgery. The former mainly aims at the mechanism of water accumulation and the preservation of auditory function, the latter is mainly the innervation of the vestibule of ear, and the function of hearing is not necessarily preserved. For the pure tone audiometry speech recognition it; 70 dBHL and 20% were the best choice for hearing preservation surgery. Only one ear with hearing should avoid surgical therapy.

   (a) nondestructive surgeries

      - endolymphatic sac operation: endolymphatic sac decompression, endolymphatic bursa mastoid drainage and endolymphatic sac subarachnoid drainage. The effective rate of all kinds of endolymphatic sac operations is about 75% [7].

- cryotherapy: semicircular canal window can reduce the canal within the lymph flow, reduce its sensitivity and selectivity is chosen to permanently reduce the vestibular function, has the dual value can control the vertigo and hearing preservation.
- three semicircular canal occlusion surgery

  It may be effective intreating vertigo in Ménière disease, mild postoperative reaction, vestibular compensation set up fast and more complete compensation.

(b) destructive surgeries

- labyrinthectomy: this method can only be used for hearing loss. Including chemical labyrinthectomy and physical labyrinthectomy. The former mainly uses amino glycoside drugs, such as streptomycin injection tympanic (Fig. 8.41), and also reports on the general use of drugs. But at present, there is no unified standard for the method, dosage, and schedule of the drug delivery. The latter mainly uses surgical methods to remove labyrinthine, which is suitable for single ear disease, long-term or recurrent symptoms, and severe hearing loss.
- Vestibular neurectomy: can effectively eliminate the serious symptoms of vertigo patients and to preserve function, but not eliminate tinnitus and ear fullness. It is possible to use the middle cranial fossa path, the posterior sigmoid sinus path and the posterior route of the labyrinth.
- Others: chordal tympanotomy (chorda tympanectomy), cervical sympathectomy (cervical sympathectomy), decompression through vestibular window such as balloon angiotomy (sacculotomy) and cochlear balloon stoma (cochleosacculotomy).

3. Meniett therapy

   In recent years, the inner ear therapy instrument (Meinert) developed in the United States can obviously relieve vertigo and improve hearing. Meniett therapy through the tympanostomy tube, will continuously low pressure pulse transmission to the middle ear cavity and its function in the cochlear window. The ear has not compressibility, low pulse energy produced a movement of perilymph, causing the endolymph inward longitudinal flow lymphatic and endolymphatic sac and local circulation and in the film lost in absorption and absorption, reducing natural endolymph, improving hydrolabyrinth, therapy of Ménière disease (Fig. 8.42) [8, 9].

**Therapeutic Evaluation**

1. Vertigo assessment

   The number of vertigo episodes in 18~24 months after therapy was compared with the number of vertigo attacks 6 months before therapy. Press: the score = number of vertigo episodes 18–24 months after therapy/number of vertigo attack 6 months before therapy by 100. It is divided into 5 levels, that is,

   - A level: 0 (complete control, unintelligible as "cure"); level
   - B level: 1~40 (basic control);
   - C level: 41~80 (partial control);
   - D level: 81~120 (uncontrolled);
   - E level: >120 (aggravated).

2. Hearing assessment: In the 6 months before therapy is the worst time for 250 Hz, 500 Hz, 1000 Hz, 2000 Hz and 3000 Hz to average a corresponding frequency threshold for 18–24 months after therapy, the minus deviation of the mean of the assessed.

   - A level: the improvement of >30 dB or the frequency threshold <20 dBHL;
   - B level: improve 15~30 dB;

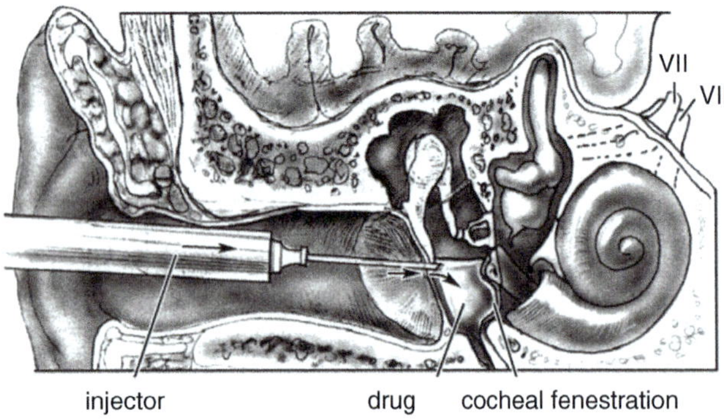


**Fig. 8.41** Chemical labyrinth excision therapy

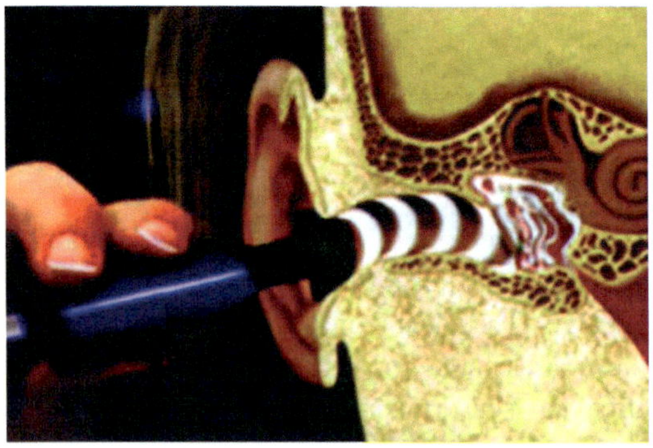

**Fig. 8.42** Meinett therapy

- C level: improve 0~14 dB (invalid)
- D level: improve <0 (deterioration).

  If the diagnosis is bilateral Meynier's disease, it should be evaluated separately.

3. Ability evaluation: The incidence of 18–24 months after therapy was compared with the 6 months before therapy. The score was equal to 18–24 months after therapy/the first half of the first half of the therapy day. It is divided into 5 levels, that is
   - A level: 0 (complete control);
   - B level: 1~40 (basic control);
   - C level: 41~80 (partial control);
   - D level: 81~120 (uncontrolled)
   - E level: >120 (aggravated).
   - Appendix: the day of onset: the sum of the day of activity limited/the sum of the days of observation. Limited day of activity refers to the days of 3 and 4 of the day's activities.
   - Activity score:
   - 0 points: any activity is not affected;
   - 1 point: mild activity;
   - 2 points: moderate activity, but no activity limitation;
   - 3 points: activities limited, unable to work, must rest at home;
   - 4 points: activities are severely restricted, all day rest or most activities cannot be accomplished [10, 11].

## 8.12 Acoustic Neuroma

Acoustic neuroma originates from the vestibular nerve (VIII brain nerve pair) the nerve cells of benign schwannoma. Originates from the nervous statoacusticus canal segment, or the inner ear nerve sheath crossing at the start of the inner ear or bottom, is one of the most common intracranial tumors, accounting for 7–12% of intracranial tumors, accounting for the cerebellopontine angle tumors 80–95%. More common in adults, the peak of the peak in 30~50 years old, less than 20 years old, children's single acoustic neuroma rare, no significant gender differences. The incidence at left ear and right ear is similar, and occasionally bilateral. Bilateral acoustic neuromas usually indicate neurofibromatosis type 2 (neurofibromatosis2), also known as central neurofibromatosis (central neurofibromatosis) or multiple bilateral acoustic neurofibromatosis (bilateral acoustic neurofibromatosis), is a kind of euchromosome dominant genetic disease.

### Clinical Manifestations

The symptoms of acoustic neuromas are mainly related to the size and location of tumor and the degree of compression to peripheral nerves, blood vessels and brain tissue. Main symptoms and signs:

1. Cochlear and vestibule symptoms: Showed unilateral tinnitus and deafness, of unilateral hearing loss, a minority of patients with sudden hearing loss as the first symptom, tinnitus for high pitched, cicadas or whistle, dizziness, vertigo and unstable sense of attack [12].
2. Headache: the frontal occipital pain is accompanied by discomfort in the large orifice of the lateral occipital bone.
3. Cerebellar ataxia: Unstable walking, horizontal tremor of the eyeball, and dysfunctional motor function.
4. Cerebellopontine angle syndrome: Symptoms and signs of nerve, facial nerve, trigeminal nerve and posterior group of brain nerve disorders, cerebellar damage and brain stem compression were the symptoms of adjacent brain nerve damage. As the disease side pain, facial twitching, facial hypesthesia, facial paralysis and eating cough, hoarseness, pharyngeal reflex disappeared or decreased; ipsilateral corneal reflexes diminish or disappear.
5. Symptoms of increased intracranial pressure Including optic disc edema, headache aggravation, nausea and vomiting, diplopia, etc.

### Specialist Examination

1. Check the audiological examination: It includes pure tone audiometry, speech recognition rate, acoustic conductivity, distortion product otoacoustic emission, cochlear electrogram, ABR latent Dynasty, etc. The pure tone audiometry showed different degrees of sensorineural deafness, the rate of speech recognition was significantly reduced, and the ABR examination showed the post cochlear lesion.
2. Vestibular function examination: the function of the semicircular canal is diminished or lost.
3. Peripheral facial paralysis: if there is facial paralysis, the electro facial electrogram should be examined.
4. Imaging examination
   (a) X-ray photography of the inner ear canal: enlargement of inner ear canal and destruction of otolith ridge.
   (b) axial bone CT: showed enlargement of inner ear canal (Fig. 8.43). There were ISO density or low-density lesions and obstructive hydrocephalus in cerebellopontine angle area.
   (c) Cranial MRI: MRI is the most sensitive and effective method at present. It shows that T1 weighted images of cerebellopontine angle area show low signal or equal signal. $T_2$ weighted images show high signal occupying lesions, and enhanced scan lesions are significantly enhanced (Figs. 8.44 and 8.45).
   (d) Cerebral angiography: can understand the blood supply of tumor and mediator embolism reduces intra operative bleeding.

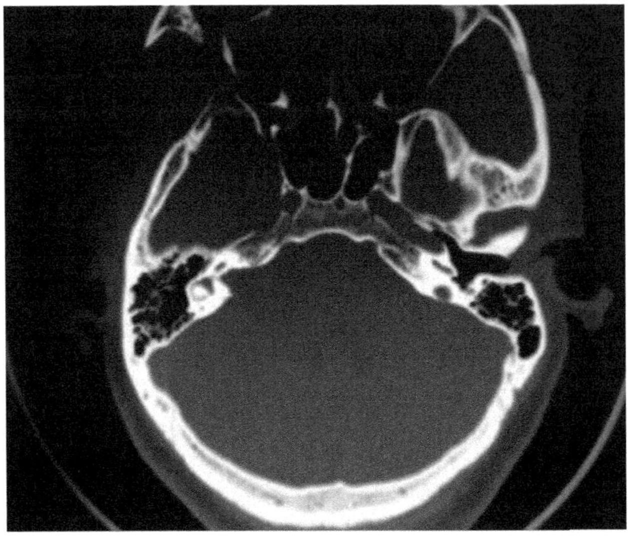

**Fig. 8.43** Axial temporal CT of right acoustic neuroma: right inner ear canal enlargement

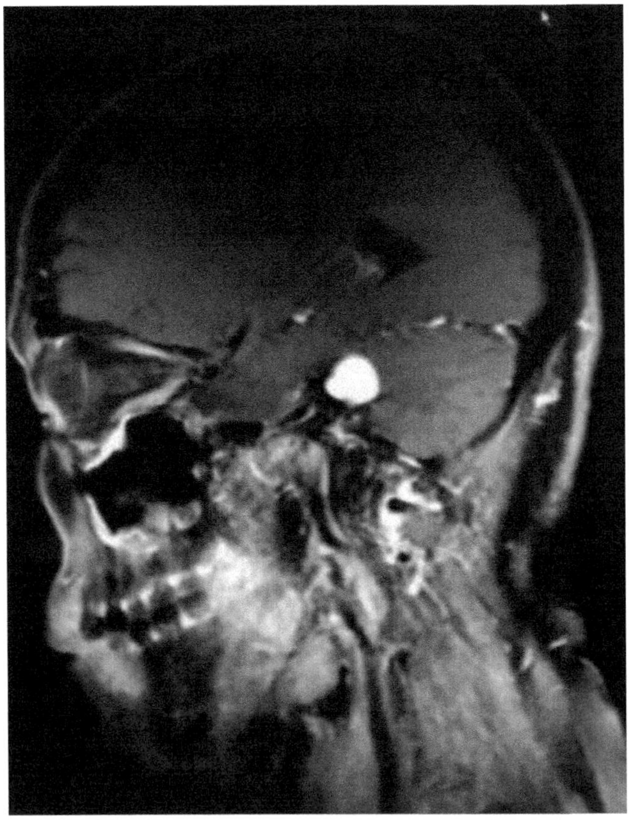

**Fig. 8.44** Weighted sagittal MRI $T_1$WI shows: acoustic neuroma

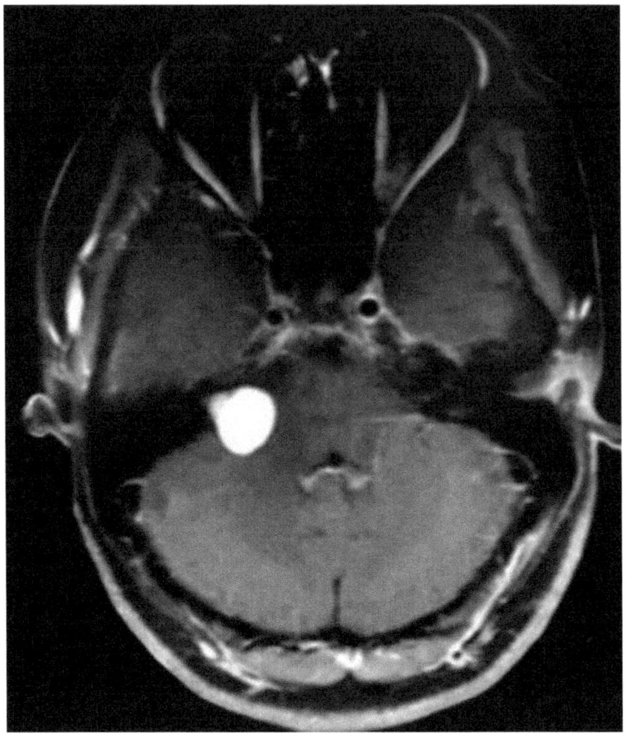

**Fig. 8.45** Weighted MRI: right acoustic neuroma

### Diagnosis and Differential Diagnosis

1. Diagnosis

   According to the results of patients with symptoms, signs, audiological examination and characteristic imaging (temporal CT and brain MRI) can be diagnosed.

2. Differential diagnosis

   This disease and facial neuroma, cerebellopontine angle meningioma, congenital cholesteatoma, arachnoid cysts, glioma, neuron inflammation, sudden deafness, and Ménière disease identification.

### Treatment

This disease is a slow but life-threatening benign tumor of the brain. There is no drug to inhibit the growth of the tumor. Surgical resection is the first accepted therapy. Small tumors by microsurgical resection, application of facial nerve and auditory evoked potential monitoring technology, function and auditory function to maximize the overall nerve.

1. Operation the approaches to acoustic neuroma surgery include:
   (a) the middle cranial fossa approach: suitable for confined to the inner ear in acoustic neuroma, and retain the residual hearing of patients.
   (b) by the way of backward Road: applicable to the main body in the cerebellopontine angle, medium size (diameter 2.5 cm) tumor resection, which is conducive to the preservation of residual hearing, not to hurt the lost structure.
   (c) labyrinthine approaches: it is suitable for severe hearing loss, facial nerve function is normal, and the tumor originates from the inner ear canal protruding

in the cerebellopontine angle pool, which is good for preserving the facial nerve function.
   (d) retrosigmoid or suboccipital approach: this approach is suitable for large auditory neuromas located mainly at the cerebellopontine angle.
2. Stereotactic radiotherapy ($\alpha$ knife, $\gamma$ knife) Suitable for surgical contraindication, no increased intracranial pressure, tumor diameter <2 cm, unwilling to accept operation, can also be the first large tumor resection and (or) ventricular shunt relieve intracranial hypertension after $\alpha$ knife or $\gamma$ knife therapy.
3. MRI continuous observation of tumor growth: it is suitable for patients with asymptomatic acoustic neuroma, aged (>70 years), unsuitable for operation or unwillingness to operate.

## 8.13 Genetic Diagnosis and Prenatal Diagnosis of Hereditary Deafness

Deafness is the most common and high incidence of deafness in human beings, with about 60% of the cases are hereditary deafness. There are about 78 million carriers of mutuated deafness gene in China with the overall carrying rate of 6%, 80% of children are born to hearing parents, and a large number of parents with delayed-onset hearing loss, mostly due to a defect in a gene polymorphism and its cause of deafness caused by environmental factors increase susceptibility to disease [13]. Hereditary deafness is mostly sensorineural deafness, which cannot be diagnosed according to clinical manifestations, and there is no effective drug therapy. Gene screening for deafness patients can, to a certain extent, clarify the cause of deafness, and guide patients and their relatives to take precautions in medication and life, prevent birth defects, control the risk of drug-induced deafness, intervene or delay the occurrence and development of deafness.

1. Genetic deafness genes could lead to the hereditary deafness, about 70% are non-syndromic deafness (non syndromic hearing loss, NSHL), and the rest about 30% are syndrome type deafness (syndromic hearing loss, SHL). The inheritance of NSHL could be expressed in a variety of genetic methods, including autosomal dominant (related chromosomal loci named DFNA), autosomal recessive (related to chromosomal loci named DFNB), X-linked NSHL (genetic linkage related chromosomal loci named DFNX), Y-linked NSHL (genetic linkage related chromosomal loci named DFNY) and maternal inheritance. Among them, 75~80% are autosomal recessive, 10~20% are autosomal dominant, X-linked NSHL is less than 2%, and a Y-linked Chinese deaf family has been reported now. Autosomal recessive deafness is mainly manifested in pre-lingual deafness, while autosomal dominant hereditary deafness is mainly manifested as post-lingual deafness [14, 15].

   In 1999, Chinese academics Xia Jiahui, etc. reported 2 unrelated autosomal dominant Chinese deafness families. A heterozygous mutation of *GJB3* was found in two Chinese deaf families, and the *GJB3* gene was cloned. As of March 2015, there were 144 loci of non syndromic hearing loss in the world, including 31 autosomal dominant genes, 56 autosomal recessive genes, and 5 X-linked NSHL genes. At present, the target of deafness gene screening has been widely carried out in China. It is mainly focused on screening of *GJB2*, *SLC26A4* and mitochondrial *12sRNA A1555G* mutations [16].
2. Diagnostic techniques and applied strategies for genetic hearing loss gene screening
   (a) Screening and diagnostic techniques for deafness genes

   There are a variety of diagnostic techniques for deafness gene screening, which are simply summarized as two kinds of indirect and direct methods.
   - Direct method

     It is the sequence analysis of the target gene directly to identify whether there is a pathogenic mutation. It includes direct sequencing, gene chip, mass spectrometric analysis and SNP typing, each with advantages and disadvantages. The purpose of direct sequencing is to determine whether the specific genes of the subject are defective. It needs to make sure that a gene is a pathogenic gene of a disease, and known mutations, and take the peripheral blood or other tissue samples (including paraffin sections) of patients (or pro-band), to detect whether there is a genetic mutation of the gene by testing. This is the most clinically practical genetic deafness gene diagnosis strategy. The most commonly used method of mutation analysis is PCR-direct sequencing, and GeneChip and the next-generation of genome wide sequencing is also widely used in the detection of cloned deafness genes [17]. For the deaf families or the sporadic patients with unclear genotype, hot spot mutation screening is the most popular method. Gene mutation screening is based on a variety of experimental technology (PCR-HELP, fluorescent PCR, IMLDR, etc.) [18].
   - Indirect method

     Chromosome haplotype analysis, is closely linked to genes or genetic markers which are often passed to offspring based on inspection and therefore the adjacent DNA is passed to the offspring, can indirectly determine the causative gene is passed to the offspring, the purpose is clear the subject whether there from parental genetic disease gene. Genetic markers for accurate positioning information which needs to clear disease genes and the disease gene is closely linked to the relationship, the samples of patients (or pro-band) and their family members in peripheral blood or other tissue specimens (including paraffin), genetic heterogeneity of the ring shadow, DNA recombination the influence of. The linkage analysis uses a variety of DNA polymorphic loci widely used in the genome, especially gene mutation sites or adjacent polymorphic loci as markers. FFLP, SSCP, AnT and other techniques can be used for linkage analysis. This method is often used in the location and cloning of a new pathogenic gene for hereditary deafness.

Due to genetic deafness with genetic heterogeneity is very strong, most of the existing detection technology for mutation to, used for screening, has no clinical specificity, and detection of hereditary deafness are standard genetic deafness gene screening and diagnosis at home and abroad and there is no unified standard [19], at present. The team led by Professor Feng Yong of Xiangya Hospital, Central South University, has filed a diagnosis of genetic deafness phenotype of the strategy based on the hope from the current hot gene screening and has gradually achieved the purpose of gene diagnosis. Figure 8.46 is a genetic diagnosis strategy for genetic deafness developed by the Xiangya Hospital of Central South University.

(b) Clinical application strategies
- Candidate gene detection based on clinical phenotype: the application range is phenotypic—genotyping of sporadic patients or deaf people. According to the database and literature reports, we have drawn the phenotype genotype spectrum of genetic deafness genes [20]. Based on genotype and phenotype characteristics of various hereditary deafness we have worked out effective gene diagnosis strategy for hereditary hearing loss, part of which is shown in Fig. 8.47 [21].
- Hot spot mutation screening

  Applied range of deafness or phenotypic and genotypic undefined sporadic patients. For patients with unclear candidate gene screening, according to different clinical needs, Professor Feng Yong's

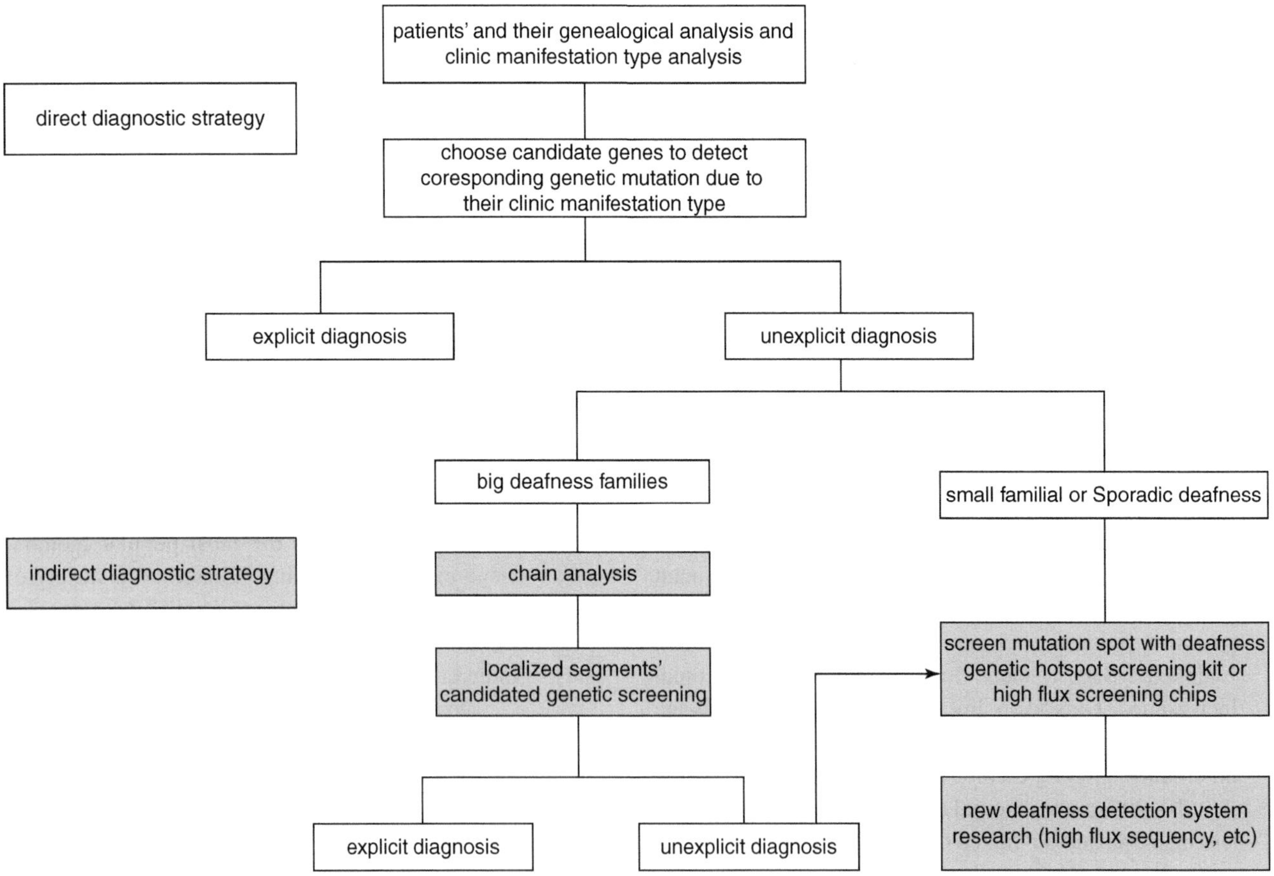


**Fig. 8.46** Xiangya hospital's genetic deafness's molecular diagnostic strategy figure

**Fig. 8.47** Xiangya hospital's genetic deafness genetic diagnosis strategy

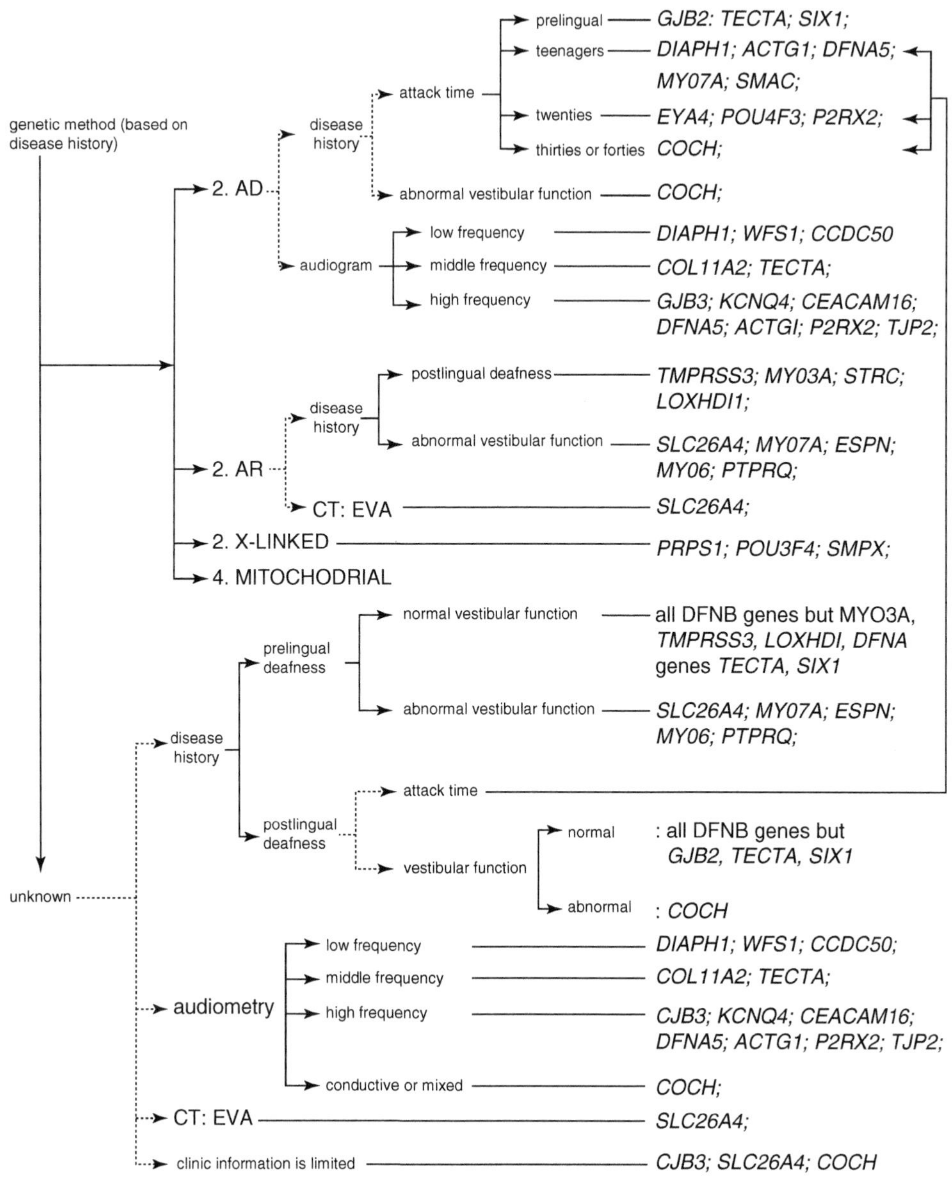


team of Xiangya Hospital, Central South University has designed various hot spot mutation kits. They are based on restriction fragment length polymorphism analysis (RFLP, which can detect 3 hot spots), fluorescent PCR Technology (detectable 14 hot spot mutations), and a new multiple band ligase Technology (IMLDR, which can detect 32 hotspot mutations) [22].

- high-throughput deafness gene diagnosis chips and copy number variation (CNVs) analysis:

Application scope is deafness gene mutuation screening in many hot spots where unclearly diagnosed patients could furthur expand the use of mutations screening, to establish a high throughput genetic deafness gene chip combined with mutation screening copy number variation for the currently known deafness mutation screening. For instance, Xiangya Hospital of Central South University [23] and Illumina company Goldengate384 chip project can detect 240 internationally recognized deafness causing mutations (including 77 dominant and 163 recessive mutations, also included 144 SNPs, of known deafness related high-throughput screening and deafness related mutation pedigree preliminary exclusion positioning. Copy number variation refers to the wide variation of human genome from deletion of 1000p (base pair) to millions of BP, insertion, repetition and complex multiple loci. The current molecular diagnosis of deafness is mainly focused on point mutation detection. There are reported copy number vari-

ants associated with deafness (WS, Usher syndrome, Teacher- Collins- Franceschetti syndrome, etc.), and CNVs has been detected in related genes. Therefore, the CNVs detection is included in the routine molecular diagnosis as a supplementary means for the detection of the clinical deafness gene, and the simultaneous detection of SNP/CNVs is realized [24].

(c) high throughput sequencing

The scope of application is to screen the genetic deafness patients without hot spot mutation, and it is also the future research direction of gene diagnosis. High throughput sequencing is based on the next-generation sequencing platform, which uses target acquisition technology to conduct high-throughput sequencing of deafness related tens or even hundreds of genes, which greatly improves detection efficiency and detection range [25]. It is suitable for finding new genes for deafness and screening for deaf patients without hot spots. Domestic and foreign scholars have cloned 8 deafness related genes (TPRN, GPSM2, CEACAM6, SMPX, HSD/7B4, HARS2, MASPI and DNMT1) using the second generation sequencing technology [26]. In addition, the development of this technology can further detect system based on the model, such as fragment enrichment technology to efficiently capture the target gene, reduce the cost of high-throughput sequencing, such as the Professor Feng Yong's team developed based on next-generation high-throughput sequencing technology "Waardenburg syndrome" and "large vestibular aqueduct syndrome" mutation detection kit.

3. Prenatal diagnosis

Prenatal diagnosis is a genetic diagnosis of a fetus with a risk of hereditary disease in the uterus before birth. By amniocentesis and chorionic villus sampling techniques, genetic and biochemical examination of amniotic fluid, amniotic fluid cells and villi were analyzed, the analysis and diagnosis of fetal chromosome and gene, is the effective way to prevent the birth of children with genetic diseases. Since the end of 1980s, PCR technology has been applied to prenatal gene diagnosis. With the development of this technology, people have received more and more attention and welcome. As far as it is concerned, it has become the most commonly used technique for genetic diagnosis of genetic disease. Various mutation gene detection methods based on this technique have become the main means of genetic disease gene diagnosis.

On the technical level, prenatal diagnosis is divided into invasive prenatal diagnosis and noninvasive prenatal diagnosis. The commonly used noninvasive prenatal diagnosis include amniocentesis, chorionic villus sampling, umbilical cord puncture, umbilical blood sampling, fetal tissue biopsy, pre-implantation genetic diagnosis; noninvasive prenatal diagnosis, including the detection of fetal cells in maternal peripheral blood by cervical exfoliated fetal trophoblast cells detection. According to the classification of the applicable stage of pre-implantation genetic diagnosis for in vitro fertilization embryo before implantation; often used in early pregnancy chorionic villus sampling (10~12 weeks), early amniocentesis (12~14 weeks), the detection of fetal cells in maternal peripheral blood (10 weeks, 15 weeks of gestation; mid pregnancy often uses the best) amniocentesis (16–18 weeks of gestation, umbilical blood sampling best) (after 16 weeks). These prenatal diagnosis methods have their own advantages and disadvantages. Amniocentesis is the most mature and widely accepted prenatal diagnosis technology because of its accuracy in diagnosis and low risk for pregnant women.

The prenatal diagnosis of hereditary deafness is currently used for members of the hereditary deafness family, which has been diagnosed by genetic diagnosis. When mother is pregnant, the fetal DNA is extracted through the above way, and then the prenatal diagnosis is made according to the genetic diagnosis of hereditary hearing loss. According to the results of prenatal diagnosis, early intervention can be done to avoid the birth of the new hereditary deafness [27].

4. The intervention system of hereditary deafness

Due to the lack of effective therapy, the three best interventions for hereditary hearing loss based on accurate gene diagnosis is the best choice. According to the result of gene diagnosis, we can intervene in deaf people of different ages. A level of intervention, specifically for the prenatal diagnosis of hereditary deafness and positive results of fetal prenatal intervention to reduce the incidence of grade two; early intervention, hearing screening and genetic screening of newborns has, according to the hearing status by effective early intervention (BAHA or cochlear hearing aids, etc.), reconstruction of hearing and speech function [28]; level three intervention, language of deaf patients, provide guidance on marriage according to audiological examination results by effective intervention (hearing aid fitting, BAHA or cochlear implantation) to establish the hearing, improve the quality of life of patients [29].

Due to the high genetic heterogeneity of genetic deafness and the fact that many pathogenic genes are not cloned, the genetic deafness detection carried out before is mostly limited to known genes or mutation sites. There are some limitations in clinical application. However, with the deepening of clinical phenotypic research on genetic deafness, the progress of molecular biology detection technology and the development of bioinformatics, the diagnosis technology of genetic deafness will continue to improve, and will eventually be widely applied in

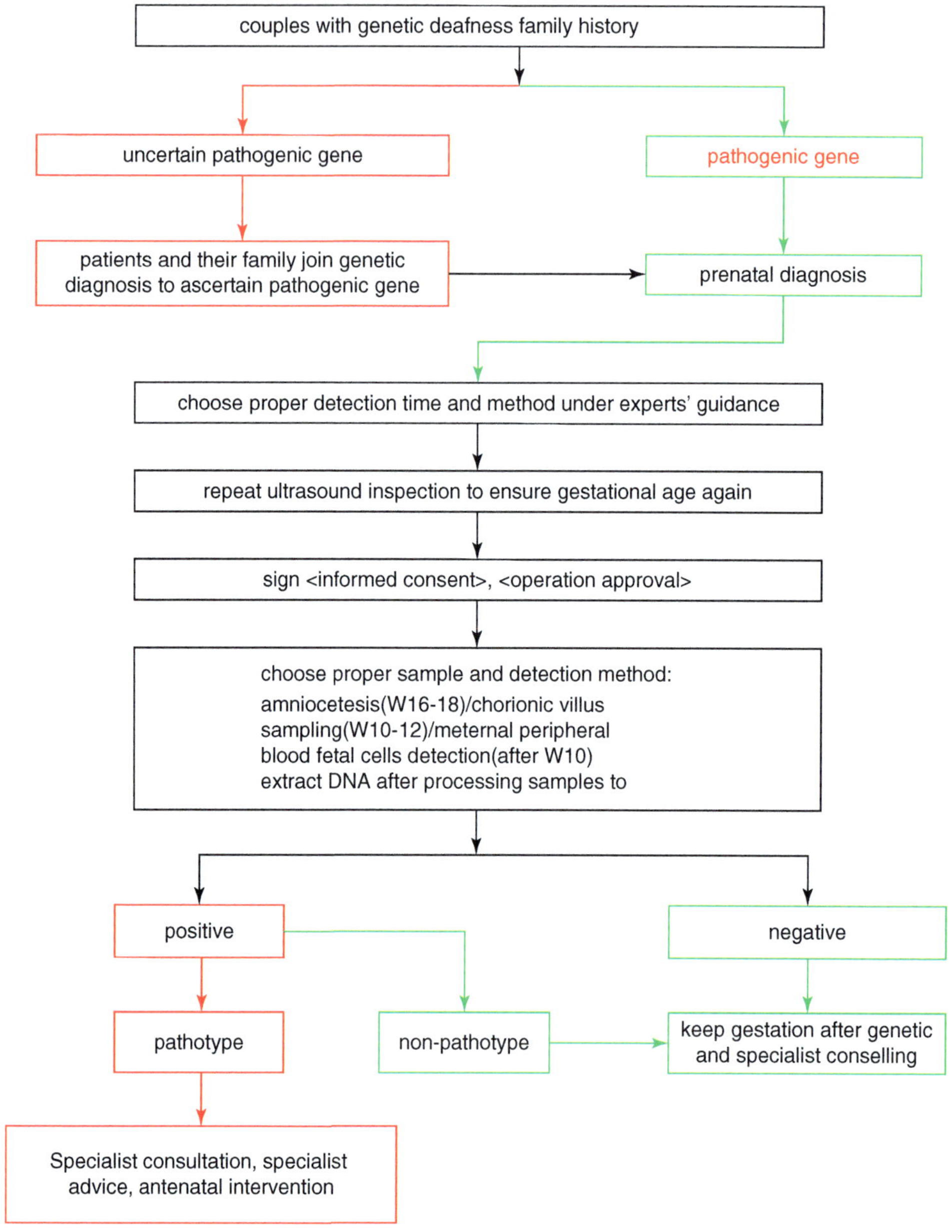


**Fig. 8.48** Prenatal genetic deafness diagnostic consultation and strategy flow

clinical practice and the prenatal diagnostic consultation and strategy flow of the genetic deafness could be made due to the information at Fig. 8.48.

## 8.14 Neonatal Hearing Screening

Newborn hearing screening can early detect congenital hearing loss, early intervention and early rehabilitation can make it deaf but not dumb and return to the mainstream society. However, universal newborn hearing screening is a systematic project, including screening, diagnosis, intervention, rehabilitation, follow-up and quality assessment, etc., which could only be accomplished by cooperation and adjustment among all the projects [30].

### 8.14.1 Summary of Newborn Hearing Screening

At 1993, the U.S. National Institutes of Health (NIH) recommended to carry out the universal newborn hearing screening. At 2000, American Joint Committee on infant hearing (JCIH) published the report, 'principles and guidelines for early hearing detection and intervention of the situation' [31], the principles and guidelines for newborn hearing screening became clear [31]. At 2007, 'situation report about principles and guidelines on early hearing detection and intervention project' [32] published by the United States JCH updated 8 structures of target hearing loss, including the definition, initial hearing screening and second hearing screening, the diagnostic audi-

tory evaluation, the medical evaluation, the early stage intervention, surveillance and screening in the medical home, the communication and information infrastructure, and strengthened the monitoring to the auditory neuropathy [32].

At 1990s, China carried out the universal newborn hearing screening project (UNHS) and developed under the support of the government. Since 2004, when the former ministry of health promulgated the 'technical gists of newborn hearing screening', UNHS had gradually spreaded at some of Chinese provinces and municipalities. At 2010, they promulagated the 2010 version of the gists to detaledly formulate the process and the quality of the newborn hearing screening. Till June, 2014, after the UNHS was widely carried out at Tibet, there are 32 provinces, municipalities and autonomous regions in total where it developped. According to incomplete statistics, recently the UNHS has been carried out at 77% of China. At some municipalities and sites in China, the goverment helps expanded the newborn hearing screening projects by researching at combining screening of the newborn auditory and the gene [33].

### 8.14.2 The Principle of UNHS

The current screening strategy for newborns in China is universal screening. The universal hearing screening refers to the application of electrophysiological detection technology to the hearing screening of all live newborns. UNHS is a systematic project, including screening, diagnosis, intervention, rehabilitation, tracking and quality assessment. Throughout the process, multi-disciplinary cooperation is always running as a vital role on accomplishment of UNHS.

The main principles of UNHS would be followed

1. General screening. All newborns in normal delivery room and NICU should receive hearing screening during hospitalization. Those who failed to pass the procedure should be rescreened at 42 days after delivery (NICU neonates should directly enter the diagnostic procedure).
2. Accept diagnosis in 3 months. To all infants who don't pass the secondary screening, auditory and medical evaluation should be performed in 3 months to ensure the existing of hearing loss.
3. Accept intervention in 6 months. All infants who have been diagnosed with permanent hearing loss should receive early intervention within 6 months old [34].

### 8.14.3 Newborn Hearing Screening Technique

Otoacoustic emissions (OAE) and automatic auditory brainstem response (AABR) are commonly techniques used during UNHS.

#### 8.14.3.1 Otoacoustic Emissions

Otoacoustic emissions (OAE) is a kind of audio energy generated from the ear, "the cochlea, the auditory ossicle chain and the tympanic membrane conduction", which are applied to the external ear canal. It reflects the function of the outer hair cells of the cochlea, but it is easy to be influenced by the function of the external middle ear. Usually, hearing loss exceeds 40 dB HL which OAE cannot record. The otoacoustic emissions technologies commonly used include the transient evoked otoacoustic emission (TEOAE) and distortion product otoacoustic emission (DPOAE). The reason why otoacoustic emission (OAE) is used for hearing screening is that it has many advantages, such as fast, accurate, objective, sensitive, noninvasive, simple and stable. But OAE also has some limitations: It can only reflect the function of the cochlear outer hair cells, the simple use of OAE screening, easily missed diagnosis of auditory neuropathy; susceptible factors of ear, ear residual fetal fat and amniotic fluid of incoming and outgoing stimulus response caused by otoacoustic emission attenuation, Create the illusion of not throughing [35, 36].

#### 8.14.3.2 Automatic Auditory Brainstem Response

AABR is an electrophysiological detection technology based on ABR. It can reflect the function from cochlea to auditory brainstem, and is relatively less affected by external and middle ear factors. Combination use with OAE can detect lesions behind the cochlea and reduce the false negative of hearing screening. However, AABR is not sensitive to low frequency hearing loss and mild hearing loss [37]. The results of hearing screening were recored as "pass" (through) or "refer" (not pass), but not "normal" or "abnormal" [38].

### 8.14.4 The process of UNHS [39]

1. Normal birth neonates are screened by two-stage screening: the initial screening was completed within 48 h after birth to the discharge, and rescreening month on both ears should be carried out within 42 days. Those who have not passed the screening should be referred to the children diagnosis centers for further diagnosis at the age of 3 months
2. Infants in the neonatal intensive care unit (NICU) were screened through automatic auditory brainstem response (AABR) before discharge, and if the newborns refer at initial screening, they should be transferred to children hearing diagnostic centers appointed by the provincial health administrative department 3 months after birth.
3. Neonates with high risk factors for hearing loss should be followed up once a year till 3. If they suspected to perform hearing loss during follow-up, they should be treated for hearing diagnosis in time.

High risk factors for hearing loss [40]:

1. The neonatal intensive care unit (NICU) was hospitalized for more than 5 days.
2. Family history of children with permanent hearing impairment.
3. Intrauterine infection caused by cytomegalovirus, rubella virus, herpes virus, syphilis, or toxoplasmosis disease.
4. Crania facial morphologic deformity, including auricle and ear canal deformity, etc.
5. The birth weight was less than 1500 g.
6. Hyperbilirubinemia meets the demand for change of blood.
7. Viral or bacterial meningitis.
8. Asphyxia neonatorum (Apgar score of 1 min, 0–4 or 5 min 0~6).
9. Premature infants with respiratory distress syndrome.
10. Oxygen in vitro membrane.
11. Mechanical ventilation was more than 48 h.
12. Pregnant women had used ototoxic drugs, loop diuretics or alcohol and drug abuse
13. In clinic or suspected to be associated with hearing disorder syndrome or hereditary diseases.

### 8.14.5 Audiological Assessment and Diagnosis

ENT doctors have the responsibility and obligation mechanism, diagnosis and therapy of combined screening institutions and ask parents to pay more attention to the early hearing diagnosis of infant, who play important role in the universal newborn hearing screening system. The diagnostic principles and procedures are as follows:

1. Newborns without passing should be diagnosed within 3 months.
2. Newborns in NICU who refer UNHS should be directly referred to the children hearing diagnostic centers for diagnosis and follow-up.
3. The hearing diagnosis should be intersected according to the test results to determine the degree and nature of hearing impairment. Children suspected of having other defects or systemic diseases were instructed to go to related departments, suspected of hearing impairment due to genetic factors, and genetic counseling for conditional health care institutions.
4. Diagnosis process
   (a) Collection of medical history.
   (b) Otolaryngology examination.
   (c) Hearing tests should include the contents of electrophysiological and pediatric behavioral audiometry, including acoustic impedance (including 1000 Hz detection), otoacoustic emissions (OAE), auditory brainstem response (ABR) and behavioral audiometry [41].
   (d) Auxiliary examination, if necessary, relevant imaging and laboratory auxiliary examination [1].

### 8.14.6 Intervention

The diagnosis of children with permanent hearing impairment should be carried out in clinical.

### 8.14.7 Follow Up

1. The screening agency was responsible for the follow-up and rescreening after initial screening. The patients who refer UNHS should be referred to the children hearing diagnostic centers.
2. The diagnosis and treatment facility should be responsible for the follow-up, diagnosis for hearing impaired children every six months (at least one time).
3. The requirements and procedures of follow-up work should be developed and included in the routine of maternal and child health care. The maternal and child health care institutions should assist the diagnosis and therapy institutions to complete the follow-up of the children diagnosed, and collect all the data of registration and preservation, instruct the community health service center to finish that well.

### 8.14.8 Rehabilitation

1. For children who use artificial hearing devices, professional hearing and speech rehabilitation training should be carried out. Check and debug regularly.
2. Parents or guardians who instruct children with hearing impairment are put on record to the relevant departments of the resident and the disabled in order to receive family rehabilitation guidance.

### 8.14.9 Quality Control

The health administrative department should organize the formulation of the assessment and evaluation plan, supervise and inspect the screening institutions and hearing impaired diagnosis institutions regularly, control the quality of every link of newborn hearing screening, find out problems and take effective measures timely.

The newborn hearing screening center or the medical institution designated by the health administrative department to undertake the hearing impairment diagnosis and therapy work should establish the newborn hearing screening database, and carry out the information management work of UNHS [42].

## 8.15 Hearing Aids

### 8.15.1 Hearing Aids Development History

Hearing aids (hearing aid) are small expansion device for hearing loss and compensation for hearing loss. Its development has gone through seven times: set the sound cylinder device, carbon, electron tubes, transistors, integrated circuits, microprocessors and digital hearing aids era.

Today's hearing aids has entered the full digital signal processing interface generation, including compression and amplification, noise reduction technology, digital feedback control technology and direction of technology, the application of these technologies, it can meet the hearing impaired. With the continuous development of digital chip technology, hearing aid technology include the latest simulation of complex wide dynamic range compression system, net noise system, dual stabilizer digital feedback control technology, intelligent system, reality adaptive directional conversion system, open ear technology, real-time data analysis system and fitting software and hardware support system, can provide users with clear, comfortable and natural listening experience. From the appearance and development of BTE, cassette, glasses, hairpin, pen, wireless and other shapes for different patients, more beautiful appearance effect. We believe that in the future, the volume of the hearing aids will become smaller and smaller, and the function will become more and more perfect.

### 8.15.2 Hearing Aids Categories

There are many ways to classify hearing aids.

1. According to their shape

   Can be divided into 5 categories: cassette, glasses, behind-the-ear type, in the ear canal type, and bone-anchored hearing aid. The glasses type BTE hearing aids, also known as ear level hearing aid, hearing aid ear level hearing aid receiving sound manner than other types of more close to the physiological state.

   (a) box hearing aid: The box hearing aid appeared earlier and larger. It looked like a miniature radio. It wore a conductor to transmit the voice output signal to the earphone before wearing it. More ordinary transistor components are used, so the price is low and the background noise is high. For the fingers gone: because the box hearing aids often friction with clothing, the sound of friction often becomes noise (Fig. 8.49).

   (b) glasses hearing aids: Only a body worn to the development process of ear level aid in transition products, microphone and receiver capable of leg in different, the signal of (contralateral routing of signal, CROS), are also in the same mirror on the legs (Fig. 8.50).

   (c) BTE: BTE hearing aids is now the most widely used, the shape of slender, rely on a hard plastic ear hook bent into a semicircular hang on the ear, can use the skin or hair color shell to hide, the amplified sound through the ear hook through a plastic the incoming sound hole in the eardrum tube (Fig. 8.51).

   (d) in the ear canal hearing aids (ITE-HA)

   It includes the ITE-HA (Fig. 8.52) and the in-the-canal HA (ITC-HA). The ITE-HA contains the gen-

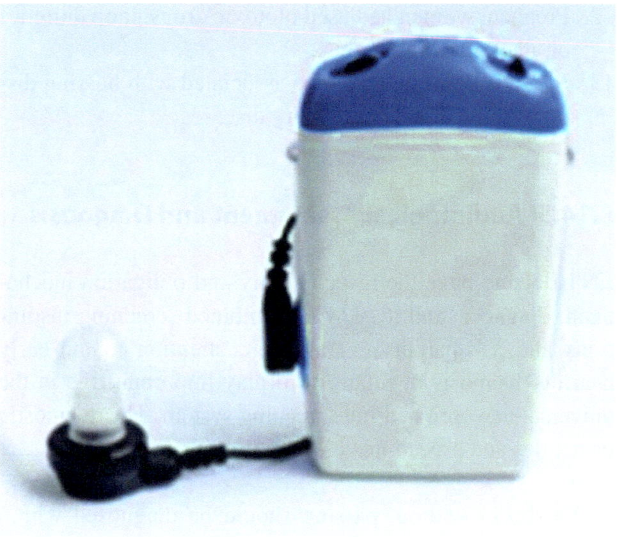

**Fig. 8.49** Box hearing aid

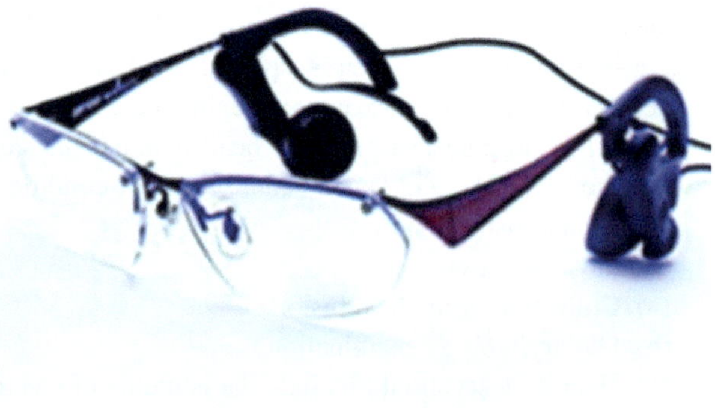

**Fig. 8.50** The eyeglass hearing aids (EG-HA)

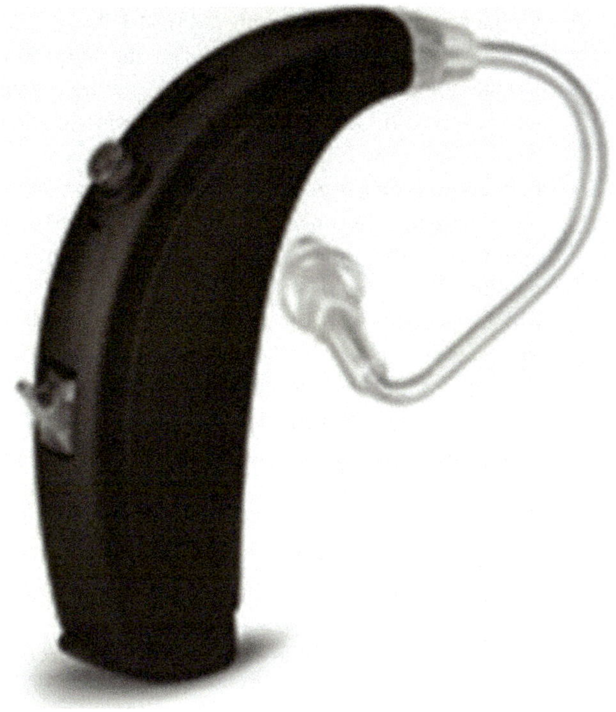

Fig. 8.51 Behind-the-ear hearing aids (BTE-HA)

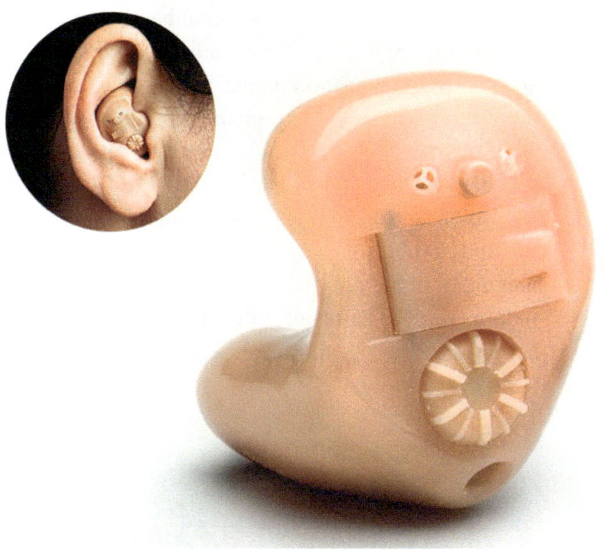

Fig. 8.52 ITE-HA

eral and the partial HA. The ITC-HA has the complete in-canal (CIC) hearing aid (Fig. 8.53). The ITE has an exquisite configuration and is custom-made. Input the aid into the cavum conchae or channel conceals without any tubes or wires. The output power of the ITE isn't high, so it is only helpful to the mild and moderate deafness.

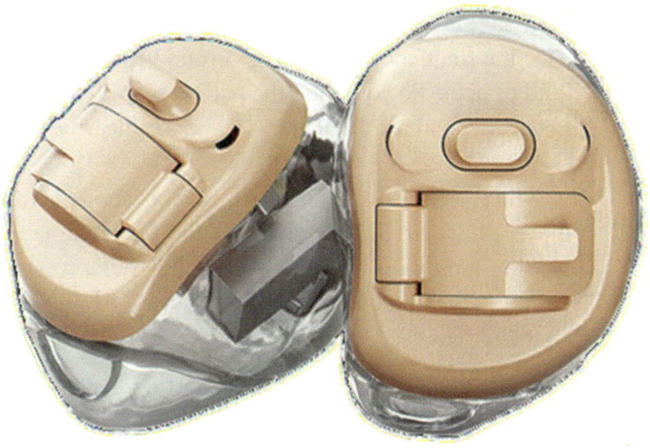

Fig. 8.53 ITC

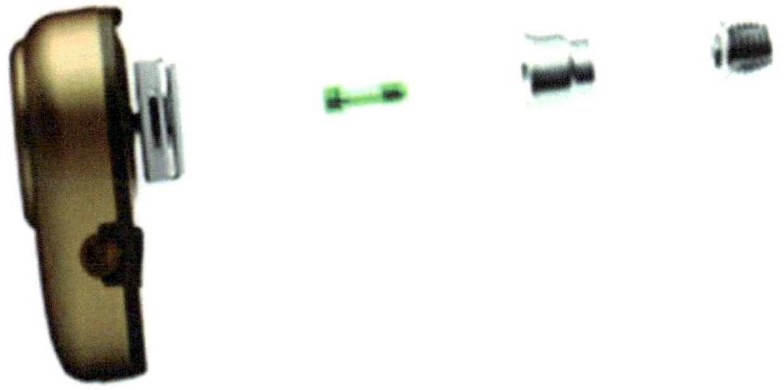

Fig. 8.54 BA-HA

(e) bone anchored hearing aids (BA-HA)

It is a surgical implanting system to treat the hearing loss, conducting the sound through the temporal bone but not the mid-ear (Fig. 8.54). The full introduction is as before (Figs. 8.31 and 8.32). The U.S FDA ratified that the BAHA could be applied on treating the conductive and mixed deafness in 1996 and on unilateral sensorineural deafness in 2002. The BAHA is used to treat the otitis media, the congenital ankylotia and the unilateral deafness who can't use the regular hearing-aids.

2. Classification due to dynamic frequency response

It can divided into two types according to the dynamic frequency response characteristics. After people measure the static frequency response of the hearing aids with several kinds of equipments, they focus more on its dynamic characteristics because that the sound we hear is in dynamic change at the frequency and the strength.

(a) Fixed frequency response hearing aids (FFR-HA)

Most of the hearing aid in market is the FFR-HA. Its frequency response is determined while being produced. The intonation button could only adjust a certain degree of the frequency response. Once the optional Personnels set the parameters of the hearing aids, the frequency response is certain no matter what kind of acoustic condition the patient is in.

(b) Level dependent frequency response hearing aid (LEFD-HA)

The typical TILL type hearing aids is applied with the K-Amp circuit, but most of the programmable hearing aids with wide dynamic range compression circuit are more matching the LDFD-HA characteristics.

3. Classification due to the effecting area

It is divided into the group hearing aids and the personal hearing aids. The personal ones fit specific personnel and the group ones are always applied to the audio-visual education, the outdoors education and especially the deaf-infants rehabilitation or school education. According to the specific function, it could be classified into three types.

(a) Fixed wired collective hearing aid (FWC-HA)

Similar to the audio spoken language classroom system: there are a master for the teacher and an extension for each student, both having a microphone and an earphone. The master computer could attach to the recorder or other assisting facilities. The information can also be shared between the master and the extension and the extensions, which causes the free discussion possible. With the advance group hearing aids, the teacher can adjust the earphone volumes according to each one's condition without any distance limit and let all of them could hear clear and moderate voice no matter where they are sitting. All above offer benefit to the spoken language teaching and improve the deaf's linguistic competence. But a coin has two sides. The disadvantages are the position limit and the possible discrepant frequency response compared to their own.

(b) Frequency modulation hearing aid (FM-HA)

The sound source passes through the frequency modulation producer (microphone-like) to be shared and accepted by one or more frequency modulation hearing aids. The FAMHA worn by the deafness not only could accept the demodulated sound signals by the 'demodulation' units, but also it can be used as a common hearing aid because of its same fitting parameters as the common ones (Fig. 8.55). The FMHA is convenient for the deafness by expanding their action area into a 100 radius and for the outdoor education of the deaf infants. The one-to-one hearing aids fit those deaf infants who have accepted the listening and speech exercise and been able to take class with normal infants in school. The teachers wear a microphone, so the deaf could hear the teachers clearly wherever they sits. Some family set the frequency modulation producer beside the TV louder to help the deaf hear the TV audio.

(c) Closed-circuit electromagnetic induction collective hearing system (CEMIC-HS)

Also called the Induction loop system (ILS). It includes the main console (the amplifier, the frequency modulation components), the coil early arranged in the indoors such as the classrooms and the family houses and the personal hearing aids with T gear (Fig. 8.56). The trans-audience, the amplifier and the frequency modulation units could emission the electromagnetic voice of the recorder, the radio, the TV and the teachers to the area the coils encircle. The deaf could turn the hearing aid to the T (tele-coil) gear to accept the distinct voice without the distance and the number of people limit through the electromagnetic induction principle in the coil-arranged indoors room. The result is directly related to the coil setting and the T gear telecoil sensitivity.

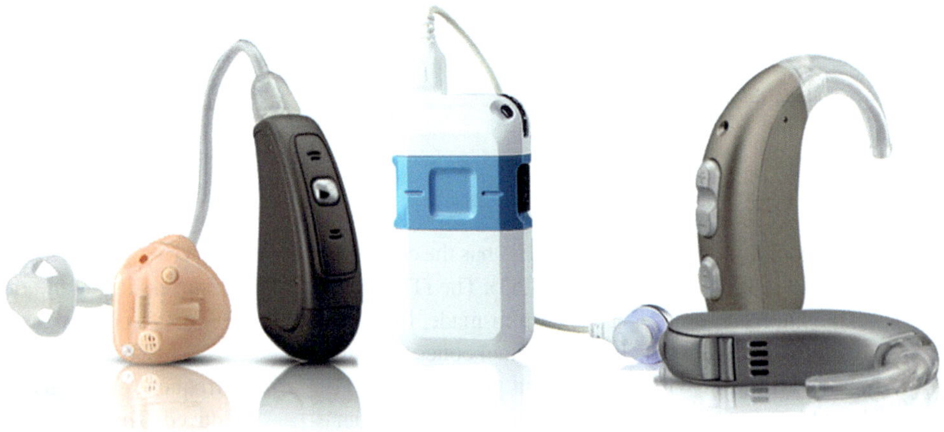

**Fig. 8.55** FM-HA

Fig. 8.56 CEMIC-HS/ILS

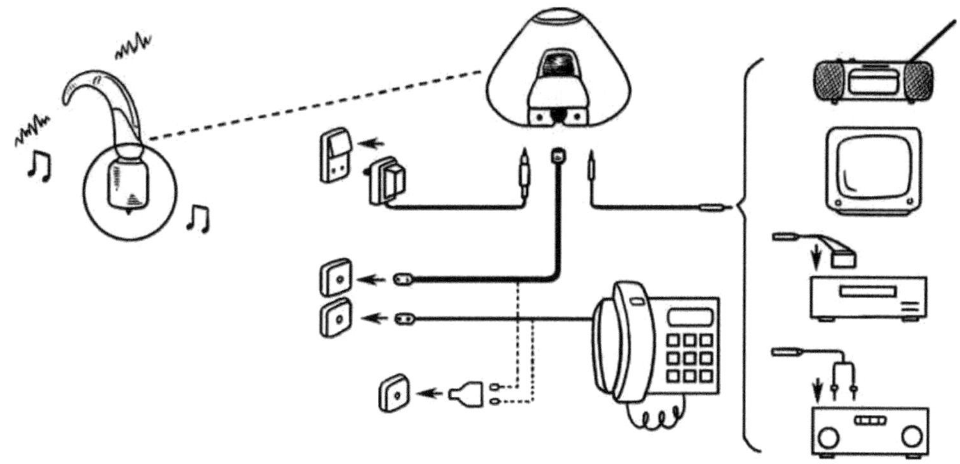

### 8.15.3 Hearing Aids Fitting

'Fitting' means that the user chooses the proper hearing aid under guideline of the professionals. Similar to the glasses, the hearing aids are also a kind of the 'fitted' auxiliary equipments for human physiologic functions.

Firstly, the hearing loss of each person varies. Cite the presbycusis examples, different deafness types, different hearing loss degrees, presence of the tinnitus, sensitivity to the voice level, audition recognition ability, etc. cause different audition difference. Different hearing loss needs different hearing aids. Actually, even to the deaf at the same property and level of the hearing disorders, the personal feeling may differ. These differences may be relative to the habits, the work environments, the subjective tolerance capacity, etc. The feeling difference cause different requirements to the hearing aids.

Secondly, there is quantity of the hearing aids brands and models, which cause that the fitting, could only be asked to be done by the professionals. Such as how the patients with severe hearing loss but sensitive to the high intensity sound choose the hearing aids? They would in-tolerate the voice while focusing on the volume up; they would not hear the voice clearly while focusing on the high intensity sound compression. Balancing the conflict is one of the main missions the professional fitting should do.

The perfect aided effect could only be achieved when the audition conditions and the chosen hearing aids' coefficient completely tally. The hearing disorders type decides the hearing aids property, and the 'fitting 'is the bridge between them. Most of the unfitted hearing aids can't achieve aided effects, possibly do harm to the remnant hearing of the wearer and even cause severer hearing loss. Due to experience above, the hearing aids should be adequately fitted by the professional fitters, then it works.

The hearing aids are the type II medical equipments in China, so there is severe licensing system on the industry service.

## References


1. Jahrsdoerfer RA, Yeakley JW, Aguilar EA, Cole RR, Gray LC. Grading system for the selection of patients with congenital aural atresia. Am J Otol. 1992;13(1):6–12.
2. Chinese Medical Association. Otorhinolaryngology Head and Neck Surgery branches otology group, Chinese Otorhinolaryngology Head and Neck Surgery journal's edition committee otology group. Otitis media clinical classification and operative type guide. J Chin Otorhinolaryngol Head Neck Surg. 2013;48(1):6–10.
3. Chinese Otorhinolaryngology Head and Neck Surgery Journal's Editors' Committee. Acute deafness diagnosis and treatment guide (2015). J Chin Otorhinolaryngol Head Neck Surg. 2015;50(6):443–7.
4. Chinese Otorhinolaryngology Head and Neck Surgery Journal of Editors' Committee, Chinese Medical Association Otorhinolaryngology Fascicle. Benign paroxymal localization vertigo's diagnostic gist and evaluation. J Chin Otorhinolaryngol Head Neck Surg. 2007;42(3):163–4.
5. Naples JG, Eisen MD. Surgical management for benign paroxysmal positional vertigo of the superior semicircular canal. Laryngoscope. 2015;125(8):1965–7.
6. Hsieh LC, Lin HC, Tsai HT, et al. High-dose intratympanic gentamicin instillations for treatment of Meniere's disease: long-term results. Acta Otolaryngol. 2009;129(12):1420–4.
7. Wetmore SJ. Endolymphatic sac surgery for Meniere's disease: long-term results after primary and revision surgery. Arch Otolaryngol Head Neck Surg. 2008;134(11):1144–8.
8. Hu A, Parnes LS. 10-year review of endolymphatic sac surgery for in-tractable Ménière disease. J Otolaryngol Head Neck Surg. 2010;39(4):415–21.
9. Ahsan SF, Standring R, Wang Y. Systematic review and meta-analysis of Meniett therapy for Meniere's disease. Laryngoscope. 2015;125(1):203–8.
10. Monsell EM, Balkany TA, Gates GA, et al. Committee on hearing and equilibrium guidelines for the diagnosis and evaluation of therapy in Ménière disease. Otolaryngol Head Neck Surg. 1995;113:181–5.
11. Chinese Otorhinolaryngology Head and Neck Surgery Journal's Editors' Committee. Ménière disease's diagnostic gist and efficacy evaluation (2006, Guiyang). J Chin Otorhinolaryngol Head Neck Surg. 2008;42(3):163.
12. Stachler RJ, Chandrasekhar SS, Archer SM, et al. Clinical practice guideline: sudden hearing loss. Otolaryngol Head Neck Surg. 2012;146(3 Suppl):S1–S35.

13. Xia J. Medical genetics. Beijing: People's Medical Publishing House; 2004.
14. Hilgert N, Smith RJ, Van Camp G. Forty-six genes causing nonsyndromic hearing impairment: which ones should be analyzed in DNA diagnostics? Mutat Res. 2009;681(2–3):189–96.
15. Rodriguez-Paris J, Pique L, Colen T, Roberson J, Gardner P, Schrijver I. Genotyping with a 198 mutation arrayed primer extension array for hereditary hearing loss: assessment of its diagnostic value for medical practice. PLoS One. 2010;5(7):e11804.
16. Zeng Y. Hereditary diseases' genetic diagnosis and treatment. 1st ed. Shanghai: Shanghai Scientific & Technical Publishers; 1999.
17. Yand TM, Blanton SH, et al. Next-generation sequencing in genetic hearing loss. Genet Test Mol Biomarkers. 2013;17(8):581–7.
18. Ruan G, Lu C, Xia J. Genetic mutation analysis technique sum. Foreign Med Genet Fascic. 1988;21(5):225–3.
19. Feng Y, He C, Xiao J, et al. Genetic deafness gene diagnostic teniques' building and origional clinical application. J Chin Mod Med. 2002;12(4):20–2.
20. Bitner-Glindzicz M. Hereditary deafness and phenotyping in humans. Br Med Bull. 2002;63:73–94.
21. Feng Y, He C, Xiao J, et al. Hereditary deafness genetic diagnosis techniques' initial establishment and initial clinical application. China J Mod Med. 2002;12:20–2.
22. Zhao J, Wu L, Feng Y, et al. Apply polymerase chain reaction-limited fragment length polymorphism technique to rapidly detect Chinese deafness personnels' genetic mutation hot spots. J Chinese Med Genet. 2009;26(5):518–20.
23. Qu C, Sun X, Shi Y, et al. Microarray-based mutation detection of pediatric sporadic nonsyndromic hearing loss in China. Int J Pediatr Otorhinolaryngol. 2012;76(2):235–9.
24. Rehm HL. Genetics and the genome project. Ear Hear. 2003;24(4):270–4.
25. Xia JH, Liu CY, Tang BS, et al. Mutations in the gene encoding gap junction protein beta-3-associated with autosomal dominant hearing impairment. Nat Genet. 1998;20:370–3.
26. Long Z, Xing E, Wang Y. Cytogenetics prenatal diagnosis techniques and norms. Chin J Pract Gynecol Obstet. 2015;31(9):811–4.
27. Liu Q. Prenatal diagnosis and prephylaxis and treatment of hereditary diseases. Chin J Pract Gynecol Obstet. 2002;18(9):514–51.
28. Yoshinaga-Itano C, Sedey AL, Coulter DK, Mehl AL. Language of early and later-identified children with hearing loss. Pediatrics. 1998;102(5):1161–71.
29. Health Ministry General Office of People's Republic of China. Infants diseases screening techniques norm. 2010 ed. 2010.
30. Han D. Newborn and infants hearing screening. Beijing: People's Medical Publishing House; 2003. p. 93–154.
31. Joint Committee on Infant Hearing. Year 2007 position statement: principles and guidelines for early hearing detection and intervention programs. Am J Audiol. 2000;9(1):9–29.
32. American Academy of Pediatrics, Joint Committee on Infant Hearing. Year 2007 position statement: principles and guidelines for early hearing detection and intervention programs. Pediatrics. 2007;120(4):898–921.
33. Haowu YH. Infants hearing screening, vol. 2014. 2nd ed. Beijing: People's Medical Publishing House. p. 177–203.
34. Huang L, Han D. Infants hearing disorder's early interfere. J Chin Otorhinolaryngol Head Neck Surg. 2011;46(3):186–9.
35. Nie YJ, Qi YS, Zhao XT, et al. Value of otoacoustic emission (OAE) technique in perinatal audiology. Chin Arch Otolaryngol Head Neck Surg. 1999;6(4):207–11.
36. Liao H, Wu ZY, Zhou T, et al. Transient evoked otoacoustic emission in healthy newborn. J Audiol Speech Pathol. 1997;5(4):184–6.
37. Li XL, Pu XK, Lu L, et al. Automatic auditory brainstem response in neonatal hearing screening[J]. CJCHC. 2008;16(1):47–50.
38. Huang L. Unscramble 2010 edition infant hearing screening technique norm. J Audiol Speech Dis. 2011;19(6):495–6.
39. Nie YJ, Cai ZH, Qi YS, et al. Research and application of newborn hearing screening model. J Audiol Speech Pathol. 2002;9:1–4.
40. Wu H, Huang ZW. Newborn hearing screening. 2nd ed. Beijing: People's Medicine Publishing House; 2014.
41. Huang LH, Han DM, Liu S, et al. Follow-up study for newborns and infants who failed hearing screening. Zhonghua Er Bi Yan Hou Tou Jing Wai Ke Za Zhi. 2005;40(9):643–7.
42. Ni D. Screening infants hearing well is otorhinolaryngologists' duty. J Chin Med. 2004;84(6):445–6.
43. Bars DM. Temporal bone cancer. Translated by Mou Z, Long H, Han D. Foreign medicine: otorhinolarngology branch. 2004;(3):186–188.

# Part III

# Rhinology

Nose is the portal of respiratory tract. It is adjacent to vital organs. It is connected with cranio-cerebral, orbital, middle ear and throat through nasopharynx, and palatal bone at the base of mouth. Nasal diseases not only affect their physiological functions, but also damage adjacent organs. With the development of electronics and photologic and the wide application of endoscopy, nasal science has made breakthroughs. On the basis of discussing the applied anatomy and physiology of the nose, this section discusses the symptoms and examination methods, common diseases, therapeutic procedures and surgeries of the nose.

# 9 Applied Anatomy and Physiology of Nose

Xin Wei and Xun Bi

## 9.1 Applied Anatomy of Nose

Nose contains external nose, nasal vestibule, proper nasal cavity and sinuses.

### 9.1.1 External Nose

External nose protrude from the center of face (Fig. 9.1). Its upper end rises up between two eyes, this is called nasion. Where the most prominent part of the lower exterior nose is called nasal apex. The interconnection piece between them is called Rhinal Bridge, whose bevel is called nasal dorsum. There are two anterior naris separated by the nasal column and their upper and lateral profiles are constituted with the nasal alar. The nasal alar is a round hump and the nasal alar flap mostly occurs in dyspnea.

Shapes of the external nose depend on the bone and the cartilage support. Upper 1/3 of the external nasal support is bony, mainly constituted with nasal bone, and lower 2/3 is formed with several cartilages. Upper nasal bone is narrow and thick, lower is wide and thin, so nasal fracture mainly occurs in the lower and it manifestates as rhinal dorsum collapse of the suffered side.

The nasal skin is thicker at the nasal apex and the nasal alar, containing plenty of the sebaceous and the sub-oriferous glands, which is also the leading sites for the nasal furuncle. The sub epithelium tissue is dense so swelling of the skin cause severe pain due to compression of the nerve endings during inflammation process. The external nose facial veins afflux at the angular veins and the venae facialis anterior. The venae facialis anterior opens to the cavernous sinus through the venae ophthalmica superior and inferior, and there aren't any venous valves, what makes the up and down circulation, such as the oppression on the nasal furuncle causes the risk of the congestion cavernous sinus thrombophlebitis. And the patients will experience headache, rigor, high fever, eyelid and tunica conjunctiva edema, protopsis, and the severe form could cause death.

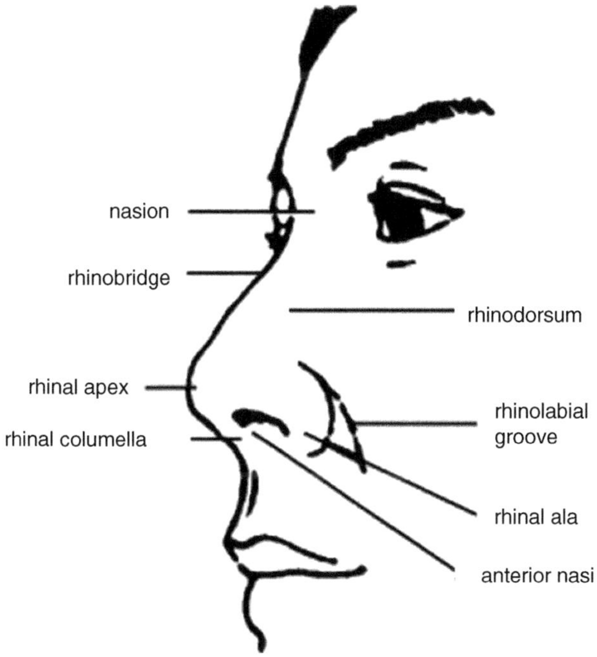


**Fig. 9.1** The external nose anatomy

### 9.1.2 Rhinal Vestibule

It starts at the anterior naris and ends at the inner nostril, which corresponds to the field surrounded by the nasal alar. The nasal column divides it into right and left parts. The rhinal vestibule is lined with skin abundant in sebaceous glands and has nasal hair (rhinothrix).

X. Wei (✉)
Department of Otorhinolaryngology Head and Neck Surgery, Hainan People's Hospital, Haikou, China

X. Bi
Department of Pediatric Surgery, The First Affiliated Hospital of Hainan Medical University, Haikou, China


Z. Mu, J. Fang (eds.), *Practical Otorhinolaryngology - Head and Neck Surgery*, https://doi.org/10.1007/978-981-13-7993-2_9

### 9.1.3 Proper Rhinal Cavum

It's also called rhinocavum (nasal cavity), which originates from the inner nostril and ends at the posterior nostril (choana). The internal wall is the septum nasi and divides the cavum nasi into the right side and the left side. The anterior and inferior parts of the nasal septum are composed of nasal septum cartilage, and the upper and posterior parts are bone osteone. Most at times, the septum nasi is slightly frank curveted or locally protruded without any symptoms to be dealt with.

The lateral cavum nasi wall has complex structures, including three echelons lining bony tissues from up to down, the superior nasal concha, the middle nasal concha and the inferior nasal concha (Fig. 9.2). The inferior nasal concha is the biggest, and it previously ends at the internal cavum nasi, inferiorly ends at the choana and also 10–15 mm to the pharyngeal opening of the eustachian tube. Hence, the swelling of the inferior nasal concha during rhinitis can not only cause nasal obstruction, but also hinder the ventilation and drainage function of the eustachian tube, resulting in tinnitus, hearing loss and other symptoms.

Between the inferior nasal concha and the lateral wall of the nasal cavity is the inferior nasal meatus, which is dome-shaped and has an opening of nasallacrimal duct at the top. The lateral wall of inferior turbinate is the thinnest 1–2 cm away from the anterior end of inferior turbinate, which can be used as the needle entry site for maxillary sinus puncture. The middle rhinomeatus locates at the infralateral middle nasal concha and it is the drainage aperture of the frontal sinus, the anterior ethmoid sinus and the maxillary sinus. Because the anatomic structure abnormality and the pathologic change of the middle nasal concha, of the middle meatus nasi and on the peripheral area are closely attached to the nasosinusitis, there is an ostiomeatal complex, including the ethmoidal infundibulum, the processus uncinatus, the ethmoidal bulla, semilunar hiatus, the middle meatus nasi, the anterior ethmoid sinus, aperture sinus frontalis, the maxillary sinus aperture and other structures.

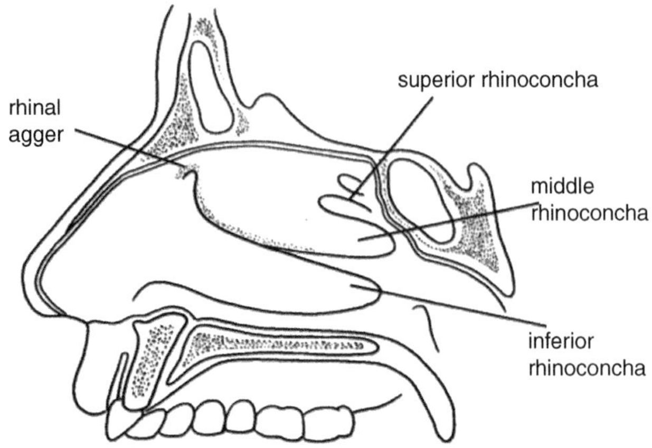

**Fig. 9.2** The nasal fossa parries lateralis anatomy

The gap between the middle nasal concha and the nasal septum is the olfactory fissure, which absorbs the airflow into the olfactory field. If the nasal septum deviates or the middle nasal concha swells it can causes the olfactory fissure obstruction and finally decreases the smell sense. The entire cavum nasi lining mucosa could be divided into the olfactory field and the respiratory region according to the mucosa features. The olfactory field locates at the middle superior cavum nasi, covered with the olfactory mucosa whose contents the olfactory glands, the olfacto cytes and the olfactory nerve, perform the olfactory function. The respiratory region is the sites under the horizontal fontal middle nasal concha in the cavum nasi. Most of the mucosa at this region is the ciliated columnar epithelium and is the continuity to the nasal sinus, the nasopharynx Eustachian tube and the middle ear cavum tympanum cavity. The nasal mucosa inflammation could spread to these corresponding positions above to cause the eustachian tube deformity and the otitis media.

There are abundant blood vessels in the nasal mucosa, especially the inferior nasal concha. There are plenty of the vascular sinuses, so it's also called the nasal concha cavernous body. Based on the main functions of these vessels, they can be divided into the capacity vessels (vein, vascular sinus), the resistance vessels (arteriole, arteriovenous ramus anastomosis) and the exchange vessels (capillary). Autonomic nerve branches innervates the blood vessels causing vasodilatation and vasoconstriction that regulate blood flow and change the volume of inferior nasal concha, which play an important role in the normal physiological function of nasal cavity (cavum nasi).

### 9.1.4 Paranasal Sinuses

The paranasal sinuses are the air-containing cavities in the craniofacial bone surrounding the cavum nasi, all open to the aperture contained with the cavum nasi. The inter sinus continues through the aperture sinus and the cavum nasi mucosa, and the inter sinus secret expels from the aperture sinus. The nasal sinus is around in pairs at left and the right sides, summing to four pairs. The sinus mucosa continues with the nasal mucosa through the ostium of the sinus, and the sinus endocrine is discharged through the ostium of the sinus. There were four pairs of paranasal sinuses (Fig. 9.3).

According to the locating skull parts, it can be divided into maxillary sinus, ethmoidal sinus, frontal sinus and sphenoid sinus.

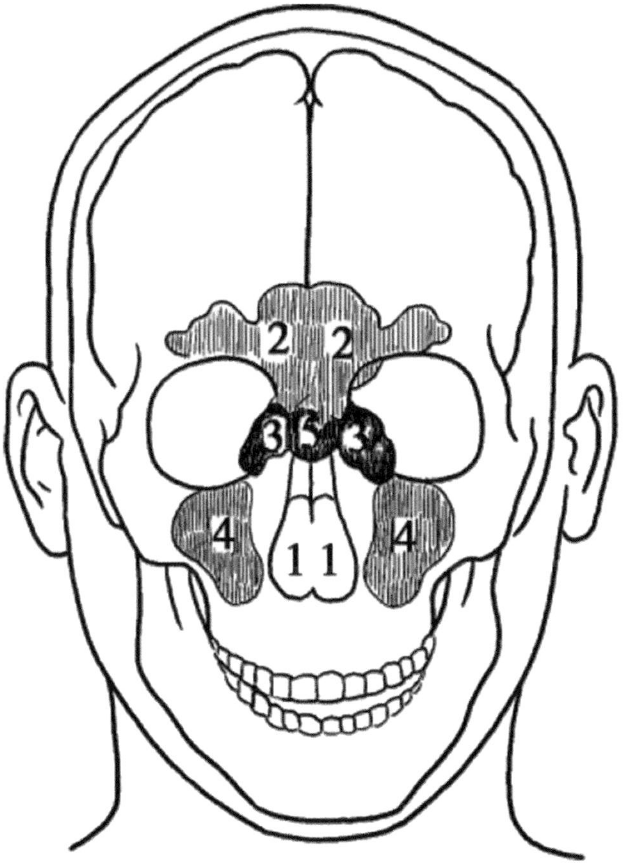


**Fig. 9.3** The nasal sinus. 1. The nasal fossa; 2. The frontal sinus; 3. The ethmoidal cellules; 4. Maxillary antrum; 5. Sphenoid sinus

The maxillary sinus locates at bilateral profile of the cave nasal and is the biggest of the nasal sinuses. The maxillary sinus's superior wall is also the inferior orbital wall, it is also where the maxillary malignant tumor invades the orbital wall to cause the protrusion of the eyeball and fracture could cause the exophthalmos. The nasal sinuses' basic wall is the maxillary bone alveolar process. The first and second molars fang (root) inflammation could evoke the odontogenic maxillary sinusitis. The maxillary sinusitis originally occurs as the maxillary sinus carcinoma at the basic wall and symptoms at its early stage are the gomphiasis, the numbness and the toothache. The internal wall of the maxillary sinus is the lateral wall of the cave nasal and its aperture is in the middle meatus nasi. The aperture locates at a high sites and the sinus cavity base is lower to the cavum nasi base, so the structures cause the intrasinus secreta drainage abnormality and finally the maxillary sinus could be easily susceptible to infection. The post-lateral wall is adjacent to the infra temporal fossa and the pterygopalatine fossa, and it is the sites where the maxillary sinus carcinoma affect this wall and invades the medial pterygoid muscle resulting in limited mouth opening.

The ethmoidal sinus locates in the ethmoid between the orbital and the cavum nasi. Its lateral ethmoid papyraceous lamina wall is adjacent to the ethmoid paper like plate. The sinus ethmoiditis could evoke the intraorbital inflammation through the papyraceous lamina. The upper wall is the ethmoid apex and upwards the anterior cranial fossa.

The frontal sinus locates in the frontal bone upwards the nose and is around in pairs at left and right. The ethmoid sinus opens to the frontal fossa through the aperture of the frontal sinus and its base decides the frontal sinus drainage according to the processus uncinatus attachment.

The sphenoid sinus is located in the sphenoid bone post-superior to the cavum nasi. Its lateral wall is adjacent to the cavernous sinus, the internal carotid and the optic canal. In the well gasified sphenoid sinus, the internal carotid and the optic canal produce the promontory, such as the sclerotin thinness and loss. The endoscopic surgery could injure the optic nerve or the internal carotid and finally causes blindness or fatal hemorrhage. Its top wall is the middle cranial fossa base and its saddle shaped, so it's also called the sella turcica. The sella turcica supports the pituitary gland. The superior wall participates in constituting the posterior part of the cavum nasi top and the posterior wall of the ethmoid sinus (sphenoid-ethmoid plate), the superior close to the septum nasi is the natural aperture of the sphenoid sinus (Fig. 9.4). The posterior wall has thicker sclerotin and is adjacent to the occipital clivus. The inferior wall is the choana upper ridge and the nasopharyngeal apex. And the pterygoid canal neuropore locates at the ossa pterygoideum roof at lateral inferior wall [1, 2].

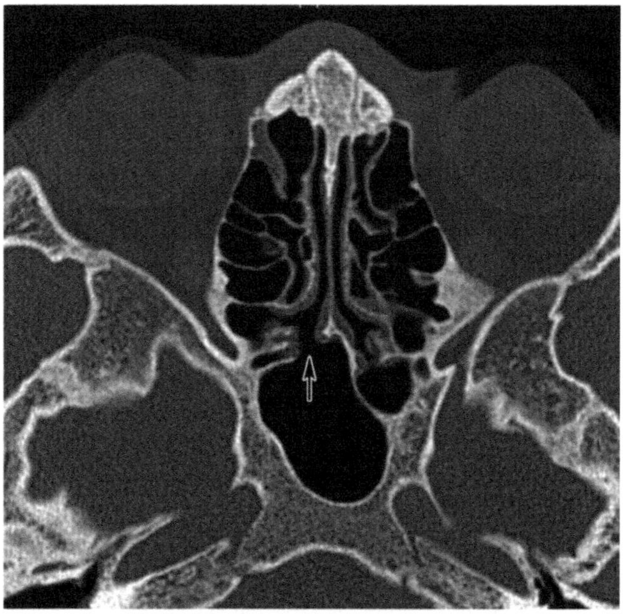

**Fig. 9.4** The nasal sinus axial CT scan. Sphenoid sinus aditus could be seen (arrow)

## 9.2 Physiology of Nose

### 9.2.1 Nasal Physiology

The nose has respiratory, olfactory, and vocal resonance functions, and it can also help in the reflex, absorption, immunity and other functions [2].

1. Respiratory

   The cavum nasi is the portal of the human respiratory channel and it helps much on the contact with the external environment.

   (a) Nasal Airflow

   The air flow into the cavum nasi is obstructed at the nasal orifice which is divides into the laminar flow and the turbulence flow. Laminar flow arcs from the upper part of the nostril to the back nostril, which is the main part of the air flow in the nostril. It is related to the air flow. It is the main part of the gas exchange in the lungs and the main air flow in the nasal cavity to regulate the temperature and humidity. Turbulence is an irregular and swirling flow formed behind the nostril. It increases the contact between the air and the nasal mucosa, which is conducive to the deposition of particulate matter such as dust on the surface of the mucosa. Laminar flow and turbulence often coexist together, but only laminar flow occurs during calm breathing.

   (b) Nasal Resistance

   The nasal resistance is produced at the nasal flap area, occupies 40–50% of the total respiratory tract resistance, helps to produce negative pressure (vaccum) at the thoracic cavity, which lengthens the air's remaining time in the alveoli during exhalation, thus increase the air exchange time. The nasal resistance is vital factors ensure the air exchange. The nasal circle changes the bilateral nasal resistance but the total resistance power keeps still. If nasal resistance decreases, such as atrophic rhinitis, lung function decreases, while increased nasal resistance, such as chronic rhinitis, can lead to inadequate nasal ventilation, affecting respiratory and circulatory functions.

   (c) Nasal Cycles

   It means the alternative contraction and expansion of the normal bilateral nasal concha mucosa capacity vessels and manifest as the corresponding alternant change at the bilateral nasal concha size and resistance. The change turns each 2–7 h but the total concha resistance remains, so the nasal cycle is also called the physiological nasal concha cycle. The cycle exists for evoking the repeated asleep turning over to help relieve the sleep tiredness.

   (d) Temperature Adjustment

   It relies on the circuitous and wide cavum mucosa surface and abundant blood supply. The cavum mucosa could adjust the inhaled air temperature similar to the common flesh to help protect the inferior respiratory channels.

   (e) Humidity Adjustments

   Glands in the cavum mucosa could secrete about 1000 mL liquid within 24 h and 70% of the liquid is used to increase the inhaled air humidity to benefit on the cilia motion.

   (f) Filtration and Clearance

   Vestibular rhinothrix resists and filtrate the large dust particles and the bacteria in air. The turbulence flow and the laminar flow both can settle the wee dust particles on the cavum mucosa. The water soluble granules are melted and the insoluble particles will move to the posterior nasal hole by the cilia motion, enter the pharynx and then are swallowed or spitted.

   (g) Mucosa Cilium System Function

   The cavum sinus mucosa is pseudostratified columnar ciliated epithelium, each of which contains 250–300 cilia whose length is about 5–6 μm and average diameter is 0.3 μm. The cillium surface covers a mucosa carpet made with the inorganic salt, the mucopolysaccharid, the macroprotein, the muramidase and water. The carpet moves posteriorly by 5 mm/min to protect the cilia and help cilia motion.

2. Olfactory Function (Sensation Odor)

   It mainly relies on the nasal olfactory mucosa and olfactory cells to play a role such as recognition, alarming, influences the appetite and emotion.

3. Vocal Resonances

   It relies on the cavum space, the sound can resonate and produce a nice sound.

4. The Nasopulmonary Reflex and the Sneezing Reflex

   Nasopulmonary reflex arc is made with the cavum mucosa trigeminal nerve as the afferent branch, the trigeminal nerve nucleus and the vagus nucleus as the central nucleus and the bronchus smooth muscle vagus nerve as the efferent branch. It is the main factors to cause the nose evoked bronchopathy.

   The sneezing reflex is a kind of afferent branch of the trigeminal nerve. When the trigeminal nerve is stimulated, series of reflex motions, such as the deep inhalation, the lifted tongue root, the severely contracted abdominal muscle and diaphragm, the abruptly opened glottis etc. These reflex causes the air abruptly emitted through cavum nasi to clear the foreign matter or stimulators in the cavum and play a protective role.

5. The Specific and Nonspecific Immunity of the Nasal Mucosa

   The substance cavum mucosa cells and glands compound and secret and the blood vessels exudate constitute the cavum mucosa immunity system, including the muramidase and the lactoferrin who has nonspecific immunity function and the immunoglobulin A and G who have specific immunity functions.

6. Nasal Mucosa Absorption Function

   The cavum mucosa membrane is about 150 $cm^2$. The subepithelial layer is rich in capillaries, venous sinuses, arteriovenous anastomotic branches and lymphatic vessels, which help to rapidly absorb the medicine into the blood circulation.

7. The Lacrimal Gland Excretory Function

   The tear could reach to the inferior meatus nasi through the lacrimal puncture, the lacrimal canaliculi, lacrimal duct, lacrimal sac and the nasolacrimal duct.

### 9.2.2 Nasal Sinus Physiology

There is still some dispute for the nasal sinus physiology; however some consensuses are also accepted as following:

1. Increase the area of respiratory mucosa, promote the warming and humidifying effect of inhaled air, and enhance the defensive function.
2. Sound resonance.
3. Lighten the head increase the buoyancy.
4. Protect important organs.
5. Preserve heat loss and adiabatic.

## References

1. Li Y, Zhou B. Practical endorhinoscopy surgery technique and application. Beijing: Peking People's Medical Publishing House; 2009. p. 1016.
2. Dalgorf DM, Harvey RJ. Chapter 1: sinonasal anatomy and function. Am J Rhinol Allergy. 2013;27(Suppl 1):S3–6.

# Symptoms of Disease and Examination Method of Nasal Disease

# 10

Xin Wei and Xun Bi

## 10.1 Symptoms of Nasal Disease

1. Nasal Obstruction

   Nasal obstruction is obstraction of nasal air ventilation and it can be divided into complete or partial obstruction, alternative, posture, intermittent, progressive aggravation and persistent, bilateral and unilateral.

   Congenital posterior nasal atresia happens to infants should be considered as the congenital nasal atresia. Most of the infant persistent nasal obstruction is often caused by the adenoid hypertrophy, the patients appear with the feature called 'adenoid face'. Unilateral nasal obstruction is more common in foreign bodies or tumors, and very few are nasopharyngeal teratomas. In adults, nasopolyps, hypertrophic rhinitis, nasal septum deviation and other manifestations can occur; unilaterally progressive aggravation is mostly the nasoma, and if it accompanies with the bloody snot, the sarcoma should be considered. The alternating nasal congestion could happen in the acute rhinitis and chronic single rhinitis. However to the intermittent nasal congestion, it appears more frequently in the patients with vasoconstrictive rhinitis or the allergic rhinitis.

   Systemic disease, such as the malformed endocrine disorders (the hypothyroidism, the diabetes, etc), the abnormal systemic diastolic disorders and longterm hypotensive drugs use, can trigger the nasal congestion. Treatments of this kind of disorders should maily focus on treatment of primary disease.
2. Rhinorrhea

   Rhinorrhea is the phenomenon that the excessive nasal secretions flow from the anterior to posterior naris (choana). Normally, the nasomucosa glands, such as the serous gland, the mucous gland, the goblet cells and the olfactory gland, could secret small amount of mucous to maintain nasal mucosa ciliary motion, adjust the inhaled air temperature and humidity. When the nasal lesion happens, the quantity and the property of the secretion could change.

   (a) Water-Based Rhinorrhea

   Secretion is rarefacted, hyaline-like, vasopercolate mucous complex secretion. Water-borne rhinorrhea secretions are thin, transparent and clear water-like. and it often is seen at the early acute rhinitis, the attack stage of the allergic rhinitis. The former (acute rhinitis), it contains deciduous epithelium cells, the macroprotein and few RBC; however at the latter (allergic rhinitis) secretion contains the eosinophils and few macroprotein. The cerebrospinal fluid rhinorrhea is also water like and non sticky can be differentially diagnosed with the water-based, cohesion less secretion and over 1.7 mmol/L glucose content.

   (b) Mucous Rhinorrhea

   It is semitransparent with macroprotein. It is mostly seen at the chronic rhinitis and chronic rhinosinusitis.

   (c) Suppurative Rhinorrhea

   The secretion is mucus-pus complex, It is caused by bacterial infection and is mainly composed of mucous epithelial cells and infiltrated polymorphonuclear leukocytes. It is common in convalescent stage of acute rhinitis and chronic rhinosinusitis. If odontogenic maxillary sinusitis is often odorous yellow-green purulent rhinorrhea.

   (d) Bloody Rhinorrhea

   It means the nasal secretion contains blood. It is often seen at the rhinal fungal infection, trauma, foreign body, nasal tumour, sinus neoplasm, nasopharyngeal carcinoma, etc. When it occurs, nasal cavity examination and nasal sinus examination are vital

X. Wei (✉)
Department of Otorhinolaryngology Head and Neck Surgery, Hainan People's Hospital, Haikou, China

X. Bi
Department of Pediatric Surgery, The First Affiliated Hospital of Hainan Medical University, Haikou, China



Z. Mu, J. Fang (eds.), *Practical Otorhinolaryngology - Head and Neck Surgery*, https://doi.org/10.1007/978-981-13-7993-2_10

and general checkup should also be done when necessary, these should be done for confirming the hemorrhage sites and causes.

(e) Epistaxis

There are plenties of causes to epistaxis, which can be local cavum disease and also general disease manifestation in pars nasalis. The epistaxis is always unilateral and sometime bilateral and differs at the quantity, the milder ones are with bloody snot and the severer ones are with the hemorrhagic shock. Repeated epistaxis may cause anemia.

3. Local Causes

(a) Trauma

The foreign body attack, the nose pick etc., can cause the traumatic epistaxis. Treat due to the quantity, the slighter ones' hemostasis should be done with simple press or cavum paddings and severe ones, such as the arterial injury, the traumatic pseudo aneurysm rupture, may cause the fetal epistaxis.

(b) Nasal Septum Deviation

It is mostly seen adjacent to the ridge or rectangular bulge or deviated convex surface, whose mucosa is thin and easy susceptible to cold air. The dry mucosa could easily cause the rupture epistaxis. The epistaxis also can be caused by nasal septum perforation.

(c) Tumor

Benign tumors, such as the vasoma, malignant cavum squamous carcinoma, nasopharyngeal carcinoma etc., can cause the epistaxis.

(d) Nasal Rhinitis

Dry rhinitis, atopic rhinitis, acute rhinitis, fungal sinusitis and others are the causes of the slight bleeding. The cavum tuberculosis, gafeira, syphilis and others can evoke epistaxis through the mucosa erosion, ulceration, granulations or perforation of nasal septum.

(e) Climate Factors

In the plateaus section, the repeated epistaxis will happen because of the dry mucosa escharosis evoked by the low humidity and the dry climate.

(f) Foreign Matter

It is mostly seen in children, and it is mostly unilateral epistaxis. Some animal nasal foreign bodies, such as the leech, can trigger the epistaxis repeatedly.

4. Systemic Factors

(a) Acute Febrile Diseases

Such as the upper respiratory channel infection, influenza, measles, Scarlet fever, typhoid fever, mumps, etc. Because of high fever, severe congestion and swelling of nasal mucosa, resulting in blood capillary rupture and hemorrhage, nosebleeds usually occur in fever stage with less amount, and most of the bleeding sites are in the anterior segment of nasal cavity.

(b) Blood Disease

- Abnormal Coagulation

  Such as hemophilia, barrier caused by plenty use of anticoagulation drugs and fibrinogenesis, abnormal methemoglobinemia, collagen diseases.

- Abnormal Platelet Quantity or Quality

  Such as thrombocytopenic purpura, leukemia, aplastic anemia etc. Such epistaxis is caused by the capillary wall damage, so it generally belongs to osmotic hemorrhage, mostly bilateral, with multiple bleeding in the shape of sieve eyes, continuous, flaky, and poor blood clot contraction.

(c) Circulation System Disease

- Hyper Angiostatin

  Hypertension, atherosclerosis, nephritis and others like excessive exertion, violent mood swings, rapid air pressure change, any of these can cause epistaxis because of elevated temporary arterial pressure. Headache, dizziness and other symptoms can appear before hemorrhage. Hemorrhage occurs abruptly but also it can stop abruptly, it is often unilateral. Chronic and acute nephritis can cause the epistaxis, and it is remarkable at the atrophic kidneys and the uremia.

- Hyper Intravenous Pressure

  Chronic tracheitis, emphysema, corpulmonale, nasal varices is also common cause of epistaxis when sever cough or asthma occurs. Epistaxis sites are often at nasopharyngeal venous plexus inferior to concha. Other causes like mitral stenosis, mediastinal tumors and superior vena cava hypertension can also cause epistaxis.

(d) Hypovitaminosis

- Vitamin C Deficiency

  It can cause reduction of collagen in vascular wall cells, vessel fragility and permeability increases, which can evoke epistaxis.

- Vitamin $B_2$ and Vitamin K Deficiency

  It is positively correlated to the prothrombin formation and if vitamin K is deficient, prothrombin time will be prolonged and epistaxis will occur easily.

(e) Liver and Spleen Disease and Rheumatism

All of them can evoke the epistaxis and the most commonly seen one is the cirrhosis. Rheumatic fever cause epistaxis during childhood.

(f) Chemicals and Drug Poisoning

Includes Phosphorus, the Mercury, the Arsenic, Benzene poisoning, etc., can damage the hemopoietic system functions and cause epistaxis. The long-term salicylate drugs' usage can cause that the prothrombin decreases and finally the wound bleeding after surgery.

(g) Endocrine Disorders Dyscrasia

Blood estrogen decreases during or several days before the menstrual period, this cause nasal mucosa hemangiectasis, so some females have the epistaxis at the menstrual period.

(h) Hereditary Hemorrhagic Telangiectasia

Arteriextasis and vasodilation occur at the frontal nasal septum, the fingertips, the tongue tips etc. may cause repeated epistaxis, which is mostly suggestive of hereditary hemorrhagic telangietasis.

The accurate cause can't be found, however the epistaxis can be controlled and unrepeated in clinic sometime, this kind of bleeding is called the idiopathic epistaxis [1].

5. Dysosmia

Scent is the sense that the odour granules (bromine) inhaled into the cavum by air approach the olfactory mucosa and stimulate the olfactory cells to evoke the nervous impulse, and the impulse conducts to the cortical center through the olfactory nerves, the olfactory bulbs and the olfactory tracts. Any sites in human scent approach can influence the olfactory function and produce the olfactory disorder.

There are three common olfactory disorders: reduced olfactory sensitivity, also known as impairment or loss of olfactory sense, olfactory allergy, and olfactory error.

(a) Impairment or Loss of Olfactory Sense

It can be divided into two types: respiratory and sensory.

- Respiratory Olfactory Impairment or Loss: it can be divided into two types: obstructive and non-obstructive. The former is caused by turbinate hypertrophy, nasal atresia, nasal polyps and nasal tumors and other causes, which obstruct airflow caring olfaction to reach the olfactory region however no airflow direction change, the latter is caused by the change of respiratory airflow direction without obstruction of nasal cavity such as tracheotomy or after total laryngectomy. This kind of situation is easy to discover during physical examination.
- Sensory Olfactory Decline or Disappearance: it can be divided into two types of peripheral and central. The former includes nerve endings of the olfactory mucosa, such as atrophic rhinitis, toxic olfactory neuritis, harmful gas damage and senile degeneration. This kind of patient has the same smell and the same reaction, which is, it can cause smell with a strong smell, however the patient can't distinguish it and think it is the same smell. Central and intracranial type, most of the skull base fracture, olfactory groove meningioma, basal meningitis, brain abscess, cerebrovascular disease etc.

(b) Olfactory Allergies

The patient's sensitivity to odor is enhanced. Slight odor is extremely intense and intolerable, and even causes headache, vomiting etc. Most of them are early manifestations of olfactory neuritis and olfactory nerve degeneration. In addition, the neurasthenia, women's pregnancy, menstruation can also appear anaphylaxis.

(c) Olfactory Errors

A kind of odor olfactory into ethylene smell, smell into olfactory odor, referred to as parosmia. Odorless sensations are known as phantom olfactory. They are common in epilepsy; neurosis; schizophrenia; and endocrine disorders.

6. Rhinogenic Headache

Rhinogenic headache due to disease caused by rhinopathy, generally divided into infectious and noninfectious.

(a) Infectious Rhinogenic Headaches

Common in acute sinusitis and its headache often has a certain location and time, such as frontal headache in the morning when acute frontal sinusitis rises, gradually aggravates and turns light in the afternoon; acute maxillary sinusitis lightens in the morning and aggravates pain in the infraorbital in the afternoon; headache aggravates when low-headed and crooked, causing congestion of nasal mucosa; and vasoconstrictor and surface anesthesia are used in nasal mucosa, can relieve headache.

(b) Noninfectious Nasal Headaches

Can be seen in atrophic rhinitis, nasal septum and nasal tumor. It's a characteristics of rhinogenous headache for many with nasal symptoms such as nasal congestion, runny nose etc.; whiles other relieving factors, such as the use of topical anesthetic for nasal septum mucosa of inferior turbinate bone spine contact, can relieve headache.

## 10.2 Examination Method of Nose

1. General Inspection Method

(a) External Nasal Examinations

When the nose and nasal cavity are checked, it should be carefully checked in order to avoid omission. Mainly watching and touching is used to do it. Observe whether there are any abnormalities in the external nose, such as deformity, such as whether the nasal ala has collapsed, whether the anterior nostril is narrow (atresia), whether the external nose is red, swollen, thickened, hardened, tenderness or nasal flapping.

(b) Nasal Vestibule Examination

Observe whether the skin of the vestibule of the nose is red, swollen, erosive, scab or chap, and the new infection are observed.

(c) Nasal Cavity Examination

Nasal examination is divided into two kinds, namely anterior rhinoscopy and posterior rhinoscopy inspection method.

(d) Anterior Rhinoscopy

The examiner puts the anterior rhinoscopy into the nasal vestibule, opens the upper and lower lobes, enlarges the anterior nostril, supports the head of the patient (examinee) with his right hand, changes the head position according to the need of examination, and examines each part of the nasal cavity in turn. First, the head position of the subjects was slightly lower (the first position), then the nasal base, inferior nasal meatus, inferior turbinate and anterior inferior nasal septum were observed from bottom to top, then the head of the subjects was inverted 30° (the second position), and the middle nasal meatus, middle turbinate, olfactory cleft and middle nasal septum were examined. Then the head of the subjects was inverted to 60° (the third position), and the upper nasal septum, nasal mound and anterior inferior nasal turbinate were observed. Pay attention to the color and swelling of mucosa, nasal secretion and characteristics, deviation of nasal septum and nasal cavity with or without new organisms. The normal nasal mucosa is light red with smooth, moist and lustrous surface. In acute inflammation, the mucosa is bright red with mucous secretions. When chronic inflammation, the mucosa is dark red, and the front of inferior turbinate is sometimes mulberry-like. The secretion is mucopurulent. The mucosa of allergic rhinitis is pale, edematous or purple, and the secretion is thin. Atrophic rhinitis mucosa atrophy, dryness, loss of normal luster, covered with pus scab, middle and inferior turbinate shrinkage. The purulent secretions in the middle nasal meatus and olfactory fissure are caused by sinus lesions.

(e) Posterior Rhinoscopy

It is used to observe the condition of septum posterior margin, nasal posterior foramen, middle and inferior turbinate posterior end and posterior nasal deformity. At the same time, the nasopharynx and eustachian tube can be observed.

2. Endoscopy

The development of nasal endoscopy has made a great change in the field of nasal medicine. Nasal endoscopy includes 0°, 30°, 45°, 70°, etc. The diameter of the endoscopy is 4 mm for adults and 2.7 mm for children.

(a) Operation Steps

- The Patient Sitting or Supine position, and The Head Fixed.
- The inspector stands on the right front of the patient facing the monitor.

(b) Mirror Method

Generally, the left hand holds the mirror and the right hand can perform biopsies at the same time. The technique of holding glasses can be used in different ways according to personal habits, however suitable for the operation of endoscopic sinus surgery.

(c) Inspection Steps

From the total nasal endoscopic nasal bottom along the parallel back slowly forward, at the same time pay attention to note the sites which have abnormalities, after passing through the nostrils, into the nasopharynx, were observed in the posterior wall of nasopharynx top and side wall, pharyngeal recess, carina, pharyngeal ostium of eustachian tube; then slowly outward from the lens endoscope, slightly upward, observe the butterfly ethmoid recess, middle meatus, nasal tip, olfactory cleft, nasal septum and nasal vestibule at exit end. It is also possible to observe the nasal vestibule, the frontend of the septum, the middle turbinate, the uncinate process, the middle nasal canal, the olfactory fissure, the sphenoid fossa and the nasopharynx.

3. Olfactory Examinations

(a) Simple Test Methods

The odorant, such as ethanol, vinegar, camphor and soy sauce, can be used as odorant. Most people are tested by smelling the odorants and compare the lowest concentration obtained by large sample statistics.

(b) Olfactory Threshold Examinations

According to certain classification gradient olfactomedin can be divided into different concentrations, The lowest olfaction threshold can be determined by the ability of the subjects to distinguish each olfactin, and the olfactory spectrum can also be drawn in $7 * 10$ small squares to make the results more intuitive.

(c) Olfactory Evoked Potential Determination

Olfactory evoked potential (OEP) is an objective and sensitive electrophysiological index for olfaction detection. It can be used to detect olfaction level in patients with hyposmia, parosmia and infantile and brain injury. It can also be used to monitor olfaction changes during operation. OEP is often used in anterior cranial fossa surgery and some nasal operations involving ethmoidal roof injury and olfactory system, causing olfactory dysfunction. The olfactory level can be objectively evaluated by using olfactory evoked potentials after operation. The decline of olfactory level may be a precursor of some diseases, such as Parkinson's disease, Alzheimer's disease, multiple sclerosis, temporal lobe epilepsy and other diseases, which are often accompanied by the decline of olfactory level in the early stage. Olfactory evoked potential can be used as a reference for the early diagnosis of these diseases [2].

4. Imaging Examination
   (a) X-Ray Plain Film
      - The nasal side is used to diagnose the fracture of nasal bone and to observe the location of nasal bone fracture, whether there is dislocation or not. This method is simple and inexpensive, because of too many overlaps; it is easy to miss the tiny fracture.
      - Sinus occipito mental position (also known as Water position) and occipital frontal position (also known as Caldwell position) of nasal sinuses mainly show the frontal sinus, maxillary sinus and ethmoid sinus, and observe the morphology and size of bone, mucosa and sinus wall bone condition. At present, the X-ray plain film of the nasal sinus is rarely used in clinical practice and is basically replaced by the CT examination.

   (b) CT Examination

      The conventional thin slice high resolution CT scanning with coronal reconstructed images at the same time, the multi planar reconstruction (MPR), can display the location, range, sinus lesion anatomy, pathogenic factors of nasal mucosa lesions, observe whether bone re-sorption or fracture, the solution of ostiomeatal complex is smooth, but also according to the characteristics of some CT sinusitis properties were determined, such as the characteristics of sinus cavity, the increased density of calcified plaques is fungal sinusitis. Nasal CT virtual endoscopy (CTVE) can clearly show nasal anatomic structure, especially ostium and nasal complex. It can also show the range of occupying lesions in nasal cavity and its relationship with surrounding structures, which is highly consistent with nasal endoscopy.

   (c) MRI Examination

      Nasal sinus MRI examination showed more clear nasal soft tissue disease than CT. If we show tumor invasion of nasal cavity and nasal sinus and its surrounding soft tissue, we can accurately judge the diffusion of tumor to the brain; observe the range and extent of space occupying lesions of the soft tissue in the sinuses, and the anatomical relationship with the surrounding muscles and vessels. In addition, MRI can also be used for guided biopsy, which is an important basis to help develop treatment plans and select surgical approaches. MRI combined with enhanced scan can usually make a more accurate differential diagnosis of benign tumors. The shortcoming is that the MRI examination cannot show the anatomical bone markers and variations well, and can be combined with the three dimensional reconstruction of CT to evaluate the tumor staging.

## References


1. Chinese Journal of Otorhinolaryngology Head and Neck Surgery editorial committee Rhinology group, Chinese Medical Association Otorhinolaryngology Head and Neck Surgery branch Rhinology group. Epistaxis diagnosis and treatment guideline (draft). Chin J Otorhinolaryngol Head Neck Surg. 2015;50(4):265267.
2. Zhang W, Zhang L. Olfactory Dysfunction's diagnosis and treatment. J Cap Med Univ. 2013;34(6):814819.

# Common Rhinal Disease

# 11

Xin Wei, Zhonglin Mu and Jugao Fang

The external nose located at the front face of the human body, vulnerable to external injuries. As the nasal airway portal, the nasal cavity is exposed to external environmental hence vulnerable to bacterial or fungal inflammation. Nasal septum deviation is one of the important reasons of nasal obstruction and epistaxis. Nasal and sinus tumors, especially malignant tumors, seriously affect the quality of life and survival of patients. This chapter focuses on common diseases of the nose.

## 11.1 Trauma of Nose, Paranasal Sinus and Adjacent Tissue

### 11.1.1 Nasal Bone Fracture

The nasal bone is located at the front and center part of the human face, which is vulnerable to trauma and fracture. Because the nasal bone is thicker and thinner, the fracture of the nasal bone is mostly located in the lower part.

**Cause**
It occurs as result of the external force, such as boxing, hard impact or car accident.

X. Wei (✉)
Department of Otorhinolaryngology Head and Neck Surgery, Hainan People's Hospital, Haikou, China

Z. Mu
Department of Otorhinolaryngology Head and Neck Surgery, The First Affiliated Hospital of Hainan Medical University, Haikou, China

J. Fang
Department of Otorhinolaryngology Head and Neck Surgery, Beijing Tongren Hospital, Capital Medical University, Beijing, China

**Clinical Symptoms**

1. Clinical Symptoms

    Local pain can cause nasal bleeding due to nasal mucosa tear. Nasal septum fracture or nasal mucosa swelling can lead to side or bilateral nasal congestion.

2. Clinical Signs

    Subcutaneous congestion can be accompanied by tenderness, nasal collapse or deviation, can touch the sense of bone friction, nasal swelling can cover up nasal deformities.

3. Imaging Examinations

    Osseous discontinuity of the nasal bone is visible on the side of the X ray, and bone dislocation, deformation, or depression can be seen in severe cases, accompanied by swelling of the soft tissue of the nose and back (Fig. 11.1). CT can not only show the direction of fracture line, the displacement of fracture fragments and soft tissue injury, but also show tiny fractures, which cannot be observed by X-ray. CT 3D reconstruction can directly show the continuity of nasal bone surface (Fig. 11.2).

**Diagnosis**
According to the history of trauma, clinical signs and imaging examination, it can be diagnosed clearly. Because of nasal bone fracture often associated with craniofacial or craniocerebral trauma, we need to perform related examinations to avoid missed diagnosis.

**Treatment**
The principle of treatment is to restore normal nasal shape and ventilatory function.

There is no special treatment for simple fractures without displaced fractures. For closed fracture of nasal bone, nasal bone fracture reduction surgery can be performed after



Z. Mu, J. Fang (eds.), *Practical Otorhinolaryngology - Head and Neck Surgery*, https://doi.org/10.1007/978-981-13-7993-2_11

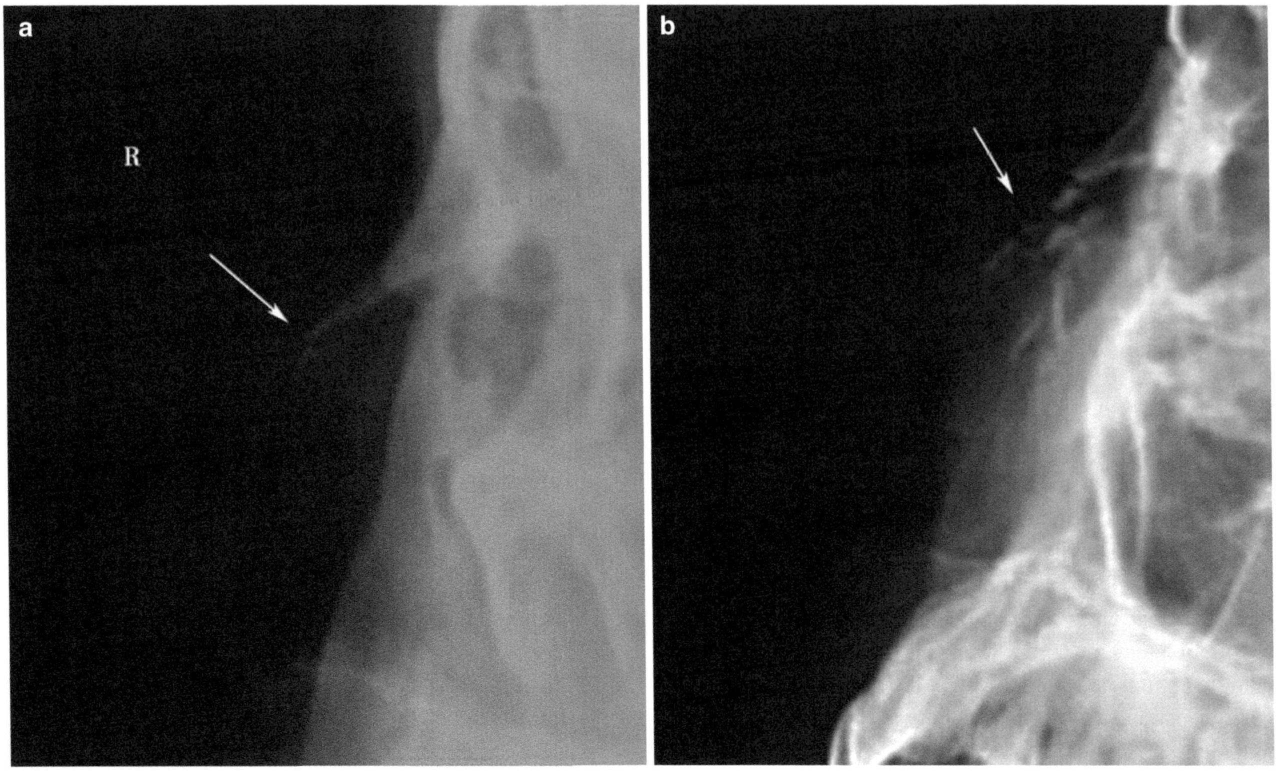


**Fig. 11.1** X-ray lateral projection displays rhinobony fracture. (**a**) Linear fracture (arrow) (**b**) Comminuted fracture (arrow)

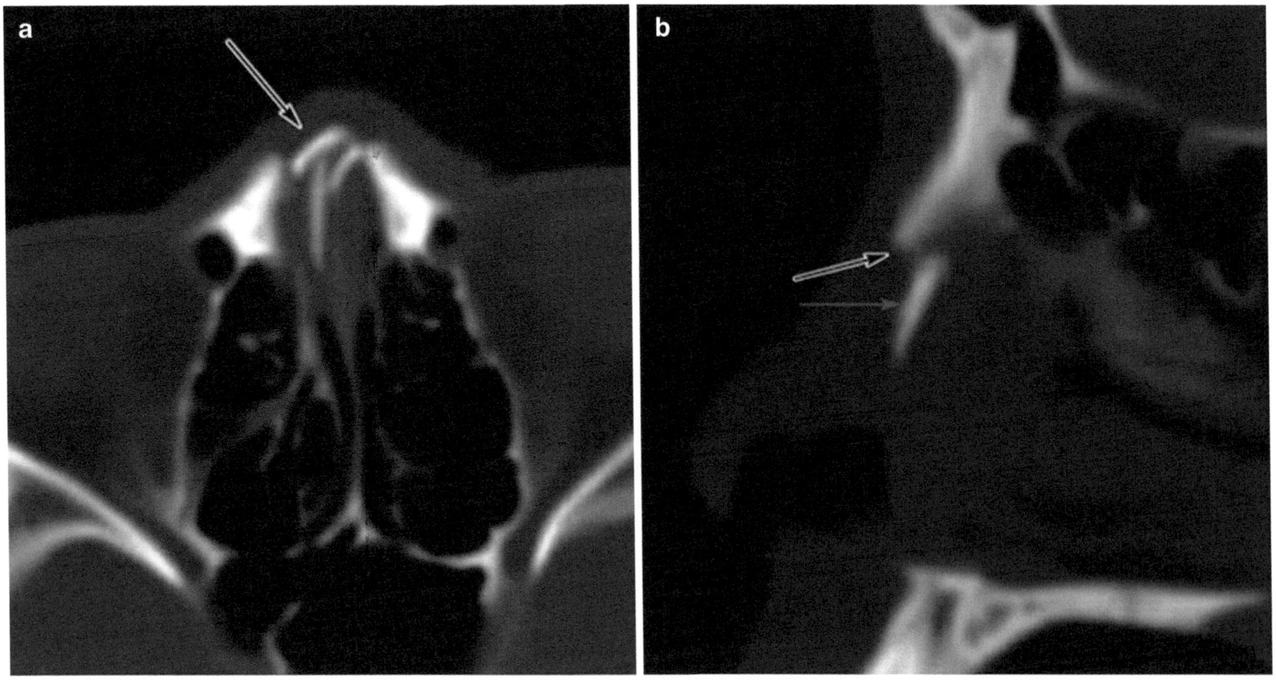


**Fig. 11.2** Rhinobony fracture CT scan manifestation. (**a**) Axial CT bone window imaging. (**b**) Sagittal CT bone window imaging. (**c**) CT 3D reconstruction (VR)

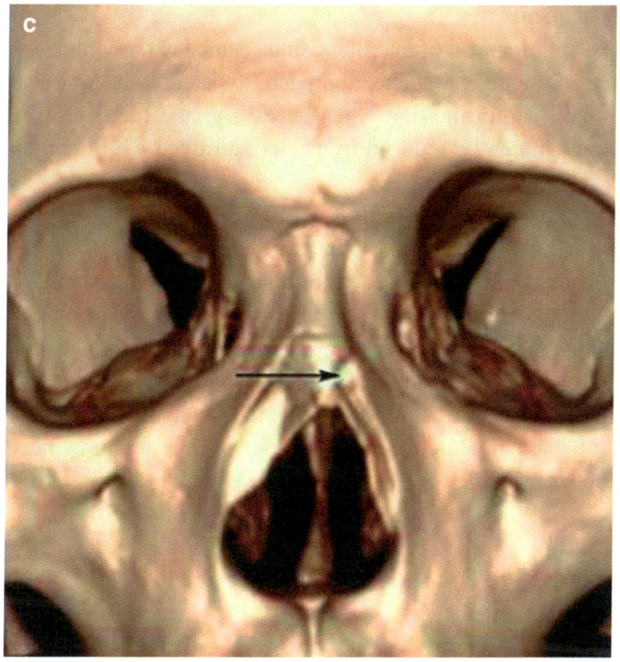


Fig. 11.2 (continued)

definite diagnosis. If nasal swelling affects judgment, patients can be ordered to perform surgery after swelling subsides, but the time is not more than 2 weeks, so as to avoid callus formation affecting reduction. Septal fracture or dislocation with clinical symptoms can be corrected simultaneously if the septum can not be reduced by itself after reduction of nasal bone fracture. For old nasal bone fracture, butterfly incision through nasal columella can be used for open reduction.

Closed reduction method: According to the patient's age and wishes, surface anesthesia or general anesthesia can be used. The length of the anterior nostril to bilateral medial canthus can be measured out with the nasal bone reductor outside the nose and marked with the thumb. The reductor is placed in the nasal cavity to the lower part of the collapsed nasal bone, which can be restored forcefully upward. At the same time, the other hand holds the nasal bone to help shape the nasal bone. Bone frictions during reduction are often audible. After reduction, carefully check whether the reduction is in place, nasal packing gauze plays a supporting and hemostasis role, 48 h after removal.

### 11.1.2 Nasal Sinus's Fracture

#### 11.1.2.1 Frontal Sinus Fracture

According to the fracture site can be divided into anterior wall fractures, fractures of the posterior wall and the bottom wall before the fracture, among which anterior fracture is the most common (Fig. 11.3), posterior wall fractures often accompanied by dura tear, with cerebrospinal fluid rhinorrhea or intracranial hematoma.

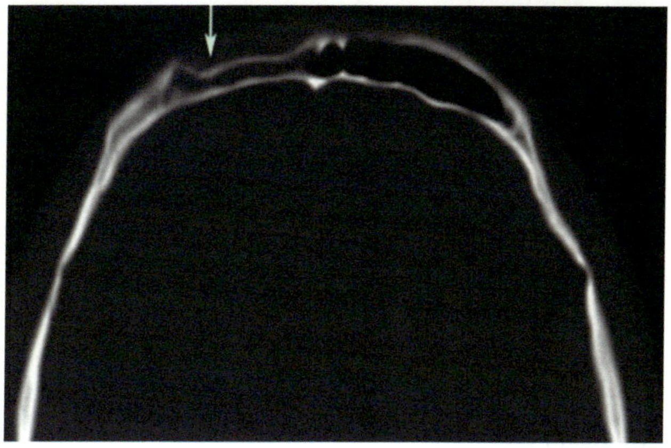

Fig. 11.3 Horizontal CT scan shows right frontal sinus's frontal wall fracture (arrow)

**Clinical Manifestation**

Anterior wall fracture is characterized by local swelling subsided after the visible forehead sag. Posterior wall fractures can be characterized by cerebrospinal fluid rhinorrhea and intracranial hemorrhage or hematoma. Basal fracture can be characterized by swelling of the supraorbital region and downward displacement of the eyeball.

**Diagnosis**

The diagnosis can be made according to the history of trauma and clinical manifestations. CT scan can identify the fracture site and scope.

**Treatment**

The principle of treatment is to restore the appearance and function of linear fracture without special treatment, and can use decongestants to keep sinus drainage smooth. Anterior depressed fracture needs open reduction surgery, which can borrow the original open wound or eyebrow arch incision, use peeler to initiate depressed fracture reduction, and fix with titanium plate. In posterior wall fractures we need to know whether there are intracranial complications, if necessary, neurosurgical assistance will be needed. If nasal fracture is unobstructed and it cannot be treated, partial stenosis can be placed T-tube. In severe stenosis, curettage of all frontal sinus mucosa will be needed together with frontal sinus tamponade with autologous fat.

#### 11.1.2.2 Fracture of Ethmoid Sinus

The ethmoid sinus is located between the skull base and the orbit. Fractures may involve the anterior skull base and cause cerebrospinal fluid rhinorrhea, ocular displacement and visual impairment, anterior ethmoidal artery and severe epistaxis or intraorbital hematoma.

**Clinical Manifestation**
This includes nasal bleeding, nasal root collapse, medial canthus widening, visual loss or Marcus Gunn pupil.

**Diagnosis**
Diagnosis can be made according to the history of trauma and clinical manifestations. CT scan can identify the fracture site and scope.

**Treatment**
Simple fracture need not be treated, Nasal packing or ligation of anterior ethmoidal artery can be used for epistaxis. Optic nerve decompression should be performed as soon as possible for patients with visual impairment.

#### 11.1.2.3 Fracture of the Maxillary Sinus

It often occurs in the anterior wall (Fig. 11.4), often a part of the compound maxillofacial fracture.

**Clinical Manifestation**
The local swelling, facial depression deformity can be seen after regression, and facial numbness can occur if combined with infraorbital nerve injury at the same time.

**Diagnostic**
Diagnosis can be made according to the history of trauma and clinical manifestations. CT scan can identify the fracture site and scope.

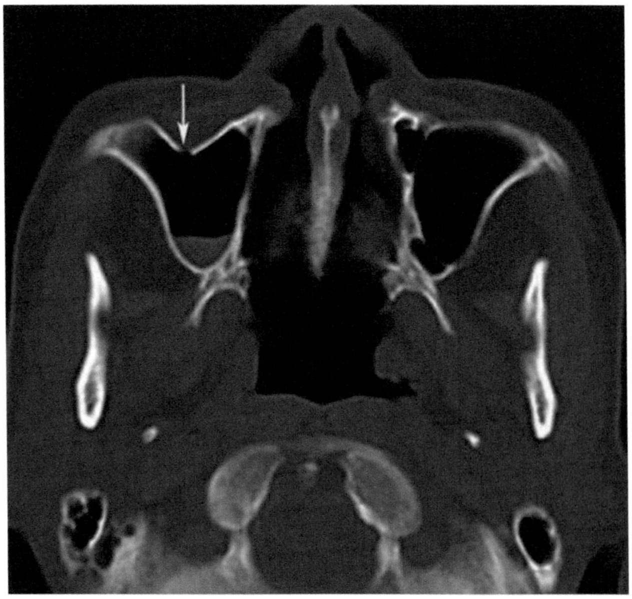

**Fig. 11.4** Horizontal CT scan shows right maxillary sinus's frontal wall fracture

**Treatment**
The anterior wall of maxillary sinus can be exposed through the Labiogingival sulcus approach, assisted with the lower orbital margin incision when necessary, and the depressed fragment can be reduced by peeler and fixed with titanium plate.

#### 11.1.2.4 Fracture of the Sphenoid Sinus

Sphenoid sinus is adjacent to pituitary fossa, optic nerve and internal carotid artery. Fractures of sphenoid sinus often involve the above structures, leading to cerebrospinal fluid rhinorrhea, visual impairment and fatal massive hemorrhage. Simple sphenoid sinus fractures are rare and often part of skull base fractures. Simple sphenoid sinus fractures need not be treated.

### 11.1.3 Eye Orbital Fractures

#### 11.1.3.1 Orbital Penetrating Fracture

It is a fracture caused by the lateral orbit injury, often accompanied by a fracture of the maxilla.

**Clinical Manifestation**
Periorbital congestion, eyelid swelling, exophthalmoses, lateral canthus displacement downward and outward, but no visual impairment and eye movement disorders.

**Diagnosis**
The diagnosis can be made according to the history of trauma, clinical manifestation, the sense of ladder-like touch of the inferior orbital wall and CT examination.

**Treatment**
The lateral eyebrow incision and lower eyelid margin incision can be made. The depressed maxillary bone is lifted and repositioned forward and outward by inserting a stripper under the zygomatic arch, and fixed with titanium plate.

#### 11.1.3.2 Orbital Fracture

It occurs when violence comes from the front of the eyeball and the orbital pressure increases, resulting in the fracture of the inferior or inner wall of the orbit, and the orbital contents break into the maxillary sinus or the ethmoid sinus.

**Clinical Manifestation**
They manifest as eyelid congestion, limited eye movement, diplopia and even vision loss or blindness. Facial numbness may occur in patients with infraorbital nerve injury.

**Diagnostic**
The diagnosis can be made according to the history of trauma, clinical manifestation, and CT examination.

**Treatment**

No nasal blow is allowed to prevent infection in orbit. At the same time, orbital contents should be returned as soon as possible and fixed. Surgical approach can be performed through inferior palpebral maxillary sinus or nasal endoscope through ethmoid sinus or maxillary sinus.

## 11.2 Acute Rhinitis

Acute rhinitis is an acute inflammation of the nasal mucosa. It is caused by virus infection and it is highly contagion. It is a part of upper respiratory tract infection, commonly known as cold and cold. It often affects the sinuses and pharynx and larynx, and is accompanied by acute sinusitis, otitis media, tracheobronchitis and pneumonia. The disease occurs frequently in autumn, winter and all seasons. All age groups are susceptible to the disease but mainly children [1].

**Etiology**

All kinds of respiratory viruses can cause this disease. The most common types of rhinovirus are adenovirus, coronavirus, influenza virus and parainfluenza virus. The main source of infection is the host. The route of transmission is mainly by droplet and fecal-aral. The most common viral rhinovirus is the main vector of the hand. When the virus infects the nasal mucosa, the local pro bacteria take the advantage of active reproduction and cause secondary bacterial infection. Blennorrhea is rhinitis secondary bacterial infection. The main pathogens were Streptococcus, Staphylococcus, pneumococcus, influenza Nakai bacteria and catarrhal coccus etc.

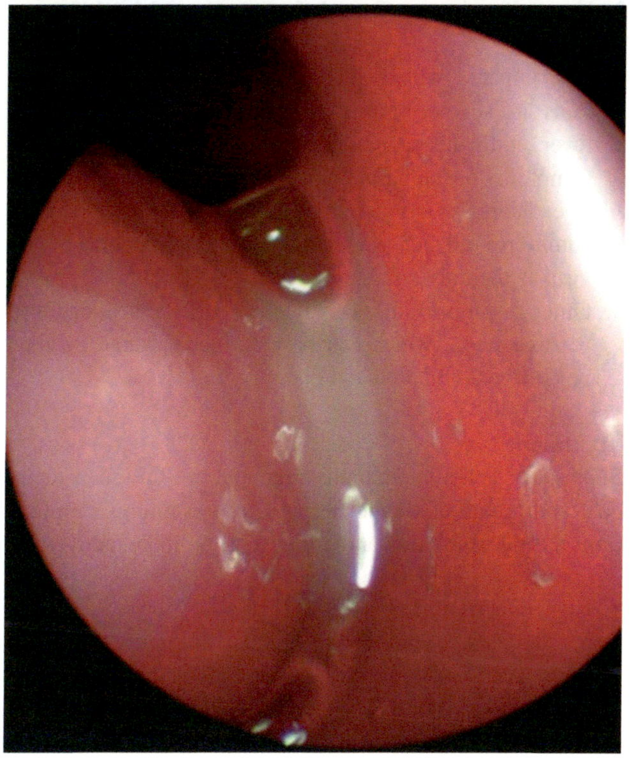

**Fig. 11.5** Sticky purulent secretion in rhinocavum

**Clinical Manifestation**

1. Early Stage (prodromal)

   1–2 days, mostly manifested as systemic acidity, dry and hot nose and nasopharynx, congestion and dryness of nasal mucosa
2. Acute Phase

   2–7 days, gradually nasal obstruction, nasal secretions increased, sneezing and nasal itching, speech was occlusive nasal sound, olfactory decline. The nasal mucosa is markedly congested and swollen. The nasal cavity is filled with mucous or mucopurulent secretions, which can turn into pus (Fig. 11.5). The patients has fever, headache, etc.
3. Convalescence

   The nasal congestion is gradually reduced and the pus is also reduced. If there is no complication, it can recover spontaneously in a few days later.

**Diagnosis**

According to the medical history, symptoms and local examination, it is generally easy to diagnose. The symptoms of acute rhinitis are similar to those of the nasal mucosa and other acute respiratory diseases. Therefore, it is necessary to differentiate.

1. Allergic Rhinitis

   The patient had a history of exposure to allergens and recurrent episodes of disease. Symptoms are mainly nasal itching, paroxysmal sneezing, a large number of clear water like mucus and nasal congestion, generally without fever and other systemic symptoms. The local examination was based on the pale edema and water secretions of the nasal mucosa, which could be accompanied by the uncinate process and the polyp of the sieve bubble. Skin prick test, nasal secretion cytology examination, excitation test and serum specific IgE antibody determination can be identified.
2. Vasomotor Rhinitis

   The cause of the disease is unknown, and the patient has more mental tension, anxiety and changes in the temperature of the environment, causing the disorder of the endocrine function. Symptoms are nasal obstruction, rhinorrhea and sneezing symptoms of a sudden onset and rapid disappearance. There are obvious incentives that can be recurred. General symptoms such as low grade fever may also occur. Local examination of the color and morphology of the nasal mucosa has no characteristic changes. Antihistamines are generally effective

3. Upper Respiratory Tract Infection Caused by Influenza Virus

   Compared with J acute rhinitis, the systemic symptoms are severe. Mainly symptoms are sudden onset of fever, chills, headache, myalgia, general discomfort. The symptoms of the nasal cavity are mild and insignificant. The diagnosis is more difficult to distinguish from the common cold hence isolation and identification of the virus is the only reliable method.
4. Other respiratory diseases include rubella, scarlet fever, pertussis, etc., which can be identified through detailed physical examination and observation.

**Treatment**

Supporting and symptomatic treatment are the main methods, and attention should be paid to preventing complications. Nasal ventilation and drainage to promote recovery.

1. Systemic Treatment

   The patient should rest in bed, drink more water and be isolated to avoid infecting others. Fever patients can take antipyretic and sweating drugs internally. Traditional Chinese medicine mainly relieves wind, relieves exterior and eliminates pathogens, such as Sangju cold tablets and Yinqiao detoxification tablets. Antibiotics can be used when bacterial infections or complications occur.
2. Local Treatment
   (a) If necessary, 1% ephedrine solution nasal drip, ventilation and drainage.
   (b) Acupuncture of Xiang point; nasal cavern; or point massage to prevent infection or complications.

## 11.3 Fungal Rhinosinusitis

Fungal sinusitis is a kind of inflammatory disease of sinuses, mucous tissue and even bone, or a response of nasal mucosa to fungi, or a fungal inflammatory disease in the nasal banquet. Fungal sinusitis can be divided into two types: invasive and non-invasive. The incidence of fungal maxillary sinusitis has a significant tendency to increase. The main pathogenic bacteria in clinic are Aspergillums (more than 80%), followed by Trichoderma, Candida albicans and spores, which are all condition pathogenic bacteria. The infection of Trichoderma is quite sinister because it is more inclined to invade the elastic intimal of the arteries and form thrombus, secondary ischemic thrombus and hemorrhagic necrosis. The obstruction of nasal drainage caused by various factors is one of the main pathogenic factors of partial fungal sinusitis. Long term use of corticosteroids, broad spectrum antibiotics and tumor drugs, radiotherapy and AIDS patients are all vulnerable to fungal sinusitis. The clinical incidence of women is higher than that of men. Maxillary sinus is susceptible to diseases and others are sinus ethmoid sinus, sphenoid sinus and frontal sinus. A single nasal sinus is often the main cause of the disease, but one side of the whole group of nasal sinus can be gradually involved [2].

**Etiology**

The most common pathogenic fungi of nasal sinusitis in clinic are Aspergillums, but mucous infection is also increasing. Although naso-cerebral mucormycosis is rare, its condition is very dangerous, its development is very rapid and its mortality rate is very high. In addition, rhizopus, Rhizopus and ploughshare fungi from rotten vegetables, seeds, excreta of fruits and animals, soil and other substances, as well as Mucor, Hamildew and Mucor are also considered to be associated with the pathogenesis of invasive fungal sinusitis. Aspergillus requires special environmental reproduction and invasion, including nasal cavity mucosa itself due to previous infection or surgical operation injury, mucosal hypertrophy, chronic bacterial sinusitis etc. Acid and high sugar environment, such as diabetic ketoacidosis, is an ideal condition for the growth of Trichoderma. Disorder of iron metabolism or excessive storage of iron is also beneficial to the occurrence of mucormycosis mucocolasosis. Trichoderma has the characteristics of vascular endothelial cells, so it is easy to destroy the blood vessels.

**Clinical Manifestation**

1. Invasive fungal rhinosinusitis

   Fungi invaded the mucosal artery, causing thrombotic arteritis, resulting in ischemic necrosis of the mucosa and bone wall. In severe cases, it involves the orbital, pterygopalatine fossa and even the anterior cranial fossa, resulting in exophthalmos, ophthalmoplegia, visual impairment, posterior orbital pain, fever, coma and death. There are bloody pus, granulation and necrotic bone defects in the nasal cavity and paranasal sinuses. There are acute invasive fungal rhinosinusitis. Sinusitis and chronic invasive fungal rhinosinusitis
2. Noninvasive fungal rhinosinusitis

   The lesions are limited to nasal cavity and sinus cavity. The sinus cavity was filled with pale green, dark brown, grey-black filthy debris-like cheese, and mucosal edema and hyperplasia.
   (a) fungal balls formed from hyphae and spores, degeneration of white blood cells and epithelial cells. They are dark brown, black mass of fungus ball granuloma which increasing compression bone wall, sinus mucosa edema and hyperplasia.
   (b) allergic reaction types: also known as allergic fungal sinusitis, often with the history of nasal polyps and asthma, after multiple sinus surgery, but the attack of

sinusitis is still repeated. Sinus cavity filling with hard brittle and sticky white brown, microscopic examination showed a majority of eosinophils, eosinophil granule free, Charcot Leyden crystal (Charcot Leyden) and fungal filaments.

**Diagnosis**

1. More common in the elderly and affects more women than men. The patient usually has a normal immune function. The incidence of unilateral sinus was the highest, followed by sphenoid sinus and ethmoid sinus, and frontal sinus was rare. The clinical manifestations are chronic sinusitis, such as unilateral nasal obstruction, purulent discharge or stench. No symptoms were found except during sinus imaging examination. The fungus ball develops larger, may have the facial protuberance and the pain, has the fewer pus and haemorrhage and the surrounding structure like the orbital involvement symptom, generally does not have the whole body symptom. CT scan of the sinuses showed an increase in uneven density of the unilateral sinuses (Fig. 11.6). High density calcification spots or spots could be seen in 70% of the sinuses, and sinus wall swelling or absorption could be observed. Generally, there was no bone destruction. CT examination of nasal sinuses is an important preoperative diagnostic reference, and the final basis is pathogenesis.
2. Allergic Fungal Rhinosinusitis

   It occur more in adults and young people with atopic constitution often accompanied by nasal polyps and bronchial asthma. The onset of this disease is hidden, slow progress, more involved in one side of the sinus. Lesion expansion and development in the sinuses, nasal and sinus dilation caused by increased bone wall compression absorption, clinical manifestations of maxillofacial side or slowly progressive uplift, painless, fixed, hard, irregular, drop increasing haze caused by compression of the eye proptosis, displacement, and restriction of eye movements, diplopia, blepharoptosis, violent sinus CT display lesions of central high density allergic mucin from shadow was uniform and ground glass (Fig. 11.7). Gomori staining showed fungal mycelia in the pathological tissue, but there was no direct invasion of the mucous membrane and bone in the sinus.

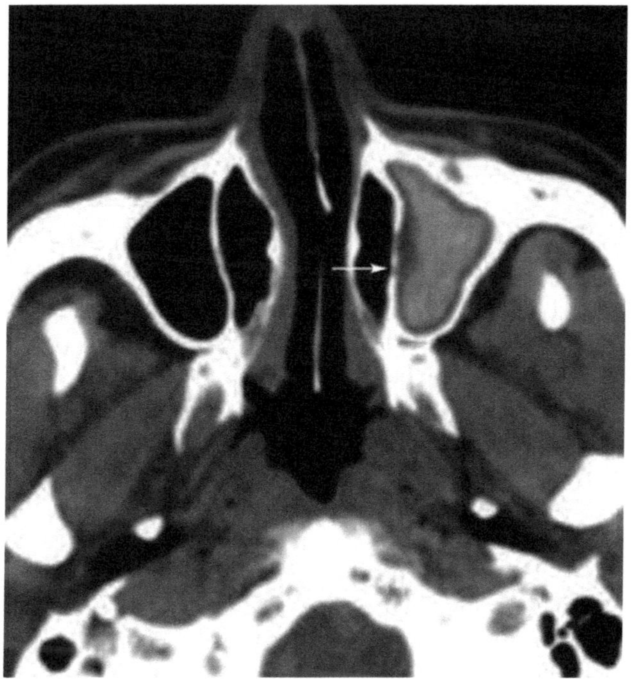

**Fig. 11.7** Left maxillary sinus fungal nasal sinusitis. Axial CT scan shows uniform frosted glasslike relatively higher density shadow in left maxillary sinus

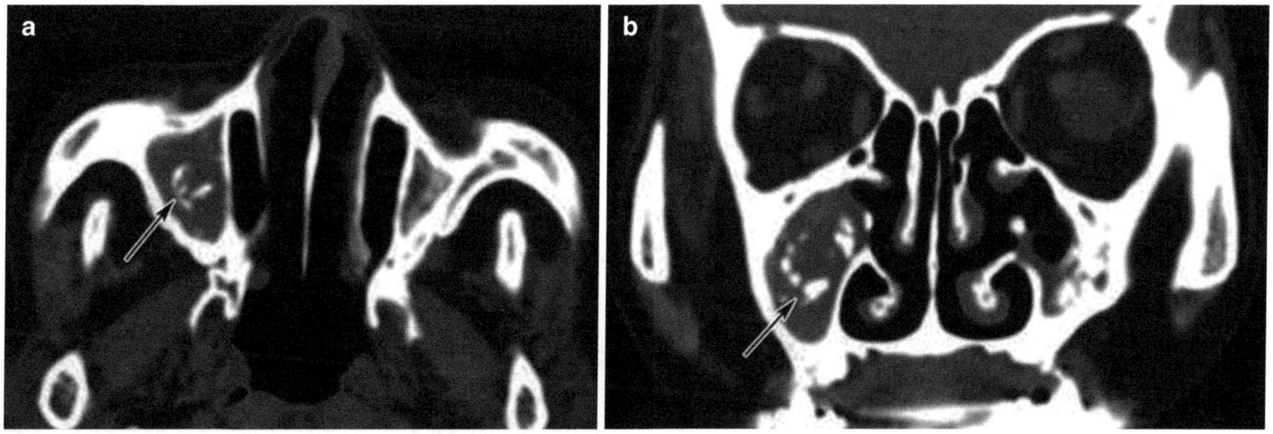


**Fig. 11.6** Right maxillary sinus fungal manifestation at nasal sinus CT scan. (**a**). Axial CT scan. (**b**) Coronary CT re-stablishment, showing internal right maxillary sinus soft tissue density shadow filling and internal mottling or sand granular calcification (arrow), but with normal sinus cavum form and no sinus wall sclerotic damage

3. Acute Invasive Fungal Rhinosinusitis

   Mostly occur in patients with low immune function or deficiency. It is commonly seen in diabetic ketoacidosis, organ transplantation, longterm application of glucocorticoids or anti-tumor agents or broad-spectrum antibiotics, radiotherapy and AIDS patients. The pathogenic bacteria are Aspergillus and Trichoderma. This type is characterized by rapid onset, rapid disease progress, dangerous condition and very high mortality rate. The clinical manifestations are fever, nasal damage and necrosis, large amount of purulent scab, swelling and pain of periorbital and cheek (invasion of the infraorbital nerve), or exophthalmos, conjunctival congestion, ocular paralysis, loss of visual acuity and orbital pain after, or waist defect, or severe headache, high pressure, frequent seizures, confusion or hemiplegia, or sleeping tip syndrome, and cavernous sinus thrombophlebitis. If it is not diagnosed in time, it can cause death within a few days. Sinus CT shows the lesions involving the nasal cavity and multiple nasal sinuses, extensive bone wall destruction, and the invasion of the face, orbit, and skull base or pterygopalatine fossa.

4. Chronic Invasive Fungal Rhinosinusitis

   This disease is characterized by slow progressive tissue invasion. The common pathogenic bacteria were Aspergillus moldis, gilligella and Candida. Patients with bloody nasal discharge or severe headache, sinus CT showed sinus involvement or bone destruction and intraoperative observation of sinus lesions and debris like material with a high content of thick pus, sinus mucosa showed degree of swelling, play dark red, crisp and easy bleeding and surface granular changes or mucosa is black, necrosis. Most of the early diagnosis and reasonable treatment can be cured. Later treatment is difficult, easy to relapse and worse.

**Treatment**

The principles of treatment for fungal rhinosinusitis are as follows

1. Early Surgical Treatment

   The invasive patients should be operated as soon as possible to remove the fungal pathogens and necrotic and irreversible pathological tissue in the nasal cavity and sinus and restore the smooth drainage of the sinuses. The mode and scope of the operation should be based on the extent of the lesion and the patient's specific conditions.

2. Drug Treatment
   (a) Antifungal drugs must be used after acute invasive fungal rhinosinusitis, and itraconazole and amphotericin B are commonly used as antifungal agents.
   (b) The use of glucocorticoids is a very important adjuvant therapy for allergic fungal rhinosinusitis after surgery.

3. Symptomatic Support Therapy

   Strengthen the resistance, restore the immune function, treat the original disease, and stop the use of antibiotics and immunosuppressive drugs. Transfusion of blood or plasma is necessary.

## 11.4 Rhinal Septum Deviation

The nasal septum deviation is a common disease in Otorhinolaryngology Head and Neck Surgery. It is caused by the deviation of the upper and lower diameters of nasal septum from sagittal plane to one or both sides, or the formation of local protuberances and nasal dysfunction. If there is no nasal dysfunction, nasal septum deviation is called "physiological nasal septum deviation". The cause of the disease is associated with trauma, dysplasia, and hypertrophy of the nasal turbinate on one side of the nasal cavity, tumor compression and hereditary factors. The higher the incidence of the disease has caused more and more attention of experts at home and abroad, according to the relevant documents at home and abroad as 12.7–81.2%. General deviation is C shape or S shape, part of a cone like protrusions called bone spines or moment condyle (Fig. 11.8) from the front to the back of a strip like protrusions called bone ridge mountain ridge. The type of nasal septum is shown in Fig. 11.9.

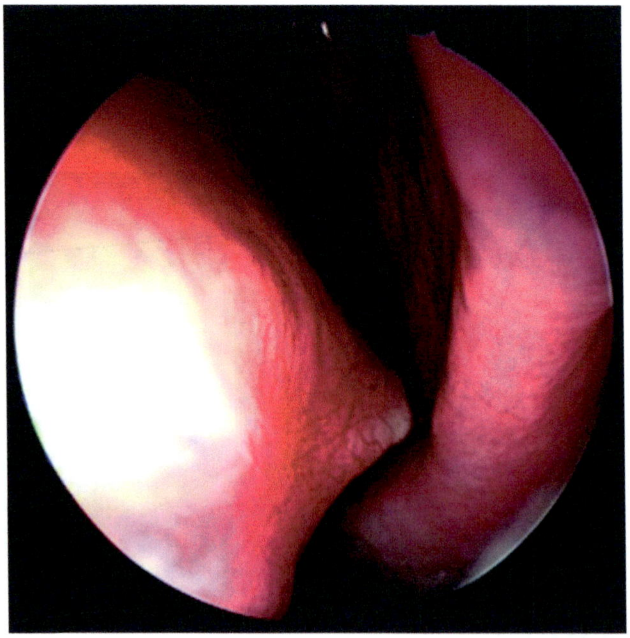

**Fig. 11.8** Rhinal septum leftwards deviation displays bone spines

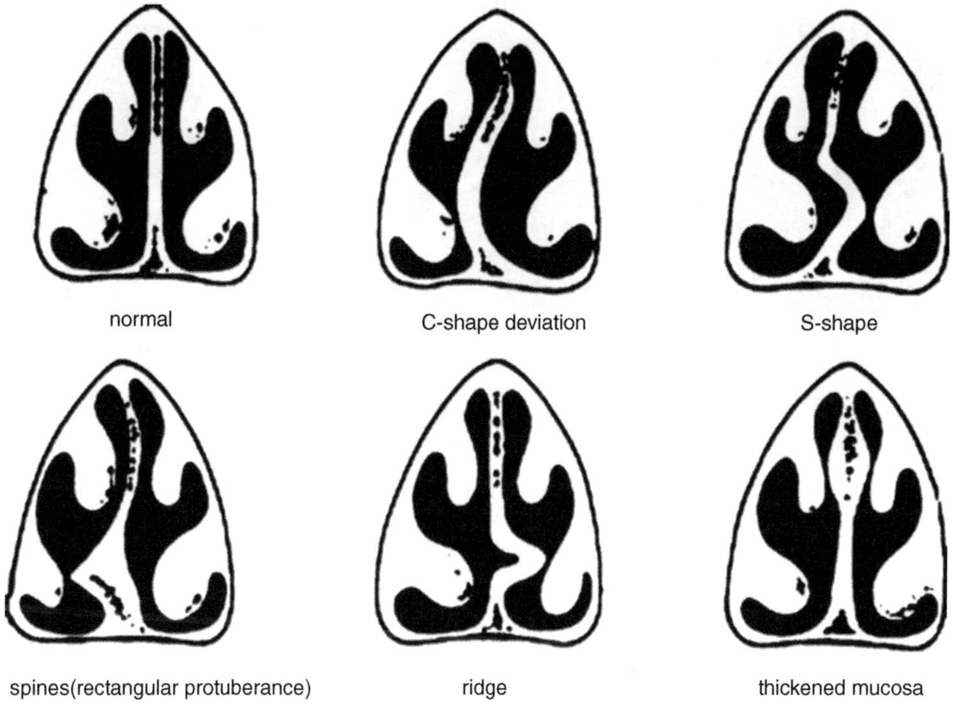


**Fig. 11.9** Rhinal septum deviation types

**Etiology**
1. The bone and cartilage of the nasal septum are unevenly developed.
2. The tumor or foreign body compress the nasal septum.
3. Trauma.
4. Children with adenoid enlargement of the nasal ventilation affect, the bottom of the nasal cavity pressure, nasal septum deviation was gradually the development state.

**Clinical Manifestation**
1. Nasal Congestion

   It is a common symptom. It is more persistent. General on one side of the nasal septum bulging is heavy, often unilateral nasal obstruction, such as the C shape deviation process, contralateral inferior turbinate hypertrophy, and also appeared bilateral nasal obstruction. S shape deviation is mostly bilateral obstruction. If patients with deviation of nasal septum suffer from acute rhinitis, the nasal obstruction is more serious, and it is not easy to recover. Severe nasal obstruction can also lead to a loss of olfaction.
2. Headache

   As part of the inferior turbinate or compression deviation of middle turbinate, can cause ipsilateral reflex headache. The nose is heavy.
3. Nasal Bleeding

   Most of them occurs on the side or ridge of the nasal septum protruding. Because of the large mucous membrane tension and thin mucosa have abundant blood supply in nasal soft tissue hence it is easier to bleed when nasal cavity is dry, blow nose and sneeze.
4. Adjacent Organs Involved Symptom

   Nasal congestion prevents sinus drainage and can induce suppurative sinusitis or fungal infection. If affects the eustachian tube ventilation drainage, it can cause the ear tinnitus, ear tightness. Long-term nasal obstruction, open mouth breathing, susceptible to colds and upper respiratory tract infections, and can occur during sleep serious snoring.
5. Nasal Septum Deviation and Bone Spine or Callus

   Hypertrophy of the inferior turbinate should be distinguished from the hypertrophy of the nasal septum. Patients with nasal septum deviation complicated by nasal deformities, such as a crooked nose, nostrils narrow.

**Diagnosis**
Combined with the history and symptoms, the diagnosis is easy. Nasal endoscopy is helpful to understand the type and degree of deviation of nasal septum, whether there are other nasal diseases at the same time, and if necessary, CT coronal scan can show the deviation more clearly, and help to understand whether there are primary lesions such as tumors in the sinuses (Fig. 11.10).

**Treatment**
Surgical correction is the only treatment. But if nasal polyp or turbinate enlargement occur at the same time, nasal polyp and turbinate surgery should be performed first. If nasal ventilation improves and nasal symptoms disappear, the deviated septum can also be untreated.

Patients with following circumstances should take operations

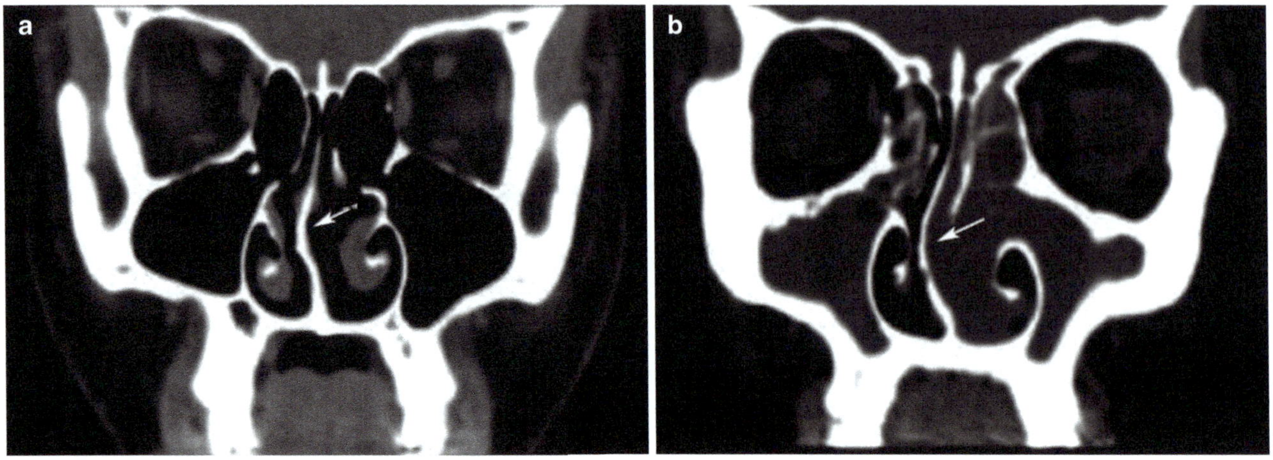


**Fig. 11.10** CT plain scan coronary reconstruction displays rhino septum deviation. (**a**) Single rhino septum C-shape deviation (arrow). (**b**) Rhino septum C shape deviation(arrow) accompanies with abundant left rhinocavum soft tissues (polyps), left frontal sinus, sphenoid sinus and right frontal sinus full of soft tissues or hydrops (chronic rhinal sinusitis) (arrow)

1. Nasal septum deviation caused by long-term persistent congestion.
2. The high deviation of nasal septum affecting sinus drainage.
3. Recurrent epistaxis caused by deviation of nasal septum.
4. Reflex headache caused by deviation of nasal septum.
5. Vasomotor rhinitis obvious nasal septum deviation (structural rhinitis).

Compared with traditional surgery, endoscopic nasal septum plasty has the advantages of good illumination, clear surgical field and easy peeling, especially for patients with insufficient exposure to posterior and high deviation, which improves the surgical effect. Three-line tension reduction is commonly used in nasal septum plasty.

Three-line tension reduction method: patients take supine position, routine disinfection and towel laying, after anesthesia is effective, make a longitudinal incision at the junction of skin and mucosa on the left side of nasal septum under a 0 degree wide-angle mirror, cut from the top of nasal septum to the bottom of nasal cavity, then lengthen from the bottom of nasal cavity to the back properly; cut mucochondral membrane and separate it by suction stripper according to the routine method, and separate it backward and upward to the back of the deviated vertical plate of ethmoid bone, and downward. Separation to the plowbone, expose the deviated vertical plate of ethmoid bone, gently press the junction of nasal septum cartilage and vertical plate of ethmoid bone with nasal septum stripper, disconnect the connection between nasal septum cartilage and vertical plate of ethmoid bone, fully free the vertical plate of ethmoid bone under the opposite mucoperiosteal, suitably bite the bone of the front of vertical plate of ethmoid bone (second tension line); Vertical excision of 2–3 mm soft tissue at the front of nasal septum cartilage. The nasal septum cartilage was separated and disconnected with a stripper under the opposite mucoperiosteal to free the nasal septum cartilage from the vomer so as to free the posterior and inferior edges of the nasal septum cartilage. The cartilage strip of the inferior end of the nasal septum cartilage (the third tension line) was removed horizontally with the middle turbinate scissors, and the deviated nasal ridge and palatine nasal ridge were chiseled downward, where the nasal ridge was often formed. The deflected vomers were bitten back at the stress sites of the septum ridge, spine and posterior deviation. Patients with chronic rhinitis and hypertrophy of turbinate were treated with inferior turbinate fracture displacement or partial resection, and those with sinusitis and nasal polyps underwent endoscopic sinus surgery at the same time. Two nasal hemostatic gauze or expanded hemostatic sponge were filled 48–72 h after operation and then removed. (Fig. 11.11).

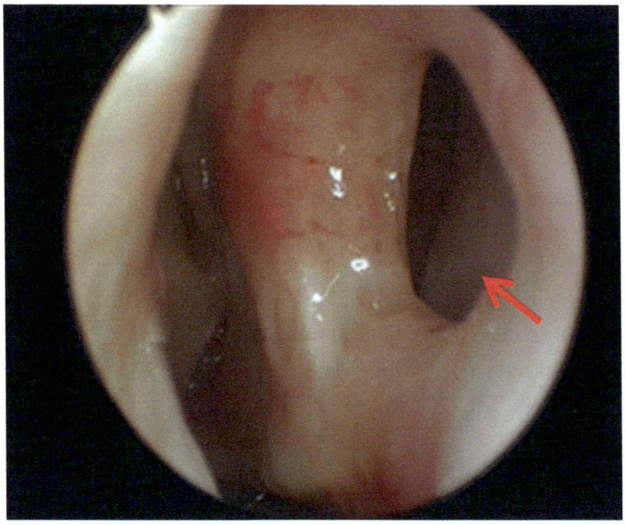

**Fig. 11.11** Perforation after nasal septum surgery (from another hospital)

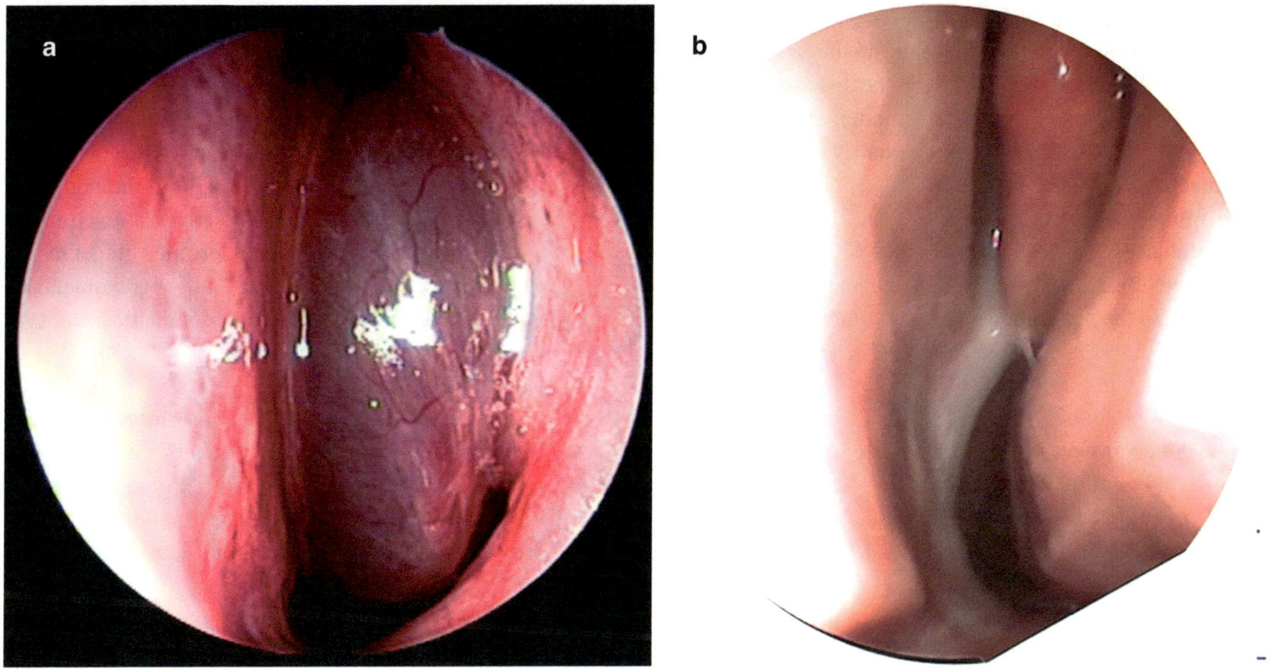


**Fig. 11.12** Nasal endoscopic examination (**a**) Left cavum rhinopolyp (**b**) Purulent secretions from the middle nasal passage

## 11.5 Chronic Rhinonasa Sinusitis

Chronic rhinosinusitis is the chronic inflammation at the nasal sinus and the nasal cavity mucosa, lasting over 12 months. The chronic rhinosinusitis media have two types:

1. Chronic Rhinosinusitis with nasal Polyp.
2. Chronic Rhinosinusitis without nasal Polyp.

The rhinal polyp preferably occurs at the middle nasal choncha free edge, ethmoid sinus, ethmoidal vesicle, ethmoid processus uncinatus, semilunar hiatus and maxillary sinus orifice and other sites. It could be caused the nasal mucosa edema, combined acting with many factors whose main cause are the allergic reaction and the chronic inflammation. It should also be differentially diagnosed from the middle meatus nasi mucosa pachynsis or the middle nasal concha, the meninx cerebrum inflation, the atrophy papilla tumor, the nasopharynx fibrous angioma and the nasal sarcoma.

**Clinical Manifestation**

1. Main Symptoms

   The main symptoms are nasal obstruction, viscous or mucopurulent runny nose.
2. Secondary Symptoms

   Include swelling and pain in the head and face, and loss of sense of smell.

   The diagnosis is based on the above two or more related symptoms, of which nasal obstruction, viscous or mucopurulent runny nose must be one of the main symptoms.

**Examination**

1. Nasal endoscopic examination

   Sticky or purulent secretions from the middle nasal concha, the olfactory fissures, the nasal mucosa congestion, edema or polyp occurs.(Fig. 11.12)
2. Imaging Examination

   CT scan of the nasal sinuses showed that the mucosa of the nasal sinuses was thickened, the ostiomeatal complex was obstructed, and there were soft tissue density shadow in the nasal cavity and nasal meatus with clear boundary, uniform density, and slight linear enhancement on enhanced scan. When the polyps filled the nasal meatus or sinus cavity, the nasal meatus or sinus cavity showed expansive changes, usually without bone destruction, occasionally with slight bone mass. Absorption or hardening, as shown in (Fig. 11.13)

The diagnosis was made on the basis of clinical symptoms, endoscopy and/or CT findings of the sinuses. In the diagnosis of chronic rhinosinusitis in children, it should first be based on symptoms and signs, and combined with the results of endoscopic examination to determine, if there is no clear diagnosis or special circumstances, CT examination is recommended.

**State Evaluation**

According to the recommendation of "Guidelines for the Diagnosis and Treatment of Chronic Rhinosinusitis (Kunming, 2012)" issued by the Rhinology Section of the Otolaryngological Head and Neck Surgery Society of the Chinese Medical Association [3]. The following methods were used to evaluate the overall condition of patients with chronic rhinosinusitis

1. Subjective general evaluation
   It is the subjective evaluation of the severity of the disease. According to VAS score, the disease was divided into (Fig. 11.14): mild 0–3; moderate >3–7; severe >7–10. If VAS > 5, the patient's quality of life is affected
2. Objective General Evaluation
   Lund-Mackay evaluation (Table 11.1) evaluates the lesion scope due to the nasal sinus CT scan. The Lund-Kennedy evaluation (Table 11.2) evaluates the state severity due to the nasal endoscope examinations.

**Treatment**

1. Drug Treatment
   (a) Glucocorticoid: it's not suggested to inject systemically or at the endosonose.
   - Endonasal Glucocorticoid: it has anti-inflammation, anti-edema, lasting at least 12 weeks
   - Systemic Glucocorticoid:
     Usually used at the chronic rhinalsinuitis with the rhinopolyp, especially the severe, recurrent rhinopolyp. It can be taken orally in a short time. It is necessary to pay attention to the contraindications of hormone use throughout the body and closely observe the possible adverse reactions in the course of medication. Chronic rhinosinusitis without nasal polyps is not recommended. Glucocorticoids are not recommended for systemic or intranasal injection.

   (b) Decyclic Lactones Drugs
   Fourteen loop decyclic lactones drugs have anti-inflammatory and immunomodulatory effects. They are mainly used in patients with chronic rhinosinusitis accompanied by nasal polyps, ineffective routine drug treatment, non-eosinophilia, normal IgE value

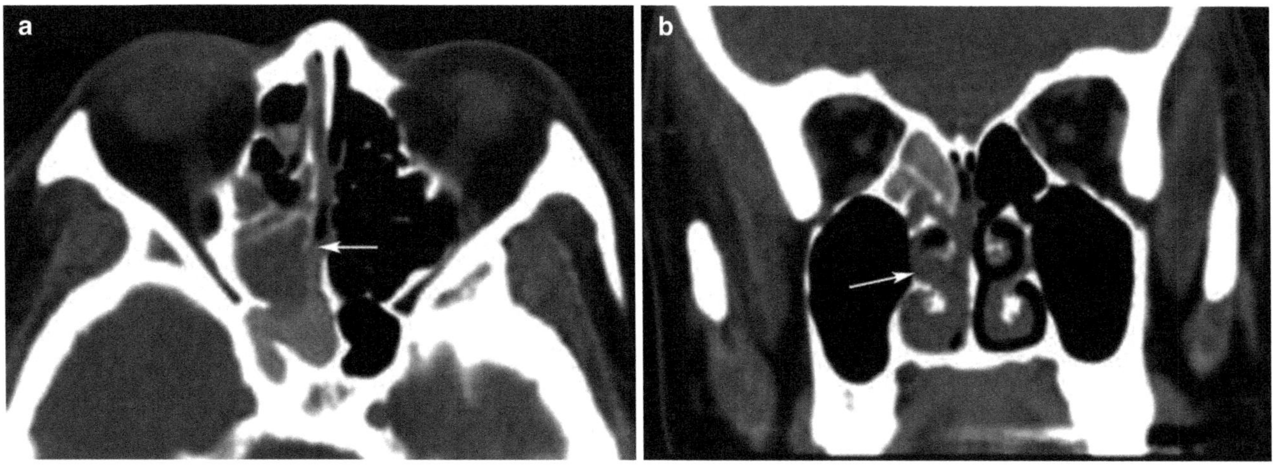


**Fig. 11.13** Plane CT scan shows the right ethmoiditis accompanying with the rhinopolyp exists. (**a**). Plane CT scan imaging; (**b**) coronal CT scan reestablishment: right ethmoid sinus and visual filled endocavum soft tissue dense shadow, no bone damage

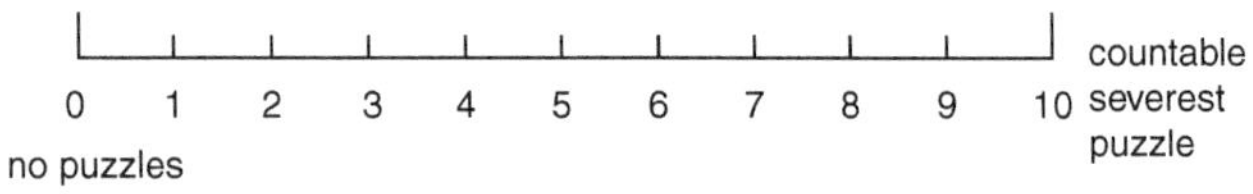


**Fig. 11.14** VAS (score 0–10)

**Table 11.1** Nasal sinus Lund-Mackay evaluation chart

| Nasosinus system | Left side | Right side |
|---|---|---|
| Maxillary sinus | | |
| Anterior ethmoid sinus | | |
| Posterior ethmoid sinus | | |
| Sphenoid sinus | | |
| Frontal sinus | | |
| Sinus Osteomeatal canal complex | | |
| Final score | | |

Gist: nasosinus: 0 = no abnormality, 1 = partial turbidity, 2 = total turbidity; 2. Sinus-oronasal complex: 0 = no obstruction, 2 = obstruction; 3. Sinus-oronasal complex: 0–12, total score 0–24

**Table 11.2** Nasosinus endoscope examination LundKennedy evaluation chart

| Characteristics | Lateral type | Base line | 3 month | 6 month | 1 year |
|---|---|---|---|---|---|
| Rhinopolyp | Left | | | | |
| | Right | | | | |
| Edema | Left | | | | |
| | Right | | | | |
| Rhinorrhea | Left | | | | |
| | Right | | | | |
| Scar | Left | | | | |
| | Right | | | | |
| Escharosis | Left | | | | |
| | Right | | | | |
| Final score | | | | | |

Gist: (1) rhinopolyp: 0 = no polyp, 1 = polyp only in the middle nasal meatus, 2 = polyp beyond the middle nasal meatus; (2) edema: 0 = no, 1 = mild, 2 = serious; (3) rhinorrhea: 0 = no, 1 = clear, thin rhinorrhea, 2 = viscous, purulent rhinorrhea; (4) scar: 0 = no, 1 = light, 2 = heavy (only for evaluation of surgical efficacy); (5) crust: 0 = no, 1 = light, 2 = heavy (only for evaluation of surgical efficacy). 0–10 on each side, with a total score of 0–20

and negative allergen detection in non-allergic chronic rhinosinusitis. It is recommended that low doses (1/2 of conventional doses) be taken orally for a long period of not less than 12 weeks.

Macrolides are not routinely used after endoscopic sinus surgery. If the nasal mucosa is persistent congestion, swelling and accompanied by purulent secretions more than 4 weeks after surgery, they can also be considered.

(c) Antibiotics Drugs

When chronic rhinosinusitis is accompanied by acute infection 4 weeks after surgery, sensitive antibiotics can be selected according to the results of bacterial culture and drug sensitivity test. Routine dosage is not more than 2 weeks.

(d) Grume Dissolution Drug (Mucosoluble)

It can dilute the secretions of nasal cavity and sinuses, improve the ciliary activity of nasal mucosa, promote the excretion of mucus and help the recovery of physiological function of nasal cavity and sinuses. It is recommended to use.

(e) Anti-allergy Drugs

Antiallergic drugs, including oral or nasal antihistamines and oral leukotriene receptor antagonists, can be used for patients with allergic rhinitis and/or asthma for a period of not less than 4 weeks. For patients with asthma, oral leukotriene receptor antagonists are preferred [4].

(f) Chinese Traditional Medicine

The traditional Chinese clinic medicine has accumulated plenty of valuable experience in clinical practice. The traditional Chinese medicine should assist to treat the chronic rhinosinusitis sinusitis according to the conditions and based on the overall analysis and diagnosis principle.

(g) Congestion Subtraction Drugs (decogestants)

They are not principally suggested. But to those who have persistent severe nose obstruction, it can be short term used with a course less than 7 days.

(h) Nasal irrigation

It's an efficient measurement for treatment of chronic rhinosinusitis and also a common assistant treatment measurement after endoscopic sinus surgery.

(i) Omalizumab for Injection

As worldwide first innovative asthma target drug, inflammatory mediators and eosinophils could be reduced by being bound with IgE, however, it could be applied to adult's patients with sinusitis and rhinopolyps accompanying with asthma in clinic [5].

2. Surgery

(a) Surgery Indications

- Obvious anatomic abnormality influences the sinus aperture canal complex or nasal sinuses drainage.
- Rhinopolyp affecting the sinus aperture canal complex or nasal sinuses drainage.
- Unsatisfied Improvement after drug treatment.
- Intracranial and intraorbital complications.

The indication of operation for children with chronic rhinosinusitis should be strictly limited, and surgery should not be performed in principle under 12 years old.

(b) Perioperative Period Management

The managment is centered on surgery. In principle, it should include a series of medication strategies and principles from 1–2 weeks before operation to 3–6 months after operation.

- Preoperative Stage (714 days)

  The principle is to alleviate the inflammatory reaction of nasal cavity and sinus mucosa, control systemic diseases, and create ideal conditions for improving the quality and safety of surgery.

- Operation Stage

  The principle of management is reasonable and minimally invasive nasal-sinus surgery.

- Post Operation Management

  Management involves anti-inflammation, reduction of intraoperative adhesion, reduction of intraoperative vesicles and polyps, maintenance of open drainage of sinus orifice, and acceleration of epithelialization of mucosa.

  Frequent nasal endoscopy and surgical intervention should not be performed after operation. Postoperative local treatment time can be limited to: the first operation cavity cleaning within 1 to 2 weeks after the operation, mainly to remove old hematocele and secretions, and then determine the interval of follow-up treatment according to the recovery of the operation cavity. The interval of each treatment is usually not less than 2 weeks, lasting for 3 to 6 months.

(c) Refractory rhinosinusitis Treatments

Refractory rhinosinusitis refers to the difficulty of clinical treatment, which is that after standardized endoscopic sinus surgery and comprehensive treatment for more than 3 months, the condition has not been effectively controlled, and persistent infection and persistent inflammatory reaction in the operative cavity. Because of its complex pathogenic factors, it is difficult to achieve satisfactory results in single clinical treatment. It is suggested that personalized comprehensive treatment should be formulated on the basis of in-depth etiological analysis.

## 11.6 Nasal Vestibular Cyst

Nasal vestibular cyst is a cystic mass located under the skin at the bottom of nasal vestibule and in the superficial soft tissue of alveolar process of maxilla, which is more common in women.(Fig. 11.15).

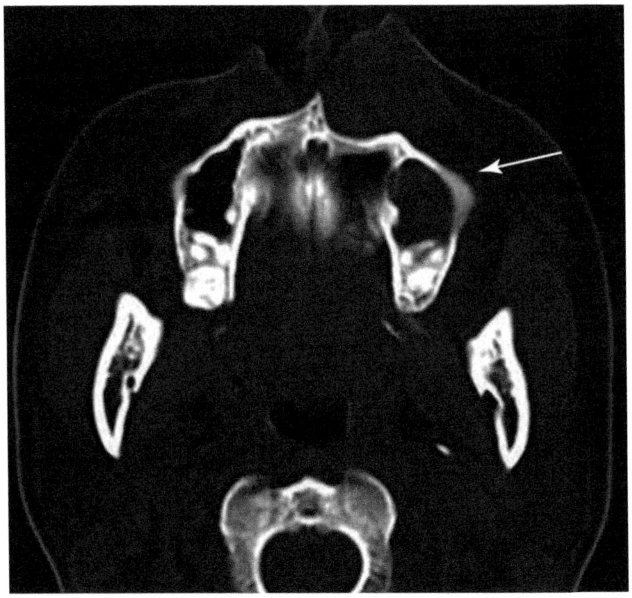

**Fig. 11.15** Paranial sinusaxial CT scan indicates the left nasal vestibular cyct (arrow)

**Etiology**

Two major theories: glands retention theory considers that it is caused by secretion retention after the cavum base mucosa mucous gland tube obstruction; facial cleft theory thinks that it is developed from the residual epithelium at the facial protrusion junctions at the embryonic period.

**Pathogenesis**

The cyst wall is composed of connective tissue containing elastic fibers and many reticular vessels, lined with ciliated columnar epithelium, cubic epithelium or flat epithelium. The cyst fluid is mostly mucous, brown and yellow, mostly cholesterol-free, and purulent when combined with infection.

**Clinical Manifestation**

The cyst grow slowly and are mostly asymptomatic in the early stage. With the enlargement of the tumors, the nasal vestibular bulge can be seen, accompanied by congestion or swelling pain on the ipsilateral side. When combined with infection, the cyst enlarges rapidly and local pain aggravates. Examination showed that the nasal vestibular area was raised, palpation could palpate and smooth elastic hemispherical tumors, local puncture could extract brown and yellow mucus, mostly without cholesterol. CT showed round soft tissue shadow in pyriform foramen area without adjacent dental lesions.

**Diagnosis**

It can mostly be confirmed due to the clinic manifestations. It should differ from the odontogenic cyst, which is secondary to the teeth lesion, often develops the unilateral superior teeth line lesion, the hydatoncus is tawny or sauce black, mostly contains cholesterol and the alveolar process fracture damage or the tooth in the hydatoncus is seen at imaging examination.

**Treatment**

It is mainly on surgery, which could enter the channel through the labiogingival groove, completely remove the cyst wall and pad the cavum after surgery. The endoscopic cyst peel method can be applied to excise the wall inserts into the nasal cavum to make a cystostomy in the nasal cavum and it is less traumatic, less time using and faster recover.

## 11.7 Rhinonasosinus Benign Tumor

### 11.7.1 Hemangioma

Hemangioma is the most common benign tumors of nasal cavity and paranasal sinus, which originates from vascular tissue and can be divided into capillary hemangioma and cavernous hemangioma. Capillary hemangioma is small, mostly occurs in the nasal septum, and can be pedicled. Microscopically, it is composed of most mature thin-walled capillaries, closely arranged in clusters or lobulated. Cavernous hemangioma is large, broad-based, soft, no envelope. It often occurs in the lateral wall of the nasal cavity and inferior turbinate. It can involve the sinuses. Microscopically, the tissues are composed of sinuses of different sizes that communicate with each other [6].

**Clinic Manifestations**

The main manifestation is the nasal hemorrhage. When the tumors are large, diplopia and headache may occur due to nasal obstruction or compression of adjacent organs. On physical examination, pedicled or broad-based dark red neoplasms can be seen in the nasal cavity, which are soft and easy to bleed. Cavernous hemangioma of the maxillary sinus can protrude from the middle nasal meatus and present as hemorrhagic polyps. Removal or biopsy can lead to severe hemorrhage.

**Diagnosis**

Diagnose according to the clinic manifestation mostly. The maxillary sinus cavernous hemangioma should differ from the maxillary sinus hemorrhage, necrotic polyps and sarcoma.

**Treatment**

Treatment is mainly by surgical excision, excising the tumor and the root mucosa. Most hemangioma could be excised under nasal endoscope. Large hemangiomas in the nasal cavity or those involving nasal sinuses or skull base which are difficult to resect under endoscopy alone can be assisted by lip-gingival incision or nasal incision according to the location of the tumors. Maxillary artery embolization is feasible before operation to reduce intraoperative bleeding.

### 11.7.2 Inverted Papilloma

Inverted papilloma is one of the most common nasal and paranasal sinus tumors in the department of rhinology. It often occurs unilaterally. The most common site of inverted papilloma is around the ethmoid sinus and maxillary sinus. Its occurrence may be related to human papillomavirus. Although the pathology is benign, the biology is invasive and malignant. It is usually considered as a borderline tumor.

**Clinic Manifestations and Gradings**

1. Unilateral nasal obstruction with the purulent snot, sometimes within blood.
2. Bilateral lesions causing smell loss.
3. Tumor enlargement can lead to headache, eye pain, diplopia and other symptoms.
4. Physical examination showed that the tumors were like multiple polyps, but the surface was not smooth, hard and easy to bleed when touched.
5. CT scan result of the cavum or nasal sinus could be soft tissue dense mass shadow with irregular shape and unclear boundary but well distributed (Fig. 11.16) producing specific 'air bubble' phenomenon because it contains air inside (Fig. 11.17) Bone resorption or hyperosteogeny can occur, which suspect the malignancy changes if the bony damage is severe. Enhanced CT scan shows slight enhancement and MR enhancement shows characteristic "brain return sign". (Fig. 11.18), and can be used to distinguish the pathological changes in the sinus cavity from tumors or retention of inflammatory secretion [7].

There are many grading method in clinic, of which the Krouse staging is the mostly common one.

- $T_1$: The lesion limits in the cavum nasi
- $T_2$: The lesion involved the medial wall and upper part of ethmoid sinus or maxillary sinus.
- $T_3$: The lesion involves the lateral wall and the inferior sites of the maxillary sinus or invades the sphenoid sinus and the frontal sinus.
- $T_4$: The lesion is beyond the range of nasal cavity and paranasal sinus or malignant change.

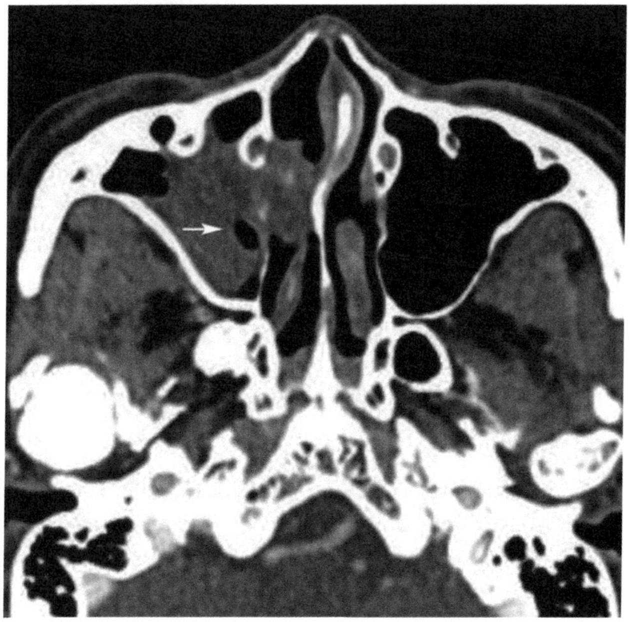

**Fig. 11.17** Axial CT scan manifest the right maxillary sinus inverted papilloma. 'Air bubble' phenomenon may occur (arrow)

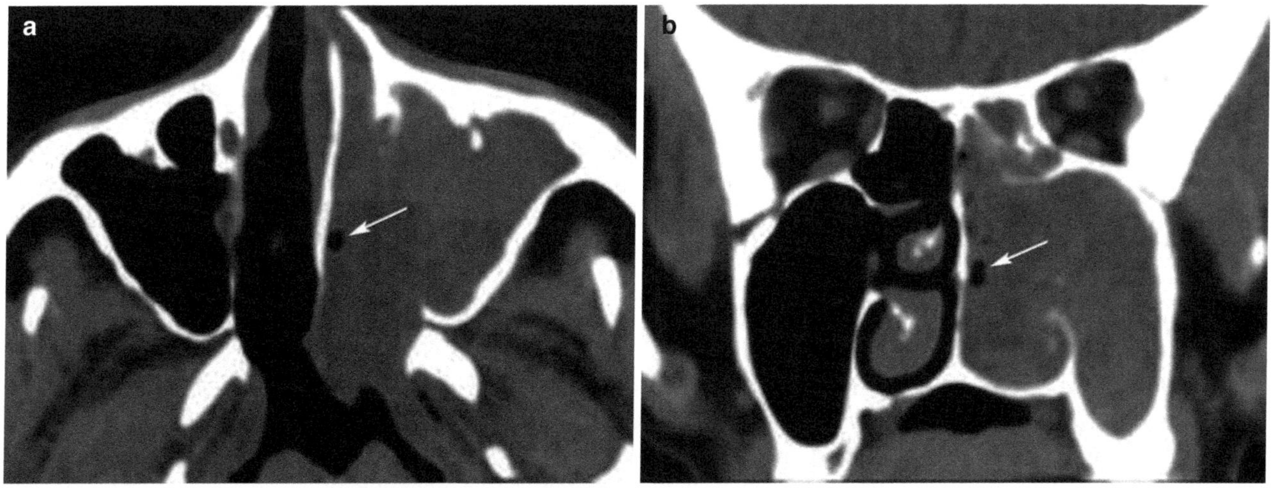


**Fig. 11.16** Entropy papilla. (**a**) Plane axial CT scans. (**b**) Coronary rebuilding. It shows the filled soft tissue dense shadow at the left cavum nasi, the ethmoid sinus and the maxillary sinus, containing low dense 'air bubble 'phenomenon (arrow), the opening of the left maxillary sinus was obviously enlarged and the bone absorption of the sinus wall was not obvious

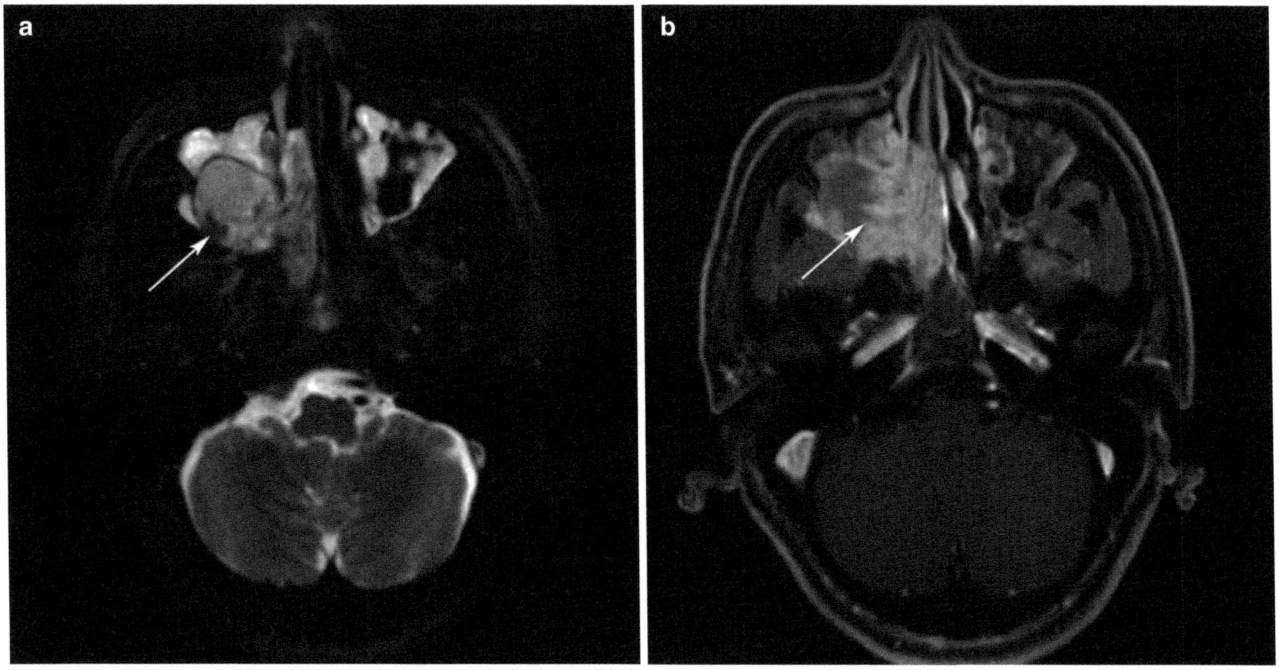


**Fig. 11.18** Right cavum nasi entropy papilla (malignant). (**a**) MR axial $T_2$WI fat saturation. (**b**) Axial $T_1$WI enhancement. The bilateral ethmoid sinus, maxillary sinus mucosa obviously thickens; the right maxillary sinus and the sphenoid sinus fills with the $T_2$ signals. An irregular soft tissue signal in the right nasal cavum and the maxillary sinus, badly distributed and appearing as a lengthened $T_2$ signal; strengthened dense lesion distinctly intensifies and manifests as 'brain gyrus sign' (arrow)

**Diagnosis**

Diagnose according to the history, physical examination and the imaging examination and differentiate diagnosis with the pathology biopsy result. If there is malignant transformation, treatment should be the same to carcinoma.

**Treatment**

Surgery is the main treatment, which requires complete excision of tumors and pathological mucosa, partial removal of bone in germinal center, and high recurrence rate is related to unclean excision. Inverted papilloma of maxillary sinus can be resected through anterior lacrimal recess and inverted papilloma of frontal sinus can be resected by Draf III operation. Malignant transformation should be treated according to the principle of resection of malignant tumors.

## 11.8 Rhinonasosinus Cancer

The relative incidence of malignant tumors of nasal cavity and paranasal sinus is relatively low, accounting for 3%–5% of all malignant tumors of head and neck; malignant tumors of maxillary sinus are the most common malignant tumors of nasal cavity and paranasal sinus, followed by malignant tumors of ethmoid sinus, malignant tumors of frontal sinus, sphenoid sinus and nasal cavity are rare; however, advanced tumors often involve all nasal cavity and paranasal sinus, and it is difficult to determine the pathological types of malignant tumors of nasal cavity and paranasal sinuses are various, including squamous cell carcinoma, adenocarcinoma, sarcoma, neuroendocrine carcinoma, olfactory neuroblastoma, adenoid cystic carcinoma, malignant melanoma, malignant tumors from small salivary glands of nasal cavity and paranasal sinuses, etc. Among them, squamous cell carcinoma, adenocarcinoma, olfactory neuroblastoma, malignant melanoma and so on are the most common, and the biological characteristics of various tumors are different. Different, lack of unified treatment norms. Most cases are concentrated in some large hospitals. It is difficult for specialists in general hospitals to master the treatment of all kinds of malignant tumors of nasal and paranasal sinuses. Therefore, a comprehensive grasp and analysis of malignant tumors of nasal and paranasal sinuses should be carried out from the basic to the clinical, in order to better design treatment programs for patients.

### 11.8.1 Nasal Cavity Carcinoma

Nasal cavity carcinoma differ at the etiology type but the clinic manifestation is similar.

**Etiology and Epidemiology**

The etiology of nasal malignant tumors is still unclear, which may be related to viral infection, chemical harmful gases and dust stimulation, family genetic susceptibility, etc.

The papilloma of nasal cavity and paranasal sinus caused by human papillomavirus infection is related to canceration of nasal cavity.

**Pathogenesis**

Cavum carcinoma is Mostly the squamous cell carcinoma, the adenocarcinoma, the olfactory neuroblastoma, the adenoid cystic tumor, the malignant melanoma (Fig. 11.19) and other tumors such as the undifferentiated tumors, the lymph epitheliumoma, the sarcoma, the granuloma malignum, the lymph tumor, etc.; the malignant archromelanoma is hard to differentiated from the nasal polyps and the nasal entropy papilla tumor. The malignant lymph coma especially the NK-T lymphoma doesn't appear the evident mass and only shows the mucosa extensive hemorrhage, erosion and escharosis.

**Clinical Manifestation**

1. Symptoms
   (a) Bloody Snot

   The early stage tumor lesion may trigger the ulceration, hemorrhage to cause the bloody snot or nasal hemorrhage. The symptoms could be cured temporarily, but it can also recur over and over again.

   (b) Nasal obstruction

   Tumors occupy one side of the nasal cavity and affect ventilation, characterized by unilateral nasal obstruction and progressive aggravation.

   (c) Epiphora

   When the tumor invades the nasolacrimal duct or lacrimal sac, it causes the obstruction of lacrimal passage and causes epiphora.

   (d) Advanced stage of tumors may involve the nasopharynx, orbit and skull base. Blocking the upper respiratory tract may cause nocturnal snoring or pathological sleep apnea, as well as visual impairment, diplopia and headache.

2. Physical Examination

   Physical examination under nasal endoscopy shows that nasal cavity has a rough surface of new organisms, can have ulcers, touch the texture is brittle, easy to bleed. Coronal CT shows malignant left nasal cavity when the tumor (Hemangiopericytoma) is large, the nose often smells bad.

**Diagnosis**

Based on the physical manifestation sign, the initial diagnosis can be done. The final diagnosis relies on the pathogenic examination result.

1. Imaging examination
   (a) CT Scan:

   Soft tissue shadow of nasal cavity can be seen, the boundary is unclear, and it is difficult to distinguish from obstructive inflammation of nasal sinuses. It can be adjacent to bone destruction. CT can assess the extent of soft tissue involvement and bone destruction of the lesion (Fig. 11.20). If skull base is involved, enhanced MR scanning is necessary.

   (b) MR Examination:

   soft tissue shadow with T1 high signal and T2 low signal in nasal cavity, and images with T1 low signal and T2 high signal in adjacent nasal sinuses (Fig. 11.21); and the extent of involvement of dura and subdural lesions can also be determined.

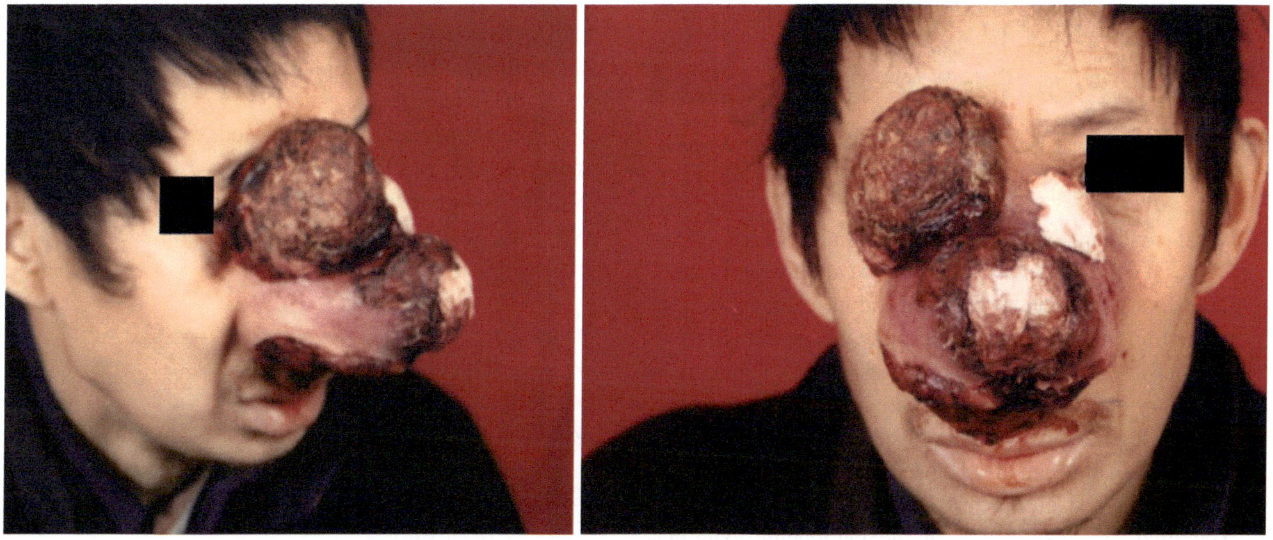

**Fig. 11.19** Cavumnasosinus malignant melanoma

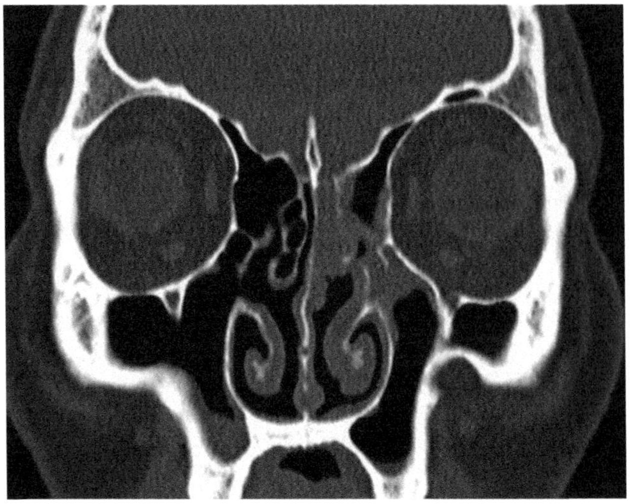

**Fig. 11.20** Coronary CT scan manifests the left cavum malignant vessel epithelium tumor

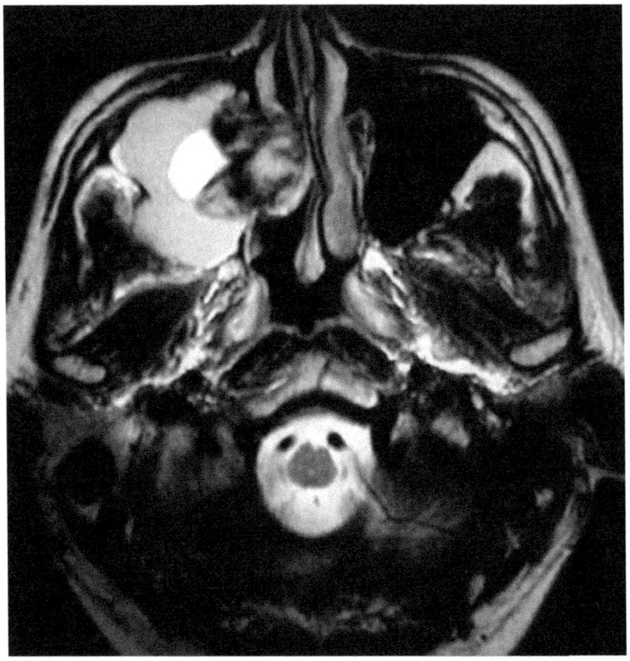

**Fig. 11.21** Horizontal MR shows the right cavum malignant melanoma

2. Nasal cavity and Nasoendoscope Examination

   Nasal cavity and nasal endoscopy can directly observe the primary location, size, shape and nasal sinus opening of the tumors by means of fiberoptic nasopharyngoscope and nasal endoscopy. For those suspected of malignant maxillary sinus tumors, nasal endoscopy can be used to observe lesions in the sinus or take biopsy; sphenoid sinus and frontal sinus can also be used.
3. Biopsy and the Cell Smear Examination

   The final diagnosis relies on the pathogenic examinations. The cavum biopsy could be applied when there is the tumor invades the cavum nasi. If it suspected as the nasosinus tumor, the biopsy or the smear under nasal endoscope and the maxillary sinus puncture examination can also be applied? To those whose pathogenic examination result is negative, diagnosis is hard to confirm and cases are regarded as the doubt cases, repeated biopsy is vital and the nasosinus exploratory section consultation can also be considered.

**TNM Grading (AJCC 2010)**

**T grading**

- $T_1$: The tumor limits at a sub-region with or without bone damage.
- $T_2$: The tumor invades two sub-regions in an area or an adjacent area in the ethmoid nasal complex with or without bone damage.
- $T_3$: The tumor invades the orbit base or intra lateral wall the maxillary sinus the palatine or the ethmoid plate.
- $T_{4a}$: Moderate advanced local disease

  The tumor invades an alternative site as following: the anterior orbit content, nasal sites or cheek skin, microinvasion at anterior cranial fossa, pterygoid lamina, sphenoid sinus or the frontal sinus.
- $T_{4b}$: Advanced stage local disease

  The tumor invades alternative site of the followings: orbit apex, the dura mater, the cerebral cells, the fossa cranii media, and the cranial nerve (except the trigeminal maxillary branch, nasopharynx or the clivus

**N gradings**

- $N_0$: Inconspicuous local lymph node metastasis
- $N_1$: Local single lymph node metastasis, maximum diameter $\leq$ 3 cm
- $N_2$: Unilateral single lymph node metastasis, 3 cm < maximum diameter < 6 cm, or unilateral multiple lymph nodes metastasis, maximum diameter $\leq$ 6 cm
- $N_{2a}$: Unilateral single lymph node metastasis, 3 cm < maximum diameter < 6 cm
- $N_{2b}$: Unilateral multiple lymph nodes metastasis, maximum diameter $\leq$ 6 cm
- $N_{2c}$: Maximum metastasised lymph node diameter > 6 cm
- $N_3$: Local metastasised lymph node completely can't be graded.

**M gradings**

- $M_0$: Inconspicuous further metastasis
- $M_1$: Further metastasis occurs
- $M_x$: Unrecognizable further metastasis

**Gradings**

- Stage 0: $T_{is}$ $N_0$ $M_0$
- Stage I: $T_1$ $N_0$ $M_0$

- Stage II: $T_2$ $N_0$ $M_0$
- Stage III: T3 $N_0$ $M_0$;$T_1$ $N_1$ M0;$T_2$ N1 $M_0$;$T_3$ $N_1$ $M_0$
- Stage IV: T4 N1-3M0-1

**Treatment**

Malignant tumors of the nasal cavity and paranasal sinus are generally treated by comprehensive treatment with operation as the main method. Comprehensive treatment was adopted according to pathological type and range of lesions. For moderate to low malignant tumors, such as squamous cell carcinoma, adenocarcinoma, adenoid cystic carcinoma, olfactory neuroblastoma and so on, if the tumors can be completely resected according to the imaging examination, they can be resected first, followed by radiotherapy or concurrent radiochemical therapy. If the malignancy of the tumors is high or the scope of the lesions is large, it is not appropriate to operate first. Radiotherapy or concurrent radiochemical therapy should be chosen first, and then surgical resection should be decided according to the situation.

1. Surgery

   Surgical treatment of nasal malignant tumors can be performed by endoscopic resection or lateral nasal incision. With the advancement of nasal endoscopy technology, more and more cases are treated by endoscopic nasal resection, which has the advantages of less trauma, better function retention, less pain and faster recovery of patients, and has achieved good results. For patients with high requirements for facial cosmetology, and difficult to resect under nasal endoscopy, the tumors can be resected by a face-in-face approach.
2. Radiotherapy

   Radiotherapy alone is not effective for nasal malignant tumors. Generally combined with surgery, preoperative radiotherapy or post-operative radiotherapy or concurrent radiochemical therapy are selected according to the condition. Chemotherapeutic drugs can be paclitaxel, cisplatin, carboplatin and so on. They can be used in combination or alone.
3. Chemotherapy

   Chemotherapy can reduce the size of mesenchymal malignant tumors or poorly differentiated epithelial malignant lesions. Because of the drug resistance of tumors, it is difficult to radically cure tumors by chemotherapy alone. Induced chemotherapy can be given for 2–3 cycles before surgery or radiotherapy to reduce the size of tumors. Or concurrent radiochemical therapy combined with radiotherapy.

**Prognosis**

The most common one is the local expansion; the less one is the lymph node metastasis and further metastasis. The overall prognosis is not bad and the survival rate of 5 years is about 75%.

### 11.8.2 Maxillary Sinus Carcinoma

Maxillary sinus malignant tumors are the most common malignant tumors of nasal cavity and paranasal sinus, accounting for about 3% of head and neck malignant tumors and about 0.2% of all malignant tumors of the whole body. Because of the concealed location of maxillary sinus malignant tumors, it is difficult to detect them in the early stage. Generally, they are found in the middle and late stages, which are difficult to treat and have poor prognosis.

**Etiology and Epidemiology**

Maxillary sinus sarcoma's etiology isn't clear from then on what may be related to adverse gas and the dust stimulations, the repeated chronic inflammation, the virus infection the hereditary susceptibility gene. Some epidemiologist found that the lumberjack and the furniture makers are easier to have the maxillary tumors, what may relate to the dust and the chemical gas stimulations.

**Pathogenesis**

The squamous cell carcinoma is the most common one, which the adenoid cystic carcinoma, the papilla tumor progression, the melanoma, the sarcoma, the carcinosarcoma, the sarcoma from the minor salivary glands such as the muco epidermoid carcinoma and the myoepithelial carcinoma, etc., and others are secondary.

**Tumor Invasion and Metastasis**

The maxillary sinus is adjacent anteriorly to the eye orbits, inferiorly to the alveolar process, inner to the cavum nasi and outer to the infra-temporal fossa and the pterygopalatine fossae. There are plenty of the neurovessels open to the encephalic by what the tumor invades the surroundings. The invasion could be forwards to the infra-orbital nerve, along which the tumor invade the sphenomaxillary fissure and the superior orbital fissure and finally approach the anterior-superior cavernous sinus to lesion the optic nerve, the oculomotor nerve and the abducent nerve; it can be backwards to the posterior-lateral wall, lesion the maxillary nerve, along which the tumor efferently invades the encephalic through the fossa ovalis and finally approach the anterior-inferior site to invade the trigerminal's other branches; it can also invade the internal carotid (Fig. 11.22).

**Clinical Manifestation**

There hypothetical line is drawn from the inner canthus to the mandible angle, which is called the Organ malignancy line. The prognosis of tumors occurring below this line is better than that occurring above this line. This may be because tumors that occur in the lower part of the body are easy to detect early.

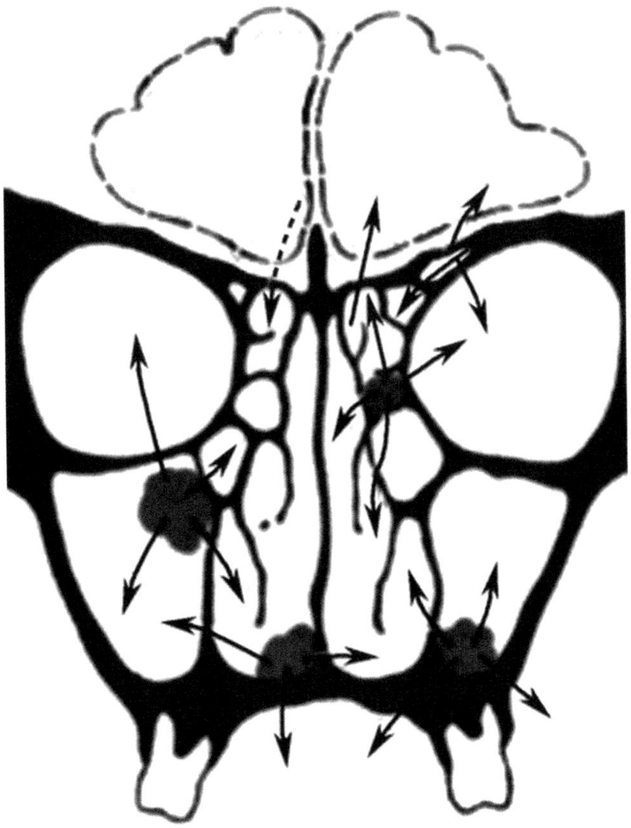

**Fig. 11.22** The maxillary sinosarcoma partial invasion imaging

1. Facial ants' Crawling Sensation

   The anterior wall of the maxillary sinus is deep in the cheek. Tumors originating from the anterior wall may involve the infraorbital nerve and the skin of the cheek, leading to facial numbness and the sense of crawling
2. Nasal congestion and Bloody Snot

   The medial wall of maxillary sinus with blood in nasal obstruction and mucus is also the lateral wall of the nasal cavity. The tumors may involve the nasal cavity in the medial wall, leading to nasal blockage and bloodshed in the mucus. They may also cause epistaxis because of the rupture of the tumors. The tumors may infect the nasal mucus and cause the odor of putrefaction.
3. Diplopia, Vision Loss and Exophthalmos

   The superior maxillary sinus wall is adjacent to the eye orbit, so the tumor could damage the superior wall to invade the orbit and cause the diplopia, the eyeball fixation, the vision loss or the exophthalmos, etc.
4. Facial Pain or Headache

   The maxillary sinus inferiorposterior wall is adjacent to the infratemporal fossa and the pterygopalatine fossa, so when the tumor extrudes the inferiorposterior wall, it could involve the maxillary nerve to evoke the persistent pain, which is difficult to alleviate. When the tumor lesions involve the pterygoid muscle, it could be hard to open mouth.
5. Toothache or Gomphiasis Defluvium

   The inferior maxillary wall is the superior alveolar process, so when the tumor lesions the inferior wall, the tumor could evoke the toothache, gomphiasis or the defluvium. Do not mistake it as a tooth lesion.
6. No positive findings at the early examinations, when the tumor invades enough sites to cause the facial swellings, the gomphiasis, the tooth percussion pain, the gingiva swellings or the hard palate tumor and sometimes the partial ulceration. The nasoendoscopic examination could show the inner metastasis of the cavum lateral wall. When the tumor inserts into the cavum through the maxillary sinus inner wall, the cavum tumor along with pseudomembrane caused by the ulceration and the infection could be seen under nasoendoscope. It can be seen that the facial skin is inflamed, tender, unclear boundary, or skin ulceration. When the upper lip is involved, it is easy to have swollen submandibular or cervical lymph nodes.

**Diagnosis**

According to the clinic manifestations and the imaging, the diagnosis could be done, but the differentiated diagnosis needs the pathological biopsy.

1. CT

   CT scan can show the sinus cavum soft tissue mass, uniform density, unclear boundary, occasional necrotic cystic change; when the mass is big in size, the sinus wall bone damage could be seen, the tumor breaks the sinus wall and invades surrounding the eye orbit, infra temporal fossa, pterygopalatine fossae and other structures around it. The tumor is obviously enhanced under enhanced scan, but the inner necrotic cystic area was not enhanced. Three-dimensional CT reconstruction could clearly show the size and extent of the tumors (Fig. 11.23)
2. MRI

   MRI could help distinguish the lesion in the maxillary sinus cavum if it is the tumor or just liquid retention. It can also help observe the maxillary bone marrow signal change at the early bone damage to judge whether there is any early bone damage or not and finally help distinguish it as benign tumor or early malignant tumor (Fig. 11.24).
3. PET-CT Scans

   The PET-CT scanning can preliminarily differentiate benign or malignant lesions, and can observe whether there is cervical lymph node metastasis and distant metastasis. It plays an important role in clinical tumor grading, but it is also more expensive.

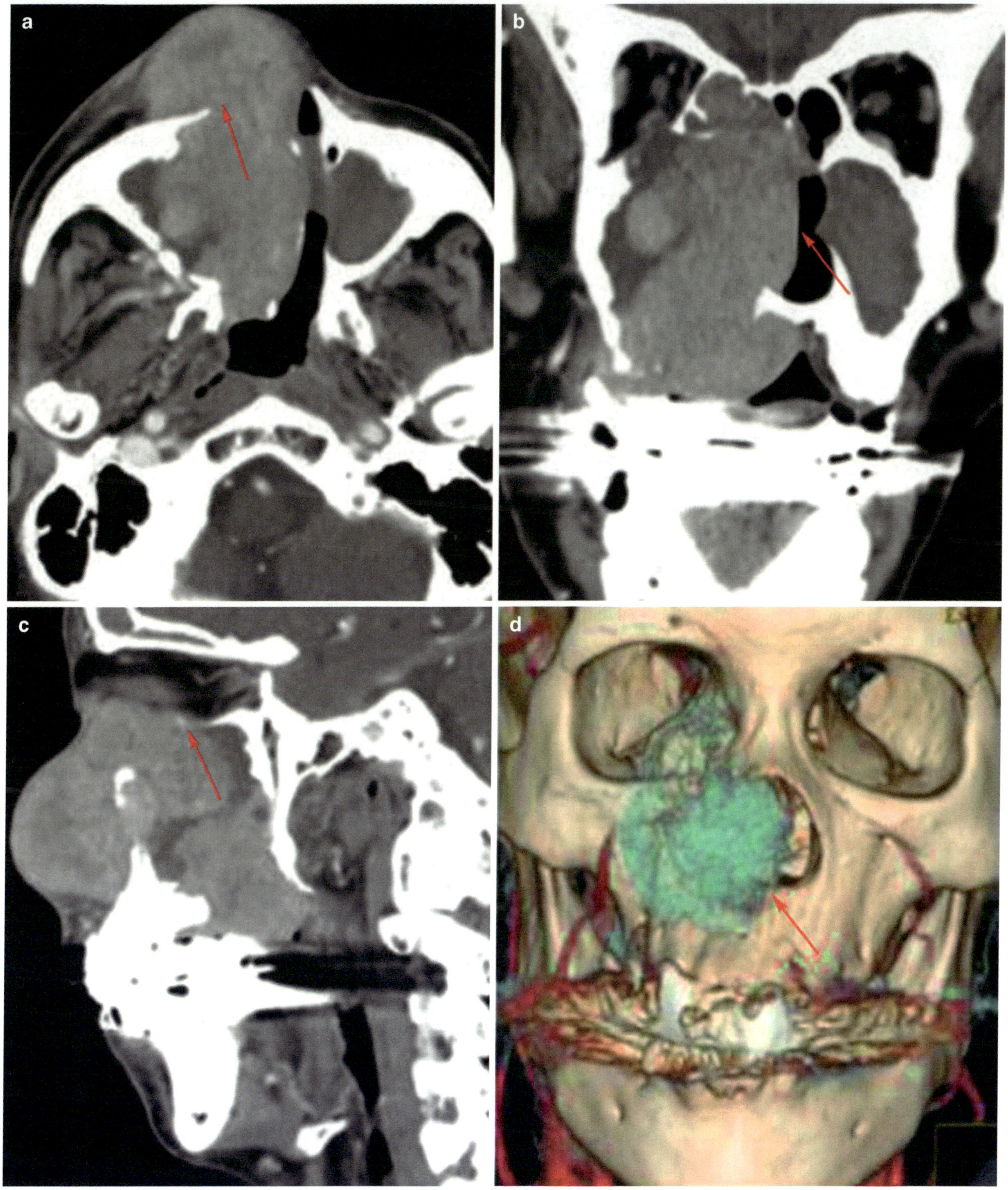


**Fig. 11.23** Right maxillary sinus cancer imaging. (**a**) Enhanced axial CT scan shows that the right maxillary sinus cavum had soft tissue mass swellings with unclear boundary and evidently strengthened. The tumor invades the right maxillary sinus anterior wall (arrow) and then the cheek subcutaneous tissue; (**b**) The enhanced CT scan coronary reconstruction imaging shows the tumor invades upwards to the right sphenoid sinus (arrow), downwards to the inferior maxillary sinus wall to invade the hard palate; (**c**) Enhanced CT scan sagittal shape. The reconstructed imaging shows that the mass invades upwards to the right superior maxillary wall and then the eye orbit (arrow), downwards to the hard palate and forwards to the nasal vestibule; (**d**) CT volume representation technique (VR) shows the right maxillary sinus bone damage and the tumor scope (arrow)

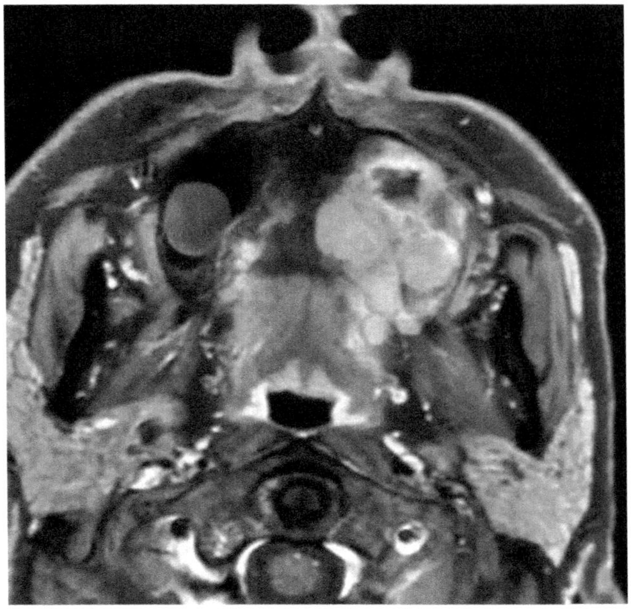

**Fig. 11.24** Horizontal MR shows left maxillary sinus adenoid cystic carcinoma

4. Biopsy

   Biopsy is the golden standard for the final diagnosis of maxillary sinus cancer. If the tumor invades the nasal cavity, it can be directly clamped. If the tumor is confined to the maxillary sinus, it can enter the maxillary sinus through the natural orifice of the maxillary sinus or through the window of the inferior nasal meatus under nasal endoscope.

**Clinical Staging**

The TNM staging of maxillary sinus carcinoma is as follows:

1. Anatomical Division

   A hypothetical line is made from the inner canthus to the mandibular angle, and the maxilla is divided into two parts: the upper (supra-structure) and the lower (infrastructure). The upper part includes the posterior part of the posterior wall of the bone and the top of the maxilla, and the rest of the infrastructure.
2. T Classification
   (a) $T_x$: Tumor cannot be identified.
   (b) $T_{is}$: Carcinoma in situ.
   (c) $T_1$: Tumor is localized in the mucosa of the maxillary sinus and has no bone destruction or erosion.
   (d) $T_2$: Tumor induced bone destruction or erosion including invasion to the hard palate and (or) the middle meatus, except the invasion of maxillary sinus posterior wall and wing plate.
   (e) $T_3$: Tumor invades any of the following areas: the subcutaneous tissue of the posterior wall of the maxillary sinus, the bottom wall of the orbit, the medial wall, the pterygopalatine fossa, and the ethmoid sinus.
   (f) $T_{4a}$: Local disease of middle and late stage. The tumors invaded anterior orbital contents, cheek skin, pterygoid plate, infratemporal fossa, ethmoid plate, sphenoid sinus or frontal sinus.
   (g) $T_{4b}$: Locally very advanced disease. The tumor invades any of the following parts: the orbital apex, the dura, the brain, the middle cranial fossa, the cerebral nerve (except for the maxillary branch of the trigeminal nerve), the nasopharynx, or the clivus.
3. N Classification
   (a) $N_0$: No local lymph node metastases.
   (b) $N_1$: Local single lymph node metastasis is important; the maximum diameter is equal to or less than 3 cm.
   (c) $N_2$: On the ipsilateral single lymph node metastases, the maximum diameter of more than 3 cm, but less than 6 cm, or on the ipsilateral multiple lymph node metastasis, the maximum diameter is not more than the 6 cm.
   (d) $N_{2a}$: On the ipsilateral single lymph node metastases, the maximum diameter was more than 3 cm, but less than 6 cm. There were multiple lymph node metastases on the ipsilateral
   (e) $N_{2b}$: There were multiple lymph node metastases on the ipsilateral side, of which the maximum diameter was no more than 6 cm.
   (f) $N_{2c}$: Ipsilateral or contra-lateral lymph node metastases, of which the maximum diameter was no more than 6 cm.
   (g) $N_3$: Metastatic lymph nodes are more than 6 cm.
   (h) $N_x$: The local metastatic lymph nodes were completely incapable of grading.
4. M Classifications
   (a) $M_0$: No distant metastasis was found.
   (b) $M_1$: Has a distant metastasis.
   (c) $M_x$: Distant metastasis can't be judged.
5. Stages
   (a) Stage0: TisN0M0.
   (b) Stage I: T1NoM0.
   (c) Phase II: T2NoM0
   (d) Stage III: T3NoMo; T1N1Mo; T2N1Mo; T3N1M0.
   (e) Stage IV A: T4aN0M0; T4aN1M0; T1N2M0; T2N2M0; T3N2Mn; T4aN2M0.
   (f) Stage IV B: T4a any NM0; any TN3M0.
   (g) Stage IV C: any T any NM1.
6. Histology Classification (G)
   (a) $G_x$: Level cannot be evaluated.
   (b) $G_1$: High differentiation.
   (c) $G_2$: Middle differentiation.
   (d) $G_3$: Is low differentiation.
   (e) $G_4$: Was undifferentiated.

**Treatment**

There is no prospective case-control study for the treatment of upper collar malignant tumors. A retrospective analysis shows that for patients who undergo resection, surgery plus postoperative radiotherapy is the best treatment mode. The 5 year survival rate of combined treatment with surgery and radiotherapy was about 56%, while the 5 year survival rate of radiotherapy alone was only about 22%. For patients who are not able to completely remove the wood after radiography, or those with orbital involvement and skull base, they can be treated by radiotherapy or chemotherapy before surgery excision.

1. Surgical Treatment

   The maxillary carcinoma T and T2 lesions are rare, most of which are T3 or T4 lesions, and the range of excision is determined according to the scope of the lesion to determine the removal of the model. But there should be a certain safety margin. The general need of frontal subtotal or full bone resection guide with hard carbon, communication of the mouth and the nasal cavity, the reflux of the nasal cavity when eating, the opening of the nasal voice when speaking; the removal of the inferior wall of the eye, which leads to the loss of the content of the shadow. Drooping caused diplopia. Therefore, if there is no immediate repair and reconstruction of the local defect after the total excision of the bone, the birth weight affects the birth of the patient life quality.

   During maxillary resection, attention should be paid to the safe margin of incision. Tumor residues are often found in the infraorbital nerve, maxillary zygomatic process, pterygoid process root and maxillary nerve stump. It is easy to have residual tumor. For the patients with the thickening of the peripheral nerve of the maxillary sinus, the frozen margin should be delivered during the operation. Repair and reconstruction of maxillary bone after resection of maxillary resection: if complete tumor resection, 1 stage reconstruction was the best. Repair and reconstruction. The method is divided into the prosthesis of puny body and the repair of autologous tissue flap. The autologous tissue flap is divided into the local pedicled tissue flap and the vascularized free tissue. According to the size of the patient's defect and the basic diseases such as diabetes, hypertension and other basic diseases, the repair method is chosen: the repair of the compound of glass is relatively simple and easy to take. But it is not easy to locally produce dense and close fitting, drinking water mouthwash is easy to reflux in the nasal cavity, and the local tissue after retraction after radiotherapy is easy to be unsuitable. Small autologous tissue flap can be used with pedicle tissue flap or free vascularized tissue flap: local pedicled tissue flap mainly has pedicle muscle. The pedicle flap, the buccal mucosa flap, the tongue flap etc. The pedicle temporalis flap is the most convenient local tissue flap. It is convenient to make transfer distance is short, for the appearance and the function of image features such as small temple, at the same time to repair the hard palate and inferior orbital wall support (Fig. 11.25).

   If there is a microsurgical skill, the condition of anastomosis of small vessels can be done. The patient has no

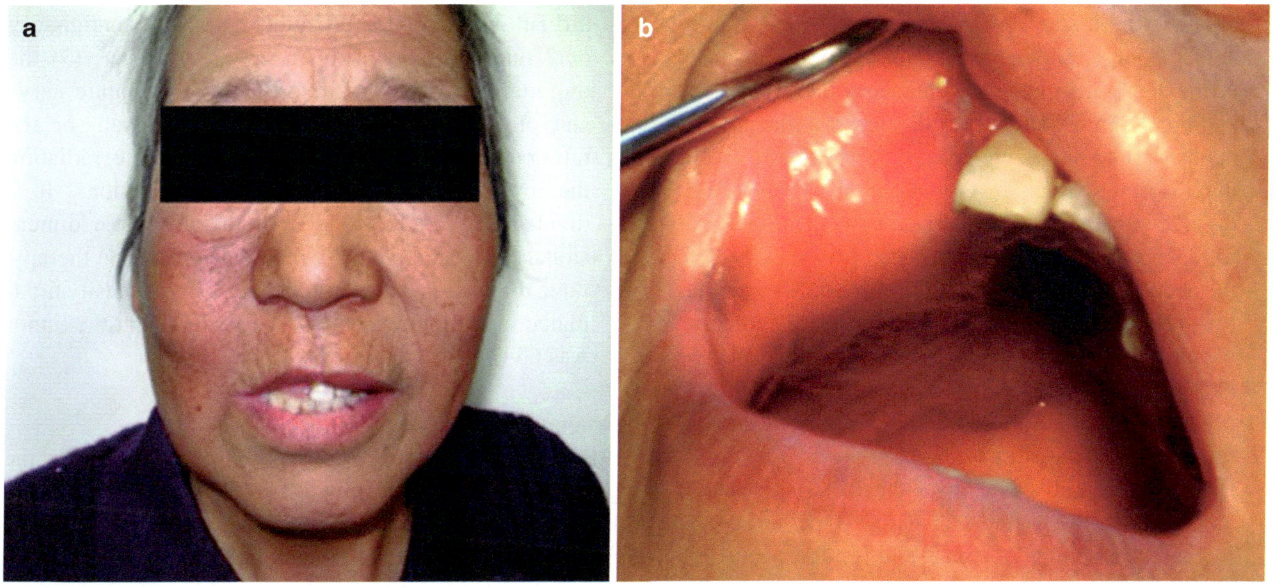


**Fig. 11.25** Posttemporoprothesis right maxillotomy. (**a**) Facial view. (**b**) Hard palate view. Suitable for repair of defect of simple hard palate flap and buccal mucosal flap, tongue flap collar, especially pedicle flap under the chin, if with the beard heavy. Or female patients can be cut 58 cm, large tissue, local defect and function of the donor area is not obvious

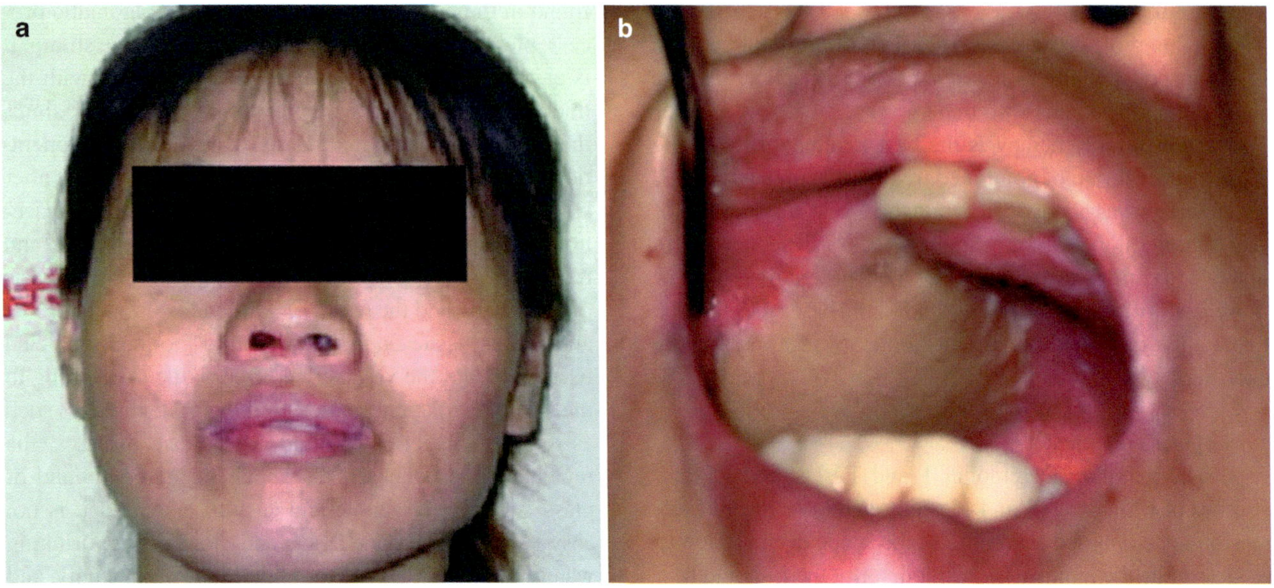


**Fig. 11.26** Postrafemoral anterior lateral flap prothesis at left maxillary sinusocancer maxilotomy. (**a**) Facial view. (**b**) Oral view

diabetes, hypertension, arteriosclerosis and other diseases. Free tissue flap is an ideal material for repair and reconstruction of maxillary defects and is suitable for all sizes of defects. Suitable for the defect weight after total maxillofacial resection free tissue flap has a anterolateral thigh perforator flap (Fig. 11.26) rectus abdominis myocutaneous flap, fibula myocutaneous flap, and forearm flap, leg flap, the iliac bone flap, the scapular flap, the pectoralis major myocutaneous flap, etc., among them, the tissue flap without bone is called the soft repair and the band bone group flap is called hard repair. It can be chosen according to the skill of the operator. The soft repair is the first preferred anterolateral thigh flap. The defect is large. The rectus abdominis myocutaneous flap or the pectoralis major myocutaneous flap was selected, and the fibula myocutaneous flap and the iliac myocutaneous flap could be preferred by hard repair. We have maxillofacial excision the defect after operation is divided into 4 types: the lower part of the maxilla defect: to repair palate and nasal base: the upper maxilla defect: the need to repair of the bandit bottom: 5. After all maxillofacial excision defect: need to repair hard and dormant support; enlarge the defect after the upper collar bone excision the maxilla, the resection may include the orbital content, the skull base, the ascending branch of the mandible, the skin of the cheek, etc. It needs to be repaired the skull base, cover the facial skin, etc. The anterolateral thigh flap can carry some muscles and increase the volume of tissue, and is convenient for cutting and making 2 groups of operators can be operated at the same time. The defects of the area are concealed and the function is not affected. The maximum of the anterolateral thigh flap can be taken to 10–16 cm, Can also repair the hard palate defect and inferior orbital wall support. For the large maxillary resection combined with orbital contents and (or) resection of skull base defects, free abdominal myocutaneous flap can provide large tissue capacity, cover, fill the defect, support the skull base, reconstruct the facial contour, etc.

2. Radiotherapy

   It is an important part of the comprehensive treatment of maxillary sinus malignant tumors, divided into preoperative radiotherapy and surgery radiotherapy Preoperative radiation therapy is generally used as: (1) the range of tumor lesions is larger and the operation is difficult to be completely removed; (2) the malignancy of 2 tumors high, the boundary is not clear; (3) the important structure of the orbital content, optic nerve and other important structures are involved, or the tumor is close to the tumor. Postoperative radiation therapy is generally used in T above lesions. It is divided into conventional radiotherapy, three dimensional conformal intensity modulated radiation therapy, three dimensional conformable real time intensity modulated radiation therapy, etc. General radiant the tumor was 65–70Gy.

**Prognosis**

The prognosis of maxillary sinus carcinoma is related to the pathological type of the tumor, the choice of treatment, the level of doctors and the compliance of the patients off. The advantage of first external irradiation and surgical treatment is to reduce tumor volume, microvascular occlusion, reduce intrao-perative bleeding and reduce cancer cells. The 5 year survival rate was about 56%. According to CT and MRI, the range of tumor was evaluated, and computer selected the optimal scheme. Recent years, the 5 year survival rate was significantly increased by the combination of surgical treatment and radiotherapy.

### 11.8.3 Ethmoid Sinus Cancer

It is rare that the malignant tumor of ethmoid is relative to the malignant swelling of the cavity and the malignant swelling of the upper superior sinus. Most of the malignancies in this region are neuroblastoma (Fig. 11.27). Squamous cell carcinoma is common, and adenocarcinoma is common in Europe, and the others are sarcoma, melanoma, adenoid cystic carcinoma, and malignant lymphoma,

In Neuroendocrine carcinoma, Olfactory neuroblastoma is a relatively inert malignant tumor. Most patients have a relatively slow course of disease and are associated with the degree of differentiation of the tumor.

Neuroblastoma that divided the tumor into 4 levels with the degree of differentiation. In 1988, Hyams proposed a grading system for olfactory neuroblastoma, which divided the tumor into 4 levels with the degree of differentiation:

- Grade I: The differentiation is best, the tumor has obvious lobule structure, the tumor cell differentiation is good, and Homer Wright type false chrysanthemum shaped group is common, not visible calcification;
- Grade II: Well differentiated, the tumor has a lobular structure, a fibrous matrix containing a blood vessel, the nucleus has an atypical nucleus, and it can be seen scattered in the nucleus., the pseudo-chrysanthemum and varying degrees of calcification can still be seen;
- Grade III: tumor differentiation is poor, tumor tissues still have lobular structure and inter vascular interstitial, and the cell nucleus cleavage is obvious, and Flexner Win is visible;
- Type Steiner real chrysanthemum shaped clusters and local necrosis, without calcification.
- Grade IV: the differentiation of tumor is the worst, the structure of lobule is not obvious, the tumor cell differentiation is primitive, the chrysanthemum is rare, no calcification is found, and the necrosis is common.

**Clinical Manifestations**

Early ethmoid malignant tumors often have no obvious symptoms, and develop to a certain extent, with blood and headache in the middle of the nose. When the nasal cavity is violated, it can have nasal congestion, and the infection can also have the purulent nose and odor with blood silk; the contents of the orbit can lead to diplopia and visual appearance descends; the late involvement of the intracranial may also have the symptoms of headache, nausea and vomiting caused by intracranial hypertension.

**Diagnosis**

The diagnosis of ethmoid malignant tumor is mainly clinical combined imaging examination. Enhanced CT can observe the range of tumors. For the invasion of the sur-

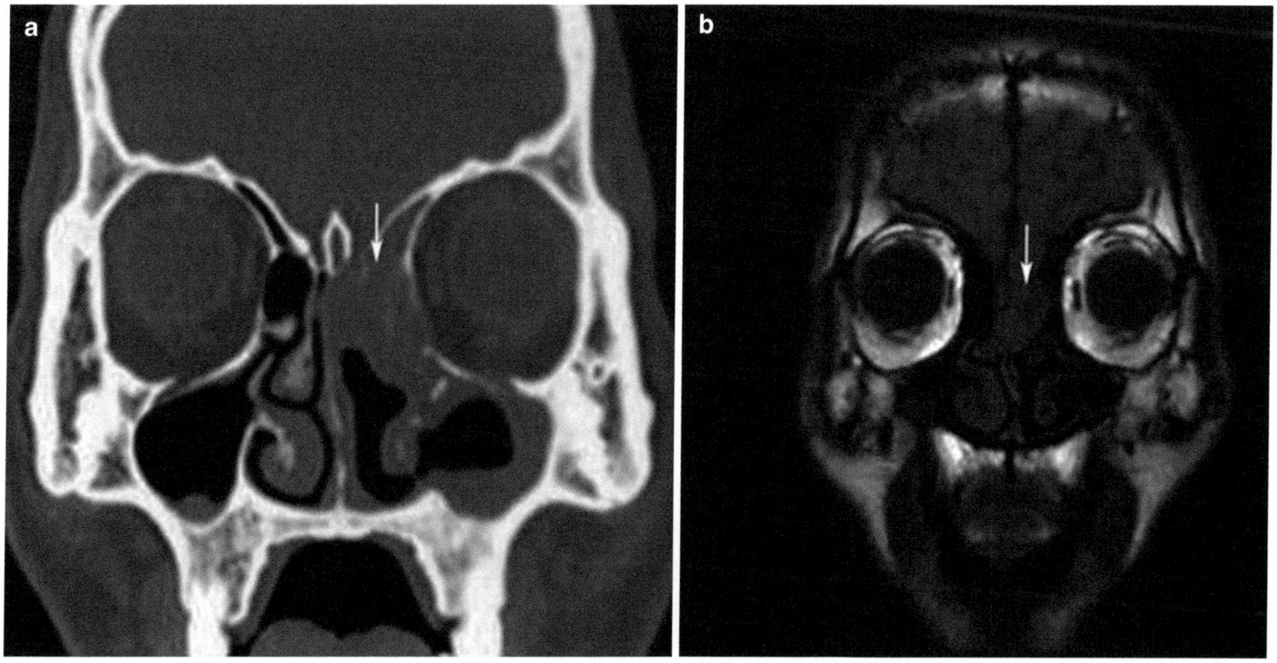


**Fig. 11.27** Left sphenoid sinus olfactory neuroblastoma (arrow). (**a**) Coronal CT. (**b**) Coronal MR

rounding bone, enhanced MR can identify the tumor or the obstructive inflammation of the sinus, and can also show the dura and brain tissue tired. Determine the diagnosis of biopsy by pathological tissue. Because of the variety of pathological types, especially small cell malignant pomegranate, it is often required to be immunohistochemica. Step classification is to guide the formulation of clinical treatment.

The TNM staging of the ethmoid Sinus malignant tumor is generally the same as the malignant tumor of the nasal cavity.

### Treatment

A malignant tumor of the middle and low degree of epithelial origin such as a malignant transformation; if the operation is considered to be completely excised, surgery and radiotherapy are generally used the assessment is not completely removed; the mode of radiotherapy plus surgery is selected. For adenoid cystic carcinoma, mucoepidermoid carcinoma and other tumors which are insensitive to radiation, the general choice is surgical excision to assist the integrated treatment of postoperative radiotherapy and for the source of mesenchymal tissue. Malignant tumors, such as various sarcomas and malignant melanoma, are susceptible to distant metastasis because of their high degree of malignancy. Chemotherapy can be selected firstly. Then surgery and the radiotherapy.

### Prognosis

The malignant tumor of ethmoid sinus is better than that of maxillary sinus malignant tumor, but the pathological type, the size of the swelling and the treatment of the patients with the malignant tumor of the maxillary sinus are better than that of the malignant tumor of the maxillary sinus 5 year survival rate was 50–65%.

## References


1. Journal of Chinese Otorhinolaryngology Head and Neck Surgery Editorial Committee Rhinology Group. Chronis rhinosinusitis diagnosis and treatment guideline (Kunming, 2012). J Chin Otorhinolaryngol Head Neck Surg. 2013;48(2):92–4.
2. Fang G, Wang C, Zhang L. Diagnostic value of CT and MRI to rhinocavum rhinosinus inverted papilloma. J Chin Otorhinolaryngol Head Neck Surg. 2015;22(8):422–5.
3. Eifan AO, Durham SR. Pathogenesis of rhinitis. Clin Exp Allergy. 2016;46(9):1139–51.
4. Montone KT. Pathology of fungal rhinosinusitis: a review. Head Neck Pathol. 2016;10(1):40–6.
5. Hennessey PT, Reh DD. Chapter 9: benign sinonasal neoplasms. Am J Rhinol Allergy. 2013;27(Suppl 1):S314.
6. Chen Y, Chai X. Suggestive progress of monuclonal antibody therapy on chronic rhinonasal sinustis accompanying or unaccompanying with rhinopolyps[J]. J Clin Otorhinolaryngol Head Neck Surg. 2018;32(10):789–93.
7. Bachert C, Zhang L, Gevaert P. Current and future treatment options for adult chronic rhinosinusitis: Focus on nasal polyposis. J Allergy Clin Immunol. 2015;136(6):1431–40.

# 12 Rhinal Treatment Procedure and Operation

Xin Wei and Zhonglin Mu

## 12.1 Rhinal Foreign Body Extraction Surgery and Lithotomy

Foreign body is one of the most common emergencies in the otolaryngology department. It is often seen in children and can be seen in adults. The foreign body of the nasal cavity is a foreign substance. The nasal cavity can be divided into two major categories: abiotic foreign bodies and biotic (animal and plant) foreign bodies. Abiotic foreign objects such as all kinds of materials, small toys (including plastic, glass, metal etc.), toilet paper and button batteries; plants such as peanuts, nuts, beans, foreign body; dynamic foreign objects such as insects and leeches are commonly found in the tropics. Sometimes when you sneeze at the time of trauma, vomiting, or eating, after surgery causes the nasal foreign body, and the small foreign body of the nasal cavity can be retained for a long time to form the nasal stone. The clinical manifestations of unilateral nasal obstruction and purulent nasal discharge complication nasosinusitis.

1. Indications and Contraindication
   (a) Indications

   Clear diseases history, typical symptoms of unilateral nasal obstruction, pus and blood tears, anterior rhinoscopy or nasal endoscopy showed nasal foreign deposit. The larger and deeper foreign body can be located by CT inspection.

   (b) The patients with severe heart disease, primary hypertension, severe hemorrhagic disease and other diseases are not tolerated or operated on foreign body can be taken after a stable condition.

2. Anaesthesia and Position
   (a) Anaesthesia

   Patients who can cooperate with anesthesia cannot be anesthetized or removed under surface anesthesia. Patients who do not cooperate can take general anesthesia. Take foreign objects.

   (b) Position

   Position was taken with the foreign body under the surface anesthesia, and the patient took the seat. In case of children, an assistant is required to fix the child's head and hand and foot to prevent the child. In the process of operation, the child does not cooperate in the operation, causing the instrument to damage the nasal mucosa or to cause the foreign body to fall into the trachea at the risk of falling into the trachea. General anesthesia tracheal intubation in supine position, no anesthesia endotracheal intubation is low head position.

3. The Procedure of Operation
   (a) In the absence of anesthetic or surface anesthesia, take the correct position, specifically in the " Anesthesia and position" Chap. 2.
   (b) First identified in the front of the nose under the foreign body position, generally located in the common meatus (Fig. 12.1). Depending on the nature and shape of the foreign body most surgical instruments. It is necessary to use a blunt foreign body hook from the foreign body to cross the foreign body and press the foreign body on the nose for the ball and smooth foreign objects at the bottom of the cavity, the foreign body is hooked forward (Fig. 12.2).
   (c) If the foreign body is too large, it can be broken into pieces and removed. Generally, it is not advocated to push the foreign body to the rear nasopharynx and take out the oral cavity. If need remove from the nasopharynx, supine head low position, prepare the

X. Wei (✉)
Department of Otorhinolaryngology Head and Neck Surgery, Hainan People's Hospital, Haikou, China

Z. Mu
Department of Otorhinolaryngology Head and Neck Surgery, The First Affiliated Hospital of Hainan Medical University, Haikou, China



Z. Mu, J. Fang (eds.), *Practical Otorhinolaryngology - Head and Neck Surgery*, https://doi.org/10.1007/978-981-13-7993-2_12

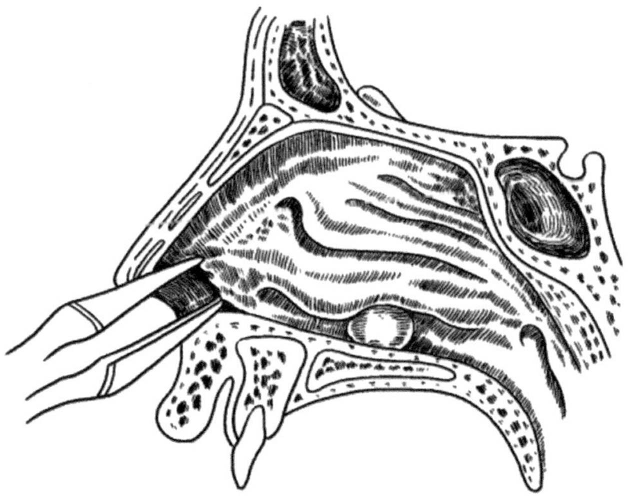

**Fig. 12.1** Foreign bodies are commonly at common rhinal canal

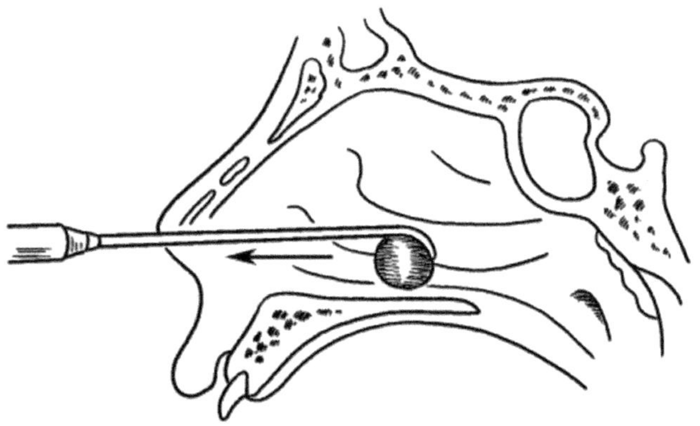

**Fig. 12.2** Hook foreign body forwards from its back

suction equipment, prevent foreign body falling or mistaken trachea.

(d) To check whether or not the injury of the foreign body and the nasal mucosa, such as the mucous damage of the blood, should be further treated.

4. Postoperative Treatment
   (a) Because the foreign body stays in the nasal cavity for a long time, the mucous membrane in the nasal cavity can be swollen obviously, complicated with sinusitis, and the antibiotic can be used properly for infection.
   (b) Observation of postoperative bleeding of the nasal cavity and hemostasis if there was bleeding.

## 12.2 Maxillary Sinus Puncture

Maxillary sinus puncture needle into the maxillary sinus cavity from the lateral wall of nasal tract, suitable for the diagnosis and treatment of acute or recurrent acute maxillary sinusitis and lesions of maxillary sinus biopsy, otolaryngology is one of the commonly used local treatment and diagnosis methods, because it is not the solution to the chronic maxillary occlusion, so it is not recommended as a treatment for chronic maxillary sinusitis.

1. Indications
   (a) Indications

      Acute maxillary sinusitis or acute recurrent maxillary sinusitis. The nature of the lesions in the maxillary sinus is unknown, and it is feasible to diagnose puncture. It is feasible to diagnose maxillary sinus malignant tumor by maxillary sinus biopsy.

   (b) Contraindications

      There are repeated nasal hemorrhage, X-ray and CT examination for suspected maxillary sinus hemangioma; serious heart disease, hypertension, severe bleeding disease cannot tolerate surgery.

2. Preoperative Preparation

   First, 1% ephedrine and other vasoconstrictor drugs are used to fully constriction the nasal mucosa and expose the nose to the nose. Avoid operation on the patient's empty stomach and prevent escape.

3. Anesthesia and Position
   (a) Anesthesia: In the nasal cavity, the surface of the nasal mucosa was anaesthetized three times with 1% tetracaine or 1% tetracaine cotton tablets were placed on the surface of the lateral wall of the lower nasal canal and the surface of the inferior turbinate for a few minutes.
   (b) Positions: the patient took the seat, and the head was straight back on the back of the chair.
4. Procedure
   (a) Take seat, head to keep the middle, in front of the nose under direct vision, the maxillary sinus straight needle (Fig. 12.3) placed under the nose of the front close to the inferior turbinate bone attachment, needle tip towards the nasal septum, the distance 11.5 cm of inferior turbinate, pointing to the ipsilateral eye lateral canthus (Fig. 12.4).
   (b) Remove the front of the nose, a hand fixed with the head, another hand thumb and index finger to puncture needle, needle, back toward the palm against the same side paropia direction, gently rotate forward, when entering the sinus cavity with a sense of frustration.
   (c) Pull out the needle ten core, connect the 20 mL syringe with the rubber tube to the puncture needle, draw back first, if there is air, it proves that the puncture needle is in the maxillary sinus. Aspiration and exploration can help diagnose the lesions in the maxillary sinus (Fig. 12.5).
   (d) Let the patient's head down to the healthy side, lay a tray on the neck and rinse slowly with sterile saline,

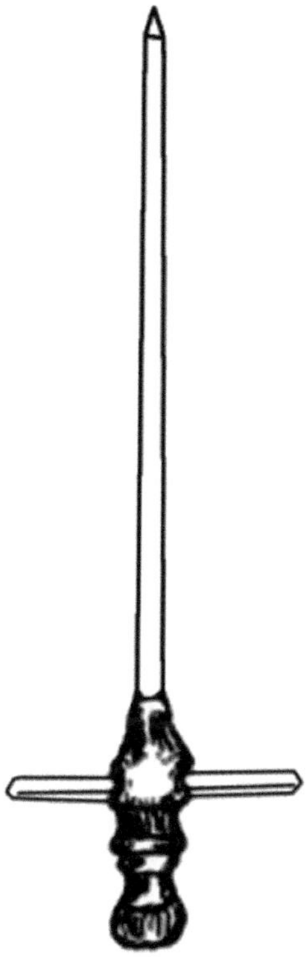

**Fig. 12.3** Maxillary sinus straight needle

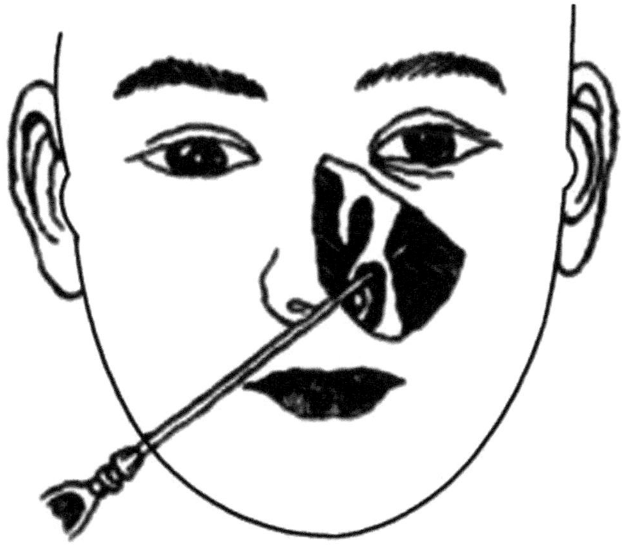

**Fig. 12.4** Needle top points to lateral canthus

until the backwash liquid is completely clear, and if necessary, we can inject appropriate amount of antibiotics.

(e) When the needle was put back, the puncture needle was pulled out. The puncture site was treated with the cotton piece to fill the blood, and the puncture was taken out after 15 min. The nature of the puncture fluid should be carefully observed and recorded. The

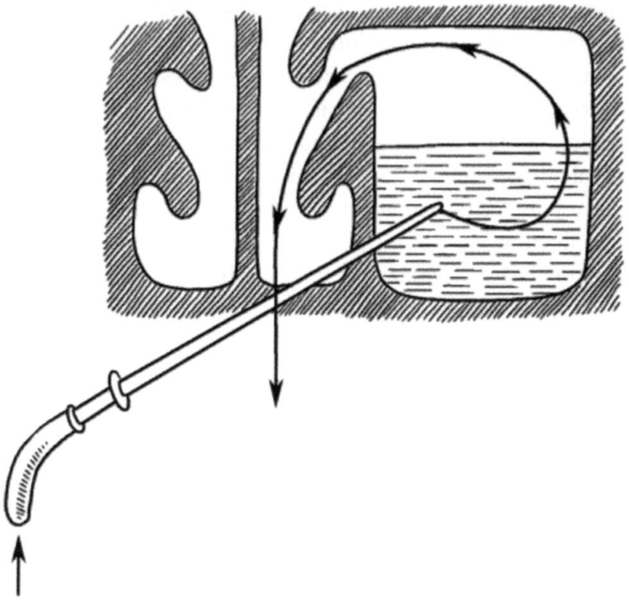

**Fig. 12.5** Aspiration Examination

yellow liquid should indicate the cyst, and the bloody secretion may be a tumor, such as pus odor, possibly itching bacterial infection.

5. Postoperative Treatment
   (a) One percent ephedrine tablets were given for 15 min under the compression of the nasal canal.
   (b) In case of facial subcutaneous emphysema or infection, anti-infection and swelling treatment should be carried out.

## 12.3 Endoscopic Rhinonasosinus Surgery

Endoscopic surgery refers to the operation of the nasal cavity, the sinus, the orbit, the skull base, and other parts of the nasal cavity, the sinus, the orbit and the skull base with the special surgical instruments under the instructions of the nasal endoscope. At the beginning of 1980s by the Austria science Messerklinger nose first, in 1985 the United States l researcher Kennedy first proposed the "functional endoscopic sinus surgery (functional endoscopic, sinus surgery, FESs)" concept, to improve and promote the modern nasal endoscopic surgery by nasal endoscopy, physicians can easily examine deep nasal cavity structure and lesions, improve the rate of early diagnosis of nasal disease combined endoscopic surgical instruments related to the past, the traditional correction of nasal septum, sinus and nasal and nasal sinus tumor resection surgery were improved, so the operation is more thorough, less trauma and complications. In addition, the surgical treatment of skull base tumors and orbital diseases also provides a nasal route may be gradually carried out by trans nasal resection of pituitary adenoma, nasal anterior skull base tumor resection, nasal cerebrospinal fluid rhinorrhea, nasal orbital tumors, nasal orbital decompression, Trans sphenoid optic nerve decompression, the nasal dacryocystorhinostomy and nasal skull base and nasocular operation, greatly reduce trauma and complications, the nasal science turn the world upside down changes, greatly promoting the development of science of the nose. Since the introduction of China in the 90 years of the Twentieth Century, it has developed rapidly in China [1].

1. Indications and Contra-Indications
   (a) Indications
      - Chronic sinusitis (which can be accompanied by nasal polyps) which is not effective by conservative treatment.
      - Rhinal sinusitis with orbital and intracranial complications.
      - Nasal diseases or symptoms caused by anatomic abnormalities
      - Nasal cavity, the foreign body of the sinuses and the foreign body of the anterior skull base.
      - Endoscopic resection of nasal vestibule, nasal cavity and sinus nasopharynx tumors or cysts (Fig. 12.6).
      - Conservative treatment of ineffective nasal bleeding.
      - Traumatic optic neuropathy.
      - The spillover caused by chronic dacryocystitis, traumatic dacryocystitis, and nasolacrimal duct disease.
      - Malignant exophthalmos.
      - Intra-orbital tumor and foreign body near the nasal side (Fig. 12.7).
      - Cerebrospinal fluid rhinorrhea (Fig. 12.8).
      - The lesion of the skull base can be removed by nasal endoscopy.
      - Parapharyngeal space occupying lesions that can be excised through nasal endoscopy.
   (b) Contra-Indications
      - All systemic diseases such as acute infectious disease, blood disease or serious cardiovascular disease, and not well controlled.
      - Invasion of a wide range of malignant tumors.
2. Operative Principles and Techniques
   (a) Master Anatomy

      Under endoscopy, we must familiarize ourselves with the anatomical structure in the stereoscopic field

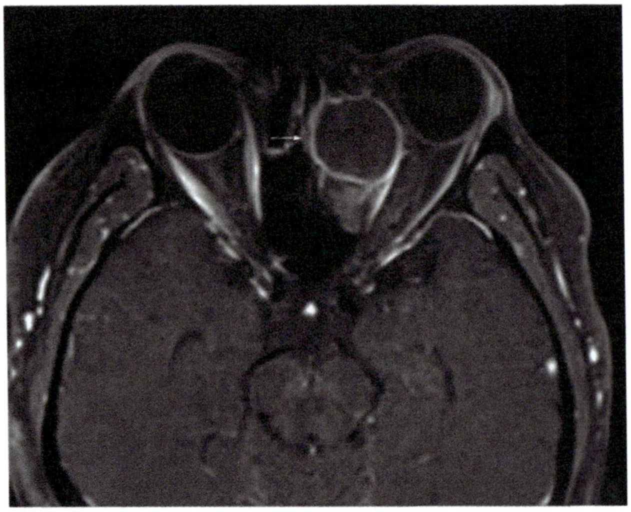

**Fig. 12.6** Rhinosinus axial MR displays left sphenoid cyst (arrow)

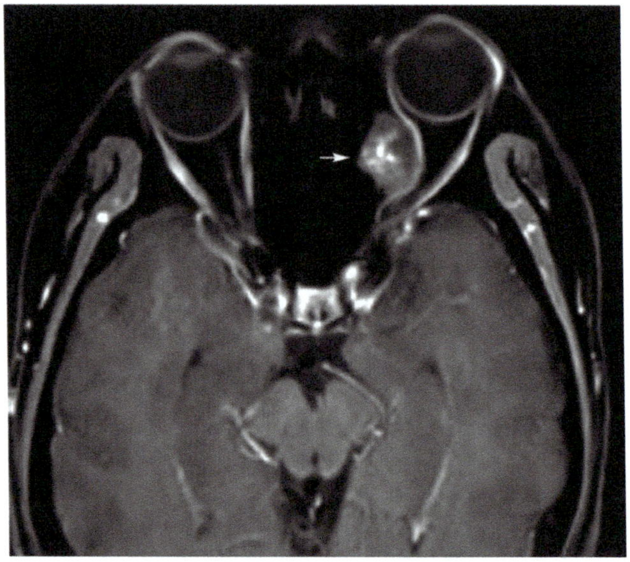

**Fig. 12.7** Rhinal sinus axial MR displays left eye orbit angioma (arrow)

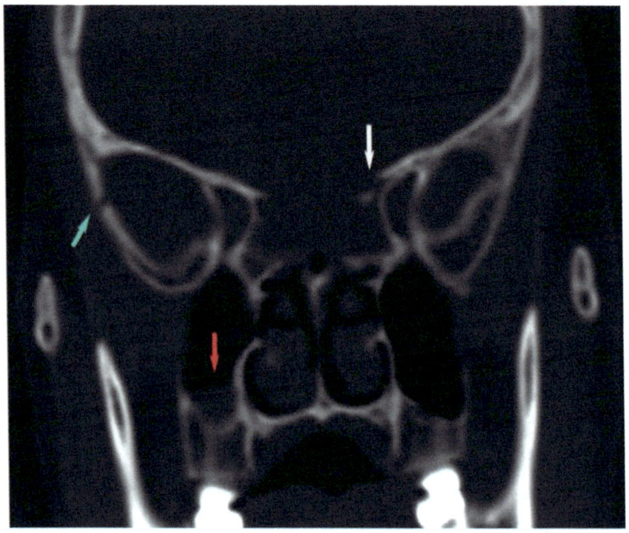

**Fig. 12.8** Postratraumatic cerebrospinal fluid rhinorrhea's rhinosinus in coronary bone window CT

of the nasal cavity before surgery. Otherwise, it is easy to cause errors or unnecessary injuries.

(b) Strict mastery of the indications and contra-indications of endoscopic sinus surgery

Especially for surgical treatment of chronic sinusitis, we should be careful. We should understand that the treatment of chronic sinusitis is mainly based on drugs and surgery. Even after receiving surgical treatment, postoperative medication is needed, even for a long time.

(c) Micro invasive concept and function remittance is soul of endoscopic surgeries

When removing the lesions and establishing the drainage channel, the normal tissue structure must be preserved, the normal mucous membrane of the nasal cavity is retained, and the bony exposure of the operative cavity must be avoided. The range of surgical excision should be determined according to the severity of the disease.

(d) We should use different angles of endoscope and apparatus according to different parts of the sinuses, so as to ensure that all operations in the field of vision, at the same time, excellent bite cutting appliances and electric suction cutting drill can minimize the damage of normal mucosa.

(e) Apply all possible means to reduce intra operative bleeding, including preoperative medication, intra operative blood pressure control, head 30 degrees of surgical position intra operative careful operation, and when the electro coagulation method, in order to ensure the correct identification of intra operative anatomic landmarks, reduce surgical complications.

## 12.4 Revised Endoscopic Paranasal Sinus Surgery

Revision endoscopic sinusitis surgery (RESS) is chronic sinusitis after more than one times endoscopic sinus surgery, there are still nasal symptoms, and need endoscopic sinus surgery again. The recurrence of nasal polyps is often represented. The main reasons are: Refractory sinusitis; the previous surgical correction of nasal septum or sinus open room of the gas is not complete, residual disease, or excessive intra operative injury of normal mucosa, leading to bone exposed granulation vesicle repeated growth, wound healing difficulties; the nonstandard postoperative medication and follow-up. RESS is more difficult than the first operation of the first operation to change or removal of the normal sinus anatomy, makes the position of re operation signs missing, increases the incidence of surgical complications; the previous surgery and the development of inflammation and hyperplasia of fibrous tissue, disease tissue resection difficult, also led to more easily in operation bleeding [2].

1. Indications and Contraindications
   (a) Indications
   - Nasal septum correction is not complete or nasal adhesion, stenosis, leading to the occurrence of nasal symptoms.
   - The stenosis of the middle nasal tract and the atresia of the sinus orifice affect the drainage.
   - The opening of the gas room is not complete, and the residual inflammation and infection are not effective by conservative treatment.
   - The recurrence of polyps.

   (b) Contraindications
   - All body diseases with acute infectious disease, blood disease or serious cardiovascular disease, and have not been well controlled.
   - Patients with cystic fibrosis, immunodeficiency or primary ciliary movement syndrome are relative contraindications.
2. Operative Principles and Techniques
   (a) Fully understand the time, type and scope of the last operation.
   (b) Before operation, three dimensional CT and endoscopic sinus examination were performed to analyze the causes of the failure of the last operation, to understand the location and extent of the major lesions, and to confirm the operation plan.
   (c) Pay attention to the normalization of drug therapy in the preoperative period
   (d) The normal nasal sinus mucosa was preserved as far as possible.
   (e) Intra operative use of all means to reduce bleeding, ensure that the operative field is clean, and make full use of fixed anatomical marks, such as maxillary sinus orifice, posterior nostril dome, and available residual anatomical marks, to minimize the occurrence of complications.
   (f) In the wood to read the film at any time to help judge, such as the image navigation is the most ideal.

## References

1. Y. Li, B. Zhou. Practical endorhinoscope surgery technique and application. Beijing: People's Medical Publishing House; 2009. p. 260–3.
2. Govindaraj S, Agbetoba A, Becker S. Revision sinus surgery. Oral Maxillofac Surg Clin N Am. 2012;24(2):285–93.

# Part IV

# Pharyngology

Pharynx locates at front of cervical vertebra; it originates from the skull base at top. The pharyngo mucosa has abundant nervous and vascular distribution. The pharynx is the common channel for respiration and digestion; so it has many physiological functions, including the deglutition, the respiration, the phonation resonance, and the middle ear pressure adjustment, the defense, etc. This part would help master the pharyngeal anatomic structures and main physiological functions by mastering its anatomy and physiology, and then emphatically discuss pharyngeal symptoms, clinic inspection methods and the diagnosis and treatment hotspots of the common pharyngeal diseases.

# Applied Anatomy and Physiology of Pharynx

# 13

Xuejun Zhou and Xun Bi

## 13.1 Applied Anatomy of Pharynx

1. Pharynx Anatomy

   The pharynx could be divided into three parts: the nasopharynx, the oropharynx and the laryngopharynx (Fig. 13.1).

   (a) Nasopharynx

   Nasopharynx opens anteriorly to the cavum nasi through the choana, and its apex is the corpora ossis sphenoidalis and the occipital bone basement and inferiorly horinzonal to the first and second cervical vertebrae. The posterior apex wall is dome, abundant lymph tissue orange slice like walelined in mucosa, which is called the adenoid, also the pharyngeal tonsils. The hypertrophy adenoid can not only obstruct the cavum nasppharynx to influence the ventilation but also obstacle the eustachian tube pharynx aditus to evoke the hearing loss. The eustachian tube pharynx opening locates at bilateral nasopharynx about 1.0 cm posterior to the inferior nasal concha, surrounds by the lymph tissue, which is called the tonsilla tubaria. The apophysis superior to the eustachian tube pharynx aditus is called the torus tubarius. A depression posteriorsuperior to the torus is called the pharyngeal recess, which is also a favor site of the nasophrtnx carcinoma. The superior recess is adjacent to the foramen lacerum, through which the nasopharync carcinoma invades the encephalic; inferiorly opens to the oropharynx, while deglutition, the soft palate rises to contract with the inferior pharynx wall, the nasopharynx temporarily departs with the oropharynx.

   (b) Oropharynx

   Oropharynx locates posterior to the oral cavity between the horizontal soft palate and the upper epiglottis border. It anteriorly opens to the oral cavity through the isthmus faucium. What is called the isthmus faucium is that what superiorly ends at the uvula and soft palate free border, inferiorly at the annular narrow site made by the dorsal tongue, the bilateral palatoglossal arch and the palatopharyngeal arch. The depression between the palatoglossal arch and the palatopharyngeal arch is called the tonsillar pit, which contains the palatotonsil (Fig. 13.2). The wale strip lymph tissue posterior to each lateral palatopharyngeal arch is called the lateral pharyngeal bands. There are also free lymph follicles under the posterior pharynx wall mucosa.

   The oral apex is called the palate. The front 2/3 is the hard palate, which is structured by the maxillary palatine process and the horizontal palatine sites; the posterior 1/3 is called the soft palate. Muscles constitute the soft palate include the velopharyngeal tensor, the velopharyngeal levator, the palatoglossus muscles, the palatopharyngeus muscles, the musculus uvulae, etc. The inferior oral cavum wall is the tongue and the oral base. The tongue is made with muscle plexus, with tough tongue back surface, covered with pseudo stratified squamous epithelium and is closely correlated with the lingualis; There is a foremen cecum at the inferior tongue, what is the embryoductusthyroglossus vestige. The posterior 1/3 tongue is the tongue lingual root, on which there is the lymph tissue mass, and the mass is called the lingual tonsil. The mucosa connective tissue protruded in the inferior tongue center and inferiorly metastasiss to con-

X. Zhou (✉)
Department of Otorhinolaryngology Head and Neck Surgery, The First Affiliated Hospital of Hainan Medical University, Haikou, China

X. Bi
Department of Pediatric Surgery, The First Affiliated Hospital of Hainan Medical University, Haikou, China



Z. Mu, J. Fang (eds.), *Practical Otorhinolaryngology - Head and Neck Surgery*, https://doi.org/10.1007/978-981-13-7993-2_13

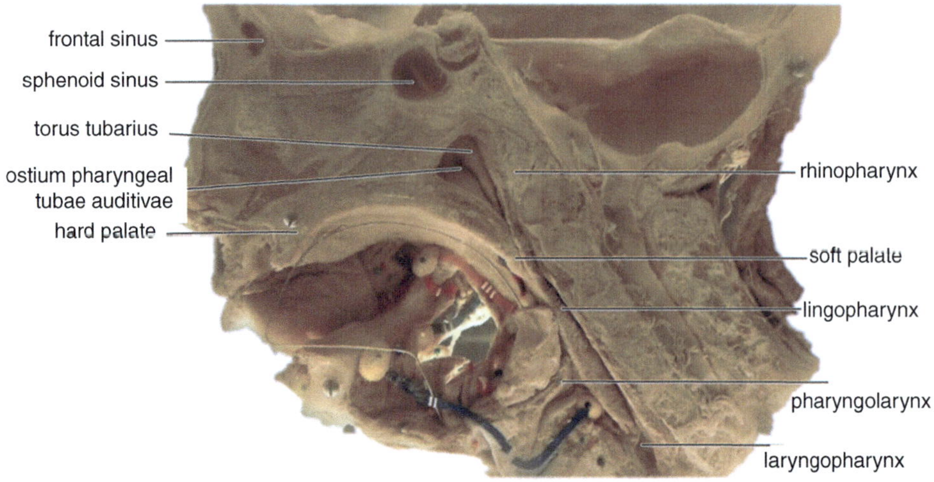


**Fig. 13.1** Pharyngeal subsections

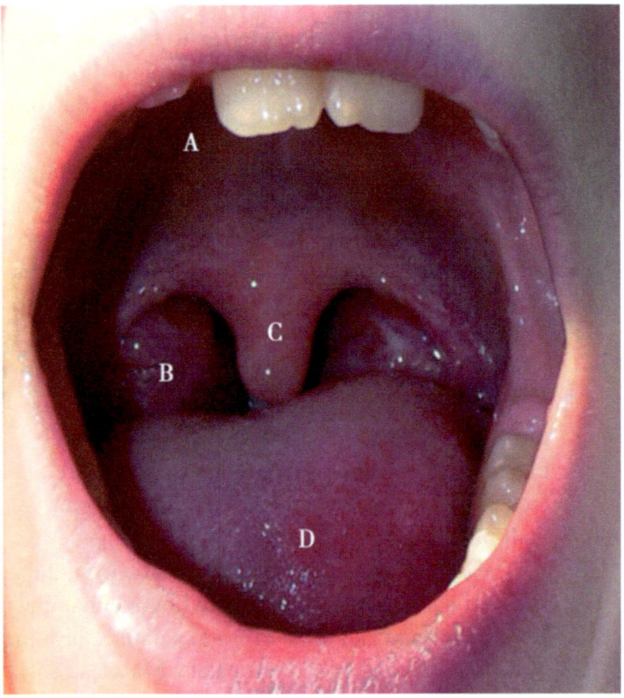


**Fig. 13.2** Oropharynx sites. A: Soft palate; B. tonsil; C. uvula; D. tongue

stitute the frenum linguae, bilateral frenum are the aditus glandula sunmandibularis. The occasional ankyloglossia could influence and suffocate the articulation.

(c) Larynopharynx

It locates between the epiglottis superior edge and the cricoid cartilage laminae's inferior edge plate, opens superiorly to the oropharynx, inferiorly to the esophagus aditus and anteriorly to the larynocavum and surrounds by the cricopharyngeus muscles. The anterior laryngopharynx has an aditus constituted by the epiglottis, the aryepiglottis fold and the arytenoid cartilage, which is called the aditus laryngis. Piriform abcesses at bilateral aditus laryngis, deep crypts, are a most common incarceration site of foreign mass. Shallow crypts at left and right between the lingual root and the epiglottis are called the vallecula epiglottica and both of them are common remaining sites of the foreign mass. Between the piriform abcesses and the at posterior cricoid cartilage laminae, there is the post cricoid space (Fig. 13.3).

2. Pharyngeal Wall Anatomy
   (a) Pharyngeal Walls

   It has four layers: mucosa, fibrin, muscle and outer membrane.

   - Mucosa

     Nasopharynx mucosa is the continuousness of the nasocavum mucosa and the eustachian tube mucosa, it has pseudostratified ciliated columnar epithelium and mixed glands in the lamina propria. The mucosa epithelium of the oropharynx and the larynopharynx are both the stratified squamous epithelium, the mucous glands exist at inferior mucosa and secret fluid to moist the pharyngeal mucosa. Plenty of the lymph tissues under the epithelium layer aggregate and substitute the inner ring of the pharynx waldeyer.

   - Fibrous Layer

     It is also called the aponeurosis layer, mainly substituted by the pharyngobasilar fascia and it is connective tissue between the mucosa layer and the muscle layer. Raphe pharyngis formed in the middle postpharyngeal line and it is the attachment site of the constrictor naris.

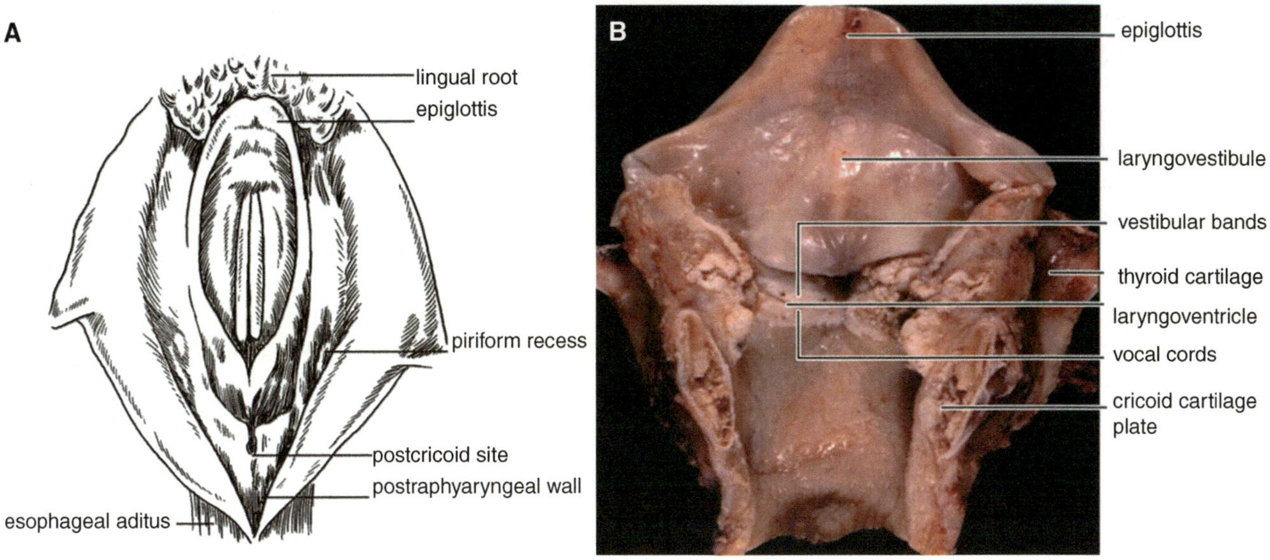


**Fig. 13.3** Larynopharynx anatomy

- Muscle Layer

  According to the functions, it could be divided into three groups:

  - Constrictor Naris

    Superior, middle and inferior constrictor naris line imbricately from above down and when the constrictor naris contracts, the pharynocavum shrink to impress the food into the esopharyngeal.

  - Levator Myopharynx

    It mainly contains the stylopharyngeus, the palatopharyngeus muscles, etc. The levator myopharyngeus could raise the throat to assist the deglutition.

  - Velopharyngeal Muscle

    It contains evator, tensor muscle, palatopharyngus, palatoglossus, uvulae, etc. It could shrink the isthmus faucium, close the nasopharynx and temporarily separate the nasopharynx and the oropharynx.

- Outer Membrane Layer

  It covers out of the constrictor naris, substituted by the connective tissue surrounding the muscle layer. It is with thin superstratum and thick substratum and also the continuity of the fascia buccopharyngeal.

(b) Interfascial Spaces

Posterior to and bilateral pharyngeal wall, there are potential areolar tissue spatia made by the neck spatia and because of its existence, the soft tissue is under coordinate accordance to achieve the normal physical function while the swollen or the neck motion. Simultaneously, because of the division by the spatia interfasciale, the lesion would be limited inside the spatia, but it offers the approach for the lesion expanding in the spatia at the meantime. The more important spatia in the pharynx are the retropharyngeal space and the parapharyngeal space.

- Retropharyngeal Space

  It locates between the prevertebral interfascia and the buccopharyngeal interfascia, its upper ending is at the skull base and the lower ending is at the mediastium, which is equivalently the first or the second thoracic vertebra, and the pharyngeal raphe seperated it into the left part and the right part. In the space, there is lymph tissues, especially at infant, but its quantity reduces and its size shrinks as people grows, so there are only few lymph nodes at adults stage, who are used to drain the lymph at tonsil, mouth, postrarhinocavum, rhinolaryngx, Eustachian tube, etc., so any site's inflammation would cause the retro Pharyngeal space infection even the retropharyngeal abscess.

- Parapharyngeal Space

  It represents the space at bilateral retroparyngeal interval, each one at one side, pyramid and peak downwards. Its upper ending is the skull base, its lower ending is the big corner of hyoid bone, its internal side separates from the sacral tonsil by the buccal pharyngeal fascia and the pharyngeal muscle, its external wall is the ascending branch of the mandible, the deep part of the pterygoid muscle and the parotid gland, and the posterior wall is the anterior fascia. The styloid process and its nearby muscles divide the gap into two parts. The forefoot is small and the medial side is adjacent to the tonsil. Inflammation of the tonsils can spread to this space; the posterior space is larger, and there are internal carotid artery, internal jugular vein, glossopharyngeal nerve, vagus nerve, hypoglossal nerve, accessory nerve and sympathetic trunk, and there are deep cervical lymph nodes. The infection can spread to this space.

3. Pharyngeal Lymph Tissue

The lymph tissue under the pharynx mucosa is abundant, of which the bigger black mass cycliclined is called the inner ring lymph, also the Waldeyer lymph ring; the outer ring lymph made by the pharynx tonsil (adenoid), the palatine tonsil, the tongue tonsil, the eustachian tube tonsil, the posterior pharynx wall lymph follicles and the lateral pharynx cord consists of the mandible angle lymph node, the inferior mandible lymph node, the submental lymph node, the posterior pharynx lymph node, etc. The inner ring lymph could be drainage into the outer ring lymph, so when the inner ring lymph tissue can't limit the pharynx infection or the tumor, it could diffuse or metastasis to the corresponding outer ring lymph node. The inner ring lymph tissue is at hyperplasia stage at childhood, and it could invoke after 10.

(a) Pharyngeal Tonsils

It is also named as the adenoid locating at the junction of the nasopharynx apex and the posterior wall, covered by the pseudostratified columnar ciliated epithelium, and with rough surface, so it is easy to retain the bacteria. The mid-fissure is the deepest one, where we could find the diverticulum depression of the residual embryo, which is called the bursa pharyngeal. The adenoid exists congenitally and invoke after 10. There isn't any connective tissues and the envelopes between the pharynx tonsil and the pharyngeal wall, so it's hard to be excised entirely.

(b) Palatine Tonsil

The palatine tonsil locates in the bilateral oropharynx tonsillar pit encircled by the palatoglossal arch and the palatopharyngeal arch and it is the oval clump lymph tissue, one at left and the other at right. It is the biggest pharyngeal lymph tissue. Its internal free surface mucosa epithelium is a squamous epithelium, it invaginate into the tonsil parenchyma and forms several branches of blunt duct irregular at depth. The blunt ducts opens abscess at the tonsil surface. so the bacteria could retain and breed at the blunt duct in the abscess and finally forms the infection 'lesion'.

(c) Tonsillar Blood Vessels and Nerves

- Arteries

  It consists of five external carotid branches. Palatine descending limb arteries, the maxillary artery limbs, distributing in the superior palatine tonsil and the soft palate; efferent palatine arteries, from the facial arteries; tonsil limb of the facial arteries; the tonsil limb of the efferent pharynx arteries, all of the four above distribute at the palate tonsil and the palatoglossal arch and the palatopharyngeal arch; dorsal tongue artery from the lingual artery and distribute at the inferior palatine tonsil.

- Veins

  There is a venous plexus out of the palatine tonsil diorama, flowing the veins to the pharyngeal veins and the lingual veins and affluxing into the jugular vein.

- Nerves

  The pharynx plexus, the second trigeminal limb and the glossopharyngeal nerve.

4. Pharyngeal Blood Vessels, Nerves and Lymph

(a) Arteries

The pharynx limb of the efferent pharynx arteries, the efferent arteries of and the tonsil arteries the facial arteries, the dorsal tongue limbs of the tongue arteries and the tonsil descending arteries are all the external carotid arteries.

(b) Veins

Open to the pterygoid venous plexus through the pharynx venous plexus and afflux into the facial veins and the internal carotid veins.

(c) Nerves

The pharynx sensory nerve and motion nerve are all from the pharynx nerves plexus made by the glossopharyngeal nerve, the labyrinth pharynx limb and the sympathetic nerve; the superior nasopharynx sensation is from the trigeminal maxillary limb.

(d) Lymph

Pharynx lymph flows to the deep cervical lymph nodes. The nasopharynx lymph firstly flows into the retro pharynx lymph node and then the efferent deep cervical lymph nodes co group. The oropharynx lymph nodes afflux into the nodi lymphatici mandibulares; the laryngopharynx lymph tubes go through the hypothyroid and afflux into the middle deep cervical lymph node cogroup adjacent to the internal carotid veins.

## 13.2 Physiology of Pharynx

Pharynx is the common channel of the respiratory and the digestion and has several complex physiological functions.

1. Deglutition

Deglutition is a reflective cooperating activity by plenty muscles. Food was inserted into the cavum pharynx through the oral cavity, the swallow reaction rises the soft palate, close the nasopharynx, contract the aryepiglotticus and the, retract the tongue, cover the laryngeal inlet with the epiglottis, and at the pharynx, it evokes the hypopharyngeal and the esophageal aditus opening, simultaneously with the pharyngeal contractor muscular contraction to oppress the food masses move down, then the food would enter the esophagus through the piriform recess, and if the pharyngomusle paralyzes, the dysphagia or the fold reflux would occur.

2. Respiratory

   The nasopharynx and the oropharynx are respiratory channels. There are abundant glands in or under the pharyngeal mucosa to help clear, humidify and adjust humidification the inhaled air while going through the pharynx sites, but its similar function in nasopharynx is better.

3. Resonance and Articulation

   The pharyngeal is one of the resonance cavities, while pronouncing, the tonsil could adjust the shape to fit the pronunciation requisitions to produce the resonance and enhanced the voice effect. It can also produce several kinds of languages with the help of the soft palate, the mouth, the tongue, the lips, the teeth etc. Corresponding change at the normal pharyngeal structures and the pharyngeal shape and size while making voice play an important role on forming a speech and articulation.

4. Defense and Protection

   The secretion from the nose, the nasal sinus and the eustachian tube could be spit out by the pharyngeal reflex reaction or be swollen to let the gastric acid eradicate microorganisms inside. Besides, the pharyngeal muscle reflex activity protects our flesh. While swallowing or vomiting, the pharyngeal muscle contracts to close the nasopharynx and the cavum larngis and eventually avoid the food or the vomitus regurgitating into the cavum nasi or being inhaled into the weasand. If foreign mass was mistakenly in the cavum pharyngis, the pharyngeal muscle can also contract to stop it falling and evoke nausea, vomiting to expel the foreign mass.

5. Adjust the Mid-Ear Air Pressure

   The eustachian tube aditus's opening is closely related to the deglutition. The aditus opens while deglutitions to balance the mid-ear air pressure and the foreign pressure to maintain the normal midear function and eventually remain the normal auditory ability.

6. Tonsil Immunity

   Tonsil locates at the aditus of the respiratory and the digestion channels and it is a positive immunity organ in infants. It contains several stagings' cyto lymph, including the B cell, the T cell, the plasma cell, the macrophage and it can produce several kinds of immunoglobin (IgG, IgA, IgM, IgE), so it occupies the main liquid immunity and effects at aspect on the cellular immunity. The adenoid is also an immunity organ though it effects less. Infants have more opportunity to touch the foreign allergen, so the adenoid enlargement is a normal condition but also it may be an immunity motion phenomenon. It would invoke.

# 14 Symptomatology and Examination Method of Pharynx

Xuejun Zhou, Zhonglin Mu, Zhiqun Li
and Rong Tu

## 14.1 Symptomatology of Pharynx

Pharyngeal symptoms are mainly caused by diseases of the pharynx and its adjacent organs, and may also be a local manifestation of systemic diseases. The main causes are sore throat, dysphagia, dysphagia, abnormal voice and reflux of diet.

1. Pharyngagia

   Pharyngeal pain is one of the most common symptoms, which can be caused by pharyngeal diseases or diseases of adjacent organs, or accompanying symptoms of systemic diseases. Acute and chronic inflammation of pharyngeal mucosa and lymphoid tissue, pharyngeal ulcer, pharyngeal trauma (foreign body, abrasion, and scald), specific infection (tuberculosis, diphtheria), malignant tumors, excessive styloid process, and some systemic diseases (leukemia, mononucleosis) can cause pharyngalgia, but the degree of pain varies. Acute inflammation, suppurative infection of pharyngeal space and laryngopharyngeal cancer are the main causes of severe pain. Pain can radiate to the ear and is reluctant to swallow food because of pain.

   There are two kinds of cases in clinic: spontaneous pharyngalgia and secondary pharyngalgia. The former occurs when there is no movement in the quiet state of the pharynx, which is usually confined to a part of the pharynx and is mostly caused by pharyngeal diseases, while the latter is caused by various activities of the pharynx, such as stimulation of swallowing, eating or tongue depressors. For example, acute and chronic inflammation of pharyngeal mucosa and lymphatic tissue, pharyngeal trauma, ulcer, foreign body, specific infection (tuberculosis, diphtheria), malignant tumors, long styloid process, carotid sheathing, cervical fibrohistitis, rheumatic lesions of pharyngeal muscles, and some systemic diseases (leukemia, AIDS) all have pharyngalgia in varying degrees.
2. Pharyngeal Paraesthesia

   It includes the unusual symptoms at pharynx, such as foreign body, obstruction, attachment, itching and other sensory abnormalities in the larynx and pharynx, which are common in organic lesions of the pharynx and surrounding tissues, such as chronic inflammation, pharyngeal keratosis, tonsil hypertrophy, uvula prolongation, tumors, reflux esophagitis, epiglottic cyst (Fig. 14.1); functional factors are mostly related to psychological

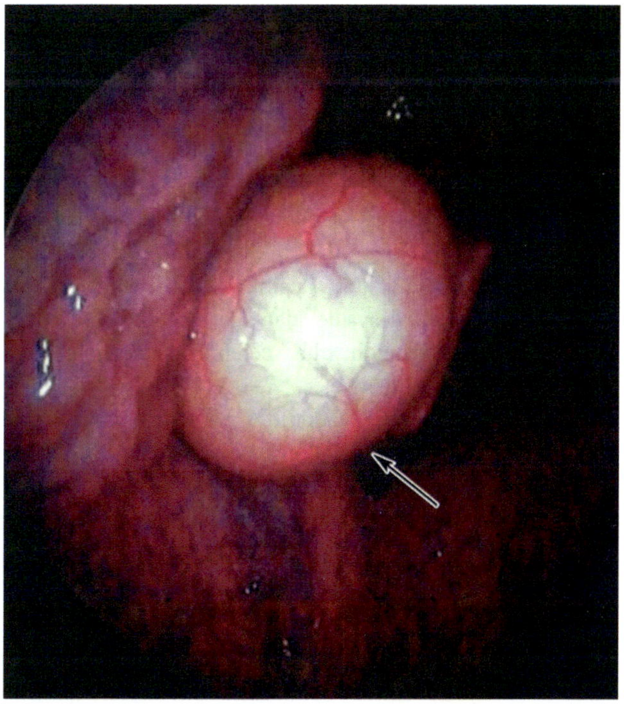

**Fig. 14.1** Epiglottic abscess (arrow)

X. Zhou (✉) · Z. Mu
Department of Otorhinolaryngology Head and Neck Surgery, The First Affiliated Hospital of Hainan Medical University, Haikou, China

Z. Li · R. Tu
Department of Medical Imaging, The First Affiliated Hospital of Hainan Medical University, Haikou, China



Z. Mu, J. Fang (eds.), *Practical Otorhinolaryngology - Head and Neck Surgery*, https://doi.org/10.1007/978-981-13-7993-2_14

factors such as fear and anxiety. It can be caused by endocrine dysfunction.

3. Dysphagia

It means the difficulty of normal swallowing function. The degree of difficulty swallowing could be briefly classified into three degrees: slight, moderate and severe. The light degree: patients can't freely swallow, choke while taking hard food, however they can tolerate a normal diet.

The patient with moderate degree can only take the semiliquid food; the patient with severe degree can take only liquid foods or can completely take in nothing.

Factors that cause dysphasia are as follows:

(a) Dysfunction

Patients with severe dysfunctional sore throat such as; acute suppurative tonsillitis, peritonsillar abscess, retropharyngeal abscess, acute epiglottis and epiglottis abscess, often suffer from dysphagia due to pain, and the degree varies with severity of pain. Some congenital malformations such as posterior nasal atresia and cleft palate, difficulty to swallow after birth.

(b) Obstruction

Obstructive pharyngeal or esophageal strictures, tumors, or foreign bodies hinder the descent of food, especially solid food, which is difficult to swallow, but liquid diet can still pass. Introesophageal obstruction such as congenital webbed esophagus, congenital esophageal stenosis, esophageal scar stenosis, esophageal foreign body, retrocervical cancer, hypopharyngeal diverticulum, estraesophageal compression such as cervical vertebral bone hyperplasia, thyroid tumors, extensive cervical lymph node metastases, mediastinal tumors, etc.

(c) Neuro Paralysis

Neuroplegic pharyngeal muscle paralysis caused by central lesions or peripheral neuritis causes dysphagia, especially when taking liquid. Such as bilateral pyramidal tract lesions, pseudobulbar palsy, extrapyramidal system damage, encephalitis, poliomyelitis, syringomyelia, cerebral hemorrhage and cerebral embolism, etc.

Children with sudden dysphagia, esophageal foreign bodies should consider. Esophageal cancer should be considered first when dysphagia occurs in middle aged and older patients and gradually aggravate. It maybe scars stenosis, dysphagia caused by emotional excitement and recurrence. Complicated symptoms also Achalasia should be considered. Complicated symptoms also have diagnostic significance, such as dysphagia with hiccups lesions, should consider at the end of the esophageal lesions, such as cancer, diaphragmatic hernia or achalasia, situation where hoarseness occurs first then there is pre-existing dysphagia, the recurrent laryngeal nerve and hypopharyngeal may be involved in laryngeal lesions. Tracheoesophageal fistula should be considered if there is a cough caused by drinking water. Postswallowing reflux, which causes cough, may be due to achalasia or food reflux in hypopharyngeal esophageal diverticulum.

4. Abnormal Sounds

The pharyngeal cavity is the common vocal cavity, and the tongue is an important organ to assist vocalization. It is closely related to the clarity and quality of voice. If there is rotation and pathological changes, the voice is ambiguous (speech clarity is extremely poor) or the sound quality characteristics are different from the original (tone color change), or the produced during sleep is not appropriate (snoring), collectively referred to as abnormal sound.

Lightness of speech and change of timbre (i.e. sound quality). When the lip, teeth, tongue and palate are defective, it is difficult or impossible to pronounce certain sounds, which leads to inarticulate speech. The patients with cleft palate and palate paralysis can not close the nasopharynx and have open nasal sounds, while the patients with adenoid hypertrophy, posterior nasal polyp, hypertrophic rhinitis and nasopharyngeal tumors have occlusive nasal sounds when the resonant cavity is obstructed. There are space-occupying lesions (abscesses or tumors) in the pharyngeal cavity. The pronunciation lacks resonance. When speaking, it is like there is content in the mouth, the words are unclear, and the crying of children is usually like that of ducks sounds.

5. Dietary Reflux

When the diet can not smoothly enter the esophagus through the pharynx and reflux to the mouth, nasopharynx and nasal cavity, it is called dietary reflux. Mostly seen in the following diseases:

(a) Pharynx

Pharyngopharyngeal muscle paralysis, retropharyngeal abscess, peritonsillar abscess, cleft palate, laryngopharyngeal tumors, etc.

(b) Esophagus

Esophageal deformity, diverticulum, stricture, dilatation, reflux esophagitis, etc.

(c) Stomach

Gastrointestinal neurosis, gastritis, gastric cancer and gastric dilatation etc.

(d) Other Diseases

Other diseases, such as endocrine disorders, brain dysfunction, hypothyroidism, primary chronic adrenal cortical dysfunction, nutritional deficiency, acid-base imbalance, can also cause gastrointestinal dysfunction and reflux.

## 14.2 Examination Method of Pharynx

### 14.2.1 General Examination

1. Pharyngeal Inspection

   The pharyngeal examinee is sitting with mouth open and breathing calmly. The examiner lifted the lips and cheeks with tongue depressor to observe whether there are bleeding, ulcers and masses on the teeth, gingiva, hard palate, tongue and floor of mouth. Then he held the tongue depressor and gently depressed the front 2/3 of tongue to observe the morphology of oropharynx; the color and luster of mucosa, whether there are congestion, secretions, pseudomembranes, ulcers and neoplasms; whether the soft palate was symmetrical and its activity; whether there is lymphatic folliclefts on the posterior pharyngeal wall and whether there are Swollen tonsil; tonsil size and palatoglossal arch, palatopharyngeal arch situation, if the palatoglossal arch is pulled open with a hook, it will be better to see the true situation of tonsil; use tongue depressor to squeeze palatoglossal arch, check whether there is cheese-like substance or pus overflow in crypt.
2. Pharyngeal Palpation

   The pharyngeal palpation patient is sitting, head slightly forward, the examiner stands on the right side of the examinee; the right hand wears gloves or finger gloves, with the index finger from the right corner of the mouth extended into the pharynx for examination. Palpation is suitable for the diagnosis of pharyngeal masses, to determine the location, size, surface characteristics, and hardness, mobility of the lesions, to check for fluctuations, fluctuations, tenderness and the relationship with the neck. Palpation can also be used to diagnose styloid process lengthening and determine adenoid size in children. However, in case of suspected pharyngeal abscess, palpation should be used carefully to avoid the risk of suffocation due to rupture of abscess and aspiration by mistake.
3. Cervical Palpation

   Cervical palpation because of the close relationship between the pharynx and the neck, cervical lymph node enlargement often indicates the existence of some pharyngeal diseases, so the neck should be carefully examined. At the time of examination, the patient sits with his arms drooping and his head slightly low. The examiner stands behind the examinee and palpates them sequentially with two fingertips. They should be done on both sides at the same time for comparison. The upper, middle and anterior cervical lymph nodes of deep cervical lymph nodes were examined along the anterior margin of sternocleidomastoid muscle to the sternum, and the posterior cervical triangle and supraclavicular lymph nodes were examined. Examination included swelling and mass, size, hardness, mobility, tenderness, adhesion and pulsation of the mass.
4. Indirect Nasopharynoscope Examination

   Indirect nasopharyngeal endoscopy examines the examinee sitting, mouth opening moderately, pharyngeal reflex sensitive person, using tetracaine for surface anesthesia before examination. Press the tongue plate on the left hand, press down the front 2/3 of the tongue, expose the back wall of the pharynx, and hold the nasopharyngoscope warming but not scalding on the right hand. The mirror is facing upward, extending from the mouth corner into the mouth, and placed between the soft palate and the back wall of the pharynx (Fig. 14.2). Do not touch the surrounding tissues, so as to avoid obstructing the examination due to pharyngeal reflex. Adjust the angle of the mirror, the back of the soft palate, the back edge of the nasal septum There are also eustachian tube pillow, eustachian tube oropharynx, pharyngeal recess and adenoids (Fig. 14.3). During examination, attention should be paid

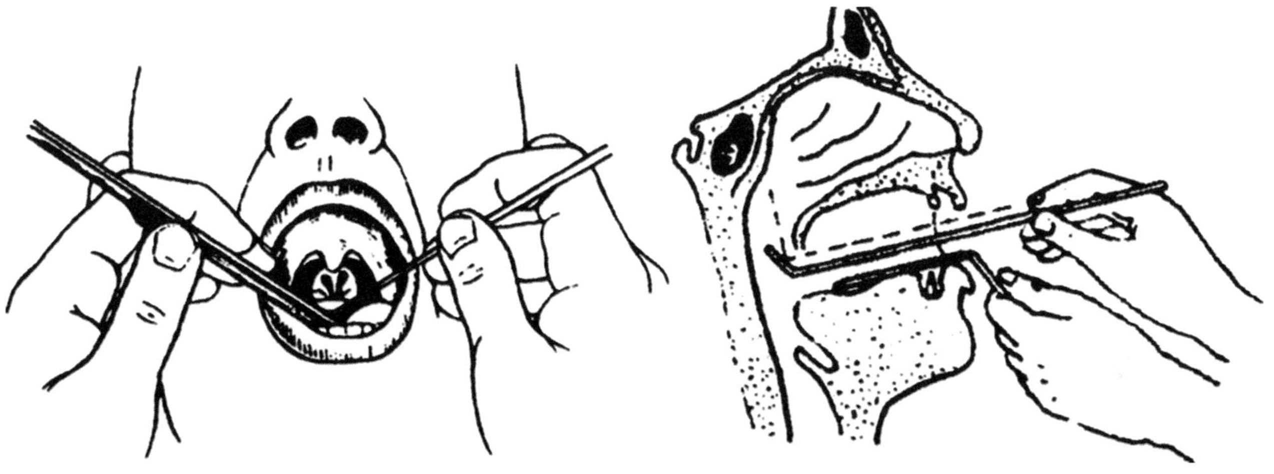

**Fig. 14.2** Indirect nasopharyngeal scope examination method

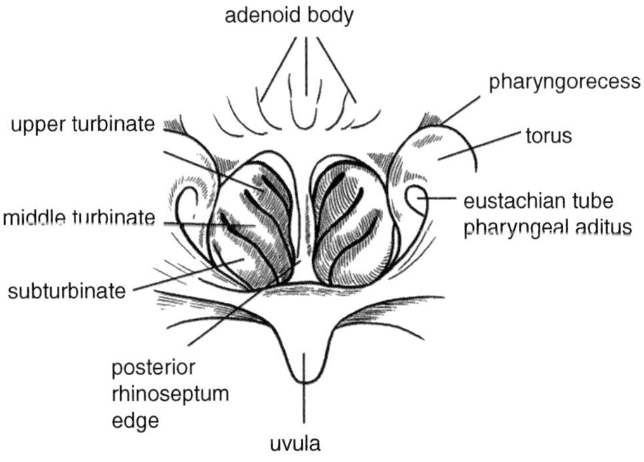


**Fig. 14.3** Common imaging under indirect nasopharyngeal scopy

to the presence or absence of congestion, roughness, bleeding, ulceration, protuberance and new organisms in nasopharyngeal mucosa.

5. Indirect Laryngoscope

   Indirect laryngoscope is the most common and convenient method of laryngopharyngeal examination in clinic. For patients with sensitive pharyngeal reflex, high tongue root and poor epiglottis elevation, the examination of laryngopharyngeal exposure is not good.

### 14.2.2 Endoscopy

1. Rigid Endoscopy

   The nasoendoscopy tube is thin. After contraction anesthesia of nasal mucosa, endoscopy is placed into the nasopharynx through the nasal base, and the tube is rotated to observe each part of the nasopharynx. The nasoendoscope tube is thicker through the mouth. It is placed in the oropharynx through the soft palate. The window at the end of the endoscope tube is made to look up at the nasopharynx.

2. Fibrous (Electronic) Endoscopy

   Fiber Endoscopy is a flexible endoscope, which can be flexible and rotative. After being introduced into the nasal cavity, it can change the angle at will and observe the whole nasopharynx with higher accuracy. Before examination, nasal endocrine should be cleaned and 1% tetracaine should be used for nasal cavity and nasopharyngeal mucosal surface anesthesia.

### 14.2.3 Imaging

1. X-Ray Examination

   X-ray examination mainly includes lateral examination and skull base examination. Because of the limited resolution, it is basically replaced by CT scan.

   Contrast examination mainly includes laryngopharyngeal (pyriform recess) angiography, which is the preferred examination method for lesions of pyriform recess. Subjects swallowed 150–200%(W/V) barium suspension for double contrast radiography. Positive, lateral and left-right oblique radiographs were taken during filling and resting periods respectively. The morphology of epiglottic valley, pyriform recess and esophageal entrance was observed. In order to better display the above structure, we can also do an improved Valsalva action, that is, after taking barium, let the examinee pinch his nose, close his mouth and hold his breath forcefully, blow up his cheek and throat, and take positive and lateral films. CT and MRI can also show the anatomical structure well, but the display function is not as good as that of angiography.

2. CT Scan

   CT scan includes plain scan and enhanced scan. The nasopharynx is closely related to the skull base, so the examination of the nasopharynx should include the skull base. The soft tissue window and the bone window should be observed simultaneously to understand the skull base and other bone structures. Because the pharyngeal structure is soft tissue, the lesions are closely related to the parapharyngeal space and cervical vessels, therefore, pharyngeal examination should be enhanced scanning, which is helpful to the localization and characterization of the lesions and the relationship with the surrounding structures, and can identify the vessels and lymph nodes.

   During pharyngeal CT scan, patients must be told to breathe slowly and calmly, not to swallow and speak, in order to avoid artifacts.

   The specific scanning methods of nasopharynx, oropharynx and laryngopharynx are as follows.

   (a) Nasopharyngeal CT Scan

   - Cross Section

     The patient is put in supine and the auditory canthus line should be perpendicular to the scanning table. The scanning range would be from sphenoid body to hard palate plane. The thickness and spacing were 5 mm. The scanning conditions were 130 kV and 160 mA. To understand the condition of cervical lymph nodes, the hyoid plane should scanned downward with 10 mm thickness and space.

     Enhanced scanning should be performed by intravenous injection of 80-100 mL iodine contrast agent at a rate of 2-3 mL/s. Continuous scanning should be started after injection of 50 mL.

   - Coronary Scanning

     Patients lie on their back, head droop, and backward, so that the line of auditory canthus is parallel to the plane as far as possible (the angle of the frame can be adjusted properly). The scanning range is from the front edge of the flange to the front edge of the first cervical spine. The thickness and interval of the lamina are all 5 mm. Since the wide application of multi-slice spiral CT, coronal scanning has gradually been replaced by coronal reconstruction of cross-sectional scanning.

(b) Oropharyngeal CT Scan
- Cross sectional scanning

Posture and nasopharynx scanning, scanning range from hard palate to upper edge of epiglottic cartilage, thickness and interval are 5 mm. To understand the lymph node status, 10 mm thickness and interval were scanned downward to the lower edge of the third cervical spine.

- Coronary

Same as the nasopharynx.

(c) Laryngopharygeal CT Scan
- Cross section

Patients in supine position, mandible elevation, first take lateral positioning film of head and neck, scanning plane parallel to vocal cord, if the direction of vocal cord can not be determined, scanning plane can be consistent with the central cervical interval; scanning range from the upper edge of epiglottis of hyoid bone to the lower part of glottis (i.e. below the lower edge of cricoid cartilage), equivalent to the upper edge of the third cervical vertebra to the lower edge of the sixth cervical vertebra; slice thickness and interval are all 5 mm.

- Coronary

Coronal scanning: Coronal images can be obtained by coronal reconstruction through cross-sectional scanning.

3. MRI

Magnetic resonance imaging (MRI) is another significant progress in imaging after CT in the 1980s. It has excellent tissue resolution, multi-directional imaging ability and various imaging sequences. It can display normal pharyngeal anatomy and lesions more clearly and comprehensively than CT. MRI images can clearly show the mucosal part and deep structure of nasopharynx. Therefore, MRI is not only helpful to detect superficial lesions, but also helpful to estimate the depth of invasion of lesions. Fat showed high signal on T1 and T2 weighted images. The parapharyngeal space of nasopharynx was surrounded by adipose tissue. The disappearance or displacement of fat tissue suggested the existence of lesions and could judge the location of lesions, which is much more sensitive than CT.

Spin echo sequence is often selected for pharyngeal imaging. Coil selection head, neck coil. The cross-section is the basic direction, and the sagittal or coronal plane is supplemented. Spin echo sequence is often used in pharyngeal imaging. T1 weighted imaging uses repetition time (TR): 400–700 ms, echo time (TE) 15–30 ms, T2 weighted imaging TR: 2000–4000 ms, TE: 60 ms, 90 ms or 120 ms. Layer thickness is 3–5 mm, matrix $256 * 256$ or higher FOV (field of view) 18–44 cm as required. In order to reduce the artifacts of breathing movement, patients should be advised to avoid swallowing during scanning, and saturated bands should be applied to the upper, lower or front of the scanning range according to different scanning directions. The parameters of enhanced scan are the same as those of plain scan.

4. Nuclear Medicine Imaging

PET-CT can be used for staging malignant tumors.

# 15 Common Pharyngeal Disease

Bo Feng, Yongjun Feng, Xuejun Zhou, Zhonglin Mu and Jugao Fang

## 15.1 Congenital and Other Pharyngeal Diseases

### 15.1.1 Congenital Nasopharyngeal Stenosis and Atresia

**Etiology**

In general, the buccal-pharyngeal membranes of newborns have been completely ruptured after birth. If the buccal-pharyngeal membranes are not ruptured, congenital nasopharyngeal atresia will occur.

**Clinical Manifestation**

No breathing or crying occurred after birth. At birth, the child's color was normal, but soon cyanosis occurred after ligation of the umbilical cord. The manifestation is neonatal nasal obstruction. Dyspnea. Cyanosis and aggravation of lactation and other symptoms of complete blockage of the nasal cavity. Examination of the pharynx revealed a thin film between the posterior margin of the soft palate and the posterior wall of the pharynx (Fig. 15.1).

**Diagnosis**

There is no airflow in front of the nostril. After contracting nasal mucosa with vasoconstrictor, the pharynx could not be accessed through nasal cavity with a thin probe, and the pharynx could not be accessed by methylene blue dripping into nasal cavity. The diagnosis can be confirmed by nasal endoscopy.

**Treatment**

Usually surgical treatment, often under nasal endoscopy through, open the atresia membrane, generally placed silica gel tube dilation for 3–6 months to prevent restenosis.

Figure 15.1 nasopharyngeal atresia.

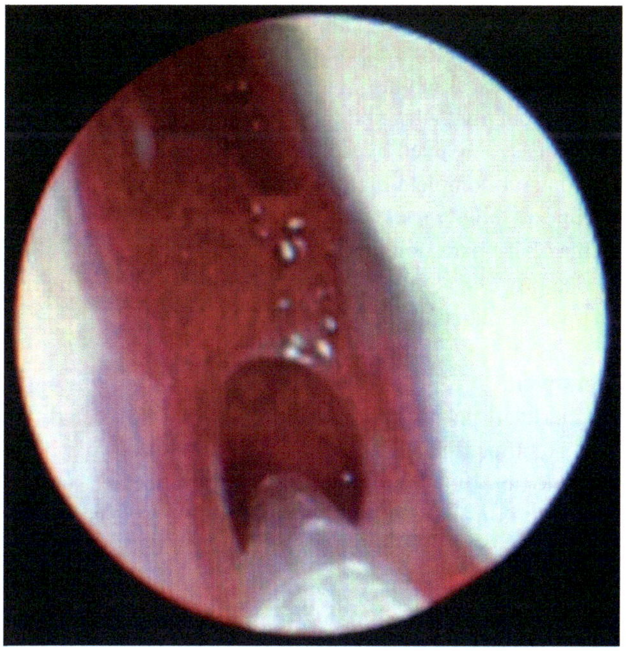

**Fig. 15.1** Nasopharyngeal stenosis

B. Feng (✉)
Department of Otorhinolaryngology Head and Neck Surgery, Chinese People's Liberation Army (CPLA) General Hospital, Beijing, China

Y. Feng
Department of Otorhinolaryngology Head and Neck Surgery, The Second Affiliated Hospital of Hainan Medical University, Haikou, China

X. Zhou · Z. Mu
Department of Otorhinolaryngology Head and Neck Surgery, The First Affiliated Hospital of Hainan Medical University, Haikou, China

J. Fang
Department of Otorhinolaryngology Head and Neck Surgery, Beijing Tongren Hospital, Capital Medical University, Beijing, China



Z. Mu, J. Fang (eds.), *Practical Otorhinolaryngology - Head and Neck Surgery*, https://doi.org/10.1007/978-981-13-7993-2_15

## 15.1.2 Cleft Palate

**Etiology**

The occurrence of cleft palate may be related to nutritional deficiency, endocrine abnormalities, viral infection and genetic factors in pregnant food. Cleft palate is a congenital developmental defect. With the growth and development, deformity changes with age. It can cause language, hearing and other functional barriers, as well as psychological barriers in social interaction.

**Clinical Manifestation**

Severe cleft palate can cause severe nutritional disorders in newborns due to inability to suck milk, or inhalation pneumonia due to dysphagia. It can be eaten if the swallowing function is close to normal through the compensatory function of the tongue. There will be characteristic open nasal sounds

**Diagnosis**

1. Soft Cleft Palate
   Only soft palate ruptures, sometimes even only uvula; usually without harelip; more often seen at female in clinic.
2. Incomplete cleft palate is also called partial cleft palate. Complete cleft soft palate with partial cleft hard palate; sometimes unilateral incomplete cleft lip, but alveolar process is often complete.
3. The unilateral complete cleft palate is completely split from the palate lobe to the incisor foramen, and obliquely outward to the alveolar process, which is connected with the alveolar cleft; the edge of the healthy side is connected with the nasal septum; sometimes the alveolar cleft disappears only with the cleft, sometimes the cleft is very wide; often accompanied by the same side cleft of the lip.
4. Bilateral complete cleft palate often occurs at the same time as bilateral cleft lip. Cracks occur in the anterior maxillary part, oblique cleft in each direction to the alveolar process; nasal septum, maxillary process and anterior lip are isolated in the center.

**Treatment**

Smaller cleft palate, such as uvula, may not be treated if it does not affect the normal physiology of the pharynx. If the physiological function of the pharynx is affected, surgical treatment is usually recommended. The cleft palate can be repaired by plastic surgery, and pronunciation training can be carried out when necessary.

## 15.1.3 Heterotypic Lingual Root's Thyroid Gland

**Etiology**

It is caused by the fact that the thyroid gland remains in the blind foramen of the tongue during the embryonic development. Figure 15.2 Heterotopic Thyroid in the Root of Tongue

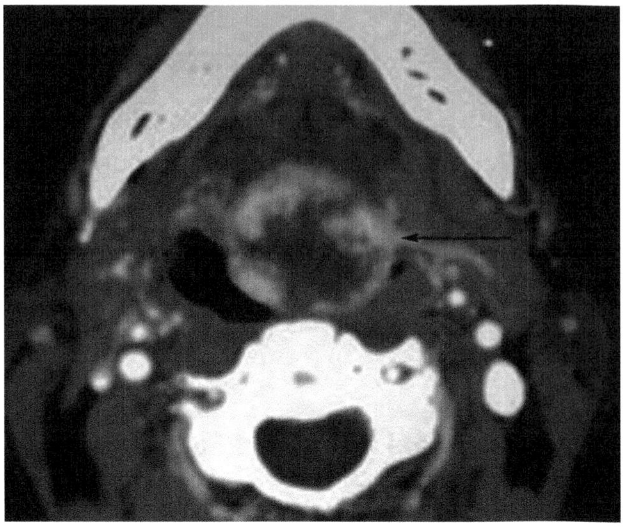

**Fig. 15.2** Heterotopic lingual root's thyroid gland

**Clinical Manifestations**

It is often manifested as a lump or discomfort in the root of the tongue, which can affect the patient's voice, swallowing or breathing. Swollen ectopic glands cause difficulty in swallowing, blocking the throat and causing the patient to have a containing sound. Specialist examination showed a pale red mass with vasodilation at the base of the tongue, which could compress the epiglottis and was moderately hard (Fig. 15.2).

**Diagnosis**

1. After taking radioisotope 131I, we can determine whether the tongue root mass is thyroid tissue by isotope scanning.
2. Depending on the typical clinical symptoms and physical examination, the diagnosis can be basically confirmed.
3. Although the thyroid tissue can be determined by puncture biopsy, it is easy to cause infection and bleeding, so it is not commonly used in clinic.

**Treatment**

When the tongue thyroid gland has little effect on function, it can be followed up. Thyroxine can be used as an alternative inhibitory therapy to reduce the volume and relieve the symptoms of tongue thyroid. Surgical treatment should be given to those who are too large and affect their functions, have tumors or cancers. Before operation, the benign and malignant lesions of the patients should be carefully evaluated, and whether there are glands in the thyroid region can be determined by iodine scan. For the patients diagnosed as lingual root goiter or nodular goiter, frozen pathology confirmed by surgery, ectopic transplantation can be adopted. Generally, one side of the submandibular gland is resected, and the thyroid pedicle of lingual root is transplanted into the submandibular gland fossa. There is often hypothyroidism after operation. We should pay attention to supplementing thyroid hormone. For patients suspected of carcinogenesis, all ectopic thyroid glands should be removed. The principle of regional lymph node dissection should refer to the treatment of papillary thyroid cancer.

### 15.1.4 Styloid Syndromes

**Definition**

Styloid process syndrome is a general term for the symptoms of pharyngeal foreign body sensation, pharyngalgia or reflex earache, head and neck pain and saliva increase caused by long or abnormal styloid process or its location and shape stimulating adjacent vessels and nerves.

**Clinical Manifestation**

1. Symptom

   Symptoms are common in adults. The onset of the disease is slow, the length of the disease is different, often tonsillar area, tongue root area pain, often unilateral, mostly not intense, can radiate to the ear or neck, swallowing aggravated, swallowing foreign body feeling or obstruction is more common, mostly on one side, swallowing more obvious, sometimes in speech, turning head or night aggravation, can also cause cough, when the carotid artery is compressed or rubbed, the pain can be from one side. The lateral mandibular angle radiates upward to the head, neck or face, sometimes accompanied by tinnitus, salivation, insomnia and other signs of neurasthenia.
2. Signs

   Physical signs palpation of tonsillar area can touch hard cords or spiny processes, patients can complain of discomfort here, and can induce sore throat or aggravation of sore throat; can be unilateral or bilateral too long.
3. Imaging Inspection

   Radiographic examination of styloid process (surface tomography) or CT plain scan and three-dimensional reconstruction can show its length, or skewed, curved and other conditions. The average length of normal styloid process is about 2.5 cm, which can be diagnosed as excessive styloid process (Fig. 15.3).

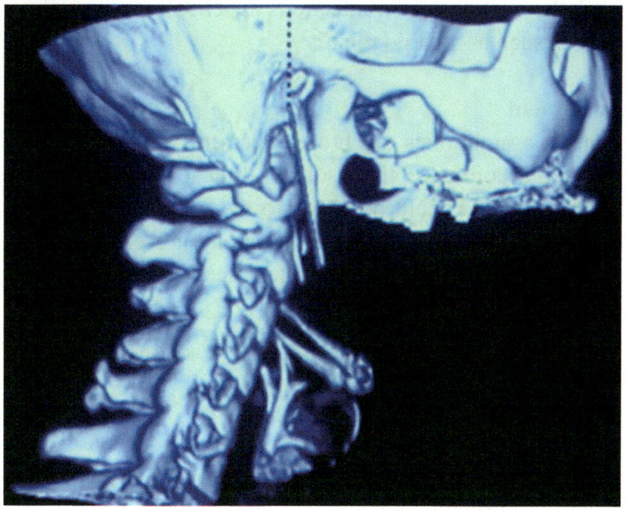

**Fig. 15.3** CT surface volume 3D reconstruction imaging displays elongated styloid process (44.2 mm)

**Diagnosis and Differential Diagnosis**

The diagnosis can be confirmed according to the symptoms, signs and imaging results of the patients. The disease should be differentiated from pharyngitis, glossopharyngeal neuritis, glossopharyngeal neuralgia and styloid process fracture.

**Treatment**

Surgical treatment was the main treatment. Indications should be based on the patient's condition. Long styloid process without symptoms or mild symptoms may not be operated on. The patient's symptoms obviously urgently require the operation. Operative methods are mostly through the oropharyngeal tonsil approach, or through the external cervical approach to cut short styloid process. Stemoidectomy can also be performed under local or topical anesthesia. In addition, it is supplemented by blocking, physiotherapy and so on.

## 15.2 Disease of Pharynx

### 15.2.1 Acute Nasopharyngitis

**Etiology**

Acute nasopharyngitis is an acute inflammation of nasopharyngeal mucosa, submucosa and lymphoid tissue, which occurs predominantly in adenoids. Usually, the symptoms of infants are more serious, while the symptoms of adults are lighter. Most of the symptoms are precursor symptoms of upper respiratory tract infection.

**Clinical Manifestation**

Children suffer from severe systemic symptoms, often with nasal obstruction and runny nose accompanied by high fever, vomiting, abdominal pain, diarrhea and dehydration, sometimes with meningeal irritation symptoms, and sometimes with systemic poisoning symptoms in severe cases; adults have mild symptoms, mainly with local symptoms, such as nasal obstruction and runny or mucopurulent. and often have a sense of dryness or burning of the nasopharynx, and sometimes have headache.

**Diagnosis**

According to the characteristics of clinical symptoms, the upper respiratory tract symptoms are obvious and the systemic symptoms are relatively mild, and the diagnosis can be made by excluding non-infectious upper respiratory inflammation such as allergic rhinitis.

**Treatment**
Sensitive antibiotics or broad-spectrum antibiotics were selected according to the results of drug sensitivity test, and glucocorticoids could be added to the patients with severe symptoms to control their condition and prevent complications in time. Local treatment, integrated traditional Chinese and Western medicine, etc.

### 15.2.2 Acute Pharyngitis

Acute pharyngitis is an acute inflammation of the pharyngeal mucosa and submucosa, which often involves the pharyngeal lymphoid tissue. Common in autumn and winter and winter and spring, can be single, often secondary to acute rhinitis or acute tonsillitis.

**Etiology**
1. Coxsackievirus, adenovirus and parainfluenza viruses are the most common viral infections, followed by rhinovirus and influenza viruses, which are transmitted by droplets and close contact.
2. Streptococcus, Staphylococcus and Pneumococcus are the most common bacterial infections, among which group A Streptococcus B infection is the most serious, which can lead to distant organ purulent lesions, known as acute septic pharyngitis.
3. Environmental factors such as high temperature, dust, smoke and irritant gases can cause the disease.

**Clinical Manifestations**
1. The pharynx is dry and hot. It has obviously sore throat and can radiate to the ear. Systemic symptoms are generally mild, including fever, headache, lack of appetite and limb soreness. If there are no complications, the course is usually about 1 week.
2. Examination showed acute congestion and swelling of pharyngeal mucosa, enlargement of lymphatic follicles in the posterior pharyngeal wall, yellow-white punctate exudates, edema of the palate and soft palate (Fig. 15.4).
3. The lymph nodes of mandibular angle are often enlarged and tender.

**Diagnosis**
According to the history, symptoms and signs, the diagnosis of acute pharyngitis is not difficult.

1. It is difficult to distinguish the pathogenic cause from bacterial or viral infection through clinical symptoms. The systemic symptoms of bacterial infection are more obvious. Viral infection symptoms are generally mild, often accompanied by runny nose and hoarseness.
2. Pharyngeal swab examination is helpful to clarify the etiology. The detection rate of group A streptococcus is as high as 90%. No bacterial growth was observed in continuous swab culture, which may be caused by viruses and other pathogenic microorganisms.
3. Blood routine and other laboratory tests.

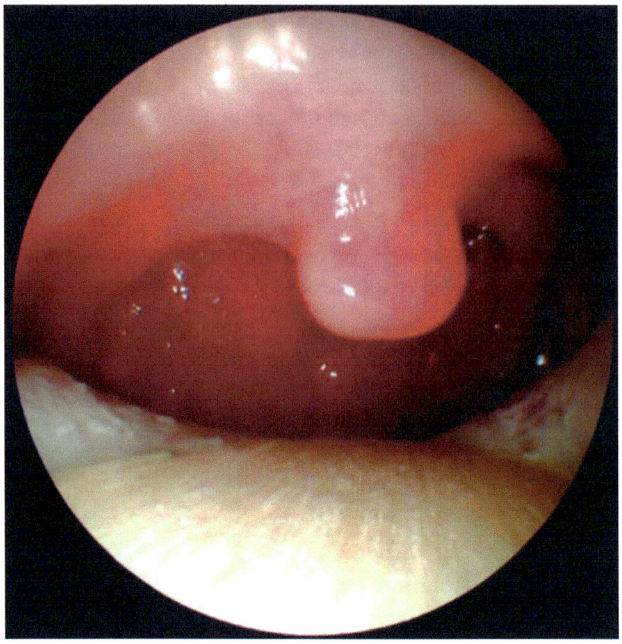

**Fig. 15.4** Acute pharyngitis

Attention to measles, scarlet fever, influenza, pertussis, poliomyelitis, encephalitis and other acute infectious diseases.

**Treatment**
1. Etiological treatment clears adjacent lesions, treats systemic diseases, quits smoking and alcohol, and prevents acute pharyngitis attacks. It is very important to strengthen physical exercise and physical fitness.
2. local treatment of local spray, Compound Tinidazole mouthwash gargle, including the tablets of metronidazole, iodine tablets and Yinhuang buccal tablets, in addition, can also used 1–3% Iodine Glycerol, 2% silver nitrate smear the swollen lymph follicles behind the pharynx. For patients with obvious sore throat, gargle diclofenac sodium gargle before meals to alleviate swallowing pain.
3. Systemic treatment of severe systemic symptoms with high fever, in addition to the above treatment, should rest in bed, drink more water and eat fluids, antiviral drugs can be intravenously administered: such as Acyclovir injection and Banlangen injection. Antibiotics were also used.

### 15.2.3 Chronic Pharyngitis

Chronic pharyngitis is a chronic inflammation of pharyngeal mucosa, submucosal tissue, lymphoid tissue and mucous glands. It is often a part of chronic inflammation and allergic diseases of upper respiratory tract. This disease is common in adults, with a long course, and its symptoms are prone to recurrence, which is not easy to cure.

**Etiology**

1. Local Factors
   (a) The recurrent episodes of acute pharyngitis relapse to chronic.
   (b) The pharynx is stimulated by inflammatory secretions of adjacent organs for a long time, such as chronic rhinitis, rhinosinusitis, allergic rhinitis, nasopharyngitis and chronic tonsillitis.
   (c) Long-term open mouth breathing caused by various rhinopathies leads to excessive dryness of mucosa and chronic pharyngitis.
   (d) Long-term addiction to tobacco and alcohol, eating spicy food, or being stimulated by dust and harmful gases can cause the disease.
   (e) Professional speakers, such as teachers, singers, waiters and other professional speakers.
   (f) Pathogenic microbial infection. Bacteriological abnormalities or pathogenic infections occur in pharyngeal secretions of some patients with chronic pharyngitis. In recent years, a small number of pharyngitis caused by gonococcal infection.
2. Systemic Factors

   Such as reflux esophagitis, respiratory allergic diseases, chronic bronchitis, endocrine disorders, autonomic nervous dysfunction, vitamin deficiency and immune dysfunction, are related to the disease.

**Clinical Manifestation**

1. Often has the pharynx foreign body feeling, the itching feeling, the burning feeling, the dryness or the slight pain feeling.
2. Often viscous secretions adhere to the posterior pharyngeal wall, causing frequent irritant cough and nausea in the morning.
3. No phlegm or only granular lotus root paste secretion coughs up. Patients with atrophic pharyngitis sometimes cough up smelly scab.

**Diagnosis**

The history and treatment of this disease should be inquired in detail. The occult lesions of nose, pharynx, larynx, esophagus, stomach and neck should be excluded, and the tonsil at the base of tongue should be enlarged. Styloid process syndrome, pterygoid hook syndrome, adverse drug reactions of some drugs and connective tissue diseases were excluded according to the situation. These diseases have similar symptoms with chronic pharyngitis. Therefore, comprehensive and careful examination should be made to avoid misdiagnosis. After a more detailed examination, the diagnosis of chronic pharyngitis was finally determined.

**Treatment**

1. Etiological treatment eliminates irritating factors, quits smoking and drinking, and avoids eating irritating food. Active treatment of rhinitis, tracheitis, bronchitis and other chronic respiratory inflammation and other systemic diseases. Improve working environment and enhance body resistance.
2. Chronic pharyngitis of traditional Chinese medicine (TCM) is characterized by deficiency of viscera-yin and disturbance of deficiency-fire, which is suitable for nourishing yin and clearing heat. Recently, watermelon cream and grass coral buccal tablets have been widely used in Chinese patent medicines.
3. Local Treatment
   (a) Chronic simple pharyngitis: to maintain oral hygiene, clinical commonly used compound borax solution, furacilin solution, 2% boric acid solution gargle. It can also contain iodine throat tablets, Mint throat tablets and the above Chinese patent medicines.
   (b) Chronic hypertrophic pharyngitis: broadly proliferated lymphatic follicles were cautered with 25–30% silver nitrate, electrocoagulation, microwave and laser, but improper use would increase mucosal scar and aggravate symptoms. Therefore, the scope of treatment should not be too wide or too deep.
   (c) Atrophic pharyngitis: Applying 2% iodine glycerin to the pharynx can improve local blood circulation and promote gland secretion. Taking vitamins regularly can promote the growth of mucosal epithelium.

### 15.2.4 Pharyngocystitis

Pharyngeal bursitis, also known as pharyngeal bursitis or nasopharyngeal cyst. The pharyngeal sac is formed by the invagination of the pharyngeal epithelium when the embryonic chordae retracts and reaches deep into the occipital periosteum. The cystic duct extends to the pharyngeal mucosa and is located in the pharyngeal tonsil or its residual lower margin. If the cyst is obstructed, cysts, nasopharyngeal cysts, nasopharyngeal abscesses and fistulas in the middle of the nasopharynx are formed.

**Etiology**

Pharyngeal bursitis, also known as pharyngeal bursitis or nasopharyngeal cyst. The pharyngeal sac is formed by the invagination of the pharyngeal epithelium when the embryonic chordae retracts and reaches deep into the occipital periosteum. The cystic duct extends to the pharyngeal mucosa and is located in the pharyngeal tonsil or its residual lower margin. If the cyst is obstructed, cysts, nasopharyngeal cysts, nasopharyngeal abscesses and fistulas in the middle of the nasopharynx are formed.

**Clinical Manifestation**

1. Posterior nostril can be seen secretions, scabs, susceptible to colds, sneezing, hoarseness, bad breath, voice clearance, cough and other symptoms.
2. Headache or head and neck pain, especially occipital pain.
3. Nasal obstruction, pharyngalgia, nasal tone and cervical lymph node enlargement.
4. Can have vertigo, tinnitus, earache, hearing loss.
5. The opening of nasopharyngeal apical sac tube is swollen, bulging or pyogenic.

**Diagnosis**

Nasopharyngeal endoscopy revealed a smooth polypoid mass on the top of the nasopharynx, sometimes covered with abscess scab. Removal of the abscess scab revealed an opening or fistula of the pharyngeal sac. The probe penetrated into the cyst cavity and secretion overflowed.

**Treatment**

Complete excision or destruction of the inner wall of pharyngeal sac mucosa to prevent recurrence. When the pharyngeal sac is small, 10–20% silver nitrate or 50% trichloroacetic acid can be used to burn the pharyngeal sac mucosa after puncture. Larger pharyngeal sac can open or open the soft palate, reveal the pharyngeal sac, cut the anterior wall of the pharyngeal sac with slender scissors, scrape the posterior wall, remove the cyst wall, if there is adenoid hypertrophy, it can be removed. Endoscopic pharyngeal sac resection has clear vision and easy operation.

## 15.3 Disease of Tonsil

### 15.3.1 Acute Tonsillitis

Acute tonsillitis is an acute nonspecific inflammation of the palatine tonsillitis. As a common disease, most of the patients are 10–30 years old, and infants and elderly people over 50 years old are rare. Generally, winter and spring are the most common diseases, which are often induced by fatigue, cold, excessive tobacco and alcohol, humidity and malnutrition. Chronic diseases, people with low physical resistance are susceptible.

**Etiology**

1. The main pathogens of infection are B-hemolytic streptococcus, staphylococcus, pneumococcus, non-hemolytic streptococcus, influenza bacilli, etc. Viral infections such as adenovirus infection, mixed infection of bacteria and viruses, etc.
2. Inducing factors such as cold, fatigue and environmental pollution can ınduce infection. In patients with chronic sinusitis, chronic tonsillitis and so on, when the body resistance decreases, hidden bacteria often multiply in large numbers and cause disease.

**Clinical Manifestation**

1. Acute onset, cold, fever, headache, poor appetite, fatigue, generally lasting for 3–5 days. Children with fever can cause convulsions, vomiting and coma.
2. Local symptoms
   (a) Pharyngeal pain is the main symptom, which is aggravated when swallowing and can be radiated to the ipsilateral ear.
   (b) Dysphagia: Children refuse to take drinking water because of pain.
   (c) Earache, tinnitus and ear tightness: If inflammation spreads to the eustachian tube, otitis media can occur.
3. Inflammation can spread to the surrounding areas, causing peritonsillitis, peritonsillar abscess, but also can cause acute otitis media, acute cervical lymphadenitis and parapharyngeal abscess. Rheumatic fever, acute glomerulonephritis, myocarditis and arthritis associated with hemolytic streptococcal infection should be paid special attention to sudden death of patients with myocarditis.

**Diagnosis**

According to the history, examination showed congestion and swelling of the tonsils were According to the medical history, hyperemia and enlargement of tonsils and purulent secretions in lacunae can be seen on examination (Fig. 15.5). The diagnosis is not difficult. Attention should be paid to the differential diagnosis of pharyngeal diphtheria, Fan Shang pharyngeal isthmitis and some hematological diseases caused by pharyngeal isthmitis (Table 15.1).

**Treatment**

1. General Treatment

   Bed rest, use warm boiled water to gargle, drink more water. Eat semi-liquid or soft foods rich in vitamins and other nutrients. Those with high fever were given ethanol bath or ice bag to cool down physically.
2. Drug Treatment
   (a) Sensitive antibiotics were selected according to clinical manifestations, pharyngeal bacterial culture and drug sensitivity (e.g. rapid detection of streptococcus).

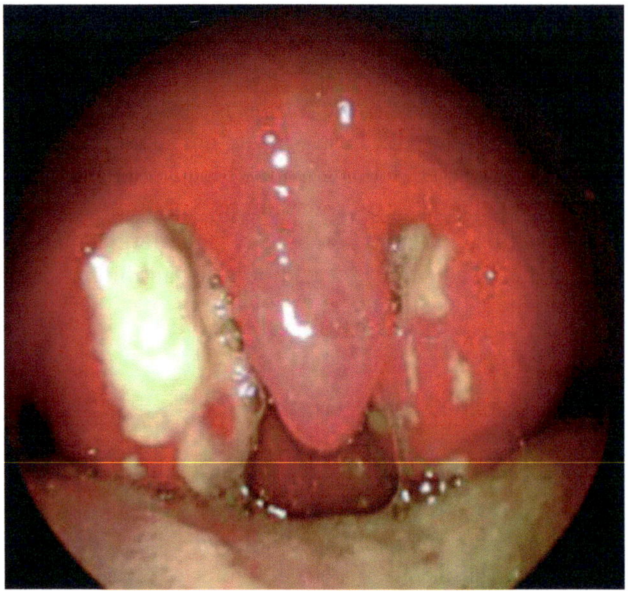

**Fig. 15.5** Congested enlarged tonsil

(b) Adequate antibiotics must be used, and the best symptoms and signs should be subsided and continued for 2–4 days. Because the tonsillar recess is branched blind canal, the depth is different, after an acute suppurative tonsillitis attack, if not completely cured; the bacteria still remain in the recess. When resistance decreases, bacteria multiply in large quantities and produce a large number of toxins, which can easily lead to the recurrence of the disease, or lead to bacterial endocarditis, myocarditis, glomerulonephritis, rheumatic fever, arthritis and other complications.

(c) Sequence of antibiotics: Penicillins are the first choice for this disease. Cephalosporins can be considered if penicillins are allergic, but cross-allergy should be paid attention to. If both of them are allergic, quinolones and lincomycin should be considered.

(d) Corticosteroids, such as dexamethasone, are added when necessary.

(e) Local use of antibiotics, such as buccal tablets, ultrasonic atomization inhalation, Chinese medicine etc.

**Table 15.1** Common acute tonsillitis differentiation diagnosis

| Disease | Pharyngache | Pharynginspection | Cervicolymph nodes and systemic condition | Lab test |
|---|---|---|---|---|
| Acute tonsillitis | Severe pharyngache, difficulty swallowing | On both sides of the tonsillar surface with yellow white punctate exudate, sometimes even easy to wipe pseudome | Lymphadenopathy and tenderness of the mandibular angle<br>The acute tolerance, high fever and chills | Smears: mostly hemolytic streptococcus, Staphylococcus, Streptococcus pneumoniae<br>Blood: a significant increase in white blood cells |
| Pharynx diphtheria | Mild pharyngache | Gray and white pseudomembrane often exceeds the range of tonsil. Any compact toughness, not easy to wipe, strong peeling easy bleeding | Cervical lymph node sometimes swollen, show "cow neck", the spirit is dispirited, the face is pale, low heat, pulse is weak, showing toxic symptom | Smear: diphtheria diphtheria<br>Blood: white blood cells generally do not change |
| Vincent angina | One side of the pharyngache, difficulty swallowing | One side tonsil covered gray or yellow pseudome wipe visible ulcers. | Cervical lymph nodes sometimes swollen in the affected side; Mild systemic symptoms | Smear: Clostridium and Spirillum Vincent<br>Blood: a slight increase in white blood cells |
| Mono increased angina | Mild pharyngache | Tonsil is red, sometimes covered with white pseudomembrane, easy to wipe | The lymphadenopathy of the whole body is known as "glandular fever"<br>High fever, headache, rash, acute sickly and sometimes hepatosplenomegaly etc.: smear negative or found in respiratory tract bacteria | Blood: abnormal lymphocytes and mononuclear cells accounted for more than 50%. Serum heterophil agglutination test (+) |
| Agranulocytosis angina | Pharyngache degrees differ | Necrotic ulcer, covered with dark brown pseudomembrane, pale and surrounding tissue ischemia. The soft palate and the gums have the same pathological changes | Cervical lymph node enlargement; septic fever, systemic failure quickly | Smear: negative or common bacteria<br>Blood: a marked decrease in white blood cells and a sharp decrease or disappearance of granulocyte |
| Leukemia angina | General painless | Early side tonsil enlargement and surface infiltration, necrosis, covered with grayish white pseudomembrane, often accompanied by oral mucosal swelling, ulceration or necrosi | Systemic lymphadenopathy, acute stage body temperature, early systemic hemorrhage, and exhaustion | Smear: negative or common bacteria<br>Blood: leukocytosis, classified as primary white blood cells and infantile leukocyte |

### 15.3.2 Chronic Tonsillitis

Chronic tonsillitis is often caused by repeated attacks of acute tonsillitis or poor drainage of crypts. It can also evolve into chronic inflammation due to bacterial and viral infections in the crypts. Acute infectious diseases (such as scarlet fever, measles, influenza, diphtheria, etc.), nasal cavity and sinus infections can also cause the disease. The most common age of onset was 7–14 years old, followed by young people, and the elderly were rare.

**Etiology**

1. Most of them are acute tonsillitis recurring and turning into chronic.
2. Some infectious diseases such as scarlet fever, influenza and measles can cause chronic tonsillitis.
3. Neighboring lesions such as nasal cavity and sinus infection may be associated with the disease.
4. The pathogenic bacteria are type A or B hemolytic streptococcus, Staphylococcus and so on.

**Clinical Manifestation**

1. There is a history of repeated attacks of acute tonsillitis, or peritonsillar abscess, susceptible to "cold", low fever, fatigue, headache, indigestion and so on.
2. Dry throat, itching, foreign body sensation, burning, slight pain, bad breath, dry cough.
3. Tonsil hypertrophy in children is characterized by irritating cough, snoring, swallowing and respiratory disorders.

**Diagnosis and Differential Diagnosis**

Diagnosis was made according to medical history, symptoms and signs. The determination of erythrocyte sedimentation rate, anti-streptococcal hemolysin O, serum mucin and electrocardiogram are helpful for diagnosis. The disease should be differentiated from the following diseases:

1. Physiological hypertrophy of tonsils is common in children and adolescents. There is no history of conscious symptoms and repeated inflammation attacks. There is no secretion retention in tonsillar recess and no adhesion with surrounding tissues.
2. Tonsil keratosis is caused by excessive keratosis of tonsillar recess orifice epithelium, and the appearance of white sharp sand particles, hard to touch, firm to adhere to, not easy to wipe off.
3. Tonsil tumors with unilateral tonsillar enlargement or tonsillar enlargement and ulceration, often accompanied by ipsilateral cervical lymph node enlargement, should consider the possibility of tumors.

**Treatment**

If there are operative indications, tonsillectomy should be performed, and the operative indications should be strictly controlled. For the lesions of tonsillitis which cause nephritis, lupus erythematosus, psoriasis and pustulosis of palm and toe, the operation should be performed as soon as possible on the premise of adjusting the general condition. Those who are not suitable for surgery may be treated with systemic or local medication. In view of the characteristics and allergy of chronic tonsillitis infection, immunotherapy and antiallergic therapy should be considered in addition to antibiotics and surgery.

### 15.3.3 Tonsillar Hypertrophy

**Etiology**

In general, when children are 6~7 years old, the tonsillar develops to the maximum and gradually atrophies after puberty. If tonsils are repeatedly infected with chronic inflammation, or malnutrition and other factors, it may cause tonsillar compensatory hypertrophy or abnormal enlargement. This disease is commonly seen in children aged 3~5 years, and adults are rare.

**Clinical Manifestation**

1. Ear symptoms: due to tonsil hypertrophy, if there are inflammatory secretions, it is easy to obstruct the pharynx and orifice of the eustachian tube, leading to acute otitis media, which can cause tinnitus, ear stuffiness or hearing loss.
2. Nasal symptoms such as hypertrophy of tonsils often cause rhinitis or sinusitis, which can lead to nasal obstruction, runny nose, mouth opening breathing, salivation, and obstructive nasal sounds in speeches, which are the main causes of snoring in children.
3. Inflammatory secretions of respiratory tract infection symptoms often stimulate respiratory mucosa, causing throat, trachea and bronchitis, so children may have pharyngeal discomfort, voice changes, cough and spitting, asthma, low fever and other symptoms.

**Diagnosis**

It is easy to diagnose according to medical history, symptoms and signs. Adhesion between the soft palate and the posterior pharyngeal wall can be seen at the mouth opening. A small passage leading to the nasopharynx is often found at the rear. The size of the passage and the upward expansion of the scar can be detected by inserting a curved probe into the opening. The extent of adhesion and the thickness of scar can be roughly detected by finger touch from the mouth. There are more secretions in the nasal cavity. Fiberoptic nasopharyngoscopy, X-ray lateral nasopharyngeal radiography, CT or MRI examination are helpful in the diagnosis of pediatric nasopharyngeal diseases.

**Treatment**

General treatment should pay attention to nutrition, prevent colds, improve immunity and actively treat primary diseases. With age, the tonsils will gradually atrophy, the disease may be alleviated or symptoms completely disappeared.

### 15.3.4 Tonsillectomy

Tonsillectomy is the best method for the treatment of recurrent tonsillectal infection and hypertrophy. Conventional tonsillectomy and plasma tonsillectomy can be used. Laser partial tonsillectomy and electrotome resection can be used. Ultrasound scalpel tonsillectomy is the most commonly used method for tonsillectomy. Currently, low temperature plasma is also used.

1. Indications
   (a) Chronic tonsillitis recurs three or more times a year.
   (b) The obstruction of upper respiratory tract caused by tonsillar hypertrophy results in severe snoring, dysphagia and poor pronunciation.
   (c) Peritonsillar abscess was operated on 2–3 weeks after acute inflammation subsided.
   (d) Tonsils cause systemic diseases and become focal tonsils, which need to be operated on when the condition is stable.
   (e) Precursor operations of Some operations, such as intraoral styloid process truncation.
   (f) Benign tonsillar tumors.
   (g) Some tonsillar malignant tumors are confined to the tonsil in the early stage, or the tonsillar fossa is not exceeded. Radiotherapy can be used to reduce the size of the tonsil, and then selective tonsillectomy and neck lymph node dissection may be performed if necessary [2]. Precautions before operation.
2. Precautions before operation
   (a) Acute tonsillitis should not be removed because the wound is prone to bleeding or secondary infection after operation.
   (b) Surgery should not be performed during menstruation and premenstrual period.
   (c) Diseases with hematopoietic and coagulation systems, such as hemophilia, aplastic anemia, leukemia, purpura, etc., should not be operated on.
   (d) Surgery should not be performed in the active stage of nephritis, hepatitis, rheumatism, tuberculosis and other diseases.
3. Surgical operation
   Tonsillectomy under local anesthesia
   (a) Local anaesthetized tonsillectomy
   Patients usually take their seats, the surgeon sits opposite the patient, and the light source is on the patient's head.

- Anetheticm medicine injection

  Injection of anesthetics: take 0.5–1% lidocaine 20 mL, add 4–6 drops of 1:1000 adrenaline solution to mix, extract half of the above anesthetics with 10 mL syringe, press the tongue depressor at the junction of 2/3 and 1/3 in front of the tongue, make the pharynx exposed clearly, and inject anesthetics 3–4 mL in the upper, middle and lower parts of the palatoglossal arch respectively; first, puncture the needle tip into the submucosa, then inject the needle. The tip penetrates around the tonsil. In addition to the anesthetic effect, the injected anesthetic can separate the tonsil from the tonsillar fossa. A little anesthetic should be injected between the upper part of the palatopharyngeal arch and the upper pole of the tonsil, and the opposite side should be anesthetized accordingly. At this time, the patient feels swollen and inconvenient to swallow. After the injection, the operation will be performed in 5 min.
- Incision: Use tonsil knife along the palatoglossal arch, 1–2 mm away from the free edge, cut from the upper pole of tonsil down to the root of palatoglossal arch, then bypass the upper pole, extend the incision and open the palatopharyngeal arch. However, it should be noted that the incision should not be too deep, only the mucosa should be incised. If the incision is too deep, the suprapharyngeal constrictor will be injured. Or cut into tonsil tissue, easy to cause bleeding and wound infection.
- Tonsillar Body Removal

  Peeling tonsils: The tonsil peeler is used to peel the palatoglossal arch from the incision of the palatoglossal arch. The palatoglossal arch and the front of the tonsil are first peeled off, and then the upper part of the tonsil is pressed downward. The upper part of the tonsil is held by tonsil gripper. At the same time, the tonsil is pressed downward with the peeler to separate it from the tonsil fossa until a small pedicle is left at when peeling, the peeler should not dig deep into the fossa to avoid damaging the suprapharyngeal constrictor or blood vessel and causing bleeding.
- Trap Extirpation

  Removal of the trap: The tonsil grabbing forceps at the tonsil trap were inserted, and the tonsil was pulled upward by the tonsil grabbing forceps. The pedicle should be pulled outward and downward by the trap, and the tonsil should also be pulled out by tightening the trap. Cotton balls were clamped with tonsil hemostatic forceps and placed into tonsillar fossa to compress hemostasis. At the same time, tonsil integrity and tissue damage would be examined. InspectionExamination:

The palatoglossal arch would be opened with tonsil hook to check whether there are bleeding in tonsil fossa, residual tonsil tissue, especially in the lower pole of tonsil triangular fold, where there are more lymphatic tissue. If not removed, it could still proliferate and hypertrophy, even produce inflammation after operation. In addition, the remnants of the lower pole can often cause postoperative bleeding. If active bleeding occurs, it must be stopped properly.

(b) Tonsillectomy under General Anesthesia

- Take supine position, open mouth with mouth opener, make pharynx exposed clearly. In order to stop bleeding, 0.5–1% lidocaine and 1:1000 adrenaline should be injected into the submucosa of palatoglossal arch and palatopharyngeal arch. The specific operation of the operation is the same as the local anesthesia tonsillectomy. But the surgeon is on the head side of the patient, so the direction of the operation is opposite to that of local anesthesia.
- During the operation, attention should be paid to keeping the respiratory tract open and preventing asphyxia. Hemostasis should be thorough to prevent bleeding after operation.
- After tonsillectomy, if adenoid hypertrophy occurs, adenoidectomy and hemostasis should be performed simultaneously. (4) Operative precautions and post-operative management

4. Operative Precautions and Postoperative Treatment

(a) Points for attention to operation

- After tonsillectomy, if adenoid hypertrophy occurs, adenoidectomy and hemostasis should be performed simultaneously. (4) Operative precautions and post-operative management

  The most common complication after tonsillectomy is bleeding, which is often caused by too little (residual) resection or too much (damaged surrounding tissues). Therefore, careful operation is needed to dissect the tonsillectomy along the outer capsule.
- Avoid slippage of grippers and tonsils falling into the trachea before tightening the trap.

(b) Postoperative Treatment

- Should observe whether there is bleeding, should tell patients to spit out all blood secretions in the mouth, do not swallow. For patients under general anesthesia, attention should be paid to frequent swallowing movements to estimate the possibility of bleeding. If there is blood vomiting, it should be checked in time to stop bleeding.
- Cold liquid diet should be taken on the first day after operation and half liquid diet on the second day, but not too hot. Soft food after 1 week and normal diet after 10 days. On the first day after operation, if the patient is reluctant to eat because of wound pain, he Gu method of acupuncture can be used for analgesia.
- The patient may have febrile reaction on the first day after operation. If the body temperature does not drop after 2–3 days, the cause should be checked and antibiotics should be added to prevent infection.
- 24h after operation with 1: 5000 Furacilin Solution mouth-washing to maintain oral hygiene.
- The wound albuginea formed 6~12 h after operation, began to fall off 5~7 days, and finished in about 10 days. The wound could heal.
- For patients who have tonsillectomy from the lesion, antibiotics are still needed to prevent infection after surgery.

## 15.4 Disease of Adenoid Gland

Adenoids, also known as pharyngeal tonsils, are a group of lymphoid tissues that attach to the junction of the apical and posterior walls of the nasopharynx and between the pharyngeal recesses on both sides, which correspond to the sphenoid body and the base of the occipital bone. If infected, the adenoids may become hyperemic, swollen or even hypertrophic.

### 15.4.1 Acute Adenoid Inflammation

Acute adenoiditis is a common disease in children. There is no difference between men and women. Adenoids disappear in adults, so it is rare to suffer from acute adenoiditis.

**Etiology**

Most of them occur in children. They are susceptible to seasonal changes and are often caused by bacterial or viral infections.

**Clinical Manifestation**

Often protuberant high fever, body temperature can be as high as 40 °C, nasal congestion is serious, such as pharyngitis is accompanied by swallowing pain. If the inflammation extends to both sides of the eustachian tube throat, there may be ear tightness, earache, hearing loss, etc. If the infection is serious, it can cause suppurative otitis media. Adenoid body is located in the same part as otorhinolaryngology, so its symptoms are diversified, but respiratory symptoms are still the main symptoms.

**Diagnosis**

1. Visual diagnosis of adenoid face, oropharyngeal mucus from the nasopharynx, common tonsil hypertrophy.
2. Palpation: there were soft tissue masses in the apex and posterior wall of nasopharynx.
3. Fiberoptic nasopharyngoscope or nasal endoscopy can be used to examine the adenoid hyperemia, the surface covered with exudates, throat wall inflammatory secretion retention.

**Treatment**

1. Patients should rest in bed, treat symptoms and use antipyretics in time. For patients with severe symptoms, antibiotics can be used to control infection and prevent complications.
2. If the adenoids are repeatedly infected in a short time, surgical removal of the adenoids should be advocated to prevent secondary damage such as autoimmune nephritis.

### 15.4.2 Adenoid Hypertrophy

Adenoid hypertrophy is pharyngeal tonsillar hyperplasia. Adenoid hypertrophy in children is often physiological. There are lymphatic tissues in the nasopharynx at birth and it proliferates with age. It usually reaches its maximum at the age of 6. Adenoid hypertrophy is called adenoid hypertrophy if it affects the health of the whole body or adjacent organs.

**Etiology**

The nasopharynx and its adjacent tissues or adenoids themselves are repeatedly stimulated by inflammation, resulting in hypertrophy and hyperplasia of adenoids.

**Clinical Manifestation**

Prominent upper incisors, poor occlusion, nasal septum deviation, etc., facial muscles are not easy to move, lack of expression, known as "adenoid facial facial features" "Acute otitis media or secretory otitis media are easy to complicate in children with corresponding symptoms and signs.

The main symptoms of adenoid hypertrophy are nasal obstruction, which is mainly due to the blockage of the posterior nostril and the eustachian tube and oropharynx, resulting in poor breathing, and can further cause ear, nose, pharynx, larynx and other symptoms. For example, children with long-term respiratory impairment lead to mouth breathing, air impact on hard palate will make hard palate deformed, high arch, facial development will deform, appear upper lip short and thick warping, mandible droop, nasolabial groove disappearance, hard palate arch, irregular arrangement of teeth, prominent upper incisors, poor occlusion, nasal septum deviation, etc., facial muscles are not easy to move, lack of expression, known as "adenoid facial facial features" "Acute otitis media or secretory otitis media are easy to complicate in children with corresponding symptoms and signs.

**Diagnosis**

1. The diagnosis should be given priority when children breathe with mouth opening and have typical "adenoid face".
2. Oral and pharyngeal examination showed that the hard palate was high and narrow. Viscous secretions were seen in the posterior pharyngeal wall from the nasopharynx, accompanied by palatal tonsil hypertrophy.
3. Anterior rhinoscopy revealed a large number of secretions and mucosal swelling in the nasal cavity.
   Figure 15.6 Electron (Fiber) Nasopharyngoscope of Adenoid Hypertrophy
4. Electron (fibre) nasopharyngoscopy revealed lobulated lymphoid tissue with longitudinal fissures on the top and posterior walls of the nasopharynx (Fig. 15.6).
5. Fingers are used for nasopharyngeal palpation. Soft masses can be palpable on the top and back walls of the nasopharynx.
6. Lateral X-ray, CT or MRI examination of the nasopharynx may also be helpful in diagnosis (Fig. 15.7).

**Treatment**

If hypertrophy is not serious, mucosal vasoconstrictors such as ephedrine nasal drops or antibiotic nasal drops can be used briefly to keep the nasal cavity unobstructed and prevent upper respiratory tract infection.

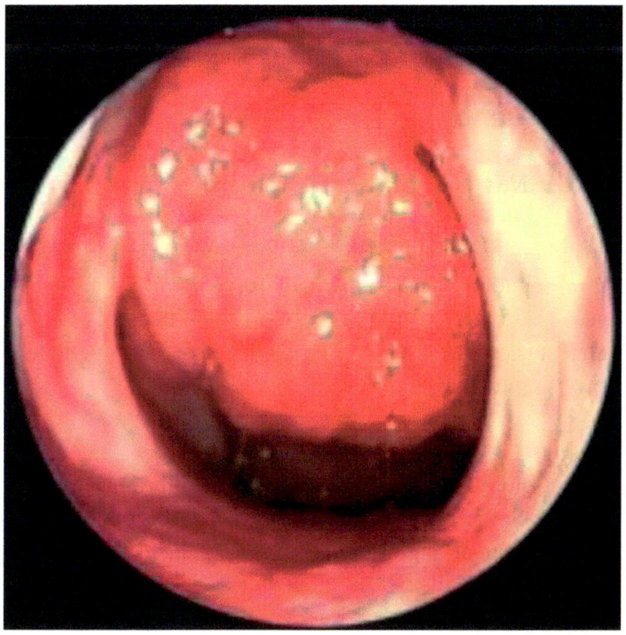

**Fig. 15.6** Electronic (fibrious) rhinopharyngoscopy indicates adenoid enlargement

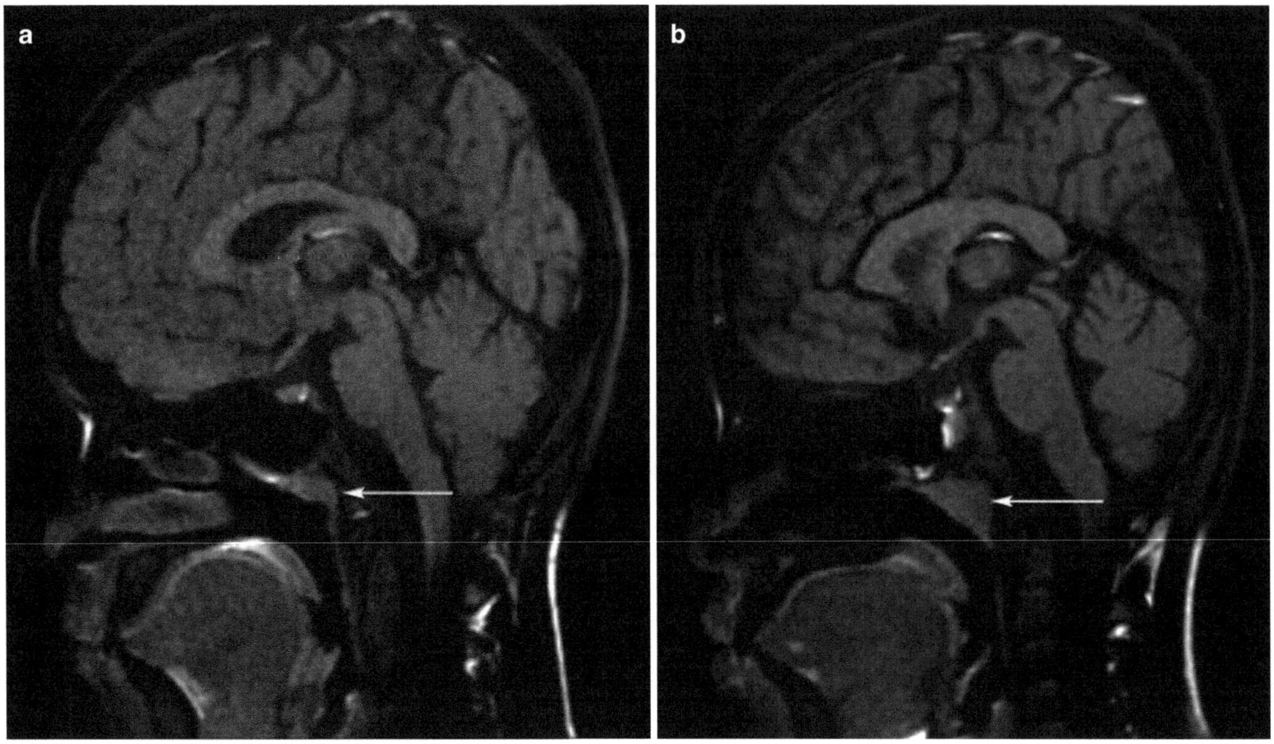


**Fig. 15.7** MRI sagittal $T_1$WI indicates adenoid enlargement. (**a**) 13-year-old male, 6 cm thick adenoids (arrow). (**b**) 13-year-old male, 12 cm thick adenoids (arrow)

If symptoms seriously affect breathing, with "adenoid appearance" or other chronic diseases such as rhinitis, sinusitis, secretory otitis media, long-term cure, then consider surgery. Adenoids are often removed with hypertrophic palatal tonsils. If the hypertrophy of palatal tonsils is not obvious and there is no obvious indication of surgery, the adenoids can also be removed alone.

## 15.5 Tumor of Pharynx and Parapharynx

### 15.5.1 Nasopharyngeal Angioma

Nasopharyngeal angiofibroma is a common benign neoplasm of the nasopharynx, which occurs in male adolescents aged 10~25 years. Pathologically, the tumors consist of vascular spaces of different shapes and sizes surrounded by fibrous tissue matrix.

**Etiology**

The etiology of nasopharyngeal angiofibroma remains unclear. Some studies have shown that the incidence of nasopharyngeal angiofibroma may be related to androgen levels.

**Clinical Manifestation**

The clinical manifestation of the disease is very dangerous, often with massive hemorrhage, and intracranial invasion tendency, so it is extremely difficult to deal with, often with the following clinical symptoms.

1. The main symptoms of recurrent epistaxis are recurrent nasal bleeding or massive oral bleeding.
2. Progressive nasal obstruction can cause obstruction of the posterior nostril on one or both sides, often accompanied by runny nose, obstructive nasal sounds, hypoplasia and other symptoms.
3. Compression symptoms of adjacent organs, such as tumors pressing the eustachian tube and oropharynx, can cause tinnitus, earache and hearing loss. If the skull base is destroyed and the cranial nerve is compressed, there will be headache and cerebral nerve paralysis. If the tumors invade the orbital, pterygopalatine or infratemporal fossa, they will cause exophthalmos, visual impairment, cheek or temporozygomatic eminence and trigeminal neuralgia. Larger tumors protrude into the pharynx, which can make the soft palate bulgy and difficult to eat.

**Diagnosis**

The diagnosis of this disease is mainly based on the patient's symptoms and imaging examination. Biopsy is very easy to cause massive hemorrhage, so it should be avoided in clinic.

1. Palpation finger or instrument can touch the base of the mass. The mass has low mobility and hard texture.

2. Indirect Nasopharyngoscope or Nasal Endoscopy

   Indirect nasopharyngeal endoscopy or nasal endoscopy revealed round or lobulated pink neoplasms with vascular striations on the surface of the nasopharynx.
3. CT Manifestation

   CT showed soft tissue density mass in nasopharyngeal cavity, with smooth and sharp outer margin and obvious and uneven enhancement. Tumors often protrude into the posterior nasal foramen, pterygopalatine fossa, infratemporal fossa and even maxillary sinus. Neighboring bone walls are compressed and absorbed, and the involved muscular spaces are not clearly visible (Fig. 15.8).
4. MRI Examination: the T1-weighted and proton density images of tumors were low and moderate signal intensities, while the T2-weighted and gradient echoes were medium and high signal intensities. There were more empty vessels in the tumors. The tumors were markedly enhanced after gadolinium contrast agent injection. Sagittal view showed that the tumors originated from the parietal and posterior walls of the nasopharynx (Fig. 15.9). The T1 weighted image of the tumor and the proton density image are low and medium signal intensity, and the T2 weighted image and the gradient echo image are medium and high signal intensity. Intratumoral vascular signal void more. The tumor was enhanced after injection of gadolinium contrast agent. The sagittal plane shows that the tumor originates from the posterior wall of the nasopharynx (Fig. 15.9).
5. Angiography can show the blood supply vessels of the tumors and determine the location of the tumors (Fig. 15.10).

   Angiography: the blood vessels of the tumor can be displayed and the tumor location is determined (Fig. 15.10).

The clinical stage of nasopharyngeal angiofibroma should be paid attention to when diagnosing the abundant blood supply vessels of nasopharyngeal angiofibroma. Fisch stage is usually used. Fisch Stage (1983):

- Stage I: The tumors are located in the nasal cavity and/or nasopharynx, with little bone destruction.
- Stage II: The tumors invaded pterygopalatine fossa, ethmoid sinus and sphenoid sinus.
- Stage III a: The tumors invaded the infratemporal fossa and orbit, with bone destruction and no intracranial invasion.
- Stage III b: The tumors invaded infratemporal fossa and orbit, with bone destruction and intracranial invasion.
- Stage IV a: The tumors invaded the dura mater, but did not invade the cavernous sinus, pituitary fossa and optic chiasm.
- Stage IV b: The tumors invaded the dura mater, cavernous sinus, pituitary fossa and optic chiasm.

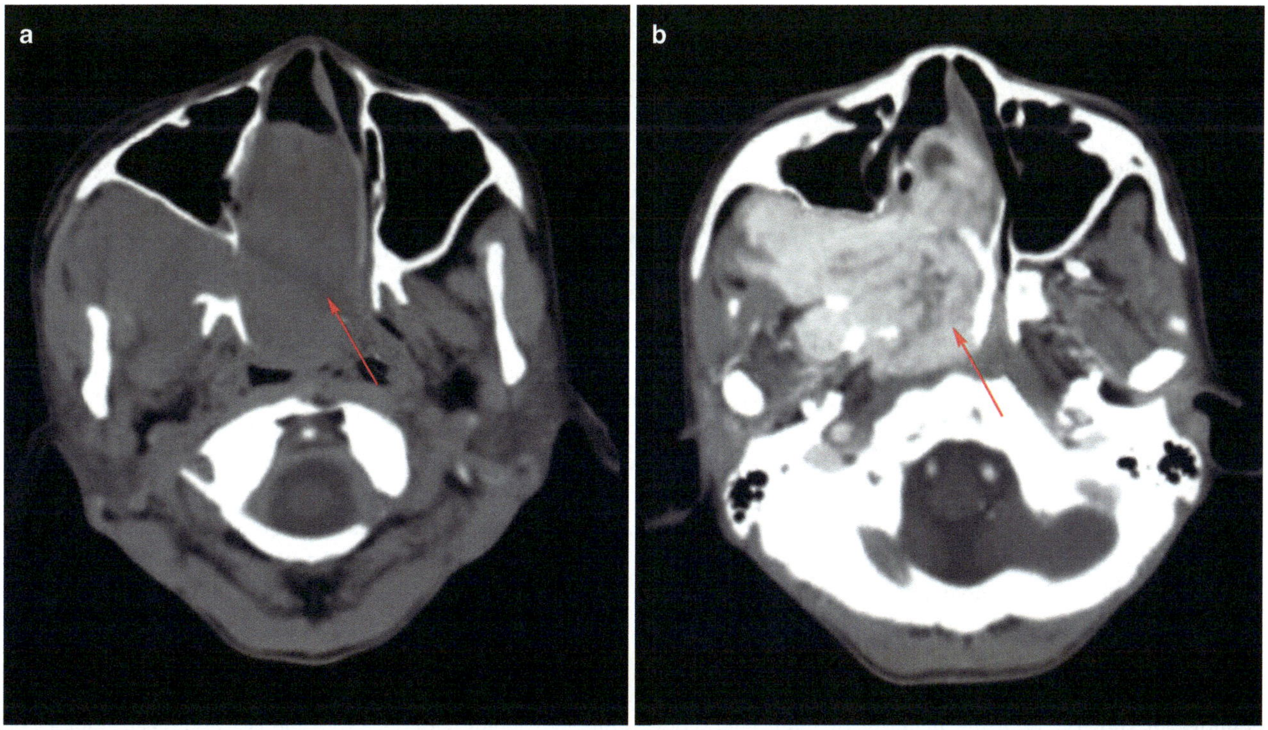


**Fig. 15.8** Rhinopharyngeal fibrious angioma. CT plain scan showed huge soft tissue mass in right nasal cavity, retropharyngeal space and infratemporal fossa (**b**). After enhancement, the mass was obviously enhanced

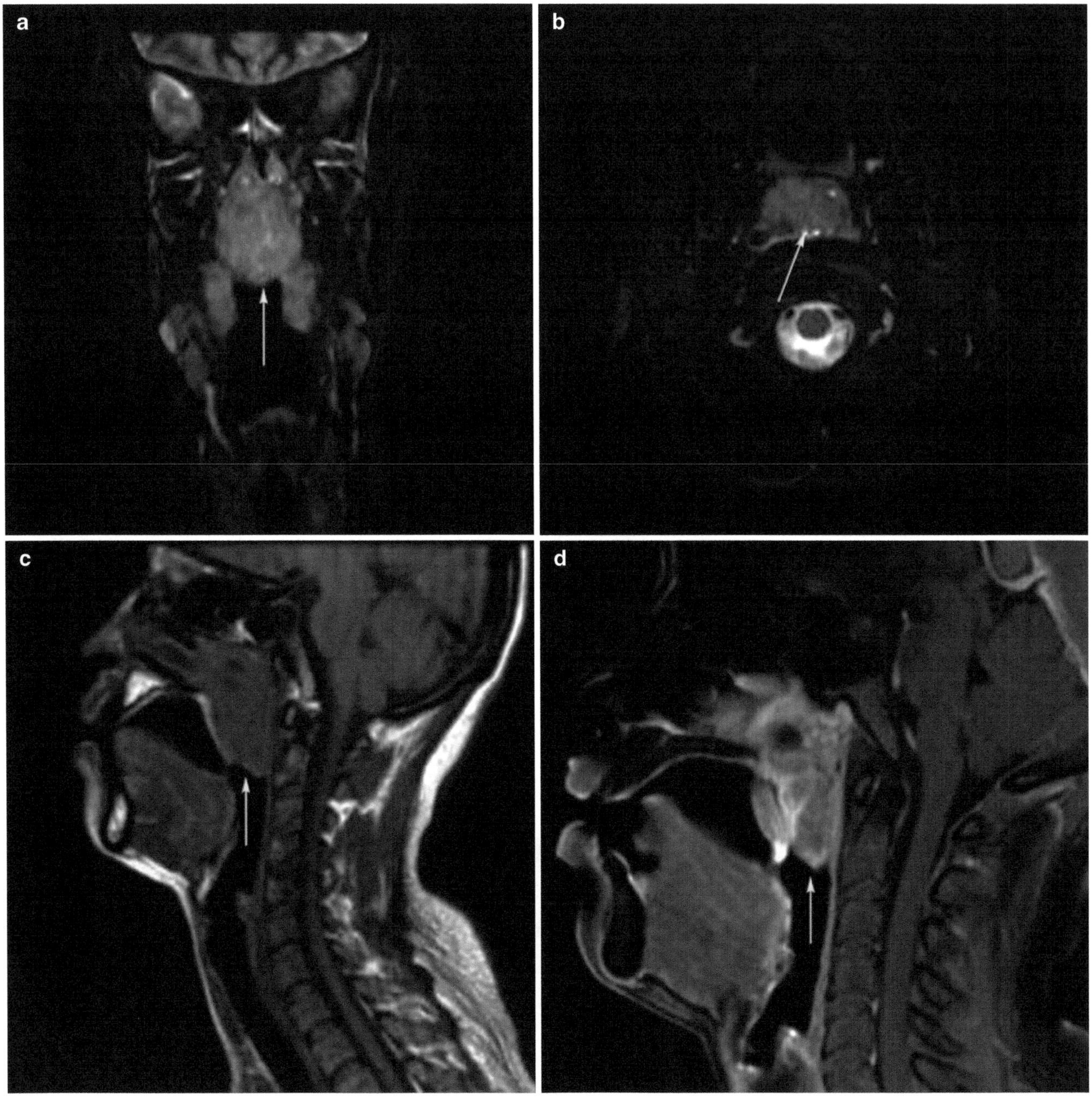


**Fig. 15.9** Rhinopharyngeal fibrious angioma MRI manifestation. (**a**) Coronary $T_2$WI. (**b**) axial $T_2$WI. (**c**) $T_1$WI plain scan. (**d**) Enhanced $T_1$WI. 4 Grams all displays a mass shadow at rhinopharynx, whose upper site approaches the rhinopharyngeal upper wall, anterior site is at posterior naris and lower site is at inferior uvula edge, and it evolves the uvula forwards, its boundary is clear and it is evidently enhanced under enhanced MRI

## Treatment

Surgical treatment is usually used. External carotid artery ligation or digital subtraction angiography (DSA) can be considered before operation to embolize the donor artery. Intraoperative controlled hypotension can also control bleeding. The traditional surgical method is hard palate resection or combined craniofacial surgery. With the maturity of nasal endoscopy, nasal endoscopic resection of nasopharyngeal angiofibroma has become the main method for the treatment of Fisch stage I, II and III a lesions. Generally, DSA responsible vascular embolism is performed 2–4 days before operation, and then nasal endoscopic surgery is performed, and controlled hypohemorrhage is often used during operation. Pressure, this method has many advantages, such as less trauma, better exposure to tumors, faster recovery of patients, no scar on the face, and so on. For patients with stage III b and IVa, combined craniofacial surgery assisted by nasal endoscopy can be used. First, intracranial and skull base tumors can be removed or cut off by

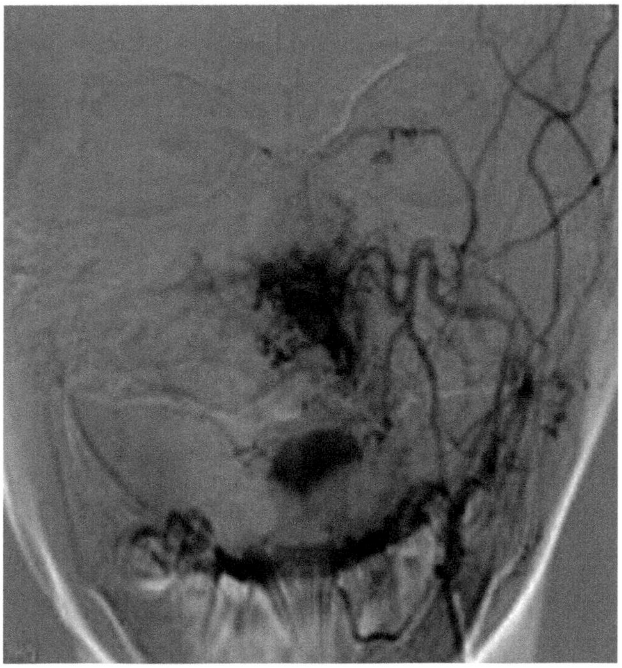

**Fig. 15.10** Angiography manifests abundant supply vessels of nasopharyngeal fibrinoma

craniotomy, and then the extracranial part of the tumors can be removed by nasal endoscopy. Or standard combined craniofacial surgery can be used to rotate the maxillary sinus and resect the maxillary bone after resecting the tumors. For patients with stage IVb, the operation should be careful to avoid uncontrollable massive hemorrhage.

### 15.5.2 Nasopharyngeal Cancer

Nasopharyngeal carcinoma (NPC) refers to the malignant tumors occurring in the nasopharynx and is one of the high-incidence malignant tumors in China, especially in the southern region, which are the first malignant tumors of the otorhinolaryngology.

**Etiology**

At present, it is believed that the occurrence of NPC is related to heredity, EB virus infection and environment.

1. Genetic Factors

   Nasopharyngeal carcinoma (NPC) has obvious family carcinomatosis and ethnic susceptibility. Many NPC patients have a family history of cancer. NPC is mainly seen in the Scandinavians descents, but rarely in the Caucasians. The descendants of high-incidence ethnic groups, such as immigrants, still have a high incidence. Studies have shown that NPC is a multi-factor hereditary tumor, and there are susceptibility genetic variations on chromosomes and genes.

2. Virus Infection

   The main factor of virus infection is EB virus. Lymphoblastic cell lines with EB virus can be isolated from nasopharyngeal carcinoma tissues, and a few virus particles can be seen under electron microscopy. Studies have shown that human papillomavirus (HPV) is also associated with the incidence of nasopharyngeal carcinoma.

3. Environment Factors

   The epidemiology researches find it that those Chinese migrate to other countries is on a Epidemiological investigation of environmental factors showed that the mortality rate of nasopharyngeal cancer decreased gradually with the genetic algebra of immigrants, and the incidence of nasopharyngeal cancer increased among white people born in Southeast Asia. Nasopharyngeal cancer can be induced by eating foods containing nitrite or nitrosamine precursors.

**Clinical Manifestation**

1. Nasal Symptoms

   The main nasal symptoms in the early stage of nasal symptoms are epistaxis, blood in sputum or bloody nasal mucus is common in the morning; if the tumor is located near the nostril, it can obstruct the nostril and cause nasal obstruction, which can be one side of the nose in the early stage, and bilateral nose obstruction in the late stage.

2. Ear Symptoms

   When ear symptoms tumors originate in the pharyngeal recess or occipital region of the eustachian tube, they invade and oppress the eustachian tube oropharynx, resulting in symptoms and signs of secretory otitis media, such as tinnitus and hearing loss, etc.

3. Eye Symptoms

   Eye symptoms of nasopharyngeal carcinoma invading the eye often cause visual impairment, visual field defect, diplopia, exophthalmos and movement limitation, and nerve paralysis keratitis. Fundus examination showed nerve atrophy and edema, etc.

4. Cranial Nerve Damage Symptoms

   The trigeminal nerve, abducent nerve, hypoglossopharyngeal nerve and hypoglossal nerve were more involved in the infiltration of nasopharyngeal carcinoma with the symptoms of brain nerve damage, while the olfactory nerve, facial nerve and auditory nerve were less involved. Tumors usually invade the fifth and sixth pairs of brain nerves first. At this time, the main symptoms are headache. If the second, third and fourth pairs of brain nerves continue to be invaded, besides the aggravation of headache symptoms, diplopia, facial numbness, blepharoptosis, blurred vision and even blindness can be accompanied. Tumors can also invade and compress the cranial nerves at the base of the skull, leading to hoarseness, cough, dysphagia and deviation of the tongue, etc.

5. Cervical Lymph Nodes Metastasis

   Cervical lymph node metastasis can occur in the early stage, mainly in the deep upper cervical lymph node group (area II). The enlarged lymph nodes are painless, hard, movable in the early stage, and adhere to the skin or deep tissue in the late stage.

6. Distant Metastasis

   Nasopharyngeal carcinoma with distant metastasis is prone to metastasis. Bone, liver and kidney are the common sites of metastasis. Multiple metastatic lesions often occur simultaneously. Patients may have chest pain, cough, liver or kidney pain, jaundice and other symptoms.

7. Cachexia

   Cachexia patients showed significant signs of emaciation, anemia, mental weakness and other systemic functional failure.

**Diagnosis**

1. Nasopharyngeal Examination

   Nasopharyngeal examination is an important examination, which should be carefully searched for suspicious points repeatedly. If the patient is sensitive to pharyngeal reflex, nasal endoscopy, electronic nasopharyngoscope or fiberoptic nasopharyngoscope can be used for examination, especially the pharyngeal recess and the posterior parietal wall. Early lesions were not obvious. Local congestion, erosion or rough mucosa with small nodules and granulation protrusions could be seen. Late tumors were generally grouped into nodular type (Fig. 15.11), ulcerative type (Fig. 15.12), cauliflower type and submucosal type (Fig. 15.13).

2. Pathological Examination

   Squamous cell carcinoma is the most common type of nasopharyngeal carcinoma, accounting for more than 95%. Other types of nasopharyngeal carcinoma include adenoid cystic carcinoma, adenocarcinoma, mucoepidermoid carcinoma and malignant transformation of pleomorphic adenoma.

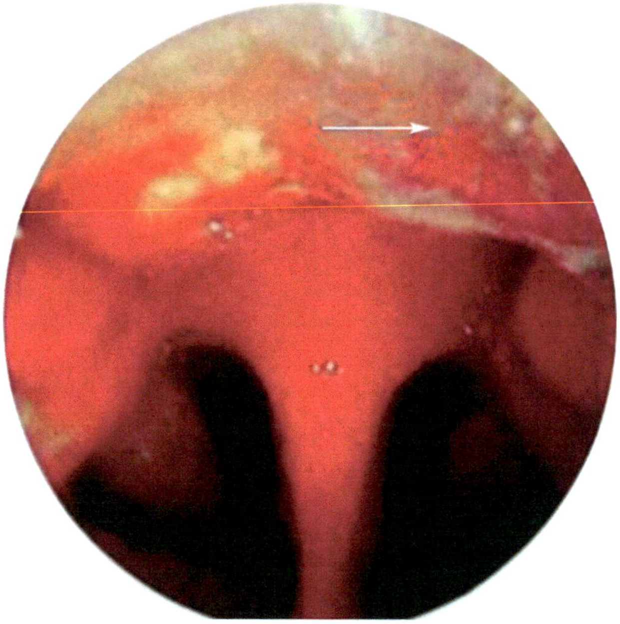

**Fig. 15.12** Ulceration type nasopharyngeal cancer (NPC)

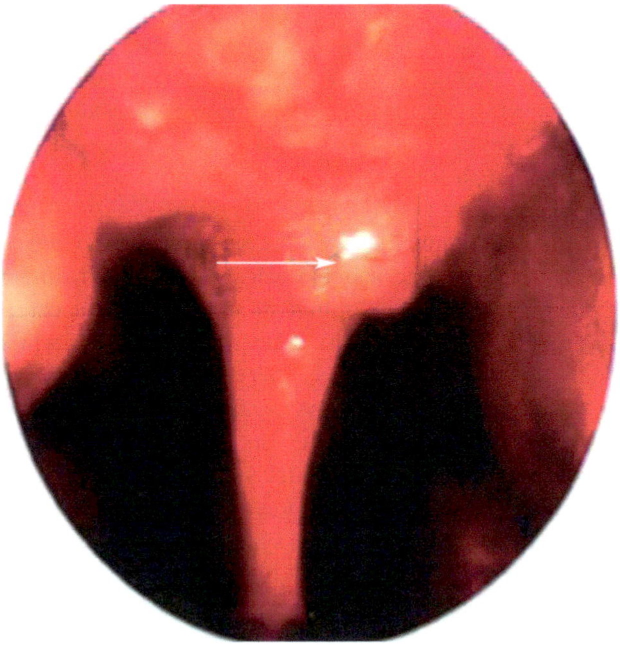

**Fig. 15.11** Nodular type nasopharygeal cancer (NPC)

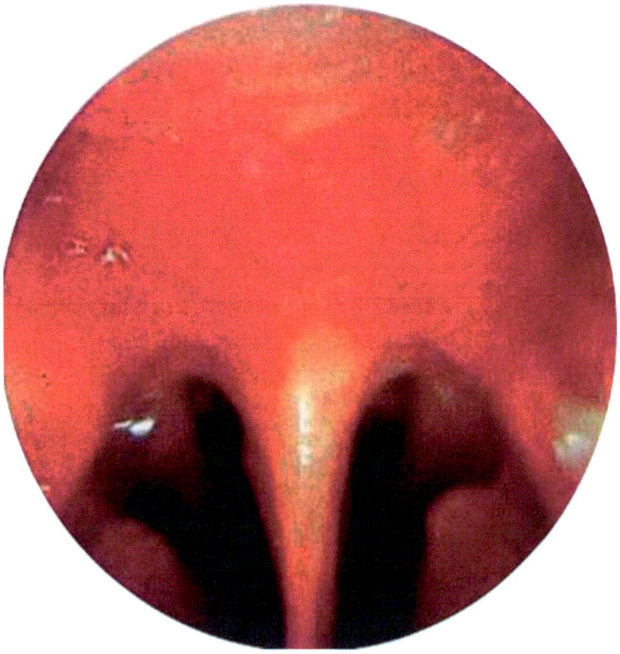

**Fig. 15.13** Submucosa nasopharygeal cancer (NPC)

(a) Biopsy

Apply the throughrhinocavum approach or the throughorocavum approach. If the biopsy is lunar, follow up diagnose to avoid omitting differentiated diagnosis.

(b) Cervical lymph node biopsy or cervical lymph node cytology puncture smear examination: cervical lymph node enlargement, and hard, should do cervical lymph node puncture smear examination. If there is no obvious suspicious lesion in the nasopharynx, lymph node puncture or excision biopsy should be considered.

(c) Cytological diagnosis of nasopharyngeal exfoliation

It is mainly used for periodic examination in the course of treatment to dynamically observe the curative effect; for recessive cancer, samples can be taken from different parts for examination.

(d) Thin needle suction cellular examination

It is very valuable for the diagnosis of metastatic nasopharyngeal carcinoma, such as cervical lymph node involvement, with the advantages of safety, simplicity, rapid and reliable results.

3. Imaging

(a) CT Scan

Nasopharyngeal carcinoma most often occurs in pharyngeal recess and parietal posterior wall, and then invades bilateral wall, parapharyngeal, nasal cavity, and oropharynx and skull base. The nasopharynx shows a mass (Fig. 15.14), involving the above sites. CT diagnosis is not difficult. When the nasopharyngeal mass is small and limited, only one side of the pharyngeal recess becomes shallow or two sides are slightly asymmetrical. CT diagnosis is difficult (Fig. 15.15). Enhanced scanning can be used to improve the display rate of the tumor. If clinical biopsy can confirm, CT examination is helpful for staging. If repeated biopsy fails to confirm, only two sides of the pharyngeal recess are asymmetrical, CT diagnosis is difficult. MRI showed that the range of tumors was better than CT.

(b) MRI

MRI examination can determine the location and extent of the tumor and the invasion of adjacent structures. For recurrent nasopharyngeal carcinoma after radiotherapy, tissue fibrosis and recurrent tumors after radiotherapy can be differentiated. Recurrent tumors are usually irregular mass, accompanied by invasion of adjacent bone and/or soft tissue structures and enlargement of lymph nodes (Fig. 15.16). Fibrosis after radiotherapy is locally thickened in massive or localized irregular patchy structure, and the boundary between fibrosis and adjacent tissues is

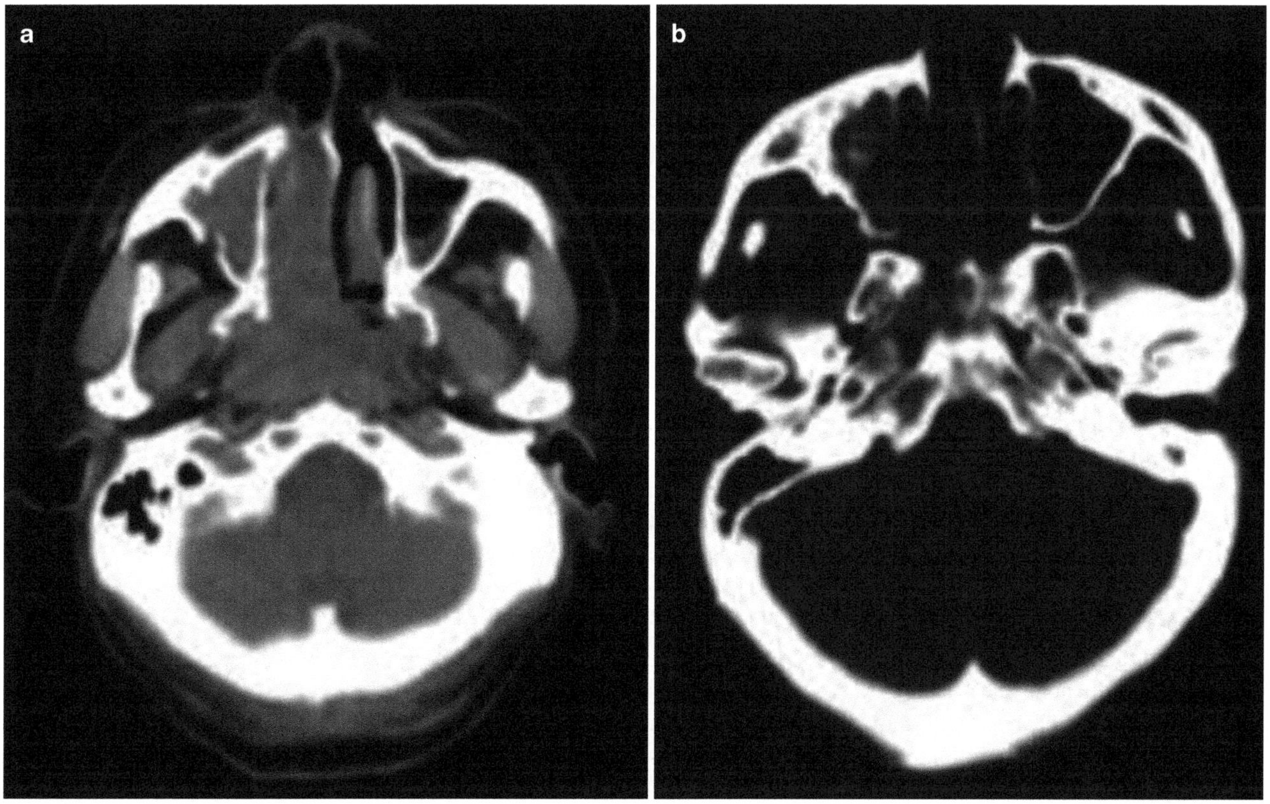


**Fig. 15.14** Late stage rhinopharyngeal cancer plane CT scan. (**a**) Soft tissue fenestra, soft tissue lump filled rhinopharynx and invades to the right rhinocavum, combined bilateral maxillary sinusitis. (**b**) bone fenestra displays the cranial base damage

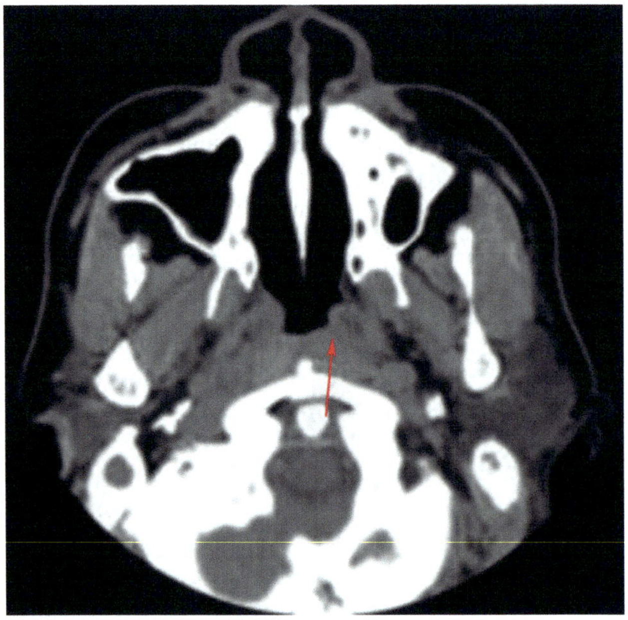

**Fig. 15.15** Early rhinopharyngeal cancer CT displayment. Only thickened mucosa (arrow), tumor boundary is unclearer than under MRI

not clear. On T1-weighted images, recurrent tumors and fibrous tissues showed low signal intensity; on T2-weighted images, recurrent tumors showed high signal intensity, while fibrous tissues showed low signal intensity.

(c) PET CT (Fig. 15.17)

4. EB virus Serological Test (EBVST)

   Serological examination of dynamic EB virus can be used as an index for diagnosis and judgment of recurrence of nasopharyngeal carcinoma after treatment. At present, many kinds of EB virus serological tests have been carried out in clinic, such as the detection of EB virus shell antigen, EB virus specific DNA enzyme and other antibodies.

5. TNM staging method proposed by the International Anti-Cancer Alliance

   (a) Primary (T) Gradings

   Tis carcinoma in situ; T0 without primary cancer; T1 tumor limited to nasopharynx or involved oropharynx or nasal cavity; T2 invaded parapharyngeal space, T3 skull base bone and/or nasal sinus, T4 tumor invaded intracranial, cerebral nerve, hypopharynx, orbital, infratemporal fossa/masticatory muscle space.

   (b) Lymphatic Metastasis (N) Gradings:

   Lymph node metastasis (N) stages: N0 without cervical lymph node metastasis; N1 supraclavicular fossa above unilateral lymph node metastasis, unilateral or bilateral retropharyngeal lymph node metastasis, lymph node maximum diameter <6 cm; N2 supraclavicular fossa above bilateral lymph node metastasis, lymph node maximum diameter <6 cm; N3a lymph node maximum diameter >6 cm; N3b supraclavicular fossa lymph node metastasis.

   (c) Distant metastasis (M) stage: M0 had no distant metastasis; M1 had distant metastasis.

Annex: clinic gradings
Stage I: $T_1N_0M_0$
Stage II: $T_1N_1M_0$, $T_2N_{0-1}M_0$
Stage III: $T_{1-2}N_2M_0$, $T_3N_{0-2}M_0$
Stage IVa: $T_4N_{0-2}M_0$
Stage IVb: any T, $N_3$
Stage IVc: any T, any N, $M_1$

**Treatment**

1. Radiotherapy

   Because most nasopharyngeal carcinoma belongs to non-keratinizing squamous cell carcinoma and is sensitive to radiotherapy, radiotherapy is the first choice in the treatment of nasopharyngeal carcinoma. Conventional in vitro high-energy radiation therapy, such as 60 Co or linear accelerator high-energy radiation therapies, is commonly used. Tissues sensitive to radiotherapy should be protected during radiotherapy. Nasopharyngeal primary lesions are mainly bilateral anterior auricular field. If nasal cavity and Paranasopharyngeal space are involved, the anterior nasal field can be illuminated. If the orbit is involved, the supraorbital field or infraorbital field can be illuminated. Lead film should be used to protect the eyes, so as not to cause radioactive cataract. The radiation range of the neck depends on the pathological changes of the lymph nodes. For those who do not touch the cervical lymph nodes, prophylactic radiation is often done on both sides of the upper cervical region. If there is cervical lymph node metastasis, prophylactic radiation is often done on the drainage area below the metastasis besides the radiation metastasis.

   (a) Continuous radiotherapy

   5 times a week, 200 cGy each time, total TD6000-7000 cGy/6–7 weeks.

   (b) Segmented radiotherapy

   Radiotherapy is generally divided into two stages, five times a week, 200 cGy each time, each stage for about 3.5 weeks. The total dose of TD6500-7000 cGy was rested for 4 weeks.

2. Drug Therapy

   It's an adjuvant therapy mainly used in middle or late stage patients or those who have not been controlled or relapsed after radiotherapy. There are three commonly used ways of administration.

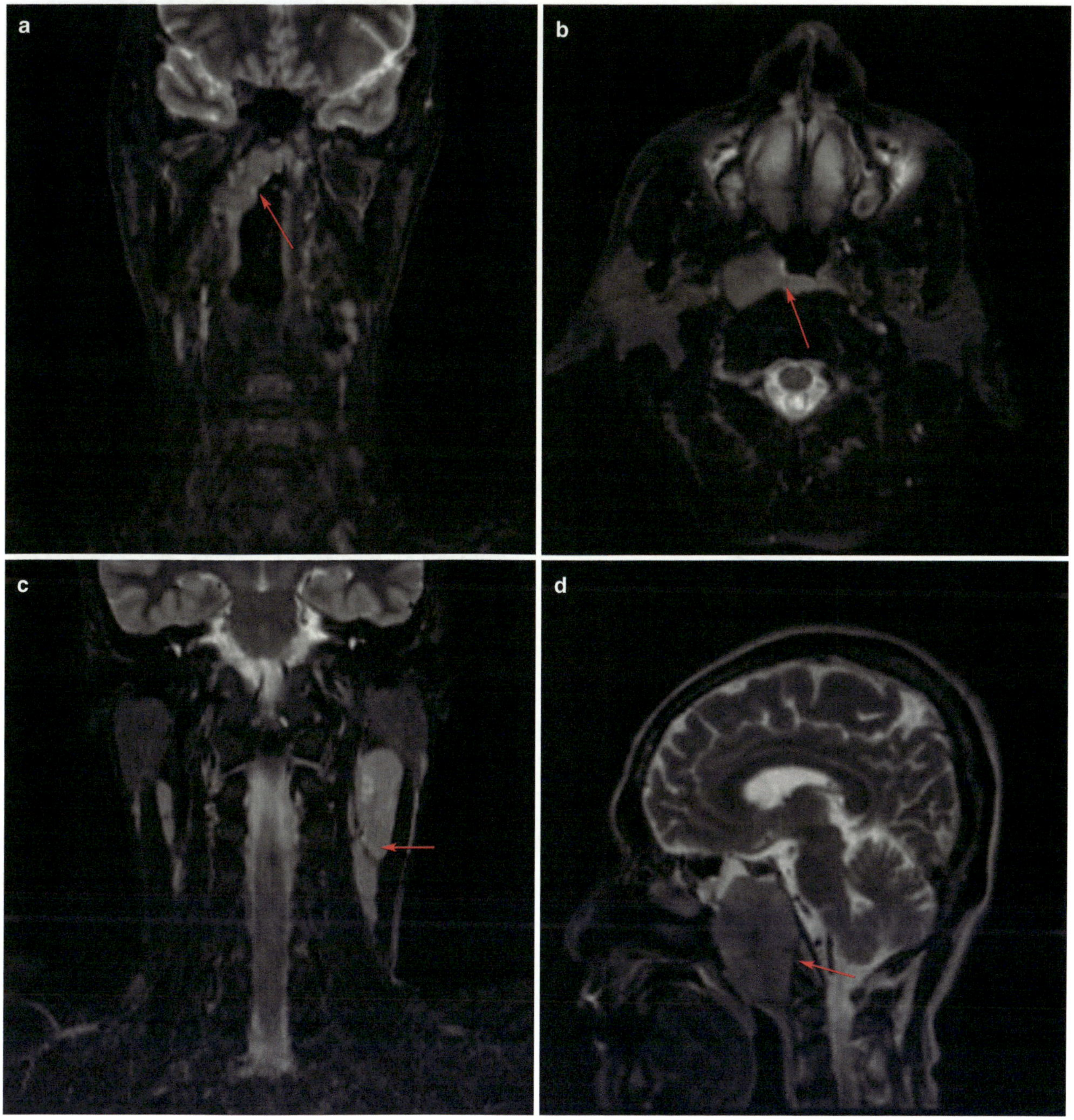


**Fig. 15.16** MRI T2WI imaging. (**a**, **b**) are from the same patient, whose coronary site and axial site imaging, display the thickened nasopharyngeal right superior wall mucosa (arrow) with clear boundary; (**c**) coronary imaging display the multiple left cervical lymph node swellings metastasis(arrow); (**d**) Sagittal imaging displays that the nasopharyngeal tumor invades the cephalic base bone (arrow)

(a) Systemic Chemical Treatment

Oral, intramuscular and intravenous injection. Common medicines are nitrogen mustard, cyclophosphamide, fluorouracil, bleomycin and cetipel. It can be used alone or in combination.

(b) Half Chemical Treatment

It is the treatment of pressing the abdominal aorta, temporarily blocking the blood circulation of the lower part of the body, and injecting nitrogen mustard rapidly from the veins of the upper limbs.

Contraindications to hemispheric chemotherapy: Hypertension, heart disease; elderly, weak, obese; superior vena cava compression; cirrhosis, large liver; severe impairment of liver and kidney function; white blood cell count less than $3 \times 10^9$/L.

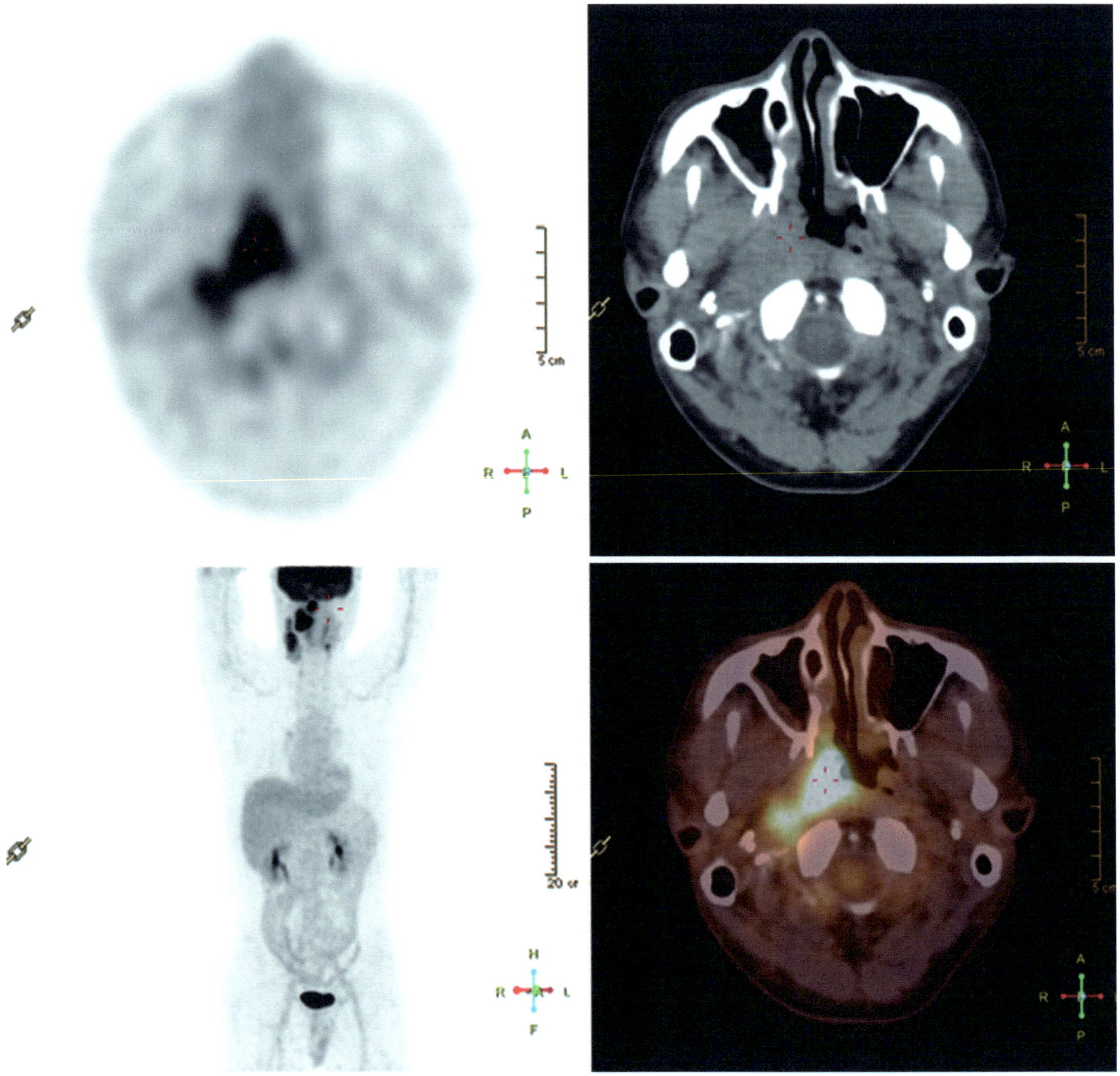


**Fig. 15.17** PET CT imaging displays nasopharyngocancer. It can be seen that the right nasopharyngeal wall is obviously thicker and the mass of FDG metabolism is increased. Considering nasopharyngeal carcinoma, the lesion invades the petrous part of the temporal bone, adjacent to the sphenoid bone and above the tonsil, and invades the tensor palatini muscle, sphenoid sinus, medial and lateral pterygoid plate, medial pterygoid muscle, posterior involvement of the right clivus; multiple lymph nodes in the parapharyngeal space, right mandible, right neck and right supraclavicular fossa. Increased FDG metabolism with lymph node metastasis

(c) Arterial intubation chemotherapy:

Can increase nasopharyngeal drug concentration, reduce systemic side effects. Superficial temporal artery or facial artery retrograde intubation was used to inject anticancer drugs. For early stage (stage I and II), including a single small case of lymph node metastasis in upper cervical deep group, late cases of brain nerve involvement, or cases of nasopharyngeal residual or recurrence after radiotherapy, all have a certain short-term effect. Commonly used anticancer drugs are fluorouracil, pingyangmycin, cisplatin and so on.

3. Induced Chemical Therapy (ICT)

Also known as adjuvant chemotherapy refers to the chemical therapy used before radiotherapy, which can reduce the load of tumors in a short period of time, alleviate various clinical symptoms caused by tumors, improve blood supply and enhance radiosensitivity. Induction chemotherapy of nasopharyngeal carcinoma is mostly used in locally advanced nasopharyngeal carcinoma or in patients with large cervical metastatic lymph nodes. The most commonly used drug is cisplatin plus fluorouracil.

4. Simultaneous Radiochemical Therapy
   Synchronized radiochemical therapy (SRT) is a combination of low dose chemotherapy and radiotherapy for tumors, especially for nasopharyngeal carcinoma, especially for advanced nasopharyngeal carcinoma, it is better to do SRT.
5. Surgery
   (a) Surgery Indications
      Non-primary treatment, only in a few cases. The indications are as follows: (1) For pathological types that are not sensitive to radiotherapy, such as adenoid cystic carcinoma, highly differentiated adenocarcinoma, highly differentiated mucoepidermoid carcinoma and malignant transformation of pleomorphic adenoma, surgery can be chosen first, followed by radiotherapy; (2) For patients with localized nasopharyngeal lesions that do not subside or recur after radiotherapy, there is no extensive bone destruction in the skull base, and the tumors do not encapsulate the cervical vascular sheath; (3) Neck The metastatic lymph nodes did not subside after 2 months of radiotherapy and showed active solitary mass. If the primary focus of nasopharynx was controlled, neck lymph node dissection was feasible.
      Surgical approaches for nasopharyngeal lesions include endoscopic resection of tumors, lateral nasal incision or nasal cone inversion, or maxillary external rotation resection. Endoscopic and transnasal resection of tumors are suitable for tumors with smaller lesions, while maxillary external rotation is suitable for larger tumors. If cervical vascular sheath is exposed during surgery, appropriate tissue coverage should be used after surgery to prevent local lesions. The wound was ruptured by infection. The covered tissue flaps included local pedicled buccal mucosal flaps, submandibular gland flaps, free forearm flaps, medial leg flaps, etc.
   (b) Contraindication to Surgery
      Extensive destruction of skull base or extensive infiltration near nasopharynx, brain nerve damage or distant metastasis; poor general condition or liver and kidney dysfunction; other surgical contraindications with poor general condition.

### 15.5.3 ParaPharyngeal Space Tumor

**Etiology**

The parapharyngeal space is located below the skull base, on both sides of the nasopharynx and oropharynx, and on the medial side of the mandible. It is a potential space. There are cervical vascular sheaths and brain nerves passing through the parapharyngeal space. The common tumors in parapharyngeal space are pleomorphic adenoma and schwannoma. The other relatively rare tumors are paraganglioma, liposarcoma, rhabdomyosarcoma and chondrosarcoma.

**Clinical Manifestation**

1. Symptoms
   Parapharyngeal space tumors with small symptoms usually have no special symptoms. Most of them are found by chance by imaging examination. When the tumors increase to a certain extent, local space-occupying compression symptoms or nerve compression symptoms occur (Fig. 15.18).
   (a) Dysphagia and dyspnea
      Tumors cause a swelling of the tonsils on one side. Tonsillectomy is often misdiagnosed as enlarged tonsils. After tonsillectomy, local swelling is still found. Imaging examinations are performed to diagnose parapharyngeal tumors. Patients may have swallowing discomfort or dysphagia. Obstructive sleep apnea syndrome may occur when the tumors increase to a certain extent.
   (b) Symptoms of cranial nerve compression
      Tumors can oppress the glossopharyngeal, vagus and hypoglossal nerves, resulting in soft palate paralysis, tongue muscle paralysis or vocal cord paralysis on one side leading to unfavorable swallowing, ambiguous language, hoarseness, swallowing and coughing.
2. Physical Signs
   (a) Unilateral tonsil or soft palate apophysis
      One side of tonsil or soft palate protrusion: smooth surface mucosa, tough texture, poor mobility.
   (b) If there are symptoms of cerebral palsy in the posterior group, there may be poor mobility of the ipsilateral soft palate, deviation of the extension of the tongue to the opposite side, fixation of the ipsilateral vocal cords, etc.

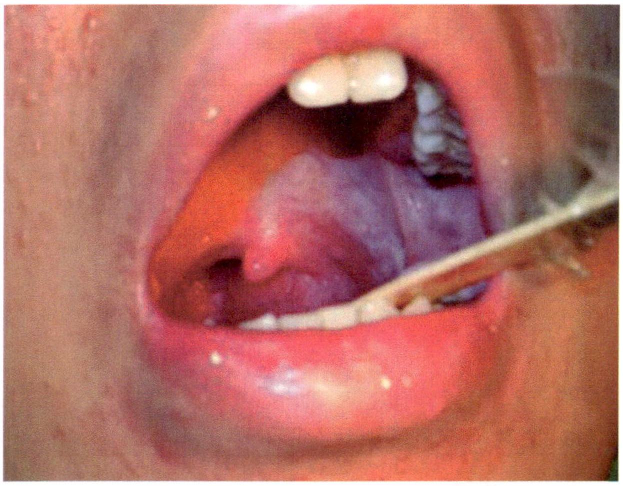

**Fig. 15.18** Lingual view of left parapharyngeal neruovagina tumor. Left infra soft tissue pharyngeal lateral apophysis could be seen

**Diagnosis**

1. CT Scan

   CT examination showed moderate density soft tissue mass in the parapharyngeal space. The lateral pharyngeal wall moved inward, the pharyngeal cavity narrowed, the boundary was clear, the tumor texture could be uneven, and the displacement of the carotid sheath was often seen under enhancement (Fig. 15.19).

2. MRI

   The soft tissue image of T1 and T2 in parapharyngeal space was clearly defined on MRI. The center may have an uneven signal. The relationship between the margin of the tumor and the surrounding tissues on MRI was better than that on CT (Fig. 15.20).

**Treatment**

Surgical treatment is the main method for benign tumors in parapharyngeal space. Surgical approaches include aperture, submandibular approach, combined neck-parotid approach, mandibular external rotation approach and maxillary external rotation approach. The size, location and origin of the tumors should be determined. The neck approach is generally preferred. If the neck approach is difficult to resect, the incision can be extended to the neck. The combined parotid approach can also remove tumors reaching the skull base.

Parapharyngeal space paraganglioma, because it encloses the carotid sheath, often requires mandibular external rotation approach resection, but also ready to resect the internal carotid artery.

Malignant tumors are usually treated by chemotherapy, radiotherapy or surgery according to their pathological types.

IV. Laryngopharyngeal Malignants

Laryngopharyngeal malignant tumors, also known as hypopharyngeal cancer, occur in the mucosal epithelium of the laryngopharynx, which is rare. The incidence of malignant tumors is about 16% in males and 6% in females. Because of the concealed location and less early symptoms, most of the visits belong to the middle and late stages. The prognosis is poor.

### 15.5.4 Hypopharyngeal Carcinoma

Hypopharyngeal carcinoma is called subpharyngeal cancer, locating on the hypopharyngeal mucosal epithelium and rarely seen. Its attack incidence occupies 16% of male cervicocranial cancers and about 6% of the females. It conceals, so there are less symptoms at early stage, the patients often come and check at mid-late stage and prognoses badly.

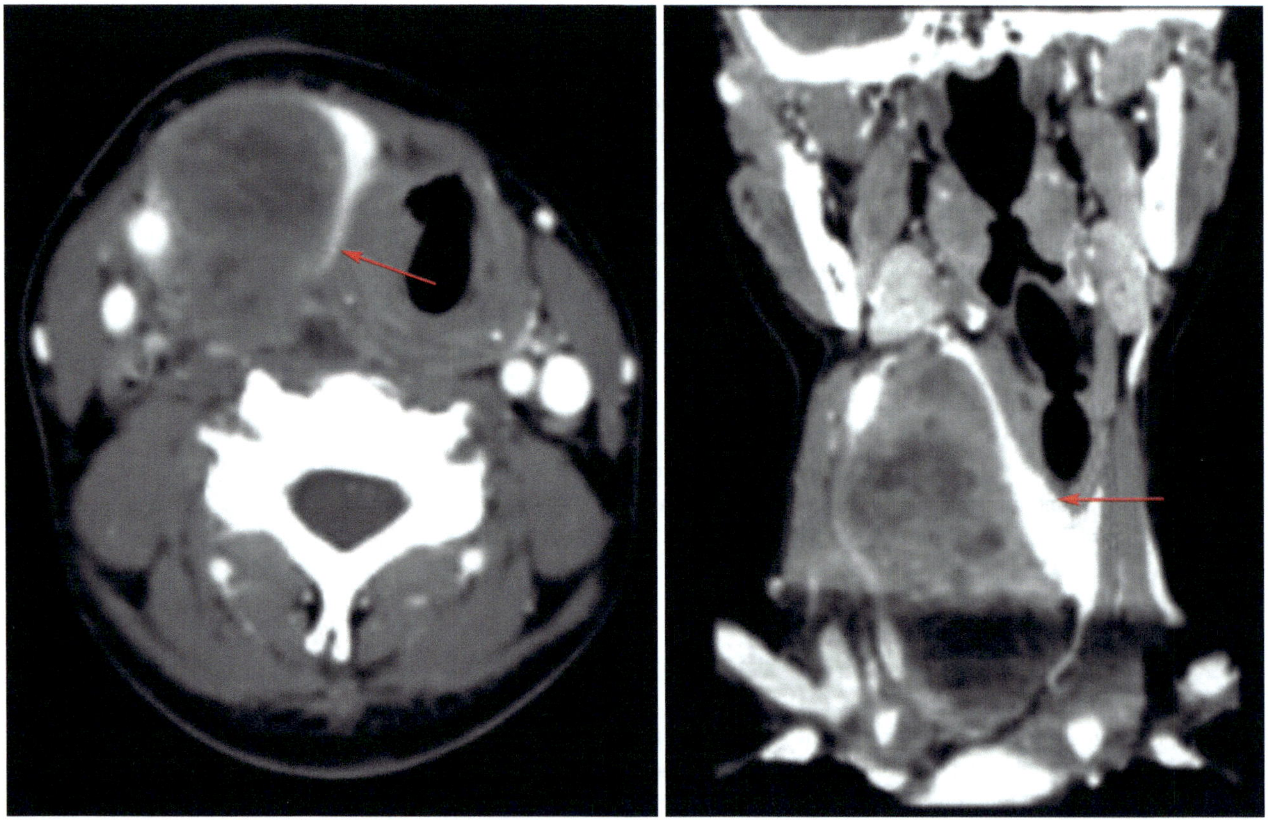

**Fig. 15.19** Enhanced CT axial scan + coronary reconstruction. The right parapharyngeal space has a huge irregular mass, and the high-density thyroid gland is compressed and moved inward (arrow point). Pathological findings showed malignant schwannoma

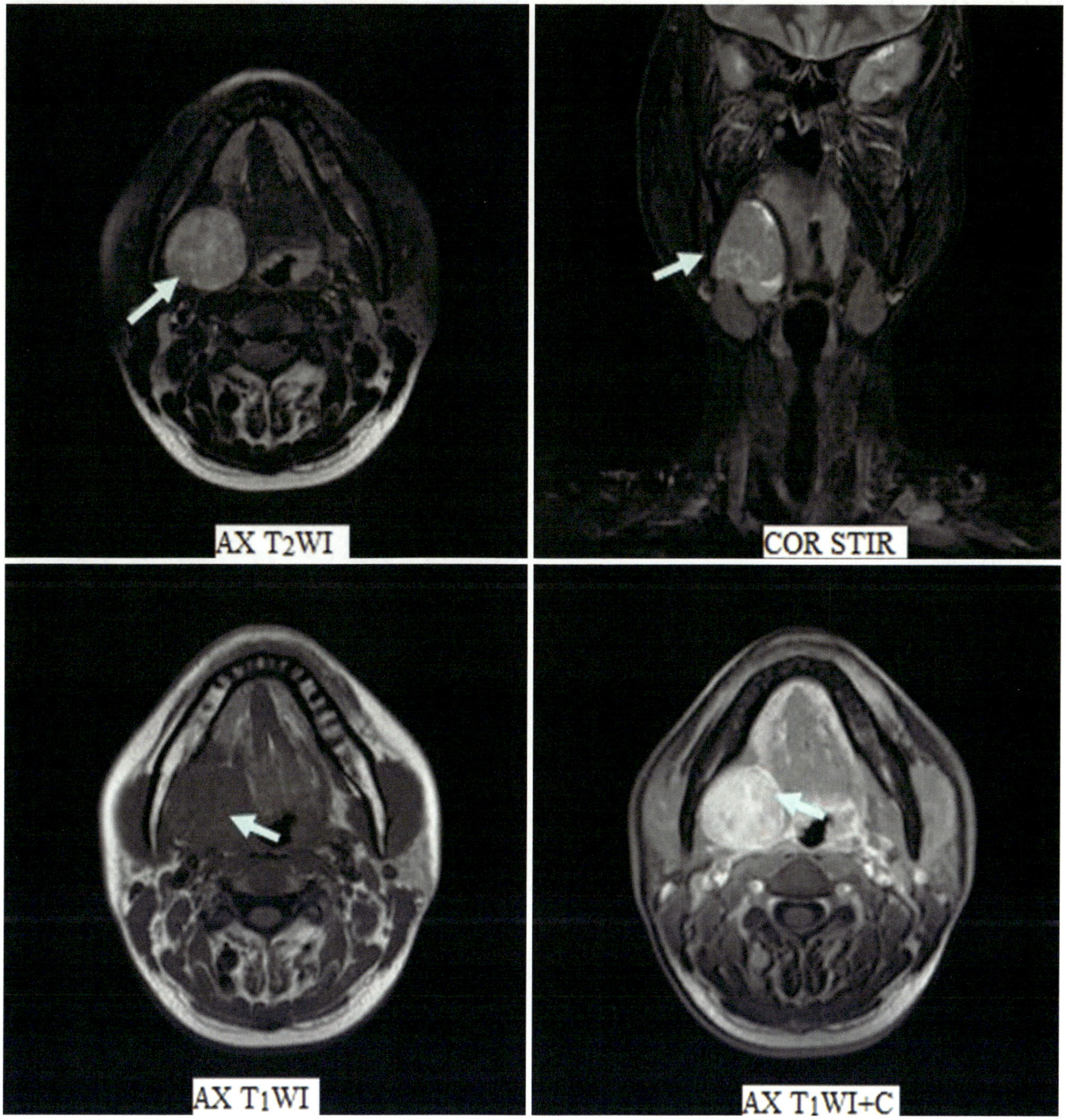


**Fig. 15.20** Axial and Coronary STIR $T_2$WI, axial $T_1$WI plane scan and enhanced MRI examination. Right parapharyngeal space round mass (arrow), with slightly higher heterogeneous signal on T2. T1 showed iso-signal and enhanced obviously after enhancement. The pathological findings were mixed tumors

**Etiology**

The etiology is unknown, which may be related to human papillomavirus (HPV) infection in pharynx, trace element deficiency, excessive tobacco and alcohol, and genetic factors. The incidence of esophageal cancer in males is higher than that in females; 20–25% of patients are complicated with middle and lower esophageal cancer.

**Pathogenesis**

Hypopharyngeal cancer generally originates from the mucosal epithelium of the hypopharynx, and squamous cell carcinoma is common, accounting for more than 98%. The degree of differentiation was more moderate or low. The degree of malignancy is higher than that of laryngeal cancer.

**Division of Hypopharynx**

1. The piriform recess is the area between arytenoid epiglottic fold, pharyngeal epiglottic fold and lateral wall of laryngopharynx.
2. The superior hypopharyngeal region is from the base of the tongue to the lateral wall of the epiglottis.
3. The posterior wall of the laryngopharynx rises from the tongue root plane to the posterior wall of the esophagus.
4. The area above the level of the esophageal entrance after the cricoid cartilage in the posterior ring area.

**Clinical Manifestation**

1. Clinic Symptoms
   (a) Foreign body sensation in pharynx
   Foreign body sensation in pharynx: foreign body sensation in pharynx is the most common and earliest symptom, which disappears when eating.
   (b) Odynophagia
   Unknown odynophagia can be radiated to the ipsilateral ear.
   (c) Dysphasia
   Dysphagia may occur when the tumors are large, and the symptoms are obvious when solid food is swallowed.
   (d) Voice Hoarseness
   When tumors involve the larynx, hoarseness can be caused by arytenoid epiglottic fold tumors and vocal cord fixation.
   (e) Cough or Bloody Snot
   Tumor stimulation of the larynx can cause cough, and tumour ulceration can cause blood in sputum.
   (f) Dyspnea
   Tumors involving the laryngeal cavity cause glottic stenosis, leading to dyspnea.
   (g) Distant Metastasis Symptoms
   Those with distant metastasis such as lung and bone may have symptoms such as cough and bone pain.
2. Physical Signs
   (a) Hypopharyngeal Neoplasm
   Cauliflower-like, globular or ulcerative neoplasms can be seen in the hypopharynx (Fig. 15.21).
   (b) Hemilaryngeal Fixation
   The tumors invade the paralaryngeal space or involve the recurrent laryngeal nerve, which can lead to hemilaryngeal fixation.
   (c) Increased Hypopharyngeal Secretions
   Saliva may accumulate in the hypopharynx when the tumors involve the esophageal entrance.
   (d) Neck Mass
   There are usually swollen lymph nodes below and behind the submandibular gland in the neck. Some patients can see a doctor for cervical mass, and even the swollen lymph nodes in the neck are metastatic squamous cell carcinoma. Only after further examination of the primary lesion can laryngopharyngeal cancer be found. Swollen lymph nodes often have a history of several weeks, no obvious pain, rapid growth, antibiotic treatment is ineffective.

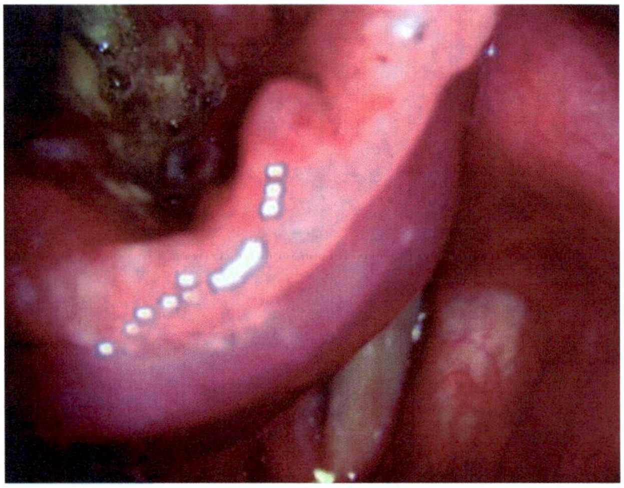

**Fig. 15.21** Right piriform recess cancer larynoscopy imaging. Cauliflower tumor constituted by the central ulceration

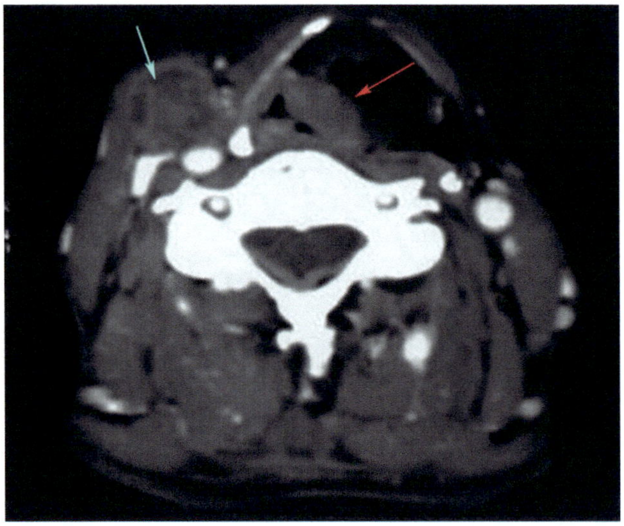

**Fig. 15.22** Laryngoscopic view of right pyriform recess cancer. Right pyriform recess carcinoma (red arrow) with ipsilateral level is visible. Lymph node metastasis in zone 3 (blue arrow)

3. Imaging
   (a) CT
   Enhanced CT examination is generally required. Soft tissue with mild to moderate enhancement in the larynx and pharynx can be seen. The boundary is not clear. It can be accompanied by enlargement of lymph nodes around the cervical vascular sheath. The enlarged lymph nodes show peripheral annular enhancement and ring-like central density reduction (Fig. 15.22), and can also be enhanced evenly (Fig. 15.23). Coronal and sagittal reconstructed images are helpful to show the anatomical relationship between tumors and surrounding tissues.

(b) MRI

Soft tissue resolution is higher than that of CT, and early invasion of laryngeal cartilage can be clearly demonstrated (Fig. 15.24). The tumors showed moderate to high signal intensity on T1WI and T2WI images, with slight to moderate enhancement after enhancement. Lymph node enlargement was also moderately high signal intensity (Fig. 15.25).

(c) PET-CT

Because of its high cost, it is generally not used as a routine means of examination. However, in patients with advanced stage, PET-CT examination is helpful to detect multiple lesions and distant metastasis. On PET-CT, laryngopharyngeal carcinoma is characterized by local hypermetabolic lesions, usually more than 6.0, accompanied by hypermetabolic lesions of local lymph nodes. Metabolic lesions less

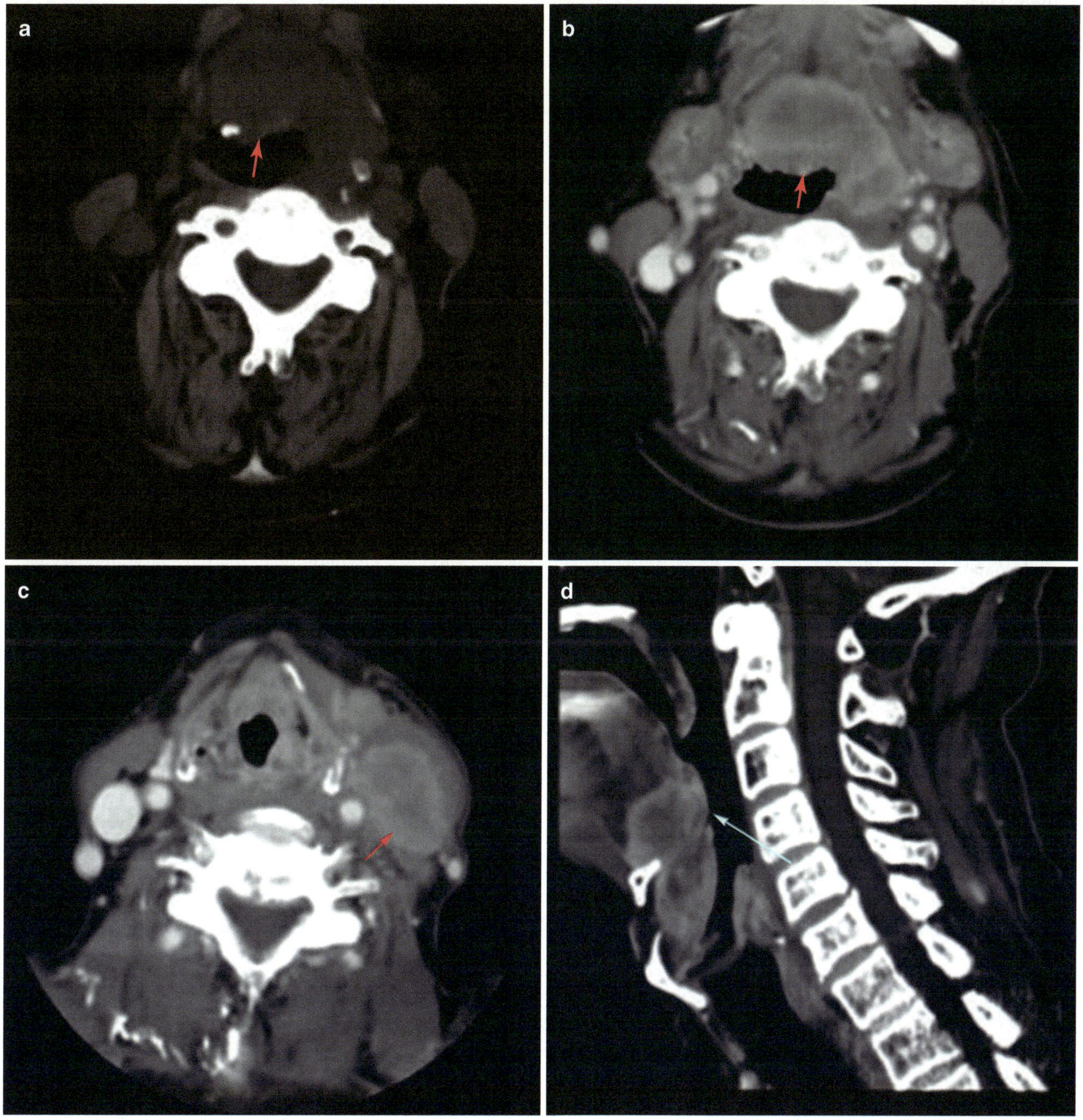


**Fig. 15.23** Oropharyngeal cancer CT scan: (**a**) Plane scanning displays the evidently thickened hypopharyngeal anterior and left wall, lesions oropharynx sites and with unclear boundary. (**b**) Obviously enhanced under enhanced scan, clear and recognizable lumps. (**c**) Simultaneous left lymphatic metastasis (red arrow); (**d**) Sagittal scan display the anterior wall lumps (blue arrow). (**d**) Coronary scan displays the large left oropharyngeal lumps (blue arrow), accompanying with lymphatic metastasis

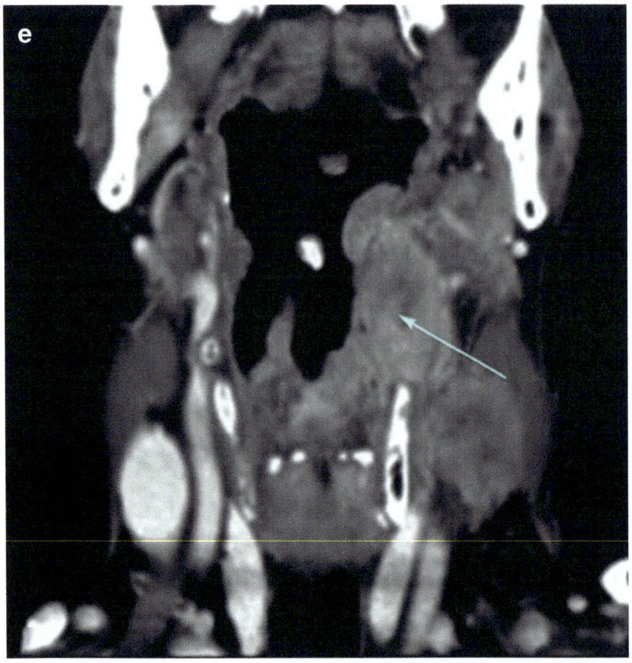


**Fig. 15.23** (continued)

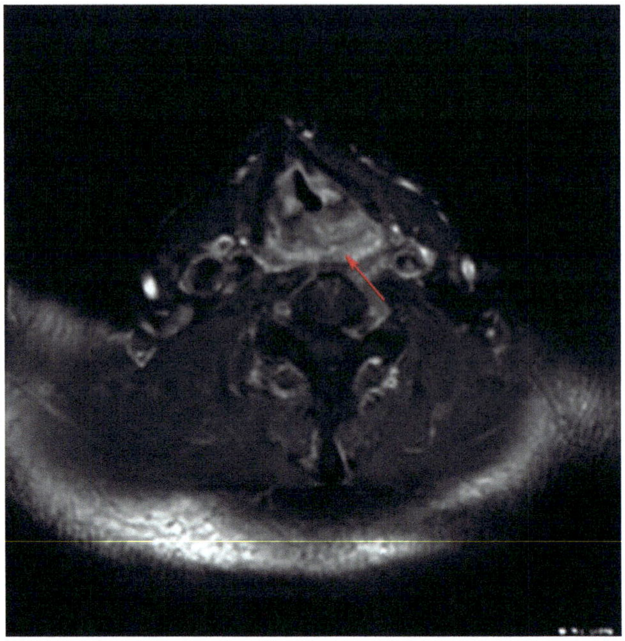

**Fig. 15.24** Oropharyng cancer MRI axial $T_1WI$ enhanced manifestation. The soft tissue mass of the pyriform recess enhanced uneven enhancement, the boundary of the soft tissue and the arytenoids cartilage was clear, the laryngeal chamber moved forward (arrow)

than 3.0 generally do not consider malignancy or change after radiotherapy (Fig. 15.26).

4. Esophagus Barium Meal Examination

   We can know the length of cervical esophagus involvement, or whether there are multiple lesions in the middle and lower esophagus. The manifestations were interruption of esophageal mucosa, local filling defect and esophageal stricture (Fig. 15.27).

5. Gastroscopy

   Electronic gastroscopy can determine the nature and extent of esophageal lesions and take pathological examination.

**Diagnosis**

According to the history and clinical examination, it is not difficult to make a correct diagnosis. Pathological examination is the final means of defining diagnosis. It is important to make correct TNM staging in the diagnosis before treatment, which is conducive to the correct choice of treatment options and the evaluation of prognosis (Table 15.2).

**Differential Diagnosis**

Laryngopharyngeal cancer should be differentiated from laryngopharyngeal papilloma, laryngopharyngeal cyst and laryngopharyngeal hemangioma.

**Treatment**

The treatment of hypopharyngeal cancer is usually combined with surgery, radiotherapy and chemical therapy.

1. Surgical Treatment
   (a) Early Lesions ($T_1$, $T_2$ lesions)

   If laryngeal function can be preserved, surgery plus post-operative radiotherapy can be selected. Surgical methods include laser excision under oral support laryngoscope, partial laryngopharyngeal excision and partial laryngopharyngeal excision. Recent oral robotic surgery has also been used in experimental applications, which can be used for partial laryngopharyngeal excision. Cervical lymph nodes require simultaneous radical or modified radical neck dissection. Radiotherapy was added after operation.

   (b) Advance lessions ($T_3$, $T_4$ lesions)

   For T3 and T4 lesions that can not be performed laryngeal function preservation surgery, surgery plus post-operative radiotherapy, total laryngectomy and partial laryngopharyngectomy, or total laryngopharyngectomy can be selected. The defect can be repaired by pectoralis major myocutaneous flap or free jejunum, free anterolateral femoral skin flap, etc. The treatment of cervical lymph nodes is the same. The lesions involving cervical esophagus can also be treated by total laryngopharyngeal esophagectomy, gastric elevation to repair cervical esophageal defect, or transverse colon, left or right colon for esophageal reconstruction. Radical radiotherapy is often needed after surgery.

**Table 15.2** Laryngeal pharynx tumor AJCC (2010 Edition) TNM staging (except for non-epithelial tumor, such as a tumor of lymphatic tissue, soft tissue, bone, and cartilage)

| | | |
|---|---|---|
| Primary tumor (T) | | |
| $T_x$ | | Primary tumor cannot be evaluated |
| $T_0$ | | Evidence of no primary tumor |
| $T_{is}$ | | carcinoma in situ |
| laryngopharynx | $T_1$ | The tumor was confined to a sub region of laryngopharyngeal anatomy and the maximum diameter of less than 2 cm |
| | $T_2$ | The invasion of more than one sub area or the adjacent anatomical dissection of hypopharyngeal area, or 2 cm < measurement of tumor diameter less than 4 cm, no fixed hemilarynx |
| | $T_3$ | Maximum diameter of the tumor >4 cm or half larynx or invasion of the esophagus |
| | $T_{4a}$ | Middle late local disease<br>Tumor invasion of thyroid/cricoid cartilage, hyoid and thyroid or central soft tissue |
| | $T_{4b}$ | Very late local disease<br>A tumor invades the anterior fascia of the vertebral body, encircles the carotid artery, or involves the mediastinal structure |
| * * Note: Central soft tissue including prelaryngeal muscle strip and subcutaneous fat | | |
| Regional lymph node (N) | | |
| laryngopharyx | $N_x$ | Regional lymph node failure assessment |
| | $N_0$ | Regional lymph node metastases |
| | $N_1$ | With a single lateral lymph node metastasis, the maximum diameter of less than 3 cm |
| | $N_2$ | With a single lateral lymph node metastasis, 3 cm < maximum diameter less than or equal to 6 cm; or the ipsilateral multiple lymph node metastasis, the maximum diameter of less than 6 cm; or bilateral or contralateral lymph node metastasis, the maximum diameter of less than 6 cm |
| | $N_{2a}$ | With a single lateral lymph node metastasis, 3 cm < maximum diameter of less than 6 cm |
| | $N_{2b}$ | The ipsilateral multiple lymph node metastasis, the maximum diameter of less than 6 cm |
| | $N_{2c}$ | Bilateral or contralateral lymph node metastasis, the maximum diameter of less than 6 cm |
| | $N_3$ | Maximum diameter of metastatic lymph nodes >6 cm |
| * Note: VII transfer is also considered the regional lymph node metastasis | | |
| Distant metastasis (M) | | |
| $M_0$ | | No distant metastasis |
| $M_1$ | | distant metastasis |
| Anatomic staging / prognosis group: | | |
| pharyngolarynx | Phase 0 | $T_{is}N_0$ $M_0$ |
| | Phase I | $T_1N_0M_0$ |
| | Phase II | $T_2N_0M_0$ |
| | Phase III | $T_3N_0M_0$,$T_1N_1M_0$,$T_2N_1M_0$,$T_3N_1M_0$ |
| | Phase IVA | $T_4N_0M_0$,$T_{4a}N_1M_0$,$T_1N_2M_0$,$T_2N_2M_0$,$T_3N_2M_0$,$T_{4a}N_2M_0$ |
| | Phase IVB | $T_{4b}$ any $NM_0$; any $TN_3M_0$ |
| | Phase IVC | Any T any$NM_1$ |
| Histology classification (G) | | |

$G_x$ Level cannot be evaluated, $G_1$ Highly differentiated, $G_2$ Differentiation, $G_3$ Low differentiation, $G_4$ Undifferentiated

2. Radiation Therapy:

   Radiotherapy alone for laryngopharyngeal cancer is less effective than surgery combined with radiotherapy. Pathological examination showed that patients with HPV positive tumors were more sensitive to radiotherapy. Radiotherapy can be used in combination with surgery before or after operation. For patients with strong desire to retain laryngeal function, concurrent radiochemical therapy can also be used. The curative effect of concurrent radiochemical therapy is better than that of simple radiotherapy. However, compared with the comprehensive treatment of surgery and radiotherapy, there is no clear conclusion on the advantages and disadvantages of concurrent radiochemical therapy for retaining laryngeal function. Paclitaxel, cisplatin and fluorouracil can be used as alternative chemotherapeutics for synchronous

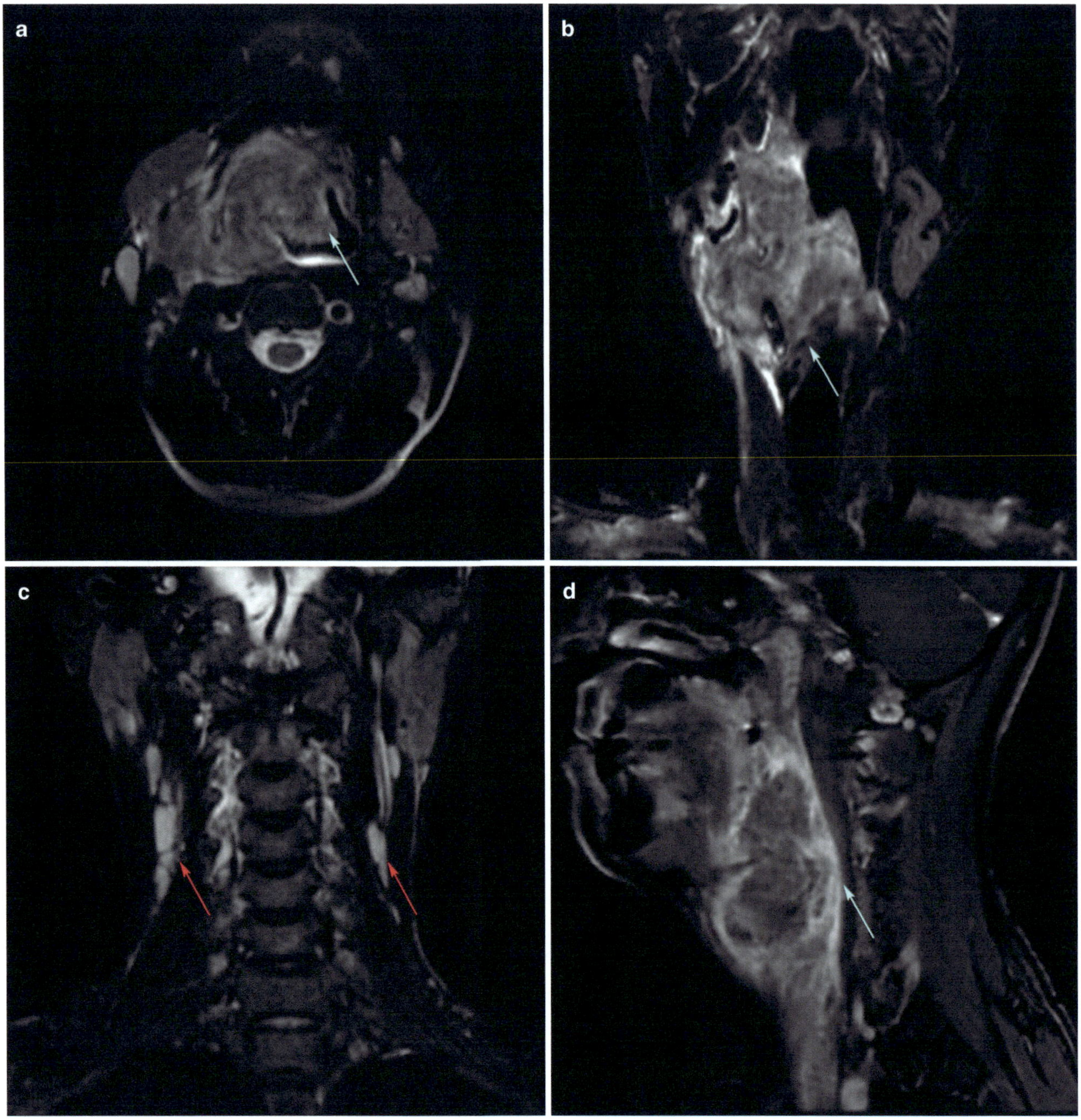


**Fig. 15.25** MRI axial and coronary $T_2$WI plain scan, sagittal $T_1$WI enhancement. (**a**, **b**) clearly showed a large irregular mass in the right pharynx, and the coronal position of the soft tissue of the parapharyngeal neck (blue arrow). (**c**) coronary scan says bilateral cervical multi-attacked elongated lymph nodes. (**d**) sagittal position of the multiple enlarged lymph nodes (red arrow) in the bilateral neck shows the relationship between the tumor and the blood vessels in the neck

radiotherapy. They can be used in combination with paclitaxel or cisplatin (or carboplatin) alone and in synchronization with radiotherapy.

3. Chemical Treatment: Chemotherapy alone has limited therapeutic effect on laryngopharyngeal cancer. It can be used in combination with radiotherapy. It can also be combined with induction chemotherapy-radiotherapy or induction chemotherapy-surgery-radiotherapy. For lesions with laryngeal function that can not be preserved in late stage surgery, induction chemotherapy can be used for 2–3 cycles, and then the curative effect can be evaluated. If the primary lesion reaches CR or PR, non-surgical radiotherapy or synchronous radiochemical therapy can be selected. If CR or PR is not achieved, surgical resection and post-operative radiotherapy can be selected. This scheme helps to preserve laryngeal function to the maximum extent while ensuring survival rate.
4. Biological Treatment: The main bio-therapeutic drugs for laryngopharyngeal cancer are monoclonal antibodies

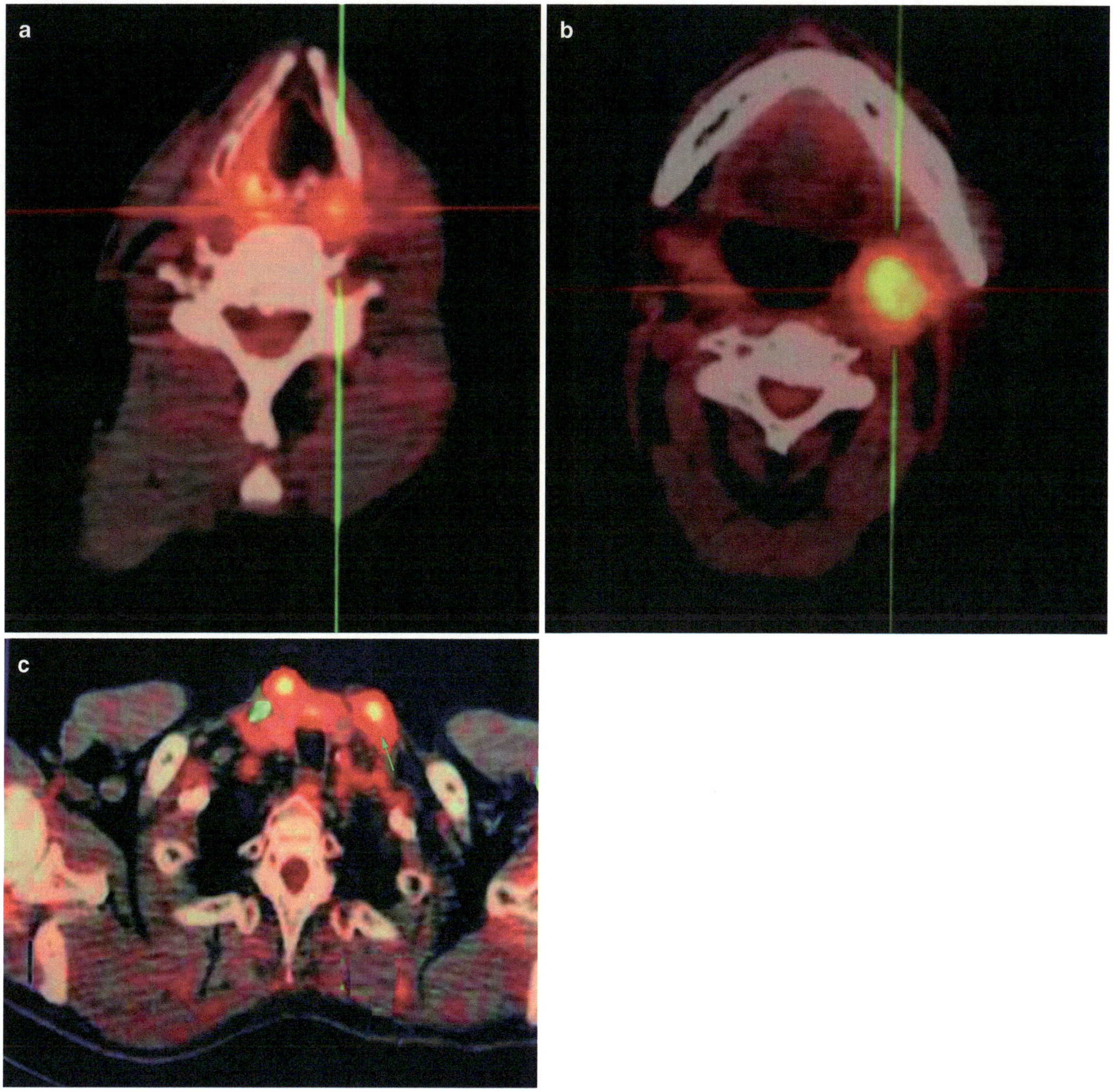


**Fig. 15.26** PET CT displays left lateral piriform recess cancer. (**a**) Plane left piriform recess glottis showed high metabolic shadow. (**b**) At the same case, the left 2 lymph node metastasis, high metabolic lesion. (**c**) High active mass in the paraplastic para space of the pharynx and multiple lymph node metastases in the supra clavicular fossa (arrow)

against epidermal growth factor and anti-angiogenesis antibodies. These drugs alone have limited efficacy and are generally combined with radiotherapy or chemotherapy. HPV16 and 18 vaccines have been widely used in Europe, and China has approved them since July 2016.

**Prognosis**

The overall prognosis of laryngopharyngeal cancer is worse than that of laryngeal cancer. The 5-year survival rate was about 40%. The 5-year survival rate of early and middle stage lesions (clinical stage 1 and 2) was about 50%. The 5-year survival rate of middle and late stage lesions (clinical stage 3 and 4) was only 20–30%.

## 15.6 Obstructive Sleep Apnea Hypopnea Syndrome

Obstructive sleep apnea hypopnea syndrome (OSAHS) refers to the frequent collapse of the upper airway during sleep, resulting in apnea and insufficient ventilation, frequent decline in oxygen saturation, accompanied by snoring, disordered

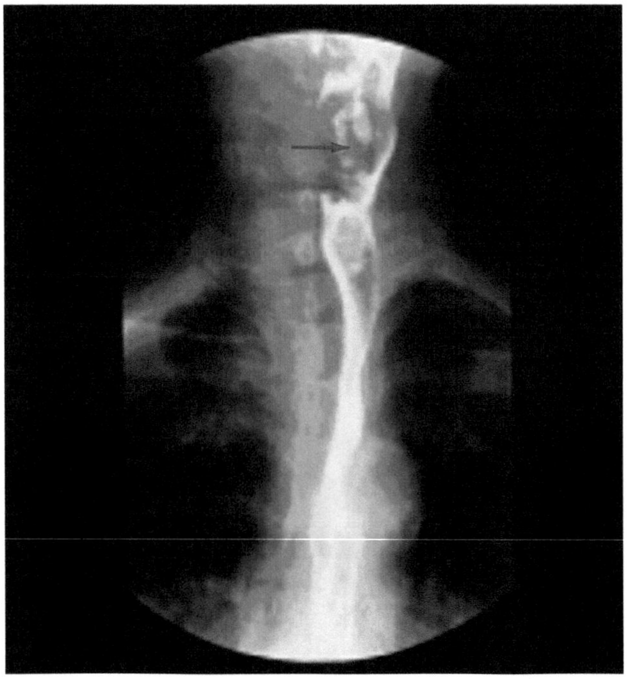

**Fig. 15.27** Esophageal barium meal inspection result says that the laryngopharyngocancer has lesioned the upper esophageal segment (arrow)

sleep structure, daytime sleepiness and so on. OSAHS is the most common form of sleep apnea. The incidence of OSAHS reported abroad ranges from 2 to 5%. OSAHS not only seriously affects the quality of life and work efficiency of patients, but also easily complicates with cardiovascular and cerebrovascular diseases. OSAHS is considered as the source of many diseases, and is receiving more and more attention.

## Etiology

1. Abnormal anatomy of upper airway leads to airway stenosis.
   (a) Nasal cavity and nasopharyngeal stenosis: including all possible causes of nasal cavity and nasopharyngeal stenosis, such as deviation of nasal septum, nasal polyps, chronic rhinosinusitis, turbinate hypertrophy, adenoid hypertrophy, etc.
   (b) Oral and pharyngeal cavity stenosis: hypertrophy of palatal tonsil, hypertrophy of soft palate, elongated uvula, hypertrophy of lateral pharyngeal wall, hypertrophy of lingual root, etc.
   (c) Laryngeal cavity stenosis: infantile epiglottis, epiglottic tissue collapse (such as laryngomalacia), etc., but relatively rare.

   Upper and mandibular dysplasia and malformation are also common and important causes of OSAHS.

2. Central Respiratory Regulation Function Abnormalities

   The main manifestations of abnormal regulation function of respiratory center are lower respiratory driving force during sleep and higher threshold of response to high CO 2, high H+ and low O 2. The abnormality of this function may be primary or secondary to hypoxic hematologic symptoms caused by long-term sleep apnea and/or hypoventilation.

3. Upper Respiratory Tract Dilator Muscle Strength Abnormity

   The abnormal muscle strength of upper airway dilator is mainly manifested in the abnormal tension of genioglossus, pharyngeal lateral wall and soft palate muscles. The decrease of muscle tension of upper airway dilator is an important cause of repeated airway collapse in OSAHS patients. The tension of pharyngeal muscles decreases with age.

   Other systemic factors and diseases can also induce or aggravate OSAHS by affecting the above three factors, such as obesity, pregnancy, menopause, hypothyroidism, diabetes and so on. Genetic factors can increase the probability of OSAHS by 2–4 times. Drinking alcohol and taking sleeping pills can aggravate the condition of OSAHS patients.

## Clinical Manifestation

1. Symptoms
   (a) Sleeps snoring

   This is the main reason for patients to see a doctor. With the increase of age and weight, the symptoms of snoring can be gradually aggravated, and there are intermittent short stops of breathing. Severe cases may have nighttime wake-up. Apnea is usually aggravated in supine position, so some serious patients can not sleep in supine position.

   (b) Daytime sleepiness

   Another major clinical symptom of the patient, with varying degrees, is mild sleepiness and fatigue, which has no obvious impact on work and life. Heavy people may have irrepressible sleepiness and fall asleep during driving or even talking. The patients fell asleep quickly and the sleep time was prolonged, but the mental and physical strength did not recover significantly after sleep.

   (c) Sexual dysfunction, increased nocturia and even enuresis may occur in some severe patients. Patients with a longer course of illness may experience personality changes such as irritability, depression.
   (d) Children may have enuresis, abnormal sleep behavior, restlessness, inattention, decreased academic performance, growth retardation, thoracic deformity and other manifestations.

(e) Patients can have memory impairment, concentration of attention, slow reaction.
(f) The patient's mouth is dry after getting up in the morning, and he often feels foreign body in the throat.
(g) Some patients may have headache and elevated blood pressure after getting up in the morning.
(h) Some patients may have a feeling of foreign body in pharynx and burning in pharynx after getting up in the morning.
(i) Complications may lead to symptoms such as night angina pectoris and arrhythmia.

2. Signs
   (a) General Features

   Most adult patients are obese or obviously obese, with short and thick neck. Some patients had obvious upper and mandibular dysplasia. Children's development is generally worse than that of their peers, with abnormal craniofacial development and abnormal thoracic development.

   (b) The Upper Airway Signs

   Pharyngeal cavity, especially oropharyngeal cavity, tonsil hypertrophy, soft palate hypertrophy and relaxation, uvula hypertrophy and excessive length; some patients can also see nasal septum deviation, nasal polyps, adenoid hypertrophy, tongue root hypertrophy, lingual root lymphatic tissue hyperplasia, pharyngeal lateral cord hypertrophy and so on.

**Diagnosis**

OSAHS should be considered for middle-aged and elderly patients who complain of snoring during sleep and daytime sleepiness if they have physical examination and obesity or have a history of hypertension and cardiovascular and cerebrovascular diseases. Life history and family history should be inquired in detail. Patients who smoke for a long time, drink heavily for a long time and/or take sedative-hypnotic or muscle relaxant drugs are more likely to have OSAHS, which usually has a family history. At the same time, careful examination of nose, throat and mouth, observation of abnormal upper airway anatomical structure, improvement of the whole body examination, hypothyroidism, acromegaly, cardiac insufficiency, stroke, gastroesophageal reflux and neuromuscular diseases may be related to OSAHS. The following will introduce several specialist examinations of otorhinolaryngology, head and neck surgery, which are of great value in the diagnosis of OSAHS.

1. Polysomnogram (PSG) is the golden standard for diagnosis of OSAHS. Polysomnography includes electroencephalogram, electroophthalmogram, electromyography, oronasal airflow monitoring, pharyngoesophageal pressure, oxygen saturation, ECG monitoring, etc. Through the analysis of the above records, we can understand the changes of the body during sleep and determine the nature (classification) and degree of sleep apnea.

   Diagnostic criteria: According to the criteria of International Classification of Sleep Disorders 3rd Edition (2014), the diagnosis can be made by PSG examination for more than 30 apnea and hypopnea episodes during 7 h of sleep per night, or sleep apnea hypopnea index (AHI) ≥ 15; 15> (AHI) >5, referring to clinical symptoms (Table 15.3).

**Table 15.3** Sleep apnea hyponea grading

| Degree | Sleep apnea and hyponea index | Lowest $SaO_2$ value (%) |
|---|---|---|
| Slight | 5~15 | ≥85 |
| Middle | 16~30 | 65~84 |
| Severe | >30 | <65 |

2. The upper airway continuous pressure measurement is performed by inserting a catheter containing a miniature pressure sensor into the nasal cavity and reaching the esophagus through the nasopharynx and oropharynx. The catheter surface contains several pressure sensors, which are located in the nasopharynx, the upper oropharynx of the lingual root, the lower oropharynx of the lingual root, the laryngopharynx and the esophagus, respectively. All the sensors show the same negative pressure changes during normal inspiration, such as hair in a certain part of the airway. The sensor above the obstruction plane has no pressure change, so it can determine the location of airway obstruction. It is considered as the most accurate location diagnosis method at present.
3. Cephalometric examinations were performed with neck CT and X-ray to locate lateral cranial films for evaluating airway stenosis caused by skeletal or other causes.
4. Endoscopy: Endoscopy can clearly observe the structure of nasal cavity, nasopharynx, oropharynx, laryngopharynx, esophagus and other parts of the structure, to understand whether abnormal function causes airway stenosis.
5. Polyvinylidene fluoride (PVDF), a new material for sensor, is a crystalline polymer with thermoelectric and piezoelectric properties. During sleep monitoring, the temperature of the mouth and nose was measured to detect the airflow of the mouth and nose, and the thoracoabdominal band (piezoelectric) was measured to assess the breathing effort. The results of the present study evaluate that the polyvinylidene fluoride sensor can be used as an alternative lead in the diagnosis of adult sleep apnea and hypopnea interpretation.
6. Percutaneous and end-of-breath carbon dioxide partial pressure detection and arterial blood detection techniques are easier to detect overnight persistent $PCO_2$.

**Differential Diagnosis**

OSAHS should be differentiated from the following diseases.

1. Simple Snoring: simple snoring at night although there are different degrees of snoring, but AHI < 5 times /h, and no symptoms during the day.
2. The upper airway resistance syndrome may appear snoring at different frequencies and degrees at night. The upper airway resistance increases, sleepiness or fatigue during the day, but the AHI is less than 5 times /h. The experimental non-invasive ventilation therapy can effectively support the diagnosis.
3. Obesity and hypopnea syndrome: patients are overweight. When awake, they have $CO_2$ retention. The partial pressure of carbon dioxide is more than 45 mmHg. Most patients can be combined with OSAHS.
4. Narcolepsy occurs mainly in young group, a daytime sleepiness, and cataplexy, sleep paralysis and sleep hallucinations, multiple sleep latency test (multiple sleep latency test, MSLT) can be used as the basis for the diagnosis. MSLT's method is to allow patients to perform a series of naps during the day to objectively determine their daytime sleepiness. Every 2 h were tested one times, and each nap lasted 30 min. The average latency time of patients to sleep is calculated. The latency time of sleep is <5 min. Somnolence is also found in patients with MSLT abnormalities. The onset of narcolepsy is also common in patients with abnormal SAHS.
5. Periodic Sleep Dynamic Syndrome during Sleep: the clinical manifestations usually involve extreme discomfort in the lower extremities during nighttime sleep, forcing the patients to move on the lower limbs or under the ground without stopping, leading to severe sleep disorders and lower limb sensation during awakening. PSG monitoring has a typical periodic leg movement, but it should be different from the legs associated with sleep breathing events.

**Treatment**

Basen on ascertaining the cause of disease and defining the diagnosis, a more targeted treatment method was selected. Generally divided into conservative treatment and surgical treatment of two methods.

**Surgical Treatment**

1. Conservative Treatment
   (a) General treatments: more than 20% of the patients with overweight should lose weight; avoid alcohol and sedative drugs, to avoid aggravating factors of upper airway obstruction, sleep posture adjustment, as far as possible to reduce the lateral tongue retropulsion apnea symptoms and obstructive sleep apnea hypopnea syndrome.
   (b) Nasal mask is positive pressure continuous ventilation treatment: during sleep, the positive pressure air is sent into the airway through a closed mask, the air velocity is adjusted to 100 L/min, and the pressure is maintained at 4~20 $cmH_2O$.
2. Surgical Treatment: according to the different level of obstruction of the different parts of the corresponding different parts of the operation.
   (a) Nasal disease: do nasal polyp extirpation, partial turbinectomy, nasal septum correction, etc.
   (b) The most classic pharyngeal disease surgery uvulopalatopharyngoplasty (UPPP) and the corresponding improved operation such as uvulopalatopharyngoplasty (HUPPP, academician Han Demin improvement, retain the uvula and functional muscle and intact mucosa, expand the soft palate resection), according to different patients is also feasible adenoid tonsil resection, etc.
   (c) The use of laser and low temperature plasma treatment.
   (d) The mandible retracted, move the mandible forward. Tracheotomy is performed in severe patients or other ineffective methods.
3. The inspire upper airway stimulation device, newly developed by the implantable upper airway stimulation device, is an implantable nerve stimulator for the treatment of moderate to severe obstructive sleep apnea syndrome. By detecting the breathing patterns of patients during sleep, the hypoglossal nerve is moderately stimulated to control the activity of the tongue and keep the airway open. Clinical studies have shown that implantable upper airway stimulator can significantly improve the quality of life of most patients, and apnea index of more than half of patients is reduced by more than 50% (Fig. 15.28) [1].

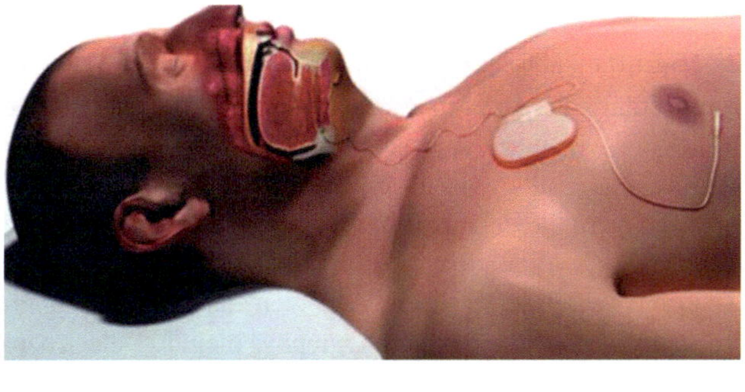

**Fig. 15.28** implant upper respiratory tract stimulation device

## 15.7 Temporomandibular Joint Disease

The temporomandibular joint (TMJ) is the only bilateral joint in the maxillofacial region, which has certain stability and multi direction activity. A variety of important activities related to mastication, swallowing, language and expression under the action of the muscles. This chapter mainly introduces the temporomandibular joint syndrome and the dislocation of the temporomandibular joint.

### 15.7.1 Temporomandibular Joint Syndrome

**Etiology**

Temporomandibular joint syndrome, also known as Costen syndrome, is the most common disease in oral and maxillofacial region. The pathogenesis is not yet clear. It may be related to mental factors, trauma factors, occlusal factors, or other systemic diseases.

**Clinical Manifestation**

The clinical manifestations of temporomandibular joint syndrome include joint swelling or pain, joint ringing and mandibular dyskinesia. The location of pain is usually around the joint area or joint, and can also be accompanied by different degrees of tenderness. Joint swelling or pain is especially evident in the chewing and opening of the mouth. The joint projectile usually occurs during the opening of the mouth, and the sound can occur at different stages of the movement of the mandible. Common movement obstruction is restricted by mouth opening, mandibular deviation in opening mouth, restricted movement of left and right side of mandible, etc. In addition, it can also be accompanied by temporal pain, dizziness, tinnitus and other symptoms.

**Diagnosis**

The main diagnostic method of the disease is imaging examination.

1. Joint X-ray Scholler position and transpharyngeal projection X-ray can be found to change the change of joint space and bone, such as atherosclerosis, bone destruction and hyperplasia, cystic change, comparison of open and closed two different states when the position of condyle, can understand the state of motion of the joint (Fig. 15.29).

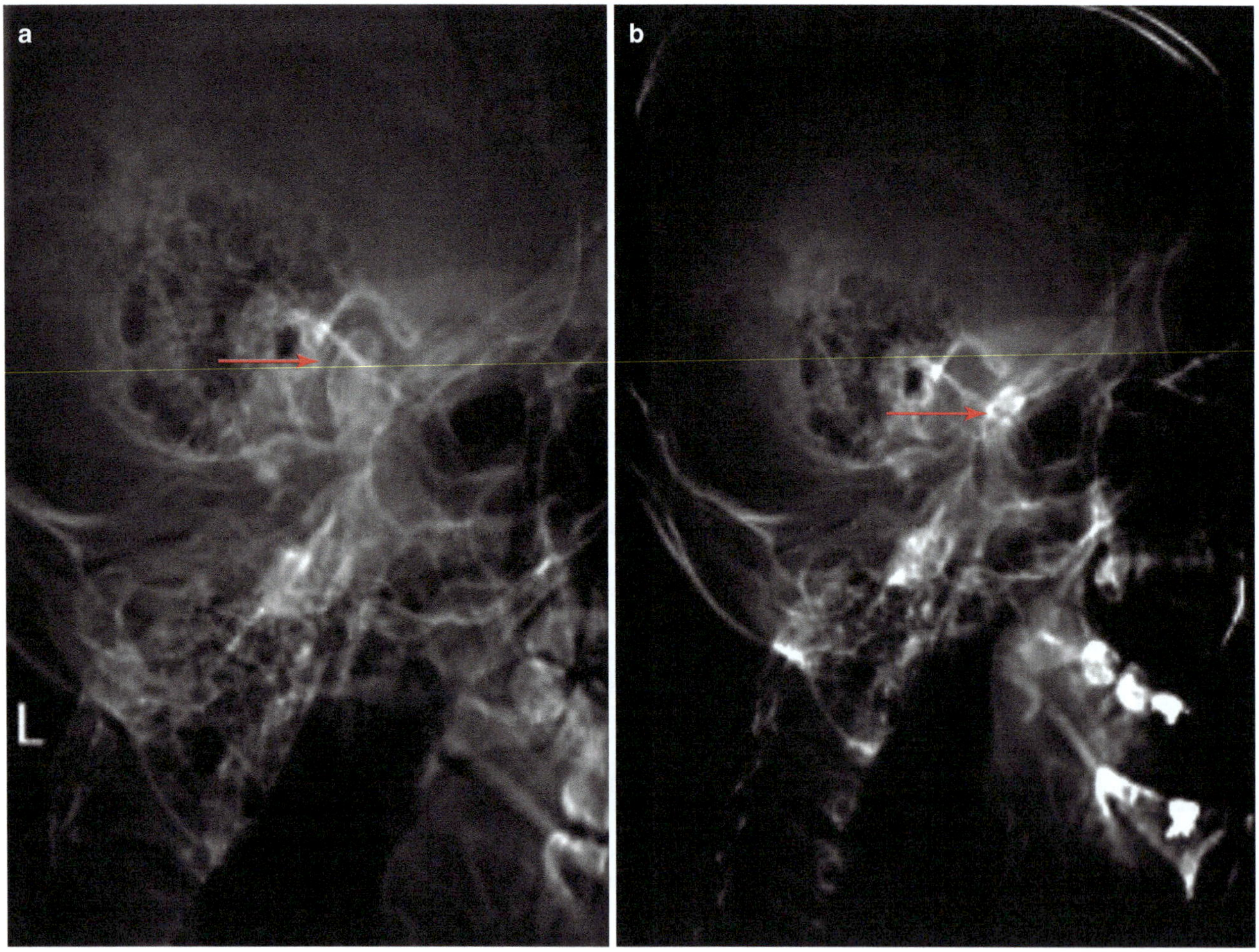


**Fig. 15.29** X- ray film of the TMJ's closed lateral position. (**a**) Closed position. The condyle is located in the articular fossa. (**b**) opening position. The condyle is located below the front of the articular fossa

2. Arthrography: superior lumen angiography is easy to use because of its easy operation, and inferior venography is seldom applied in China. Because of the application of MRI, this technology has been rarely used.
3. Spiral CT Scan: spiral CT scan, CT and 3D reconstruction, high resolution, can be around six aspects of the anatomy of the joint (Fig. 15.30), found that the fine structure changes of articular hard tissue. It is of significance to the diagnosis of joint disease.
4. MRI Examination: through high resolution MRI images, we can detect the status of soft tissue such as joint disc and muscle, and provide important information for diagnosing temporomandibular disorders (Fig. 15.31).

**Treatment**

1. Remove the influence of mental factors.
2. Correction of occlusal relationship.
3. Correct bad habits, such as excessive mouth opening, unilateral chewing, etc.
4. Physiotherapy.
5. Drug therapy or blocking therapy should be used when necessary.

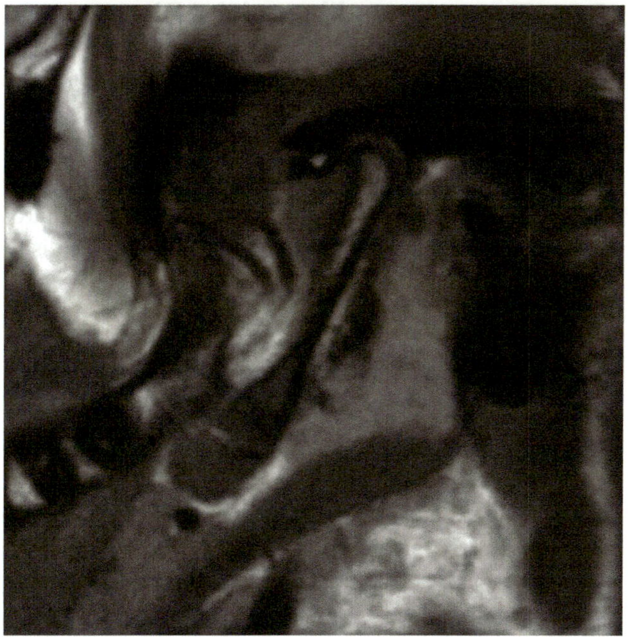

**Fig. 15.31** MRI $T_1$WI sagittal representation of the temporomandibular joint and its articular disc and surrounding muscles

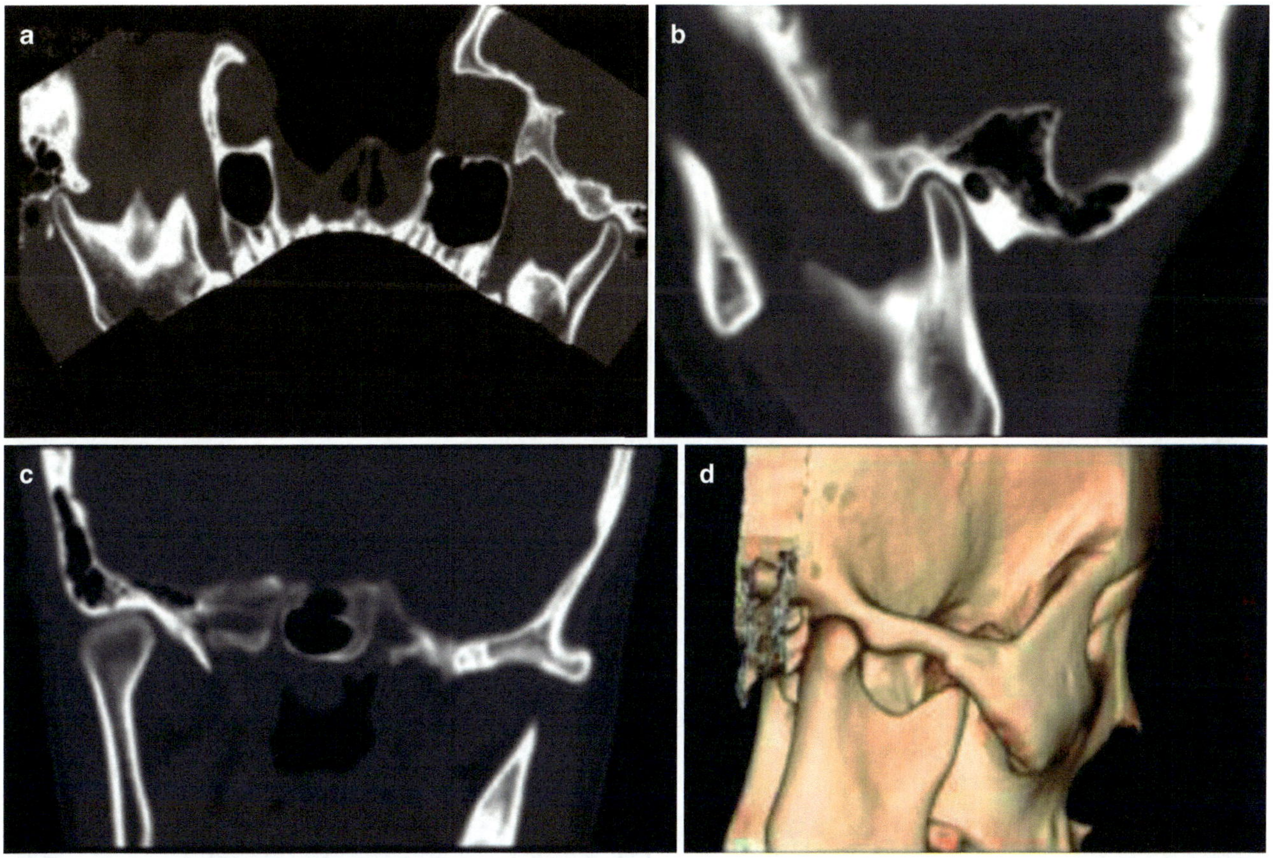


**Fig. 15.30** Reconstruction of normal temporomandibular joint. (**a**) Coronal plane to display bilateral temporomandibular joint. (**b**) Sagittal reconstruction of temporomandibular joint. (**c**) routine coronal reconstruction, showing the right temporomandibular joint. (**d**) surface volume and display stereoscopic image of temporomandibular joint

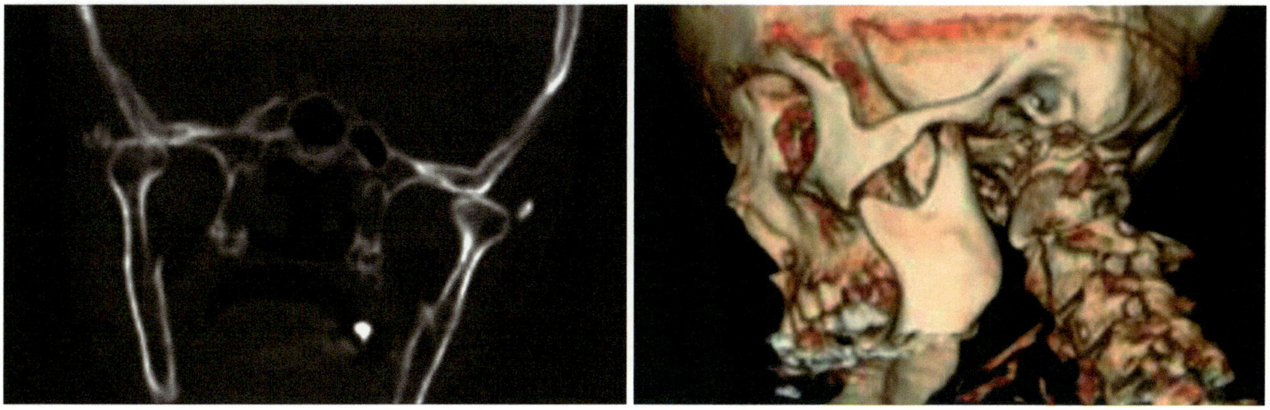

**Fig. 15.32** 3D reconstruction of CT coronal and sagittal position in recurrent dislocation of the temporomandibular joint. It can be seen that the joint nodule becomes flat and the condyle is in the posterior subluxation, which is a manifestation of recurrent dislocation

### 15.7.2 Dislocation of Temporomandibular Joint

When the dislocation of the temporomandibular joint refers to the large opening, the condyle is completely separated from the articular fossa, joint nodule or articular disc and cannot return to the normal position.

**Etiology**

1. Acute Dislocation: acute dislocation is divided into two types: endogenous dislocation and exogenous dislocation. Endogenous dislocation is common in the joint dislocation of the joint without external force, such as laughter, chewing or long opening. Exogenous dislocation is common in the dislocation of the temporomandibular joint caused by external force shock, such as oral tracheal intubation, and the use of openings.
2. Recurrent Dislocation: if the improper treatment of acute dislocation, there may be repeated or habitual dislocation. The pathological features of the joint capsule, the joint ligament and the joint disc are obviously relaxed.

**Clinical Manifestation**

1. Acute Dislocation: unilateral dislocation of the patient showed no closure, and the midline of the mandible was biased toward the healthy side. The language of the patients with bilateral dislocation is unclear, saliva Exodus, mandibular protrusion, the forehead lower, and the face shape correspondingly longer. Examination showed bilateral condyles in the articular tubercle chug out under the cheekbone below, beak. The pain of the joint area and the masticatory muscle was obvious, especially in the reduction.
2. Recurrent Dislocation: recurrent acute dislocation of the symptoms, the patient dare not open the mouth. Reset is easier.

**Diagnosis**

1. Acute Anterior Dislocation: the diagnosis is relatively simple. It often occurs in the large mouth movement or when the mandible is opened, and the joint capsule is obviously relaxed. The X- ray shows the condyle in the upper part of the articular tubercle.
2. Recurrent Dislocation: a history of recurrent dislocation of the disease. Joint capsular laxity and articular disc attachment and avulsion were seen in arthrography. The condyle and joint nodules became flat except for the anterior dislocation of the joint. CT is clearer (Fig. 15.32).

**Treatment**

The most important treatment for the disease is manipulative reduction, usually without anesthesia. After manipulative reduction, the patient is ordered to limit the opening of the mouth for 2 weeks. If the effect of manual reduction is not good, the sclerosing agent can be injected into the joint capsule. Surgery should be performed if necessary, such as joint capsule and ligament reinforcement, joint nodule excision, and joint nodule increase. Recently arthroscopy can examine and perform an operation; it is clear vision, small trauma to get good results [3].

## References


1. Maurer JT, Heyning PVD, Lin HS, et al. Operative technique of upper airway stimulation: an implantable treatment of obstructive sleep apnea. Oper Tech Otolaryngol Head Neck Surg. 2012;23(3):227–33.
2. Mesher D, Cuschieri K, Hibbitts S, et al. Type-specific HPV prevalence in invasive cervical cancer in the UK prior to national HPV immunisation programme: baseline for monitoring the effects of immunisation. J Clin Pathol. 2015;68(2):135–40.
3. Long X. Diagnosis and treatment of temporomandibular joint diseases. Wuhan: Hubei Scientific Technology Publishing House; 2002.

# Part V
# Laryngology

Larynx locates on the midcentral cervix, opening upwards to pharynx and downwards to trachea. It is the respiratory tract aperture, assuming the breathing, the articulation, the deglutition and other important physiology functions. This part will firstly explain the pharyngeal applied anatomy and physiology to help master its anatomical structures and main physiologic functions, laryngeal symptoms and clinic examination methods and finally emphatically discuss about the diagnosis and the treatments of the congenital laryngeal diseases, the laryngitis, the neurolarynx diseases and laryngoma.

# Applied Anatomy and Physiology of Larynx

# 16

Zhonglin Mu, Xiaofeng Wang and Jihong Huang

## 16.1 Applied Anatomy of Larynx

The cold larynx is located in the middle of the anterior neck, under the hyoid bone, the upper part is the upper edge of the epiglottis, and the lower part is the lower edge of the cricoid cartilage, which corresponds to the third to fifth cervical vertebrae in adults. It includes cartilage, muscle, fibrous connective tissue and the mucosa [1].

1. Laryngeal Cartilage

   It contains nine cartilages, which combine to constitute the laryngeal scaffold. There are three individual cartilages, including the thyroid cartilage, the cricoid cartilage and the epiglottis cartilage; there are also three pairs of six cartilages, including the arytenoid cartilage, the corniculate cartilage and the Wrisberg's cartilages.

   (a) Thyroid Cartilage

   Thyroid cartilage is the largest cartilage in the larynx. The anterior angle of the male thyroid cartilage is small, showing right or acute angle. Adults have prominent laryngeal knot in the neck, which is the main sign of the second sexual characteristics of men. In women, the laryngeal nodule is not obvious because of its obtuse angle. Each side of the posterior margin of the thyroid cartilage plate has an upper and a lower angle. The inner side of the lower angle and the posterior and outer side of the cricoid cartilage form a cricothyroid joint (Fig. 16.1).

   (b) Cricoid Cartilage

   It located below thyroid cartilage and above the first tracheal ring. It is the only complete cricoid cartilage in the larynx. It is very important to keep the larynx and the duct unobstructed. Its anterior part is narrow, cricoid cartilage 4, and posterior part is cricoid cartilage plate (Fig. 16.2).

   (c) Epiglottis Cartilage

   The epiglottic cartilage is located in the upper part of the larynx and is leafy. Epigloth can be divided into tongue and larynx, soft tissue of tongue is loose, swelling is obvious when inflammation. The mucosa between the tongue surface and the root of the tongue forms the plica of the epiglottis of the tongue, with a depression on each side. It is called the vallecula epiglottica, which is the foreign body easy to hide (Fig. 16.3). The epiglottis of infants is curled [2].

   (d) Arytenoids Cartilage

   It's located at the outer edge of the cricoid cartilage plate, one on the left and one on the left, and resembles a triangular pyramid. The anterior end of the base is the vocal cord process with attachment of the thyroarytenoid muscle and the vocal cord process; the lateral end is the myoid process with attachment of the posterior cricoarytenoid muscle and the lateral cricoarytenoid muscle. The arytenoid joint is formed between the base and the cricoid cartilage. The arytenoid cartilage slides and rotates along the outer edge of the cricoid cartilage plate, leading to the adduction or abduction of the vocal cord.

2. Laryngeal Membrane and Anadema

   Fibrous ligaments are interconnected between cartilages of the larynx and surrounding tissues of the larynx (Fig. 16.4).

   (a) Thyrohyoid Membrane

   It's an elastic fibrous ligament between the upper margin of the thyroid cartilage and the lower margin of the hyoid bone. The middle and bilateral parts of

Z. Mu (✉) · X. Wang · J. Huang
Department of Otorhinolaryngology Head and Neck Surgery, The First Affiliated Hospital of Hainan Medical University, Haikou, China



Z. Mu, J. Fang (eds.), *Practical Otorhinolaryngology - Head and Neck Surgery*, https://doi.org/10.1007/978-981-13-7993-2_16

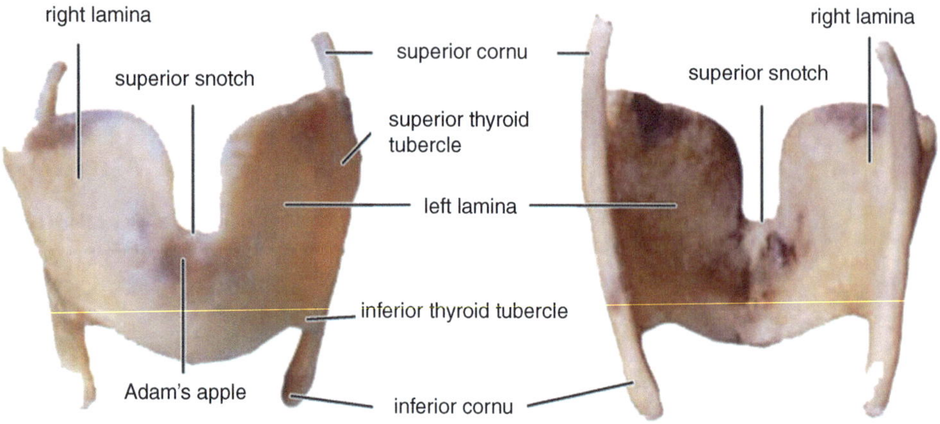


**Fig. 16.1** Thyroid cartilages

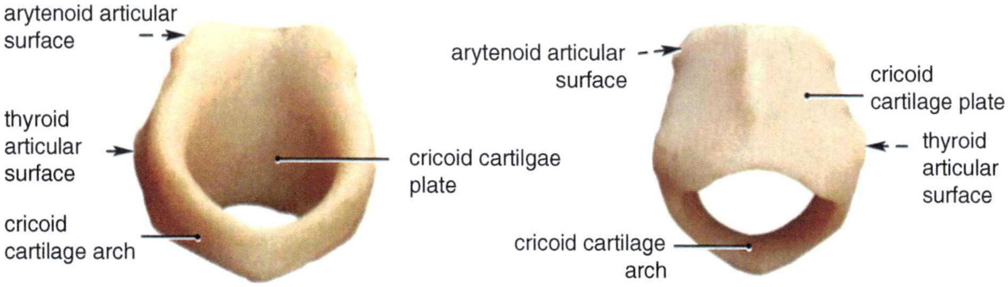


**Fig. 16.2** Cricoid cartilage

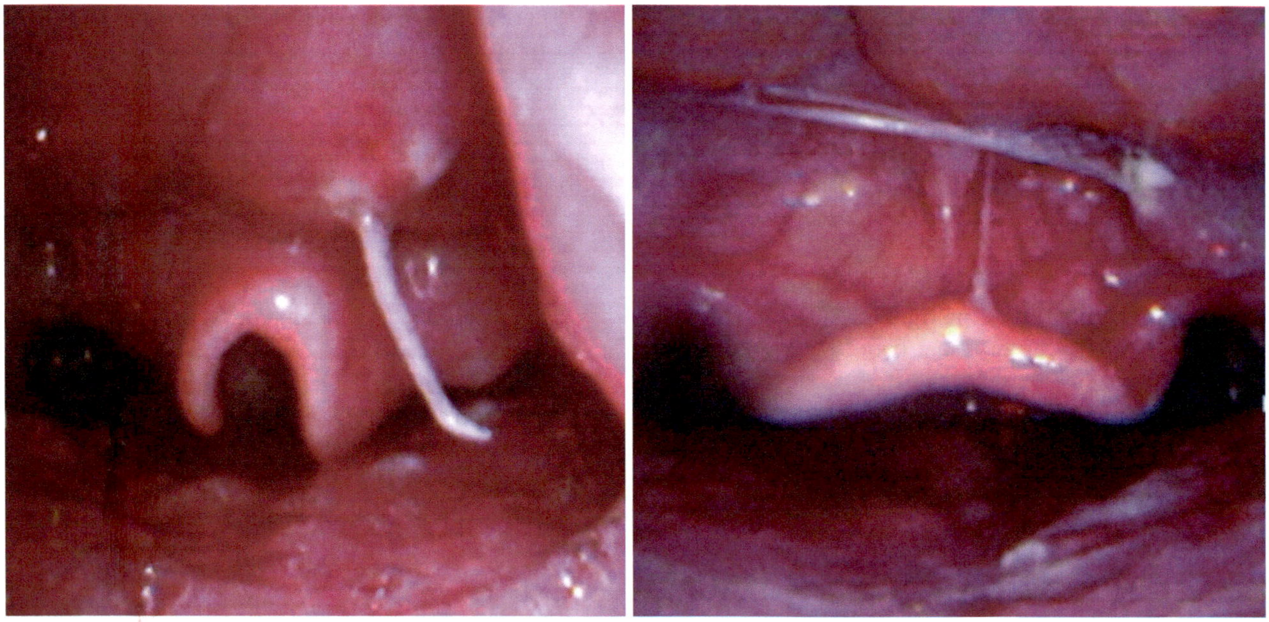

**Fig. 16.3** Epiglottis cartilage and fishbone

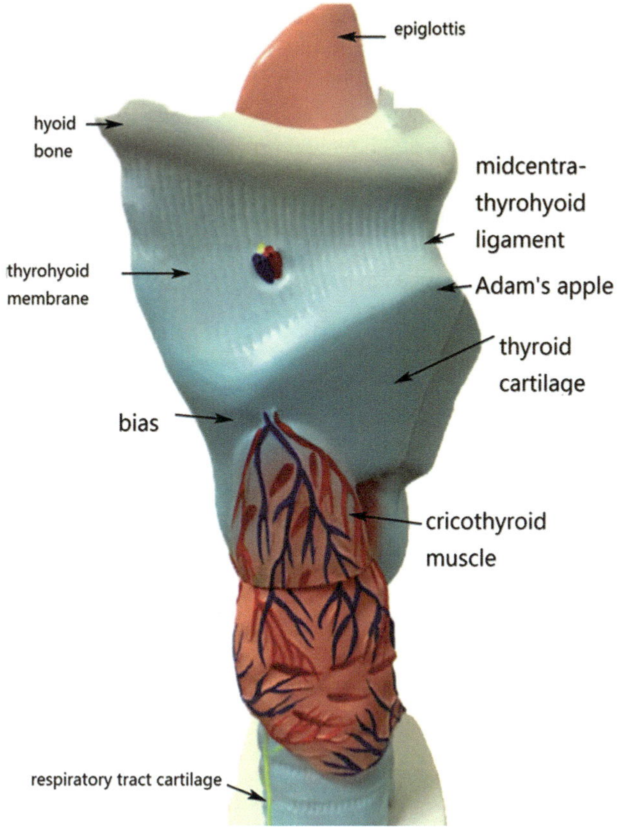


**Fig. 16.4** Laryngomembrane and anadema diagram

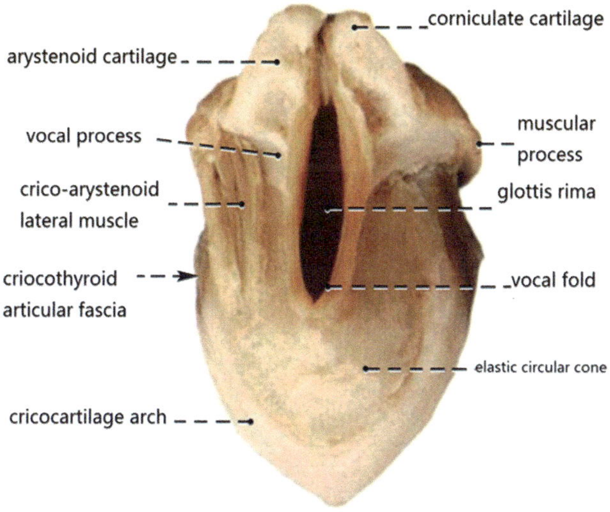


**Fig. 16.5** Elastic pyramid anatomy sample diagram

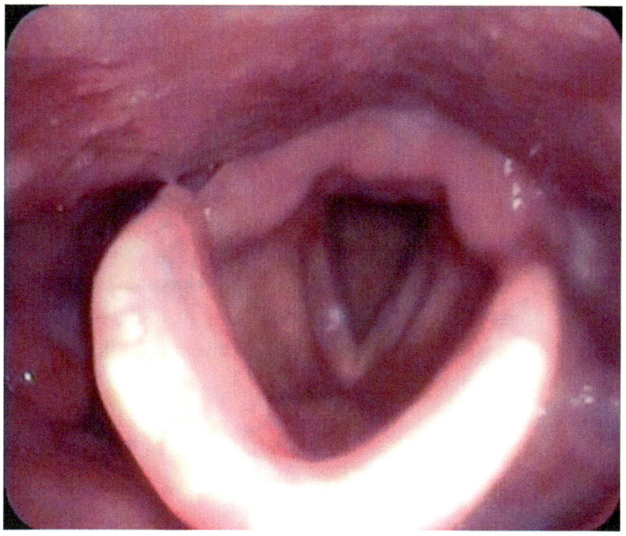

**Fig. 16.6** Normal glottis structure

the periosteum are called the median ligament of the thyroid hyoid bone and the lateral ligament of the thyroid hyoid bone, respectively. The internal branch of the superior laryngeal nerve, the superior laryngeal artery and the superior laryngeal vein penetrate into the larynx from both sides of the thyrohydrohyoid periosteum.

(b) Laryngeal Elastic Membranes

It's a broad elastic tissue, one left and one left. It is divided into two parts by the laryngeal ventricle. The upper part is called a square membrane and the lower part is called an elastic cone (Fig. 16.5). Elastic cone, also known as triangular membrane, attaches downward to the middle and anterior part of the upper edge of cricoid cartilage to form cricothyroid membrane (Fig. 16.6).

## 16.2 Physiology of Larynx

Larynx has four physiological functions: respiratory, phonation, deglutition and breath closure.

1. Respiratory

An unobstructed and intact laryngocavum structures, especially the interaction of the cricothyroid cartilage, is the basis of normal breathing. The glottis rima's reflex adjustment can control the amount of gas exchange into the lungs and adjust the blood and the alveolar $CO_2$ concentration.

2. Phonation

   Phonation function larynx is a vocal organ. There are many theories about the mechanism of laryngeal phonation. At present, it is generally believed that the vibration sound produced by airflow passing through vocal cords during lung expiration. When phonating, the vocal cord moves toward the middle line, the glottis closes, and the exhaled airflow in the lungs impulses the vocal cord to produce a pitch sound, which is then resonated through the pharynx, mouth and nose, and articulated by the tongue, soft palate, teeth and lips, thus producing various sounds and languages.

3. Deglutition

   Larynx acts in deglutition Whiles deglutition, the larynx rises, the epiglottis inclines to the postinferior to cover the laryneal aperture, the vocal cords close, then the food enters the esophagus along with the bilateral piriform recess and avoids straying into the inferior respiratory tract; the laryngeal cough reflex could expel the foreign mass strayed into the inferior respiratory tract by the defense reflex bucking.

4. Suspending Breath

   When series of the pleural pressure and the abdominal pressure motions, such as defecation cough delivery, etc. The vocal cords adduct to tightly close the glottis and then the breathing suspends to complete the motions by increasing internal cavum pressure.

## References

1. Peng Y, Wang H. Local anatomy. 5th ed. Beijing: People's Medical Publishing House; 2001.
2. Mu Z. Laryngology surgery anatomy. In: Liu Z, editor. Modern laryngology surgery. Beijing: Military Medical Publishing House; 2001.

# Symptomatology and Examination Method of Larynx

17

Yongjun Feng, Desheng Xian, Rong Tu and Jianghua Wan

## 17.1 Symptomatology of Larynx

1. Dyspnea

   Respiratory movement is regulated by the respiratory center. Maintaining normal respiratory function mainly depends on rhythmic respiratory movement, smooth respiratory tract, intact pulmonary blood circulation and alveolar gas exchange function. Anything above can cause dyspnea. Physiological dyspnea may occur during excessive exercise and fatigue. Obstruction of the throat, trachea, bronchi and bronchioles, hypoxia, acid-base imbalance, lung lesions and retention of lower respiratory secretions can all cause dyspnea.

2. Hoarseness

   It is a common symptom of laryngeal diseases; the mild type may only cause a lower and thicker tone but the severe type cause the patients' hoarseness. Patients with severe hoarseness can only be able to whisper and even lead to aphasia. Attention should be paid to the time, degree, nature, intermittent or persistent occurrence of hoarseness, whether there are incentives, and whether it continues to worsen. The main reasons for hoarseness are as follows.

   (a) Laryngeal Diseases

   - Congenital Abnormality

     Congenital laryngeal web, laryngocele, laryngeal cartilage deformity, etc.

   - Laryngitis

     Consist of acute and chronic laryngitis, laryngeal tuberculosis, and laryngeal syphilis. Laryngeal diphtheria is often characterized by vocal weakness, pseudomembranous formation and mucosal swelling.

   - Vocal Cord Polyp, Vocal Nodules and Vocal Crypt

     Vocal cord polyps, nodules and cysts: In order to cause hoarseness, the degree of hoarseness is related to the location and size of its growth. Small related, generally progressive sound, into persistence.

   - Tumor

     Papilloma, fibroma, hemangioma, laryngeal cancer, etc. Benign tumors such as papilloma and laryngeal fibroma may appear slowly.

     Progressive vocal clarity, while hoarseness of malignant tumors such as laryngeal cancer is progressively aggravated in a short period of time.

   - Laryngeal Metabolic Diseases

     Such as laryngeal amyloidosis.

   - Trauma

     Various causes of laryngeal trauma affect vocal cord or cricoarytenoid joint activity.

   (b) Vocal Cord Motion Nerve Damage

   Labyrinth is long, therefore, trauma, surgery, tumor invasion at any sites between the jugular foramen and the recurrent laryngeal nerve could cause peripheral laryngeal paralysis; cerebral hemorrhage, cerebral infarction, intracranial tumors and others can cause the central laryngeal paralysis. Check the detail on Section Four chapter eighteen.

   (c) Hysteria Hoarseness

   It is usually acute, which can occur from whispering, dysphonia to complete aphasia. The vocal cords are normal. They can't approach the middle line when pronouncing, showing a triangular glottic fissure. But the patient's cry, laugh and cough were normal and loud. Hoarseness recovers quickly and is prone to recurrence. Closure and other suggestive treatments are effective.

Y. Feng (✉)
Department of Otorhinolaryngology Head and Neck Surgery, The Second Affiliated Hospital of Hainan Medical University, Haikou, China

D. Xian
Department of Otorhinolaryngology Head and Neck Surgery, The First Affiliated Hospital of Hainan Medical University, Haikou, China

R. Tu · J. Wan
Department of Medical Imaging, The First Affiliated Hospital of Hainan Medical University, Haikou, China



Z. Mu, J. Fang (eds.), *Practical Otorhinolaryngology - Head and Neck Surgery*, https://doi.org/10.1007/978-981-13-7993-2_17

3. Dysphagia

   The pharynx and larynx under the control of central nervous system and pharyngeal plexus participate in and coordinate swallowing activities. Any link of disease can lead to dysphagia. Dysphagia caused by oral, pharyngeal or laryngeal diseases is mainly caused by swallowing pain or mechanical disorders. Dysphagia caused by pharyngeal diseases is the main cause of oral and pharyngeal diseases. Oral diseases mainly include lesions that hinder swallowing, such as neurovascular edema, tongue tumor infiltration, eruption of the third molar, etc. The laryngeal diseases that cause dysphagia are as follows.

   (a) Inflammation
      - Acute inflammation such as acute epiglottitis or epiglottic abscess.
      - Invasive and ulcerative laryngeal tuberculosis can cause pain and difficulty in swallowing when it invades epiglottis, arytenoid fold and arytenoid cartilage.
      - Laryngeal perichondritis and laryngeal edema cause dysphagia due to swelling and pain of arytenoid cartilage and piriform recess.

   (b) Laryngoma

      Late stage laryngeal tumors invade the larynx, ipsilateral piriform recess, arytenoid epiglottic fold and other places. When ulceration and infection occur, dysphagia often occurs. When laryngeal and posterior ring cancers invade the esophageal orifice, dysphagia becomes more serious.

   (c) Neurolaryngeal Paralysis

      Laryngeal nerve paralysis such as laryngeal nerve damage, loss of protective reflex when eating, food and saliva often mistake into the trachea, cough, dysphagia, often complicated by aspiration pneumonia.

4. Laryngalgia

   Laryngeal pain is a common symptom. The degree of laryngalgia varies according to the nature, course, extent and individual tolerance of laryngeal lesions. Light cases occur only when talking, swallowing or coughing. Severe sore throat can be persistent and intense pain. Patients can often refuse to eat, saliva flows out of their mouth, and even cause malnutrition and disturbance of water and electrolyte balance. The nature of laryngeal pain is blunt pain, dull pain, traction pain, needle-like pain, knife-like pain, tear-like pain or pulsatile-like pain. Laryngeal pain can occur alone or with other symptoms, such as cough, dysphagia, dyspnea, hoarseness, laryngeal ringing, etc. The common laryngeal diseases causing laryngeal pain are as follows.

   (a) Acute Laryngitis

      Such as acute laryngitis, acute epiglottitis, laryngeal mucosal ulcer, laryngeal perichondritis and laryngeal abscess, can cause severe pain in the larynx. Acute laryngeal inflammation can sometimes be accompanied by local tenderness. When swallowing, the larynx moves, aggravating the pain and radiating to the ear.

   (b) Chronic Laryngitis

      It is a nonspecific inflammation of the larynx. It usually has no pain, sometimes only mild dry pain and swelling pain, and is often aggravated when excessive voice is used. Laryngeal tuberculosis is a special type of laryngeal infection with severe pain and radiation earache. Patients with chronic laryngitis often feel slight pain and discomfort in the larynx, accompanied by a sense of dryness.

   (c) Laryngoma

      Benign laryngoma and early laryngosarcoma don't cause pain very much; the terminal tumors or the tumor ulceration accompanies with inflammation may cause pain very much.

   (d) Laryngeal Trauma

      Laryngeal trauma includes foreign body injury, severe contusion, laryngeal cartilage fracture and mucosal tear. Laryngeal pain can also be caused after radiotherapy. Compressive ulcer may occur behind cricoid cartilage and arytenoid cartilage after long-term nasogastric tube stimulation. Over-time intubation of laryngeal anesthesia or too thick intubation, pressure of the laryngeal mucosa, can form ulcers, as well as direct anterior conjunction laryngoscopy and tracheoscopy examination injury of the laryngeal mucosa, can cause laryngeal pain, swallowing aggravated, and radiate to the ear.

   (e) Laryngeal Joint Lesion

      Such as the cricoarytenoid arthritis, which often accompanies with systemic rheumatoid arthritis, gout, etc.

5. Laryngeal Stridor

   Laryngeal stricture. Inhalatory laryngitis refers to narrowing from the nasal cavity to the supraglottic region; exhalative laryngitis refers to narrowing under the vocal cord, which is produced by trachea and bronchus; dual laryngitis refers to those who both inhale and exhale, narrowing in the vocal cord region or in its lower part. Laryngeal ringing is often accompanied by different degrees of inspiratory obstruction, expiratory obstruction or respiratory obstruction. The larynx can touch the sense of vibration, which can cause dyspnea, hypoxia, and cyanosis and so on.

   The common causes of wheezing are scar stenosis caused by laryngeal deformity, trauma and physical and chemical injury, foreign body in larynx and trachea, or special infectious diseases such as laryngitis, allergic laryngeal edema, Laryngeal Benign and malignant tumors, laryngeal spasm and vocal cord paralysis.

6. Hemoptysis and Haematemesis

   Hemoptysis refers to the bleeding of respiratory organs in the larynx and below, which is discharged from the mouth by coughing. There are usually scratchy throat, cough out blood or sputum with blood, and when the amount of hemoptysis is high; foam blood is spout from mouth or mouth and nose. Suffocation can occur if larger blood clots are blocked. The cough is alkaline, and blood stains often remain in the sputum after a few days.

Hematemesis is reflex nausea caused by upper gastrointestinal bleeding stimulating the stomach. Blood is vomited through the mouth. Upper abdominal discomfort, pain and nausea often occur before hematemesis. Hematemesis can be bright red, dark red or coffee, mixed with food residues. A large amount of rapid hematemesis can lead to acute massive blood loss and endanger life.

(a) Common Etiologies of Hemoptysis
  - There are bleeding foci in the upper respiratory tract lesions, such as bleeding of tongue root, tonsil, nasopharynx, nasal cavity and sinus, nasal and sinus tumors, fungal infection of nasal cavity and sinus, etc.
  - Laryngeal lesions, laryngeal cancer, laryngeal papilloma, laryngeal tuberculosis, laryngeal hemangioma, laryngeal ulcer, laryngeal syphilis and laryngeal leprosy.
  - Tracheobronchial lesions Tracheitis, Bronchitis, Bronchiectasis, Tracheal neoplasms, Tracheal foreign bodies.
  - Pulmonary tuberculosis, lung cancer, lung abscess and so on.
  - laryngotracheal trauma.

(b) The common causes of hematemesis are as follows; esophageal cancer, esophageal perforation, esophagitis, esophageal foreign bodies, esophageal ulcer, esophageal varices, gastroduodenal ulcer, gastric tumors, small intestinal diseases, cirrhosis, blood system diseases, parasitic diseases, uremia, and some acute infectious diseases

## 17.2 Examination Method of Larynx

1. Regular Examination
   (a) Special Laryngeal Examination

   Laryngeal specialist examine first by observing whether there are abnormalities outside the larynx, whether the size are normal, whether the position are in the anterior middle of the neck, whether the two sides are symmetrical. Attention should be paid to whether there is swelling, tenderness, deformity in the larynx and whether there are enlarged lymph nodes or subcutaneous emphysema in the neck. During palpation, the thumb and index finger are used to hold the laryngeal body and move toward both sides. The sense of friction and movement of the normal laryngeal joints can be touched. If the lesion involves the inner laryngeal joints, this feeling often disappears.

   (b) Indirect Laryngoscope Examination

   Indirect laryngoscopy is the most common and convenient examination methods. The patient should sit down well, head is slightly tilted, mouth is opened and tongue is stretched out. The doctor should adjust the frontal mirror light to focus it on the uvula, package the anterior 1/3 tongue with medical gauze to avoid lower incisor's injury to the glossodesmus, pinch the anterior tongue with left thumb(superjacent) and medius (inferior) to push the tongue to the anteriorinferior. With the help of the index finger push the upper lip and press against the above teeth to handle the fixation. Then hold the indirect laryngoscope in a right holding-pen-gesture and slightly warm the scope mirror to leave it unfoggy. However take caution to the temperature to avoid scalding the mucosa membrane. Insert the laryngoscope into the pharynx, turn the mirror to the anterior-inferior and adhere the mirror back tightly to the uvula, push the soft palate to the superior, avoid nausea for contacting the post pharyngeal wall. The investigators should slightly rotate and adjust the mirror plane angle and position according to requisitions. Firstly, investigate the tongue root, the lingual tonsil, the epiglottis vallecula, the post pharyngolaryngeal wall, the lateral pharyngolaryngeal wall, the epiglottis lingual and free surface, the arytenoid cartilage, bilateral piriform recess, etc.

   Order the subjects to phonate 'Yi" to rise the epiglottis up to help observe the laryngoepiglottic surface, the arytenoepiglottic folds, the interarytenozone, the ventricular zone and the vocal cords and their occlusion cases.

2. laryngoendoscope Examination
   (a) Hard Endoscopy

   Hard tube endoscopy is placed in oropharynx through the mouth, so that the aperture at the end of the tube can observe the nasopharynx upward and the throat downward.

   (b) Electric (Fibrous) Endoscopy

   Clear the rhinal secretions before examination, and anesthetize the nasopharyngeal mucosa membrane and rhinocavum with 1% tetracaine, then insert through rhinocavum; patients with thicker tube or rhinocavum stenosis could orally take mucous anesthetics, then insert the tube through mouth and clearly observe the complete pharynx and larynx by changing angles.

   (c) Frequency-flash Laryngoscopy

   The fundamental frequency of the sound examined by strobolaryngoscope is transmitted to the arc lamp through laryngeal microphone, audio amplifier and differential frequency generator. The arc lamp emits intermittent beams at the same frequency, so that the frequency of the flash is consistent with or maintains a certain difference with the frequency of the vocal cord vibration regardless of the fundamental frequency. In this way, the rapid vibration of the vocal cord can be imaged as a relatively slow, visual motion image or still image, and the vibration process and regularity of the vocal cord can be observed. Small mucosal lesions can be detected by frequency-fash Laryngoscopy, which is helpful for early detection of vocal cord cancer, vocal cord polyps, vocal nodules, vocal cord leukoplakia, vocal cord paralysis, et al. [1].

3. Voice auditory Examination

Vocalization is one of the important functions of larynx, and laryngeal diseases often have dysphonia. Voice acoustic detection can be divided into two kinds: subjective auditory examination and objective acoustic examination.

(a) Subjective

The Japanese Acoustic and Speech Medical Association has formulated GRBAS as the auditory evaluation of hoarseness, G (overall grade) as the comprehensive degree of hoarseness; R (rough) is rough, when the vocal cord swells and softens, bilateral vibration is uneven, such as vocal cord polyps are prone to this type; B (breathy) is breathy, vocal cord closure is incomplete, exhaled airflow is large, easy to appear this type, such as Vocal cord paralysis can occur in this type; A (asthenic) is a weak type, vocal cord thinning, lack of tension, relaxation and softening can occur in this type, vocal cord paralysis sometimes this type; S (strained) is a tense type, when the vocal cord hardens, forced vocal cord can occur in this type, vocal cord cancer mostly present this type. Each type of GRBAS is divided into 4 degrees: 0 is normal, 1 is mild, 2 is moderate, and 3 is severe. Because auditory evaluation belongs to subjective evaluation, the subjective judgment of each evaluator will be different, so three professionals are required to judge independently and take the average value as the result.

(b) Objective

Acoustic frequency spectrum only applies the electronic measurement and analyses parameters to objectively offer acoustic estimate to the voice (Fig. 17.1).

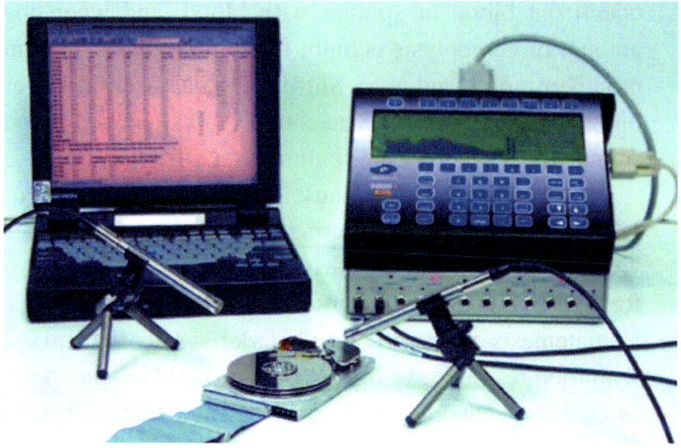

**Fig. 17.1** Acoustic frequency spectrum

- Frequency

  Frequency is the innate frequency of the vocal vibration, expressing with unit 'HZ', which means vocal vibration times/second. The frequency parameters' most representative one is the fundamental frequency ($F_0$). $F_0$ could be influenced by the age and gender more than other factors. At actual applications, estimate according to different normal value of the control groups.

- Vocal Range

  Vocal range is the frequency range between the highest and lowest voice and the highest voice contains the actual highest voice and the highest falsetto, therefore human vocal range has the actual vocal range and the falsetto vocal range. and the vocal range sets the octave or semitone (sound interval between two $\sqrt[12]{2}$ frequencies) as its unit.

- Intensity

  It is a physical unit related to the voice loudness sense, which is always expressing with unit 'dB'. The more the inferior glottis pressures the more the vocal vibration range and the higher the intensity is.

- Formant

  It is produced at the resonance cavum between the vocal cords and the mouth and lips, of all which locations could control the cavum room. The resonance apex's frequency and its overtone determine

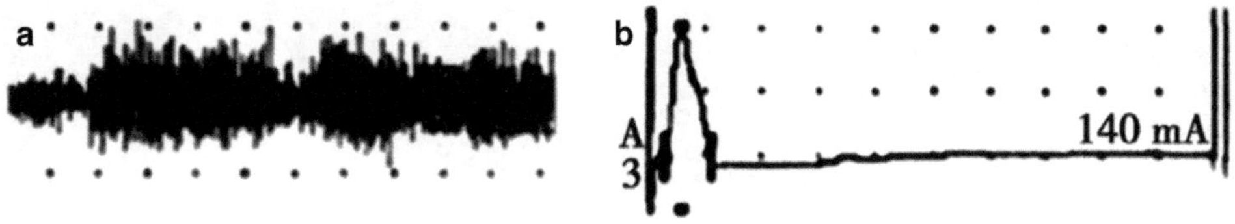


**Fig. 17.2** Myolaryngoelectrograph. (**a**) Vocal spasm electro discharge. (**b**) Induced vocal muscles electric motion principles

the tone quality and the timbre; therefore the resonance apex effects acoustic examination well.

- Perturbation

  It is divided into the jitter and the shimmer. The jitter is the micro variation along with the acoustic signals circles. As researches say, the acoustic perturbation is positively correlated to the vocal vibration rules, the vibration range, the mucosa fluctuation and the glottis occlusion conditions [2].

4. Myolaryngoelectrograph

   It is an examination measurement for researching the laryngeal muscle cells and the neurobioelectric motion to help judge the laryngeal neuromuscle system function condition which offers the neuron lesion orientations, damage condition diagnosis, the surgery neuron supervision and prognosis judgment in clinic laryngeal and acoustic diseases and others as scientific evidence (Fig. 17.2). During examination, insert the recording electrode into the corresponding intra laryngeal muscles and spontaneous and evoked potentials can be recorded, the qualitatively and the semiquantifcation could help judge the neuro muscle damage conditions and then recognize that the vocal dyskinesia is singly caused by the arthro-dyskinesia, the lesioned muscle and other semi mechanical causes or the laryngeal neuron damage or both.

5. Medical Imaging

   It plays an important role on laryngeal diseases diagnosis and recent imaging examination methods include the regular X-ray examination the CT scan and the MRI examination.

   (a) X-ray Examination

   Commonly, the due lateral imaging is mainly used to diagnose the laryngometal and animal bone foreign bodies and it is also the commonly applied imaging.

   (b) CT

   It includes cross-sectional scan, enhanced scan and three-dimensional reconstruction. In laryngeal trauma, plain scan and three-dimensional reconstruction can show whether there is fracture or dislocation of laryngeal cartilage, whether there is avulsion of laryngeal mucosa, submucosal hematoma and obstruction of laryngeal cavity after trauma. When displaying various benign and malignant tumors, plain scan, enhancement and three-dimensional reconstruction techniques can be used to determine the extent of tumor involvement and whether there is paraglottic structural invasion: distinguishing the antecedent and consequence relationship between cervical lymph nodes and primary cervical masses (Fig. 17.3).

   (c) MRI

   It is more better than CT in displaying soft tissue and inferior to CT in displaying laryngeal cartilage. Therefore, at present, the main role of MRI in laryngeal examination is to determine the extent of lesions, especially to show the boundary of tumors and the extension of tumors up and down, the invasion of primary and minor early tumors in the intralaryngeal muscular system, the relationship with surrounding tissues, and the metastasis of cervical lymph nodes, which are superior to CT imaging. It is mainly used for laryngeal cancer, which can not be found under endoscopy, and for intralaryngeal tumors which grow under normal mucosa. Estimation of the tumor's prognosis and prognosis is critical (Fig. 17.4).

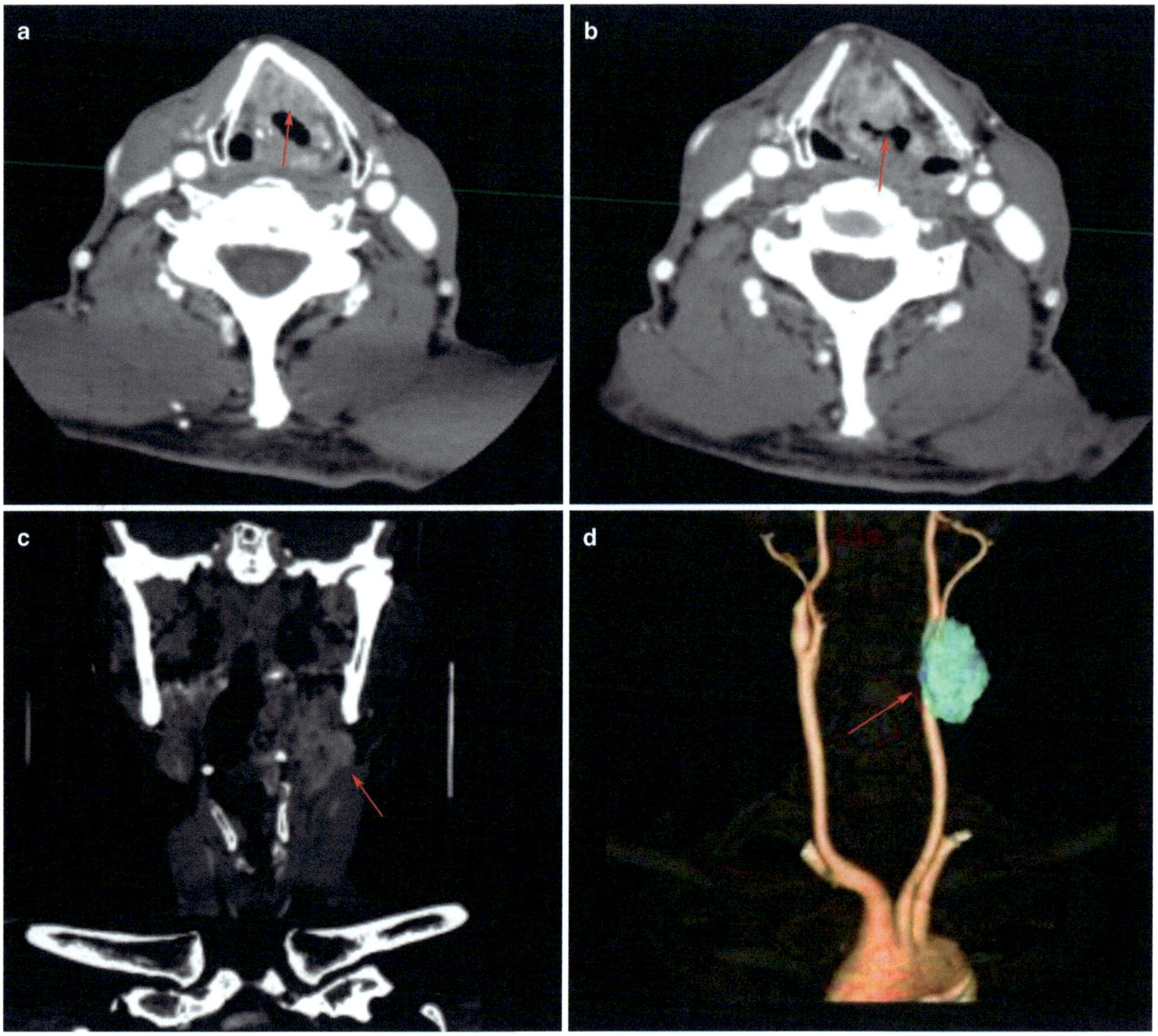


**Fig. 17.3** Laryngeal caner enhanced axial CT scan and coronary rebuilding and CTA manifestations. (**a**, **b**) Enhanced axial CT scan: In the same patient, the left glottic and subglottic region laryngeal cancer (arrow point), anterior commissure and right glottic region (**c**, **d**) were shown. Coronal reconstruction and CTA was enhanced for another patient, indicating that the tumors involved the left epiglottic Valley and parapharyngeal space. The enhancement was obvious (arrow point). CTA showed the relationship between the tumors (blue-green) and the carotid artery

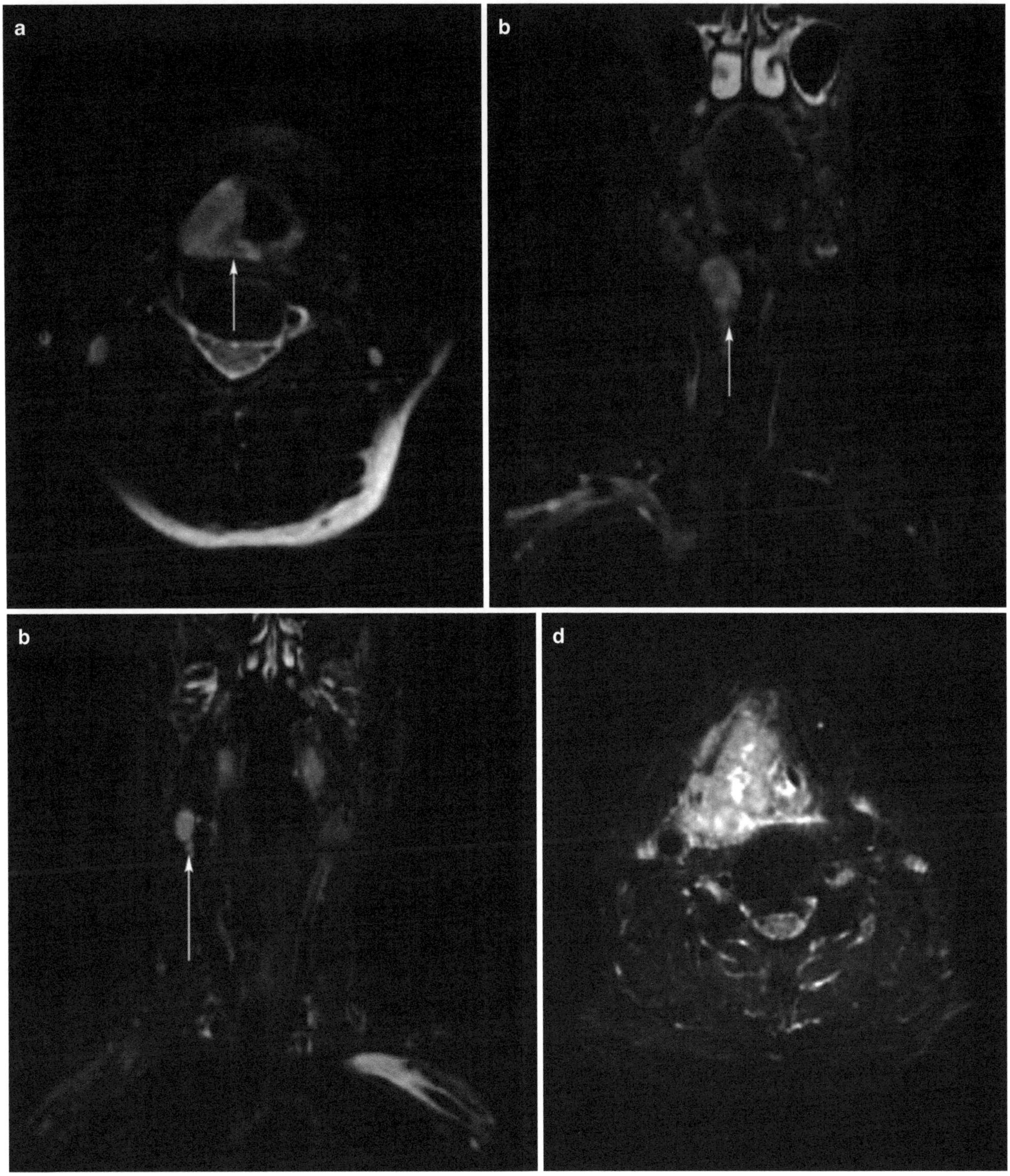


**Fig. 17.4** Right laryngocarcinoma MRI examination plain $T_2$WI scan. (**a**, **b**) Display right glottic neoplasm, involving right thyroid cartilage (white arrow). (**c**) Right cervical lymph node swelling (white arrow). (**d**, **e**) Display right glottic neoplasm. (**d**) Axial position imaging show the involvement at the thyroid cartilage and its peripheral soft tissues and pre vertebral space. (**e**) Display involvement at supra glottic portion and infra glottic portion

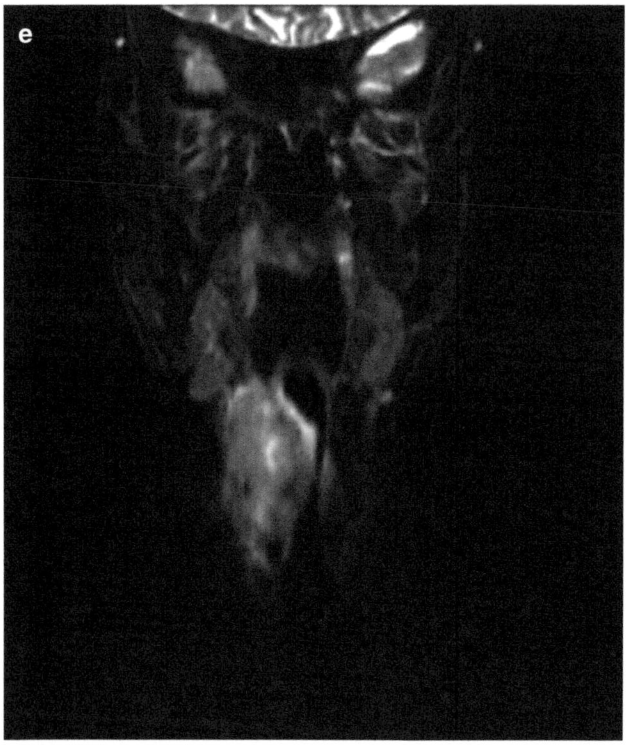


**Fig. 17.4** (continued)

## References


1. Xie J. Application of Stroboscopy at Acoustic Surgery. Sinoforeign Health Abstract. 2012;9(1):421.
2. Zhou Y, Zhang F. New Progression at Laryngeal Phonation Function Detection and Evaluation. J Audiol Speech Dis. 2006;14(5):395397.

# 18 Common Laryngeal Diseases

Zhonglin Mu, Xuejun Zhou, Jugao Fang and Yongjun Feng

## 18.1 Congenital Laryngeal Disease

### 18.1.1 Congenital Laryngeal Cyst

**Summary**

The pathogenesis of congenital laryngeal cyst is not clear. The causes include the abnormal development of the gill fissure, the dysplasia of the larynx, the obstruction of the laryngeal air bag and the mucous duct, and the theory of the ectopic thyroid. Histologically, most congenital laryngeal cysts are confined to respiratory epithelium, while others include stratified squamous epithelium, columnar epithelium, cuboidal epithelium and some mixed epithelium. In more than half of the cases, diffuse or aggregated lymphatic tissue can be observed. At present, congenital laryngeal cysts are divided into two things types: type I, cyst confined to the laryngeal cavity (Fig. 18.1), type II, cyst extending to the larynx. The latter can be further divided into type IIa derived from embryos and type IIb derived from inner and mesoderm [1].

**Electronic Supplementary Material** The online version of this chapter (https://doi.org/10.1007/978-981-13-7993-2_18) contains supplementary material, which is available to authorized users.

Z. Mu (✉) · X. Zhou
Department of Otorhinolaryngology Head and Neck Surgery, The First Affiliated Hospital of Hainan Medical University, Haikou, China

J. Fang
Department of Otorhinolaryngology Head and Neck Surgery, Beijing Tongren Hospital, Capital Medical University, Beijing, China

Y. Feng
Department of Otorhinolaryngology Head and Neck Surgery, The Second Affiliated Hospital of Hainan Medical University, Haikou, China

**Clinical Symptoms**

Symptoms are mainly determined by the size and location of the cyst, as well as the age of the patient. These symptoms include respiratory obstruction, wheezing, and intermittent crying etc. The laryngeal cyst often has no clinical symptoms, and the larger one can obstruct the airway, such as laryngeal stridor, dyspnea, anoxia, asphyxia, etc.

**Diagnosis**

A preliminary diagnosis can be made according to the symptoms, and the laryngoscopy is required for a clear diagnosis. Direct laryngoscopy can be performed in children, indirect laryngoscope, hard laryngoscope or electronic (laryngoscope) examination can be performed in adults, and imaging examination of larynx airway and neck can also be performed in adults. A fixed mass, which is not connected with larynx and does not change with respiration, can be observed. Direct laryngoscopy with empty needle aspiration and liquid or gas can confirm the diagnosis. If its volume changes with respiration, it shrinks when inhaling, and increases when it drums vigorously and it communicates with the laryngeal ventricle, it should be diagnosed as congenital laryngeal cyst.

**Treatment**

Congenital laryngeal cysts are preferred to be excised. The larynx type of the congenital laryngeal cyst, if the symptom is mild, can be treated by the age of the larynx. Resection can be performed under endoscopy and completely removed the wall of the capsule. Tracheotomy is required for patients with severe airway obstruction. There is no need for surgery for larynx cyst without obvious symptoms. If the infection is infected, an antibiotic can be used to treat the inflammation


Z. Mu, J. Fang (eds.), *Practical Otorhinolaryngology - Head and Neck Surgery*, https://doi.org/10.1007/978-981-13-7993-2_18

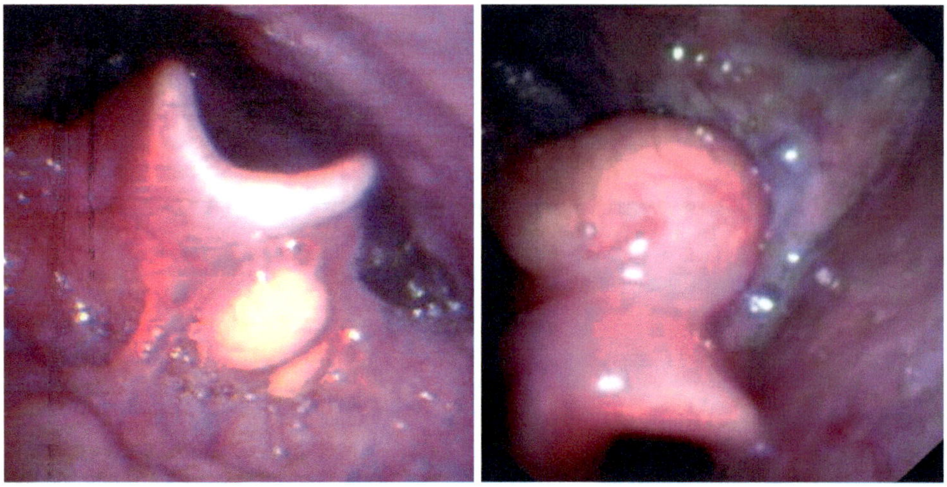

**Fig. 18.1** Epiglottis cyst

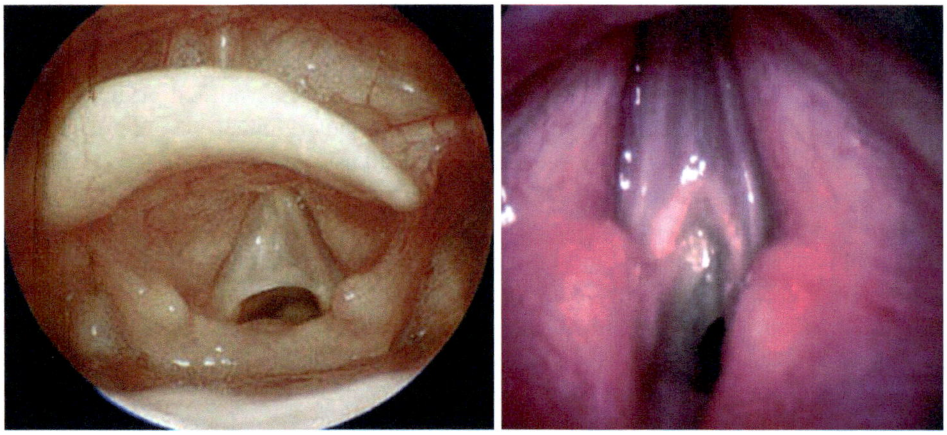

**Fig. 18.2** Laryngeal web

before the operation is removed. If the larynx type is larger than the cyst, it can be excised by external cervical approach.

### 18.1.2 Congenital Laryngeal Webs

At birth, there is a membrane like tissue in the larynx, which is called the congenital laryngeal web or the laryngeal septum.

**Etiology**

The congenital laryngeal web is the membrane of the larynx (Fig. 18.2), which is produced in the laryngeal cavity of the embryonic development period. Can be divided into supra glottic and glottic laryngeal web and sub glottic laryngeal web, the majority of the glottis laryngeal web, seldom occurred in the sub glottic, who rare occurred in the supra glottic. Most of the anterior 1/3–2/3 of the glottis are closed. The laryngeal web is a fibrous tissue membrane, which covers the epithelium up and down, and its thickness also varies from person to person.

**Clinical Manifestation**

1. The clinical manifestations of congenital laryngeal web in infants vary with the size and position of the laryngeal webs.
   (a) When the laryngeal web is large, can cause neonatal asphyxia and death.
   (b) In the middle of the larynx, there is a hoarse voice, a breathing dyspnea and an inhalation soft tissue depression.
   (c) People with smaller larynx webbed are usually asymptomatic when they are quiet. They can have a sounding throat, dyspnea or a weak cry when crying.
2. Adults and children usually have no obvious symptoms of laryngeal web. They are prone to fatigue when hoarseness or phonation which occurs occasionally. They may have difficulty breathing when they are active or have respiratory tract infections.

**Diagnosis**

1. The diagnosis can be made according to the symptoms and laryngoscopy.

2. According to the degree of obstruction of the airway, the laryngeal web can be divided into four levels.
   - Grade I: airway obstruction is less than 30%, and web is thin.
   - Grade II: airway obstruction 30–50%, accompanied with sub glottic stenosis.
   - Grade III: airway obstruction 50–75%, accompanied with obvious sub glottic stenosis.
   - Grade IV: complete obstruction of the airway and sub glottic.
3. The disease should be identified with sub glottic obstruction, congenital larynx, congenital tracheal malformation, congenital thymus hypertrophy, and congenital mediastinal large vascular malformation.
4. Children and adults should be identified with diphtheria, lupus, syphilis, tuberculosis, trauma and surgery.

**Treatment**

1. Neonatal congenital laryngeal web caused by asphyxia, immediate laryngoscopy, confirmed after the insertion of bronchoscopy, to achieve first aid and expansion of the role. A satisfactory respiratory and vocal function can be obtained after the dilatation no longer recurs.
2. infants have not yet fully webbed neck fibrosis, after treatment can no longer recurrence, it is confirmed, whether or not have difficulty breathing, should as soon as possible under direct laryngoscope laryngeal dilation.
3. Laryngeal webs of older children and adults have fibrosis and thicker tissue, which requires surgical treatment. There are direct laryngoscopes, supporting laryngoscope, endoscopic laryngeal webbed resection or laser resection, laryngeal fissure, laryngeal webbed resection, laryngeal model expansion, etc.
4. The principle of the treatment of laryngeal web caused by trauma, surgery and intubation is the same as that of the congenital laryngeal web.

### 18.1.3 Congenital Laryngeal Wheezing

Congenital laryngeal wheezing is due to the larynx caused by the softening of the laryngeal cartilage, the soft and relaxed laryngeal tissue, the collapse of the tissue and the small cavity of the throat.

**Etiology**

The causes can be caused by the softening of the laryngeal cartilage, the prolapse of the arytenoid cartilage, the curl or hypertrophy of the epiglottis, and the weakness of the tissue structure.

**Clinical Manifestation**

At birth or shortly after birth, infants have persistent laryngeal ringing and "three concave signs" of suprasternal fossa, supraclavicular fossa and costal space depression. Laryngeal sounds vary in size. Attacks can be indirect or persistent. Symptoms are obvious when crying or eating, and asymptomatic when sleeping or quiet. People with severe symptoms may have difficulty breathing.

**Diagnosis**

If the symptoms are obvious, the initial diagnosis can be made with persistent laryngeal ringing and the sign of "three concave signs". Direct laryngoscopy is feasible for definite diagnosis. Direct laryngoscopy for congenital simple laryngeal wheezing showed that the laryngeal tissue was soft and relaxed. Upper laryngeal tissue curled in the larynx when inhaled and blew out when exhaled. If the laryngeal sound disappeared when the laryngeal tissue would be disgusted or extended to the vestibule with direct laryngoscopy, the diagnosis could be confirmed.

**Treatment**

Patients with mild symptoms can be observed, pay attention to nutrition, actively supplement calcium, use antibiotics rationally in patients with co-infection, and patients with obvious difficulty in inhalation breathing can be treated by tracheotomy or endoscopic removal of congested tissue.

### 18.1.4 Congenital Malformation of Laryngeal Cartilage

The congenital malformation of laryngeal cartilage is generally divided into three types: epiglottis, malformation of thyroid cartilage and malformation of cricoid cartilage.

**Etiology**

1. Epiglottis malformation often causes obstruction of larynx when inhaling, causing wheezing or dyspnea. Generally, no epiglottis can cause clinical symptoms. The two epiglottis often causes wheezing or dyspnea, and the bifurcation of epiglottis usually does not cause clinical symptoms.
2. Thyroid cartilage malformation thyroid cartilage can make the inhalation of cartilage collapse, causing wheezing and obstructive dyspnea, serious can cause laryngeal obstruction or even suffocation.
3. In the embryonic stage of cricoid cartilage malformation, the cricoid cartilage gradually joined in the midline at the ventral and dorsal sides. Congenital laryngeal fissure is

formed if the joint is not good and there are fissures. Congenital laryngeal atresia is also caused by congenital hyperplasia of cricoid cartilage.

**Clinical Manifestation**

1. Epiglottis malformation often causes obstruction of larynx when inhaling, causing wheezing or dyspnea. Generally, no epiglottis can cause clinical symptoms. The two epiglottises often cause wheezing or dyspnea, and the bifurcation of epiglottis usually does not cause clinical symptoms.
2. Thyroid cartilage malformation can cause cartilage collapse during inhalation, resulting in laryngeal ringing and obstructive dyspnea. In severe cases, laryngeal obstruction or even asphyxia may occur.
3. Cricoid cartilage malformation causes congenital laryngeal cleft due to poor fusion; congenital hyperplasia of cricoid cartilage or dysplasia causes obstruction and even asphyxia of the larynx.

**Diagnosis**

A preliminary diagnosis can be made according to the history, clinical symptoms, the diagnosis results for laryngoscopy, because direct laryngoscopy may aggravate airway obstruction occurs, it is not clinically selected, usually choose indirect laryngoscope carefully observe patients supraglottic, epiglottis, vocal cord, laryngeal dysplasia is not.

**Treatment**

1. Deformity of epiglottis: general no symptoms and no need for treatment. Such as the epiglottis bifurcation, breathe easily into the throat, causing difficulty in breathing, free part in laryngoscopy resection of epiglottis; if the epiglottis is too large, easy to inhale absorbed into the throat, cause dyspnea in laryngoscope under partial resection of epiglottis; if the epiglottis too small, it is generally asymptomatic and does not need treatment, but the diet should not be taken too hastily to avoid coughing.
2. Abnormality of thyroid cartilage: tracheotomy is practicable when larynx and obstructive dyspnea are caused.
3. Abnormality of the cricoid cartilage: emergency tracheotomy is required when it causes dyspnea or asphyxia after birthing.

## 18.2 Inflammatory Disease of Larynx

### 18.2.1 Acute Epiglottis

Acute epiglottitis is an acute inflammation mainly in the supraglottic region, also known as supraglottic laryngitis. Inflammation is usually confined to the lingual surface of the epiglottis, or extends to the arytenoid fold, arytenoid cartilage and ventricular zone, but rarely to the vocal cord and the lower glottis (Fig. 18.3). The disease can occur all year round, mostly in early spring and late autumn. Acute onset and rapid progress of the disease is an important disease causing asphyxia in acute upper respiratory inflammation.

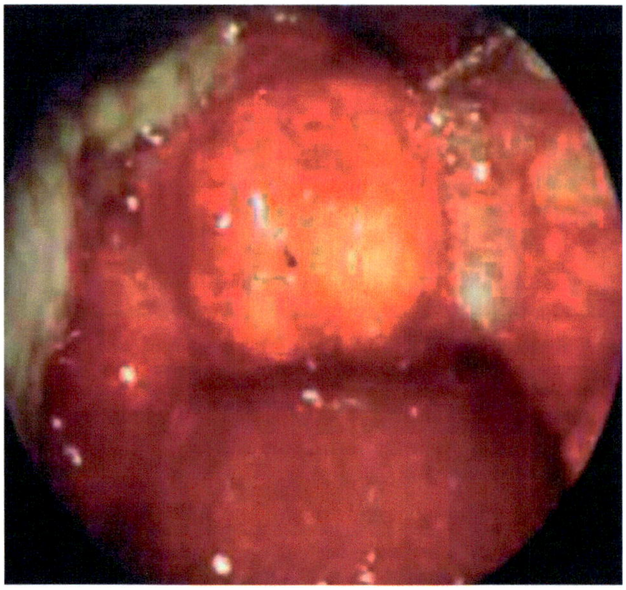

**Fig. 18.3** Acute epiglottis

**Etiology**

The most common causes of the disease are Haemophilus influenzae type B, Staphylococcus, Streptococcus, Streptococcus pneumoniae, Moraxella catarrhalis, Diphtheria-like bacilli and mixed infection with the virus. Secondary infections, foreign body trauma, irritating food, accidental ingestion of chemicals, inhalation of hot or toxic gases and various radiation damage caused by allergy are also the pathogenic factors of the disease.

**Clinical Manifestation**

1. The onset of acute and sudden infants often occurs at night, with a history rarely exceeding 6–12 h. They suddenly feel throat pain or respiratory obstruction in the middle of the night, and their condition progresses rapidly.
2. Fever and chills can occur in adults before the onset of illness. Most of the patients have body temperature of 37.5–39.5° C and a few can reach above 40° C, accompanied by restlessness.
3. Dysphagia is first manifested by sore throat, laborious swallowing, salivary exudation and refusal to eat. Laryngeal pain can be radiated to the jaw, neck, ear and back. The vocalization is normal.

4. Rapid progress of dyspnea: epiglottis congestion, high swelling and deformation, make throat smaller, often cause inspiratory larynx, dyspnea, and can cause laryngeal obstruction and suffocation within 4–6 h.

**Diagnosis**

1. Acute Infectious Epiglottitis: the pain worse acute pharyngache, swallowing, oropharyngeal examination without special disease, or oropharyngeal inflammation although it is not enough to explain the symptoms, consideration should be given to the acute epiglottitis, and indirect laryngoscopy. Pharyngache and dysphagia was the most common symptom of acute epiglottitis in adults, dyspnea, wheezing, hoarseness and salivation occur in critically ill patients. Adult acute epiglottis have slow and rapid onset of. Obstruction of the respiratory tract is mainly seen in the rapid onset, early in the course of the disease, usually within 8 h after the onset of the disease. Early diagnosis is very important because of life threatening. After definite diagnosis, we should carry out the culture of pharynx, epiglottis secretion and blood bacteria and drug sensitivity test, and choose sufficient and sensitive antibiotics.
2. Acute Allergic Epiglottis: Based on symptoms and signs should be asked whether the allergic disease history and family history, generally not difficult to diagnose. The differential diagnosis of both of them is shown in Table 18.1.

**Treatment**

This disease needs early diagnosis and early treatment.

**Table 18.1** Acute inflammative epiglottitis and acute allergic epiglottitis's differentiated diagnosis

| | Acute inflammative epiglottitis | Acute allergic epiglottitis |
|---|---|---|
| Etiology | Bacterium | Allergic reaction |
| Manifestation | Laryngoache | Laryngeal obstruction sensation |
| Pressing pain | At hyoid bone and thyroid bone | None |
| Body temperature | Rise | Normal |
| Lab test | Leukocyte quantity increases,so is neutrophile | Leukocyte decreases or remain normal level,eosnophils increases |
| Local inspection | Epiglottic redness and swelling | Epiglottic edema |
| Treatment | Antibiotics (main) | Glucocorticoid (main) |
| Prognosis | If patients accept antiinflammation treatment actively, prognosis would be good | Sudden asphyxia may occur, and death would happen if don't rescue in time |

1. Anti-infection is often combined with enough sensitive antibiotics and hormones. It can be either intravenous or topical (nebulize or sprayed into the throat).
2. If an abscess is formed, the abscess can be cut under the endoscope, and oxygen is paid attention to, and the aspirator can suck the pus in time.
3. The breathing should be closely observed, and the tracheotomy bag was placed beside the bed. The obstruction of the larynx was aggravated and the tracheotomy was performed in time.
4. Pay attention to oral cleanliness and etiological treatment.

### 18.2.2 Acute Laryngitis

Acute laryngitis refers to acute diffuse catarrhal inflammation in the subglottic area based laryngeal mucosa, also known as acute catarrhal laryngitis, acute respiratory infection is one of the common diseases, accounting for otolaryngology head and neck surgery diseases from 1% to 2%.

**Etiology**

1. Adult Acute Laryngitis
   (a) Infection: It is the main cause of infection, mostly after cold, secondary bacterial infection on the basis of viral infection. Common infectious bacteria are Staphylococcus aureus, Streptococcus hemolyticus, Diplococcus pneumoniae, Moraxella catarrhalis, and influenza bacilli and so on. The positive rates of Moraxella catarrhalis and Haemophilus in adult acute laryngitis secretion culture were 50–55% and 8–15% respectively.
   (b) Laryngeal Trauma: inhaling harmful gases (such as chlorine, ammonia, sulfuric acid, nitric acid, sulfur dioxide, nitric oxide, etc.) and excessive productive dust can cause laryngeal mucosal injury, cause inflammatory substances to exudate, and make laryngeal mucosa swollen and hyperemia. The incidence of acute laryngitis in areas with high concentration of dust, sulfur dioxide and nitric oxide in the air is higher than that in other areas. If the foreign bodies or instruments directly damage the mucous membrane of the larynx, the mucous tissue can be edema.
   (c) Occupation factors such as the use of voice more teachers, actors, salesman, vocal improper or excessive use of the voice, the disease incidence rate is often higher.
   (d) Other: too much alcohol, cold, fatigue caused by lower body resistance easy to induce acute laryngitis. The air humidity changes suddenly, the indoor dry heat is also the inducement. Some studies have suggested that the disease is also related to regional and racial factors.

2. Children's Acute Laryngitis
   (a) Chang Jifa was in acute rhinitis and pharyngitis. Most of the virus is caused by the virus, and the most easily separated is parainfluenza virus (2/3). In addition, there are adenovirus, influenza virus, measles virus etc. After the invasion of the virus, the conditions for secondary bacterial infection were provided. Most of the bacteria infected are Staphylococcus aureus, Streptococcus, Diplococcus pneumonias, etc.
   (b) Children with malnutrition, low resistance, allergic constitution, crowded teeth and chronic diseases such as chronic tonsillitis, adenoidal hypertrophy, chronic rhinitis and chronic sinusitis are easy to induce laryngitis.
   (c) Children's acute laryngitis can also be a prodromal symptom of acute infectious diseases such as influenza, pneumonia, measles, chickenpox, pertussis, scarlet fever, etc.

**Clinical Manifestation**

1. Adult Acute Laryngitis
   (a) Hoarseness is a major symptom of acute laryngitis, more sudden, light sound tone lose round and clear, tone becomes lower and thicker, loudness reduction. Severe patients have hoarseness, dysphonia, even only whispering or completely silent.
   (b) Larynx Pain: there is slight pain in the throat and trachea of the patient. The throat pain is aggravated when cough or sounding. It can also be accompanied by throat discomfort, dryness and foreign body sensation. It can aggravate when cough.
   (c) Increased Cough and Larynx Secretion: at first dry cough without sputum, spasticity, and obvious at night. Later accompanied by bacterial infection with sticky purulent secretions, because thicker, often not easy to produce adhesion on the surface of the vocal cords and aggravating hoarseness.
   (d) General Symptoms: the general symptoms of the general adult are mild and the children are heavier. They can have chills, fever, fatigue, lack of appetite and other symptoms.
   (e) Rhinitis, Pharyngitis Symptom: because the acute laryngitis is mostly acute rhinitis or the acute pharyngitis descending infection, therefore often has the nose, the pharynx's corresponding symptom.
2. Children's Acute Laryngitis
   (a) More acute onset, fever, cough, hoarseness.
   (b) In the early stage laryngeal spasm, hoarseness is not severe, manifested as paroxysmal barking cough or dyspnea, the sticky cough up sputum, repeatedly attack may occur persistent laryngeal obstruction symptoms, such as croup cough, inspiratory stridor. Also the sudden onset of severe hoarseness in children with nocturnal sudden and frequent cough, the sound of a bluff.
   (c) In severe cases, there is an obvious depression in supraclavicular fossa, rib space, sternal fossa and upper abdomen, cyanosis or agitation, slow breathing, 10–15 breaths per minute, and shallow and fast breathing in late stage. If not treated in time and further developed, cyanosis, sweating, pallor, breathlessness, even respiratory and circulatory failure, coma, convulsions and death may occur.

**Diagnosis**

1. Adult Acute Laryngitis: according to the history and laryngoscopy, the diagnosis is not difficult.
2. Children with Acute Laryngitis: according to history, seasonal and specific symptoms such as hoarseness and laryngeal stridor, barking cough, inspiratory dyspnea, preliminary diagnosis. An indirect laryngoscopy for children with a larger age can be used. If a feasible fiberoptic laryngoscope or an electronic laryngoscope examination (Fig. 18.4) is available, the diagnosis of the laryngeal mucosa and vocal band activity in the sober and natural state can be determined. The monitoring of blood oxygen saturation also helps to judge the condition of the disease.

**Treatment**

1. Adult Acute Laryngitis
   (a) Early use of sufficient broad-spectrum antibiotics and glucocorticoid with significant congestion and swelling.
   (b) To give oxygen, spasmodic and phlegm to keep the respiratory tract unobstructed, using ultrasonic atomization of water and oxygen, inhaling or via nasal oxygen. Mucosal dry, add mint, compound tincture of benzoinetc. 0.04% Dequalinium chloride aerosol sprays.

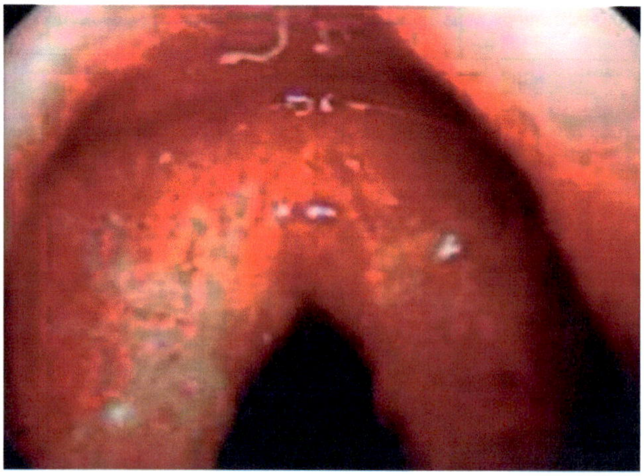

**Fig. 18.4** Acute laryngoedema

(c) Vocal Cord Rest: no sound or less voice.

(d) Nursing and General Support Therapy: regulate indoor temperature and humidity at any time, keep indoor air circulation, drink hot water, and pay attention to loose stool, smoking and alcohol.

2. Children's Acute Laryngitis

(a) The key to the treatment is to relieve the obstruction of the larynx and to use effective and sufficient antibiotics to control the infection. At the same time, glucocorticoids were given, prednisone orally, 1–2 mg/(kg. D), dexamethasone intramuscular injection or intravenous infusion 0.2–0.4 mg/ (kg. D), budesonide suspension 2 ml inhalation. Among 64 children with Acute Laryngitis Treated by various antibiotics alone, 10 cases (15.6%) needed tracheotomy, while only 5 of the 87 cases with glucocorticoids were required for tracheostomy.

(b) To give oxygen, spasmodic and phlegm to keep the respiratory tract unobstructed, and can be inhaled by water oxygen, ultrasonic atomization or through nasal oxygen. If the subglottic dry scab or pseudomembrane and viscous secretions, after the treatment can't relieve dyspnea, can be sucked out by direct laryngoscopy or clamp.

(c) For critically ill patients, intensive care and supportive treatment should be strengthened. Attention should be paid to the balance of body nutrition and water electrolyte, so as to protect lung function and avoid acute heart failure.

(d) Quiet rest, reduces crying, and reduces oxygen consumption.

(e) Tracheotomy should be performed in patients with severe larynx obstruction or the symptoms of larynx obstruction that are not relieved after drug treatment.

## 18.2.3 Chronic Laryngitis

Chronic laryngitis is a chronic nonspecific inflammation of the mucous membrane of the larynx. It can be divided into three types: simple laryngitis, chronic hypertrophic laryngitis and chronic atrophic laryngitis.

**Etiology**

1. Acute laryngitis relapse into chronic laryngitis, virus, bacteria and fungi and other infections can lead to chronic laryngitis.
2. Excessive voice and inappropriate sound production. Chronic laryngitis is commonly seen in many vocation occupations such as teachers and singers. Excessive voice can cause laryngeal mucosal epithelial congestion and exudation, resulting in chronic larynx inflammation.
3. Infection of adjacent organs, stimulating the mucous membrane of the larynx to form a chronic laryngitis. The infection of the nasal, sinus, pharynx, trachea, bronchus and lung is one of the important reasons for the production of chronic laryngitis.
4. Chronic laryngitis can be caused by long-term inhalation of exogenous stimulants such as smoking, dust, harmful gas or working in a high temperature environment.
5. Gastro-esophageal reflux or laryngopharyngeal reflux can cause reflux laryngitis.

**Clinical Manifestation**

1. Hoarseness: the most important and most common symptom of chronic laryngitis. The voice of the patient is low and cannot be pronounced for a long time. Usually the morning with severe symptoms, gradually ease; there are patients with early morning mild symptoms, however, worsening hoarseness after phonating. The degree of hoarseness in the patient was different, however a rare person who had completely lost his voice.
2. Throat secretions increase, cough cough due to pharyngeal foreign body sensation or sputum, atrophic laryngitis patients can cough bloodshot sputum or scab.
3. Larynx Discomfort: discomfort, such as stabbing pain, burning sensation, foreign body sensation, drying feeling, etc.

**Diagnosis**

Symptoms such as long-term hoarseness (more than 3 months) and laryngeal discomfort are usually diagnosed by indirect laryngoscopy or fiberoptic (electronic) laryngoscopy.

1. Chronic Simple Laryngitis: under the microscope, the laryngeal mucosa is congested and swollen, with slight swelling. The vocal cord loses its original Pearl White and turns to pink, with its edge blunted and its vibration weakening when it is voicing. Small vessels and sputum were dilated on the surface of the mucous membrane. The sputum was often made of mucous silk between the glottis.
2. Chronic Hypertrophic Laryngitis: the mucous hypertrophy of the larynx is seen under the microscope. It is chronic hyperemia, usually symmetrical. The mucosa of the inter-ventricular zone and the inter-ventricular zone is more obvious. The anterior part of the vocal cords is not observed under the indirect laryngoscope because of the hypertrophy of the ventricular zone. The vocal cord is thickened and the edge is blunt, and the glottis cannot be completely opened when it is serious.
3. Atrophic Laryngitis: the larynx mucous membrane can be seen dry, thinning and shiny, and the skin of the larynx mucosa can be scab, and the skin can be shallowly erosive. The atrophy of the inner laryngeal muscles and vocal cords can cause the closure of the glottis to form a fissure.

**Treatment**

1. Remove the Cause: it is the key to the treatment of chronic laryngitis. The active treatment of nasal cavity and nasal sinuses, oral and pharyngeal lesions, systemic disease should be treated; strengthen labor protection; avoid contact sensitization leads to chronic allergic pharyngitis; get rid of bad habits, develop good health habits; appropriate physical exercise, enhanced physique, keep healthy and have a regular routine, maintain a good attitude so as to improve their overall immunity.
2. Avoid Long Term Overuse of Sound: full vocal band rest is the most important treatment. In the acute attack period, the sound should be absolutely forbidden. After the inflammation is controlled, a correct training method should be carried out.
3. Atomization inhalation and physiotherapy can inhale gentamicin and dexamethasone to relieve laryngeal discomfort
4. Surgical Treatment: vocal cord edema or excessive hypertrophy. The patients with ineffective etiological treatment may consider excision of the lesion under the laryngoscope. The patients with chronic laryngitis with atypical hyperplasia of mucous membrane or having a tendency to change malignancy should be treated with surgery. Bilateral vocal cord lesions, especially near commissure, postoperative deep breathing; anterior commissure lesions can be staging operation, to prevent the emergence of laryngeal adhesion.

## 18.3 Benign Hyperplasia of Larynx

### 18.3.1 Vocal Nodules

Vocal nodules occur in children, called yelling nodules, and are a smaller fibrous nodular lesion of chronic laryngitis.

**Etiology**

1. The vocal nodules with inappropriate or excessive vocal cords are usually found at the junction of 1/3 of the front of the vocal cord free edge, because it is the midpoint of the vocal cords membrane. The amplitude of the vocal cords membrane is maximum and vulnerable to vibration. It can also produce strong centrifugal force. Frequent impact here during vocal production results in dilatation of interstitial blood vessels, enhanced permeability and increased exudation. Under centrifugal action, exudates gather along with the vocal cords vibration during vocal cords vocalization. There are vibrant nodules and subepithelial blood flow is easy to slow down. The distribution and structure of blood vessels are special, and the upper and lower directions of vocal cord muscles are interlaced. Twisting motion can occur during vocal production, which makes the blood supply change extremely complex.
2. The Upper Respiratory Tract: cold, acute and chronic laryngitis, rhinitis and sinusitis can cause vocal nodules, especially on the basis of the improper use of the voice.
3. Gastroesophageal Reflux: it is reported that gastroesophageal reflux in patients with vocal cord nodules is significantly higher than that of normal people.
4. Endocrine Factors: Is more common in children than in women, and tended to subside by adolescence. The incidence of adult females is higher than that of males. It is rare to be over 50 years old, which may be related to endocrine factors.

**Clinical Manifestation**

The main symptom was hoarseness. In the early stage, the voice is slightly lighter, rough or basically normal, mainly because of the fatigue of pronunciation, frequent use of voice, good or bad, intermittent hoarseness; hoarseness often occurs when pronunciation is high, accompanied by delays in pronunciation and changes in tone color; some patients may not have obvious voice changes in daily conversation, but when singing, the voice range becomes narrower, voice limitation and other obvious manifestations may occur. The condition continues to develop, hoarseness aggravates, and can develop from intermittent to sustained, and also occurs when the voice is low. Hoarseness prevents actors from singing or teachers from giving lectures. Hoarseness is related to the size and location of vocal nodules.

**Diagnosis**

A preliminary diagnosis can be made according to the symptoms and local examination. At the initial stage of laryngoscopy, there were secretions attached to the vocal cords before and at the 1/3 junction and the vocal cords gradually raised and formed a clear nodule. The nodules are generally symmetrical, with a larger side, smaller opposite side or only one side. The nodules of the vocal cords can be limited in small protuberances and can also be thickened in the broad base shuttle form (Fig. 18.5).

**Treatment**

It is mainly vocal cord rest, vocal training, and surgery and drug treatment.

1. Vocal Cord Rest: early vocal cord nodules, after proper vocal cords rest, closed vocal cords, often variable or vanished. Even if a larger knot does not disappear, the sound can also be improved. If the vocal cords rest for 2–3 weeks still have not become smaller, other treatment measures can be taken.

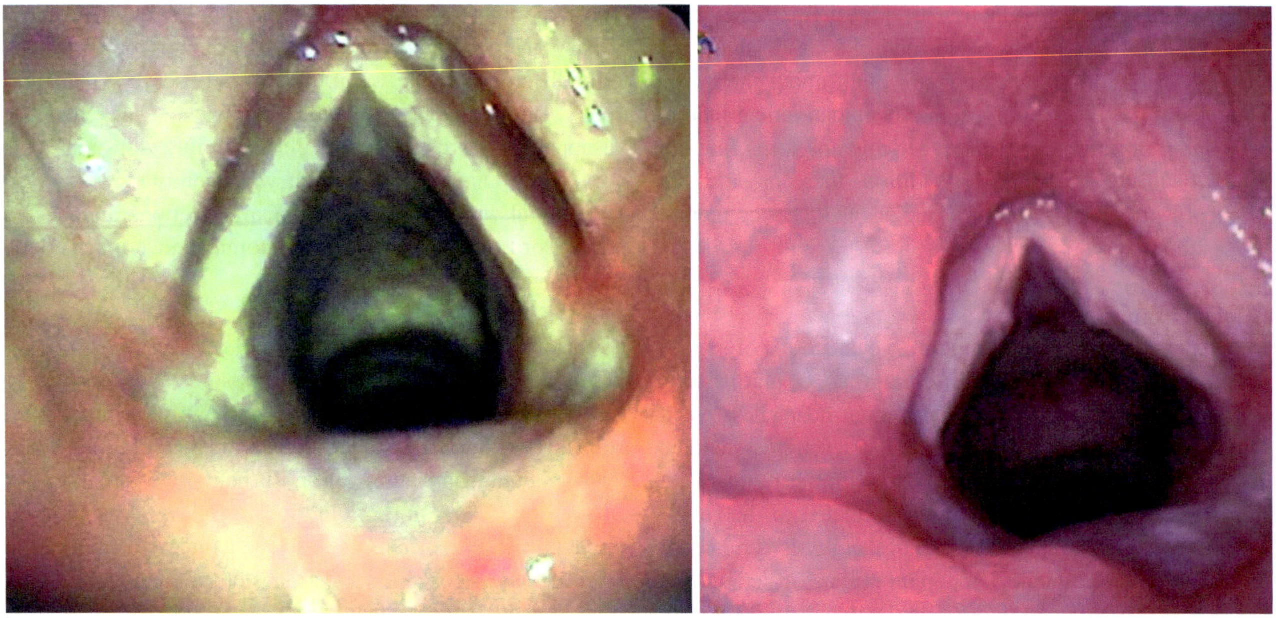

**Fig. 18.5** Symmetric Summary of the Front and Middle 1/3 Junction of Vocal Cord Free Margin

2. Vocal Training: the early smaller vocal cords, after a period of sound training, often disappear by themselves. Vocal training can be adjusted by the airflow, changing the vocal habits and better use of resonance cavity and other methods to improve the efficiency of each organ sound, vibration, resonance, coordination of breath, articulation and other functions, change the original sound with improper habits, ease the tension of the larynx, and ultimately achieve scientific sound.
3. Surgical Resection: large nodules, hoarseness and laryngeal web or obvious, can be removed. The larynx microforceps would be stripped under the surgical microscope, and the laser could be vaporized. Be careful not to damage the vocal cords. After the operation, we should still pay attention to the correct method of phonation, otherwise it relapse and the glucocorticoid should be used properly. Children's nodules are carefully operated on, and the correct method of vocal sound can disappear spontaneously to puberty.

Besides, smoking, alcohol consumption, spicy and stimulating foods should be restricted, coffee and strong tea should be avoided, and the pathogenic factors such as irritating gas and dust should be avoided, especially around the vocal cords.

### 18.3.2 Vocal Cord Polyps

Laryngeal polyps are called vocal polyps, and most of the laryngeal polyps are vocal polyps. The following is the main discussion of vocal polyps.

**Etiology**

At present, the pathogenesis of vocal cord polyps is not clear, and the main pathogenesis is the following.

1. The Theory of Mechanical Trauma: the mechanical action of excessive or improper voice can cause vocal cord vascular dilatation, and local edema is caused by the increase of permeability. Local edema aggravates trauma when vocal cord vibrates, and forms polyps, and further degeneration and fibrosis.
2. Circulation Disorder: animal experiments show that the vibration of the vocal cords when submucosal blood flow is slow, or even stop, a long time can cause excessive vocal cord blood flow continued to decline, local circulation and hypoxia, the increased capillary permeability, local edema and plasma fibrin exudation, severe vascular rupture of hematoma, inflammatory exudate, the final gather precipitate the formation of polyps in the vocal edge; if the reflux disorder, basilar venous and lymphatic polyps gradually widened, the formation of polyps or polypoid degeneration.
3. Inflammation Theory: there is a study that vocal polyps are localized chronic inflammation resulting in mucous congestion and edema.
4. Compensatory Theory: glottis closure may cause polyposis thickening of the vocal cords to strengthen the vocal cord closure, which is mostly diffuse polyposis. In recent years, clinical observations have also confirmed the existence of compensatory polyps.
5. Other Theories: reduce the vocal mucosa superoxide dismutase activity may be related to the formation of pol-

yps; autonomic dysfunction of parasympathetic nerve excitability hyperthyroidism may be associated with polyp formation; some scholars think about the occurrence of vocal cord polyps and local anatomical factors, tongue short, tongue back arched and epiglottis function easily laryngeal polyp. In addition, there are also the theory of vascular nerve barrier and the congenital genetic theory.

**Clinical Manifestation**

Hoarseness is the main symptom, vocal cord polyp size, shape and position of the different tone change, hoarse degree is also different. Mild intermittent hoarseness, vocal fatigue, sounds rough, high difficulty, or even hoarse voice. The size of polyps has nothing to do with the fundamental frequency of pronunciation, which is related to the roughness of the sound quality. The size of the glottis is related to the fundamental frequency. The giant polyp, located on both sides of the vocal cord, can be completely silent, even causing dyspnea and wheezing. Hanging on the person for glottic polyps induced cough.

**Diagnosis**

A preliminary diagnosis can be made according to the symptoms and local examination. A fiberoptic laryngoscope or an electronic laryngoscopy is required if a definite diagnosis is needed. The laryngoscopy shows a smooth, translucent or non-pedicle new creature in the middle of the vocal cords. Polyps are mostly gray or pale red, occasionally purple red, often in the size of green beans or soya beans (Fig. 18.6). The vocal cord polyps are often seen on one side and can occur simultaneously on both sides. The vocal cord polyp with pedicle can move up and down with the air flow, and sometimes it is concealed in the subglottic cavity, and it is easy to ignore. Under the dynamic laryngoscope, the periodic difference of the vocal cords was observed. The symmetry, amplitude, the mucosal wave weakened or disappeared, and the closed phase of the vibration were weakened. Diagnostic attention was identified with vocal cyst, vocal cords leukoplakia, vocal secretions attached to vocal cord and vocal cord carcinoma, and confirmed by pathological diagnosis.

**Treatment**

A polypectomy with good glottis exposure can be performed under indirect laryngoscope, which is mainly surgical resection, supplemented with corticosteroids, antibiotics, vitamins and ultrasonic atomization. If the polyp is small or has a pedicle and does not join in the front, the polypectomy of vocal cord polyps can be performed under the television fiberoptic laryngoscope. Local anesthesia cannot cooperate with patients. Under general anesthesia, tracheal intubation can remove polyps by supporting laryngoscope and suspension laryngoscope. Conditional microsurgical resection or laser microsurgical resection is feasible. The old body weak, the cervical spondylosis and the whole body condition poor, can be excised under the fiberoptic laryngoscope or the radio frequency, microwave treatment.

To avoid the damage of vocal cord muscle in surgery, if bilateral vocal cord polyp, especially near commissural lesions, should do side, both sides at the same time with surgery, should take a deep breath to prevent adhesion. It is difficult to distinguish between the early tumor and the initial polypoid, and the pathological examination should be sent after the resection. The occasional vocal cord polyp coexisted with larynx cancer.

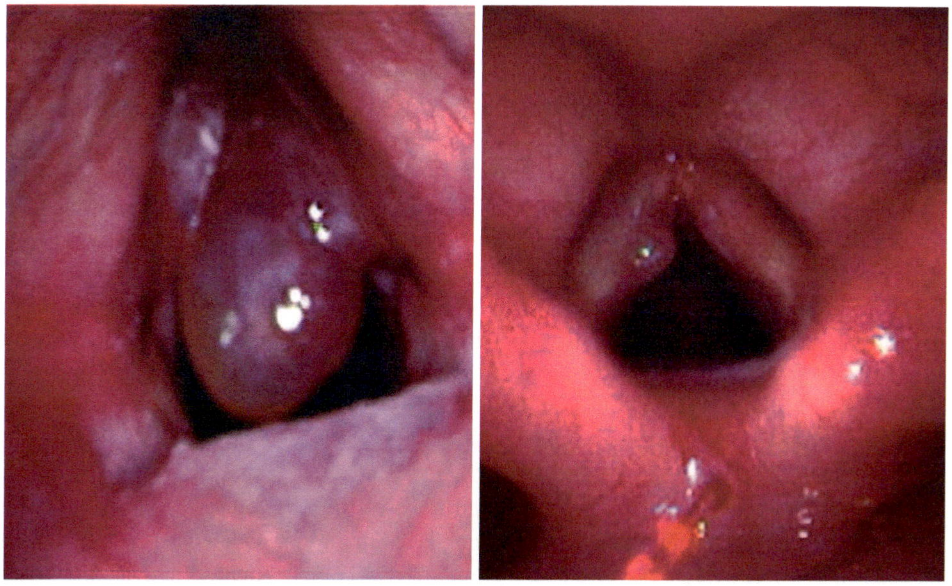

**Fig. 18.6** Vocal cord polyps

## 18.4 Neuropathy of Larynx

It could be divided into the motor neuron disease and the sense nerve disease.

### 18.4.1 Laryngeal Motor Neural Disease

When the laryngeal motion nerve damage occurs, vocal dyskinesia may happen, which include the vocal fold abduction and adduction barrier or myotension flabbiness. The left recurrent laryngeal nerve has a long process and it is close to the flavor lesion tissues and organs, therefore, the left vocal paralysis is commonly seen in clinic.

**Etiology**

According to the neuro damage sites, it could be divided into the central and the peripheral type, and the latter one is the more common type.

1. Central Type

   Bilateral cerebral cortex laryngeal motion Centre has correlated nerve bundles with bilateral nucleus ambiguus, therefore, each lateral muscle all accept bilateral cranial impulses and eventually cause the cortex lesion caused laryngeal paralysis rarely seen in clinic. The cerebral hemorrhage, the foundation basement aneurism, the postcranial fossa inflammation, the oblongata and the pons tumor can all evoke the vocal paralysis. It could be differentiated diagnosed by cranial CT scan or MRI examination.
2. Peripheral Type

   It includes the laryngeal paralysis caused by the lesion at any labyrinth regions after leaving the jugular foramen before dividing into the recurrent laryngeal nerves. The cranial fundamental base fracture, the thyroid surgery, varieties of the cervical and the laryngeal trauma, the benign and the malignant laryngeal, cervical or cranial basal tumor compression,the mediastinal or the esophagus metastasis tumor, the rhinopharyngeal cancer's invasion to the cranial base, the pulmonary apex tuberculosis adhesion, the pericarditis and the peripheral neuritis can all evoke the vocal paralysis. By the imaging and the endoscopy, the lesion can be found or the differentiated diagnosis can be ascertained (Table 18.1).

**Clinic Manifestations and Examinations**

1. Unilateral Incomplete Paralysis

   It is mainly the vocal extension disorders, who manifest unobviously. Unilateral vocal line is close to the middle under laryngoscope, extension can't be done while inhaling, however the vocal motion can be finished while phonating (Fig. 18.7).
2. Unilateral Complete Paralysis

   The affected side vocal cords' extension and adduction function disappears. The vocal cords fix in the paracentral sites, the ante-verted arytenoid cartilage, the lower affected side vocal than the unaffected side and the closed vocal and the hoarseness and weakened voice while phonating can be found during investigating (Figs. 18.8 and 18.9).
3. Bilateral Incomplete Paralysis

   It is rare, mostly due to thyroid surgery or laryngeal trauma. Both sides of the vocal cords cannot be abducted but close to the midline. The glottis is small fissures. The patient can be asymptomatic when he is calm, but he often feels difficult to breathe when he is physically active. Once there is an upper respiratory tract infection, severe dyspnea can occur.
4. Bilateral Complete Paralysis

   Bilateral vocal cords both locate at the paramid site; without any adduction ability and any abduction ability;

**Table 18.1** Relationship between the vocal muscles and the dominant nerves

| Vocal muscles | Muscular functions | Dominant muscles | Vocal paralysis | Vocal paralysis positions |
|---|---|---|---|---|
| Posterior cricoarytenoid muscle | Extentor, monitoring to open glottis | Recurrent laryngeal nerve dominates, post current laryngonerve lesion is more commonly seen | Extension disorders is the most common manifestation | When the extentor paralyses, the vocal cords fix in the mid-center |
| Arytenoid muscle, lateral cricoarytenoid muscle | Abductor muscle, monitoring to close glottis | Recurrent laryngeal nerve dominates | Abduction function disorder | Abduction impairment while phonating, glottis dysraphism |
| Thyroarytehoid muscle,cricothyroid muscle | Thyroarytehoid muscle: Shorten and loosen the vocal cords while contracting and lengthen and tensen the vocal cords while relaxing? | Suplaryngeal nerve dominates the cricothyoid muscle and the recurrent laryngeal nerve dominates the thyroarytehoid muscles | Cricothyoid muscular paralysis: is the vocal cord loosens and contracts in length and size, the unilateral affected glottis deflection occurs; thyroarytehoid muscular paralysis: if the vocal cords loosens and lengthens, unilateral unaffected glottis deflection occurs. | Suplaryngeal nerve unilateral paralysis can display that the vocal anterior commissure deflects to the affected side and the abduction and the adduction are both normal |

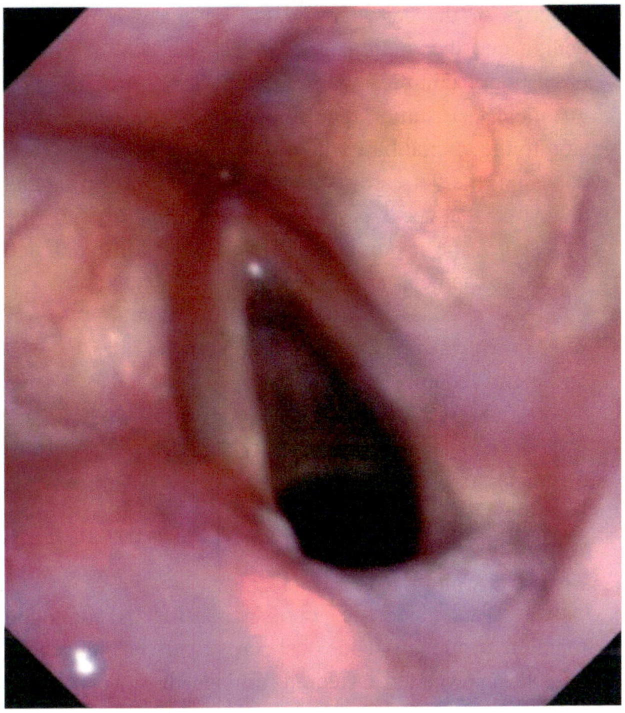

**Fig. 18.7** Left vocal extension paralysis, fixing at the mid-central site (inhaling diagram)

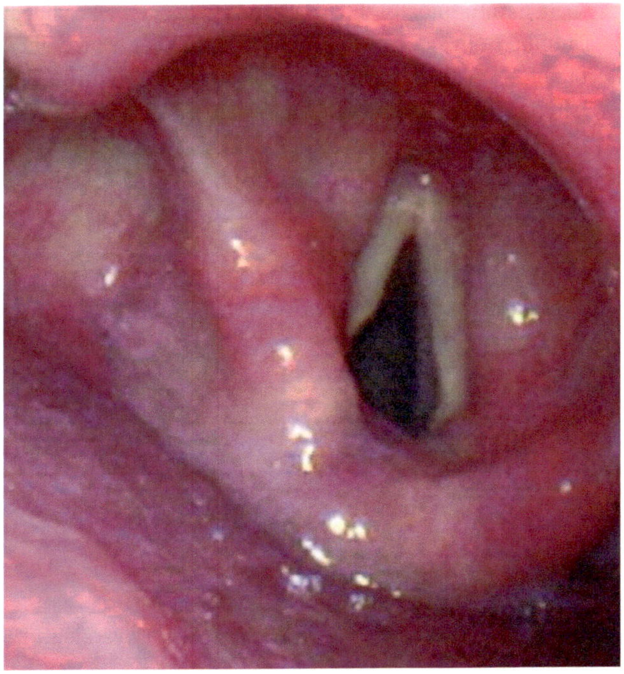

**Fig. 18.8** Completely paralyzed left recurrent laryngeal nerve (mid-central vocal cords)

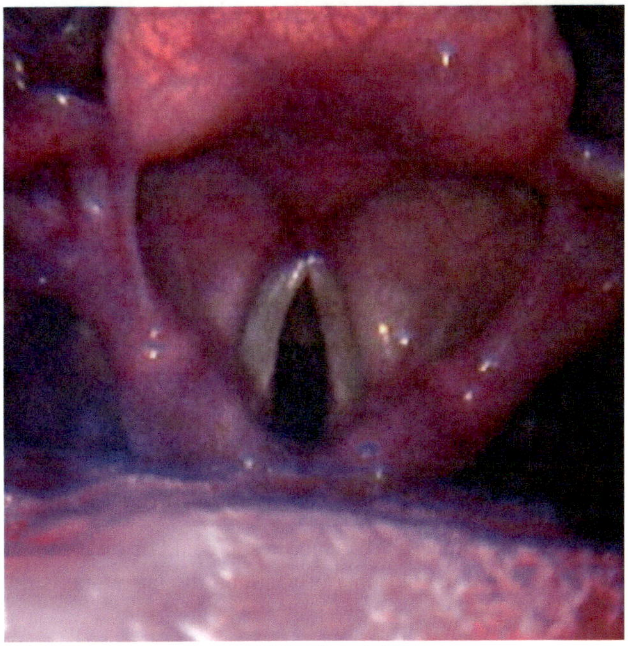

**Fig. 18.9** Left laryngeal recurrent complete paralysis and superior laryngeal nerve paralysis. (Para-median vocal cord) Left vocal cord tension is reduced and arched

hoarse and weak phonation; normal respiration, however food or saliva could be strayed into the lower respiratory tract and cause bucking.

5. Bilateral Vocal Cords Adduction Paralysis

   Bilateral adductive paralysis of vocal cords is more common in functional aphasia. Vocal cords cannot be adduction during vocal production, but cough sounds (Fig. 18.10).

**Diagnosis**

According to the history, clinical manifestations, indirect laryngoscopy, endoscopy and laryngeal electromyography, the diagnosis can be made. Among them, laryngeal electromyography is of great significance for differential diagnosis. In the patients with recurrent laryngeal nerve palsy, the motor unit potential of the affected cricothyroid muscle and the contralateral internal laryngeal muscle are normal, and the recruitment potential would be disturbed or slightly active; in the patients with complete nerve injury, the motor unit potential of the affected cricothyroid muscle and the posterior cricoarytenoid muscle rested without recruitment potential; in the patients with incomplete nerve injury, the normal motor unit potential of the affected cricothyroid mus-

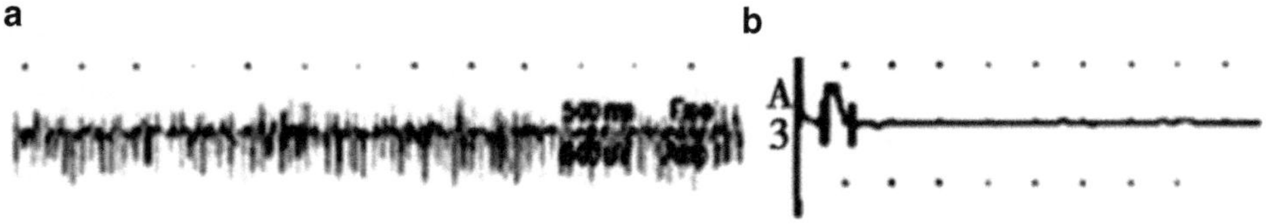


**Fig. 18.10** Laryngorecurrent nerve incompletely damaged patients' affected side thyroarytenoid electromyogram. (**a**) Raising potentials (longitudinal graduation: 500 μV; transverse graduation: 500 ms) (**b**) induced neuropotential: stimulating the affected laryngorecurrent nerve, stimulation intensity: 14.0 mA (longitudinal graduation: 1 mV, transverse graduation: 10 ms)

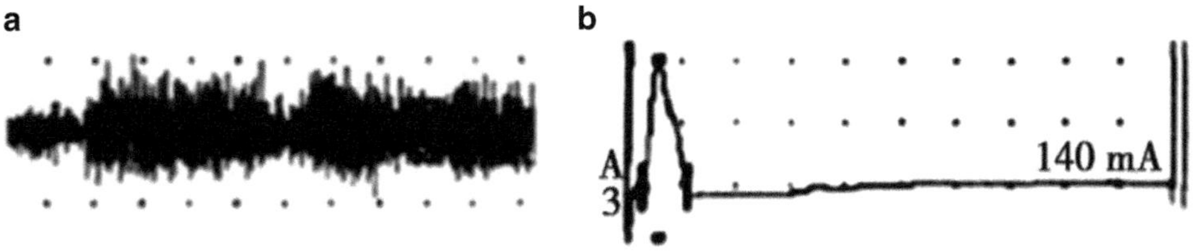


**Fig. 18.11** Cricoarytenoid articulardyskinesia patients' thyroarytenoid electromyogram. (**a**) Raising potentials (longitudinal graduation:500 μV; transverse graduation: 500 ms) (**b**) induced neuropotentials: stimulating affected side recurrent laryngeal nerve, stimulation intensity:14.0 mA (longitudinal graduation:1 mV;transverse graduation:5 ms) [2, 3]

cle and the posterior cricoarytenoid muscle are mixed with denervation potential or regeneration potential, and the recruitment potential was presented. Simple or mixed phase range in the affected side (Fig. 18.11).

**Treatment**

1. Unilateral Lesion

   To the unilateral incomplete paralysis, if phonation and respiratory function is fine, apply drug therapy like the neurotrophic drugs, the glucocorticoid, the vasodilator drugs, etc.; to the unilateral complete paralysis, if the compensatory doesn't effect for a long time and patients ask for improving phonation at the meanwhile, sublaryngomucosally inject Teflon, soluble collagenous fiber or fat to expand the vocal cords and finally draw close to the midline.
2. Bilateral Lesion

   To the bilateral extension paralysis, if dyspnea occurs, apply the tracheotomy then correct surgically, such as the arytenocartilage excision or the vocal out shift surgery. The type I thyrodectomy and other operations can also be applied.
3. Most available method to restore the vocal automatic motion and rebuild the laryngeal function is laryngoneuroreinnervation surgery: neuroanastomosis, re-innervation and neuromuscular transplantation.

### 18.4.2 Laryngeal Sensory Nerve Disease

It mainly contains the laryngohypersensitivity, the laryngoparaesthesia, the hypolaryngosis, the laryngoanesthesia etc. The laryngosensory nerve disorder mostly accompanies with dyskinesia, therefore single sensory nerve disorders is rarely seen. The laryngeal hypersensitivity is the enhanced sensitivity to the common stimulations, such as when the food and saliva contract the larynx, it may cause the bucking and the laryngospasms; the laryngeal paraethesia is the spontaneous throat itchy, burning sensation, pain, dryness, foreign mass sensation or other abnormal sensations. Laryngosensory nerve diseases are mostly evoked by the labyrinth reflex caused by the acute or chronic laryngeal inflammation, the long-term alcohol and (or) tobacco addiction and the adjacent organ diseases; they are also commonly seen in the patients who have the neurasthenia, the hysteria, the anemia, the climacteric, etc. as well the personnel who use larynx more, such as singer, teacher, ticket seller, etc.

**Etiology**

It is commonly caused by the chronic stimulation, the long-term alcohol and (or) tobacco addiction, the adjacent organs lesion, such as the rhinal sinusitis evokes the manifestations by the labyrinth nerve reflex; and the hysteria, the menopause period, the neurasthenia and the personnel who use throat more.

**Clinical Manifestation**

The main manifestations are itching of larynx, foreign body sensation, tingling sensation, ant crawling sensation, discomfort sensation and swelling sensation. Individual sensation is different, mainly foreign body sensation in pharynx, so coughing and swallowing frequently are performed. Even a slight irritation causes a stronger cough.

**Diagnosis**

Initial diagnosis could be made based on the disease history and the clinic manifestations; however the differentiated diagnosis requires a direct or indirect laryngoscopy. However, there are no obvious abnormalities under laryngoscope.

**Treatment**

1. Etiologic treatment: such as removal of adjacent organ lesions, rhinitis, sinusitis, dental disease, etc.
2. Mental: Elimination of mental burden should be considered when specific lesions can not be found in psychotherapy.
3. Closure of superior laryngeal nerve, bilateral mandibular angle and strengthening of neuronutrition when necessary.

## 18.5 Benign Laryngeal Tumor

### 18.5.1 Laryngeal Papilloma

Laryngeal papilloma is a benign tumor of the larynx, which is more common in clinic. Although laryngeal papilloma is histologically benign, it has the characteristics of multiplying and easy recurrence, which can easily cause respiratory obstruction. Multiple operations can cause laryngeal stenosis and dysphonia.

**Etiology**

Currently, human papilloma virus (HPV) infection and chronic irritation are considered to be related, especially HPV16 and HPV18 [4].

**Clinical Manifestation**

The mostly common manifestation is progressive hoarseness. When the tumor is relatively big, the laryngostridor even the aphonia may happen and the severe tumor may cause dyspnea.

**Diagnosis**

The typical symptoms were progressive hoarseness, wheezing and dyspnea. Combined with the history of disease and laryngoscopy, multiple or single reddish or dark red, uneven surface, cauliflower or papillary tumors can be initially diagnosed (Fig. 18.12), and confirmed by pathological examination. Much attention should be paid to multi-site involvement, even spread out of the larynx. CT scan is helpful for diagnosis (Fig. 18.13).

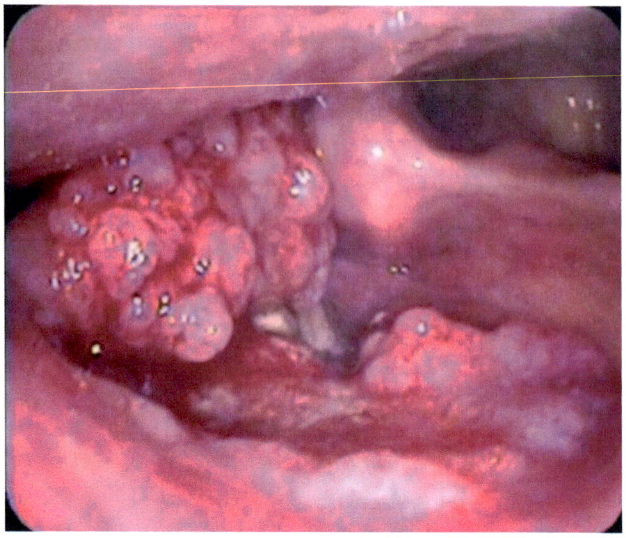

**Fig. 18.12** Laryngopapilla tumor

The right vocal cord is thickened, with nodular protrusions (shown by red arrows), and the surgical pathology is right laryngeal papilloma.

**Treatment**

Commonly, it needs operation and assist with drugs including several antiviruses and the immunity treatment among which the interferon can help adjust the immunity system function against the virus and inhibit the cellular proliferation and eventually decrease the relapse. When the laryngostasis is bit severe, firstly apply the tracheotomy and then extirpation surgery or laser excision. Recent years, America and European Union are approved to use the HPV vaccine to inject at the younger age to prevent the HPV infection.

### 18.5.2 Laryngeal Angioma

**Etiology**

Laryngeal hemangioma is usually congenital, and is common in children. Larger laryngeal hemangiomas are highly dangerous.

**Clinical Manifestation**

In infants Children often occur in the subglottic region, often asymptomatic, and paroxysmal dyspnea occurs when crying. Figure 18.14 Hemangioma of the right larynx.

Whiles in adults it often occurs in the glottic region or supraglottic region. Common symptoms include hoarseness, cough and hemoptysis.

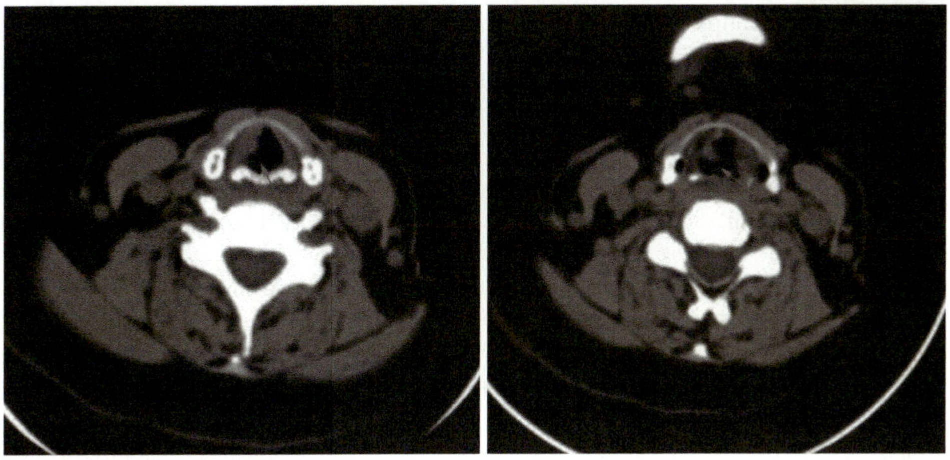

**Fig. 18.13** Right laryngopapilla tumor axial plane CT scan

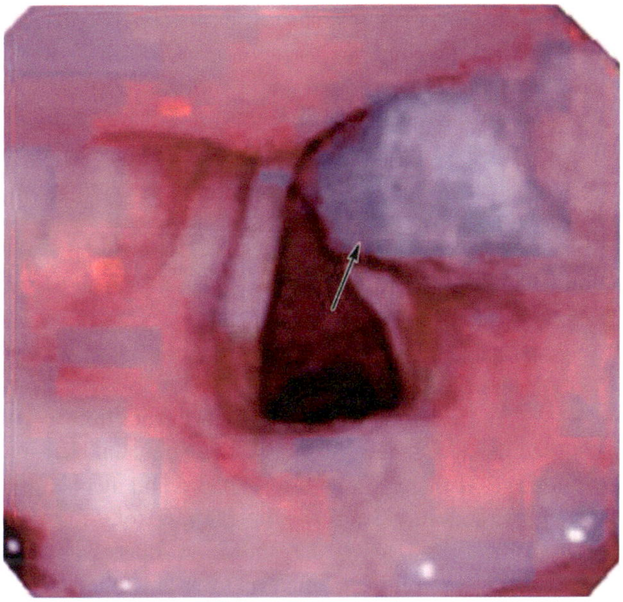

**Fig. 18.14** Right laryngeal angioma

**Diagnosis**

The tumors in infants are mostly small and asymptomatic. Larger tumors can be delayed to the neck and appear purple-blue subcutaneously. Severe tumors can cause hemoptysis, laryngeal obstruction and even asphyxia. Laryngoscopic examination showed that the tumors were soft as sponges and diffused under the mucosa of the ventricular band, laryngeal chamber and arytenoid epiglottic fold. They were dark red with uneven surface (Fig. 18.14). Adult laryngoscopy showed that tumors grew in the vocal cords, pedicled or sessile, red or light purple, with varying sizes, and could also occur in other parts of the larynx. MRI plain scan can help to clarify the extent of tumors and their relationship with surrounding tissues. Tissue biopsy is not recommended for this disease, which can easily lead to massive hemorrhage.

**Treatment**

If the tumor is relatively bigger and accompanies with hemoptysis, it is suitable to apply the tracheotomy and excise the tumor under the laryngeal fissure or the laser surgery or the frozen surgery under the self-retaining microlaryngoscope. Notice on hemostasis to avoid the blood flowing into trachea and bronchus.

### 18.5.3 Laryngeal Fibroneuroma

**Etiology**

Neurofibroma is a benign neoplasm commonly seen in skin and subcutaneous tissue. It originates from the supporting connective tissue of nerve sheath cells and mesenchymal tissue. It can occur in any part of nerve trunk and nerve end. Laryngeal neurofibroma occurs in the larynx.

The pathogenesis of neurofibroma is not clear, mainly due to genetic factors. In 1987, the National Institutes of Health (NIH) established that neurofibroma is related to gene mutations of autosomal NF1 (peripheral neurofibromatosis) and NF2 (central fibromatosis), which are associated with autosomal dominant inheritance.

**Clinical Manifestation**

Its main early manifestation is the laryngeal foreign mass sensation, and the dilation sensation may occur when the tumor magnifies. If the tumor continues enlarging, the tumor may involve the vocal cords and cause hoarseness or coughing even dyspnea.

**Diagnosis**

Its physical signs are not obvious, common examinations can't help diagnose, therefore, consulting cautiously the family history could differentiate diagnosis. The tumor mostly occurs at the arytenoepiglottis folds, and it may be seen at the ventricular bands. Under the indirect laryngoscope, single or multiple enveloped round dense lumps. The immune-histochemical S100 and positive DSE can help diagnose.

**Treatment**
It is benign, developing slowly; therefore, surgical excision is the main treatment.

## 18.6 Malignant Laryngoma

Laryngeal carcinoma is the second commonly seen cervicocranial cancer, most of which is the squamous cell cancer, which occupies over 95%.Other pathogenic types contain the sarcoma, the sarcocarcinoma, the neuroendocrine carcinoma, the adenocystic carcinoma, the malignant lymphoma, etc.

**Etiology**
Its exact etiology isn't entirely clear, which may be tobacco, drinking, air pollution, human papillovirus infection, genetic factors, microelements deficiency etc. Recently, most scholars suggest to divide the cervicocranial squamous cell cancer into the HPV related and the HPV uncorrelated head and neck squamous cell carcinoma (HNSCC), currently, there are nine valent HPV vaccines in Europe and the United States for the prevention of HPV related head and neck cancer. The laryngocancer morbidity differs all over the world, and its ordinary annual incidence is 2/0.1 million 5/0.1 million, however at those high prevalence area, such as Poland, Italy, Bulgaria, northeast and north China, etc., its annual incidence is 34/0.1 million [5].

Laryngeal original embryonic base combines the bilateral sided to the midline during developing, therefore, the left and right larynx have a relative anatomy barrier in the mid-line. The early tumor limits unilaterally. Based on the contents, larynx is constituted with the cartilage support, the muscles, the nerves and the epimucosal tissues; mucosa is the pseudo stratified firbrocolumnar epithelium of the upper respiratory tract, having the mucus secretion function. Based on the structure, larynx is constituted with epiglottis, ventricular bands, vocal cords, arytenoepiglottis folds, etc. From up to down, larynx is divided into supraglottis, glottis and subglottis sites; there is ventricle of larynx between the ventricular bands and the vocal cords, upper from whose bottom there is the ventricular bands, the epiglottis, the pre-epiglottis interval and the arytenoepiglottis folds, all above also locate at the supralaryngeal sites, therefore, where they locate is called supraglottis; bilateral vocal cords and the anterior and the inferior commissure locates at the glottis plane, therefore, where they are is called the glottis area; sites from the inferior free vocal cords edge till the inferior cricocartilage edge are called the subglottis area. and mucosa and submucosal structures differ from other areas. At the supraglottis area, mucosal membrane is related thicker, the submucosal tissue is loose and the lymph tissues are abundant, all of which also cause the supraglottis area is related easier to happen the lymphatic metastasis; at the glottis area, the submucosa lacks the lymph tubes, therefore, at this area is not easy to happen the lymphatic metastasis; the subglottis mucosa is similar to the glottis area, under the subglottis mucosa is cartilage and lacks the submucosal tissues.

**Pathogenesis**
Laryngeal cancers occupy 95% of the squamous cell cancers which originate from the epimucosa, and they can also be the sarcomas those originate from the muscles, the cartilage, or the neuroendocrine carcinoma, etc. most of those above are exogeneity cauliflower and a few are ulceration invasion; supraglottis laryngocancer could invade through the anterior commissure, the paraglottis intervals or the arytenoepiglottis folds to the glottis area; the laryngocancers which originate from the laryngeal ventriculus could simultaneously extend to the upper and the lower and constitute the transglottic laryngocancer. According to research, the ulcerative laryngocancer has higher invasiveness than the exogeneity cauliflower laryngocancer.

**Clinical Manifestation**

1. Symptoms
   (a) Hoarseness
   At the laryngocancer which originate from vocal cords, hoarseness is the manifestation at its early stage. If there is long term tobacco and alcohol history and the hoarseness doesn't restore for over 1 month, the laryngeal examination is necessary, and during examination, if neoplasms are found at the vocal cords, biopsy is timely vital. When the moderate or late supraglottis or subglottis laryngocancer involves the vocal cords, the hoarseness may occur as well.
   (b) Pharyngeal Foreign Mass
   It is often the early manifestation of the supraglottis laryngocancer, it lessens while deglutition and the deglutition obstruction sensation may occur when the tumor is related bigger; When the supraglottis cancer involves the tongue root; the deglutition pain occurs and radiates to the ipsilateral ear.
   (c) Cough and Blood Strained Snot
   Tumors evoke coughing, the tumor surface breaks up and bleeds, which may cause the bloodstrained snot and at the late stage, the tumor invades the peripheral blood vessels and cause hemorrhage.
   (d) Dyspnea
   At late laryngeal cancer, the tumor obstructs the glottis, causing the laryngostenosis, and finally evokes dyspnea. Most manifestation is inspiratory dyspnea.

2. Laryngoscopy
   (a) Laryngeal Neoplasm

   Under the indirect or fibrous laryngoscope, rough dull red tumor, rising from the laryngomucosa, could be seen; there may be ulcers on the tumor surface or accompanying with bloody secretion adhesion on the tumor surface. Moderate advanced laryngocancer may be with vocal fixation (Figs. 18.15 and 18.16).

   (b) Laryngeal Swellings

   Supraglottis laryngeal cancer or advanced laryngeal cancer often has lymph node enlargement at the anterior and inferior mandibular angle. If the lymph node enlarges, it will not shrink after 1 week of anti-infection treatment. In addition, patients with hoarseness should be suspected of laryngeal cancer and undergo a comprehensive examination (Figs. 18.17 and 18.18).
3. Imaging
   (a) CT

   Enhanced CT can show the tumors and metastatic lymph nodes more clearly. Soft tissue with slight enhancement in the laryngeal cavity is seen. There are no clear boundaries. If lymph node metastasis occurs, there may be enlarged lymph nodes in the 2–4 regions of the neck. On enhanced CT, there may be "ring-like" changes with decreased central density and enhanced margins (Fig. 18.19).

   (b) MRI

   MR imaging has a higher resolution than CT in soft tissue. It can observe the changes of thyroid cartilage bone marrow in early stage to determine the small invasion of thyroid cartilage. It is of certain significance for early glottic carcinoma to have cartilage involvement in anterior commissure. On contrast-enhanced magnetic resonance imaging, the tumors

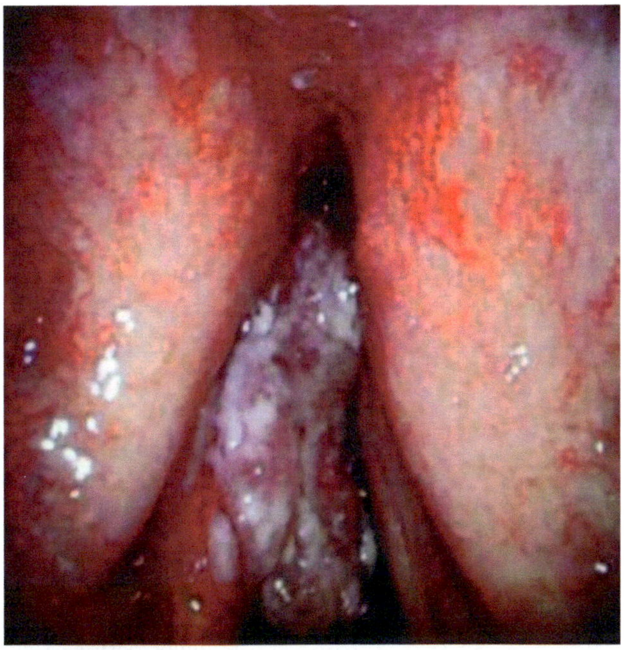

**Fig. 18.15** Right vocal cords cancer, involving the anterior commisure

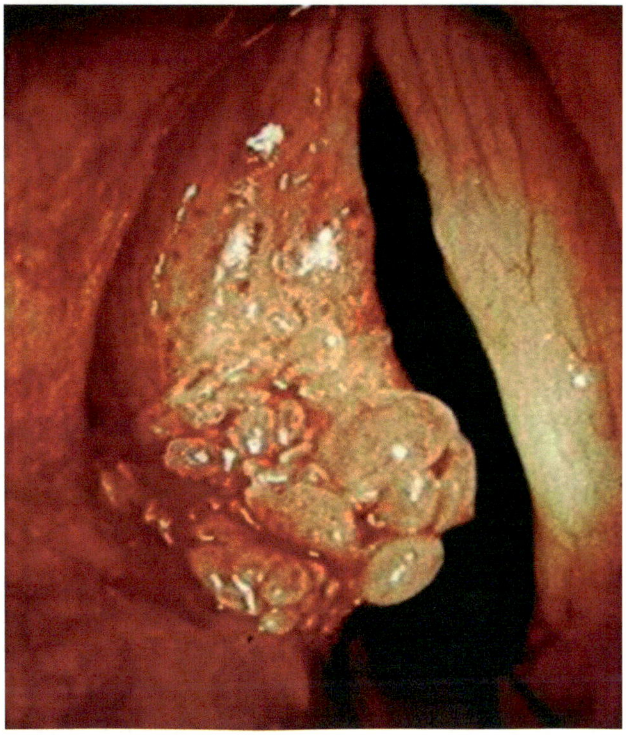

**Fig. 18.16** Left vocal cords cancer

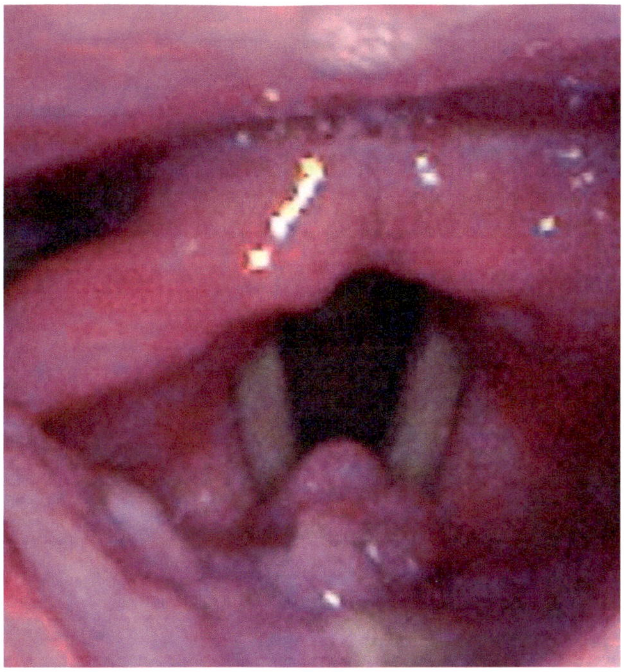

**Fig. 18.17** Laryngeal neoplasm

showed slightly to moderately enhanced high-intensity images on T1 and T2 weighted images (Fig. 18.20). Bone marrow signals of thyroid cartilage also changed when thyroid cartilage was involved.

**Diagnosis**

Accompanying with clinic manifestations and imaging examination results, it's not hard to diagnose the laryngocarcinoma, however the differentiated diagnosis still need the pathologic biopsy result.

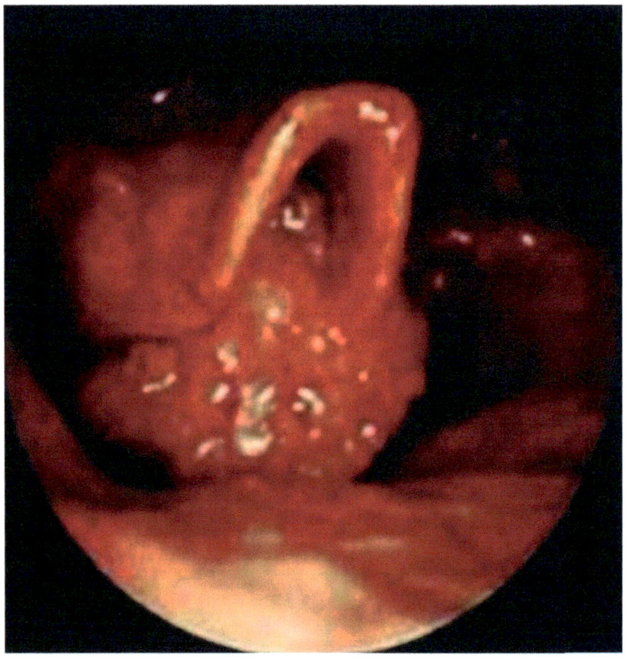

**Fig. 18.18** Supraglottis laryngocancer under laryngoscope

1. TNM Gradings (Table 18.2)
2. Differentiated Diagnosis
   (a) Laryngopapilla Tumor

   Laryngopapilla tumor is evoked by the human papilla tumor virus infection commonly and it manifests as mulberry like dark red neoplasm (Fig. 18.21) and often without ulcers. The tumor is large, however there is no vocal fixation existing. Tumor biopsy can help ascertain the laryngopapilla tumor.

   (b) Chronic hypertrophic laryngitis and vocal hyperplasia

   Chronic hypertrophic laryngitis can cause the hypertrophic vocal cords, manifesting as uniform hypertrophic dark red vocal mucosa, with (or without) rough membrane and it needs biopsy to ascertain diagnosis.

   (c) Laryngeal Tuberculosis

   It displays the laryngeal mucosal ulcerations and the ulcer edges may slightly rise up because the ulcerations are almost deep. Typical clinic manifestations are that the evident laryngalgia and aggravated pain while deglutition.

   (d) Laryngeal Amyloidosis

   It often has long-term history, slow lesion progression. Its clinic manifestations are similar to the laryngeal cancer and its laryngoscopy could be laryngocavum dark-red tumor with various heights, related-more pervading and with unclear boundary.

   (e) Vocal Leukoplakia

   It is the leukoplakia produced at the vocal epimucosal keratinized hypertrophy and overly keratinization (Fig. 18.22) and it is often recognized as pre-cancer lesion, which need to be cautiously observed.

**Fig. 18.19** Enhanced axial CT scan displays left vocal cords cancer. (**a**) Tumor lesions left vocal cords and anterior commissure (arrow), no thyroid cartilage lesion; (**b**) left cervical lymphatic swellings, evidently enhanced peripheral sites and relatively badly enhanced center, 'ring-like' change (arrow)

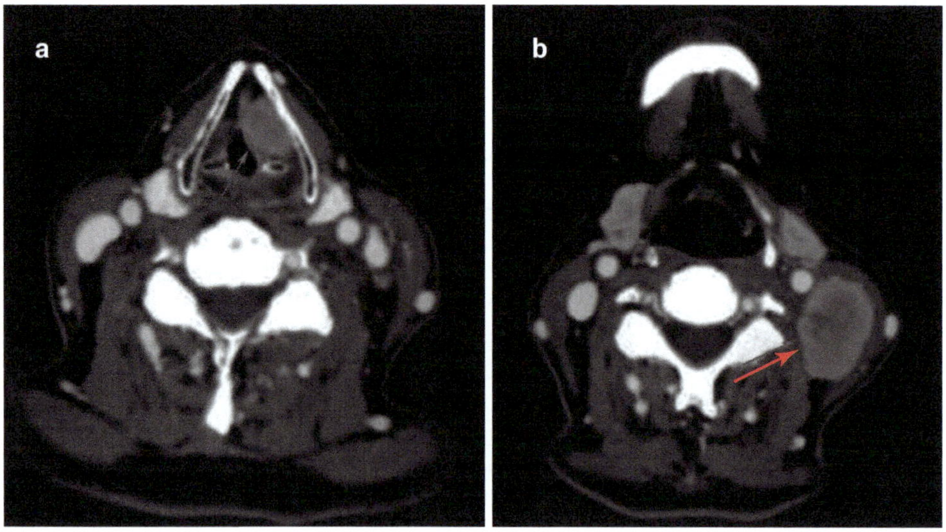

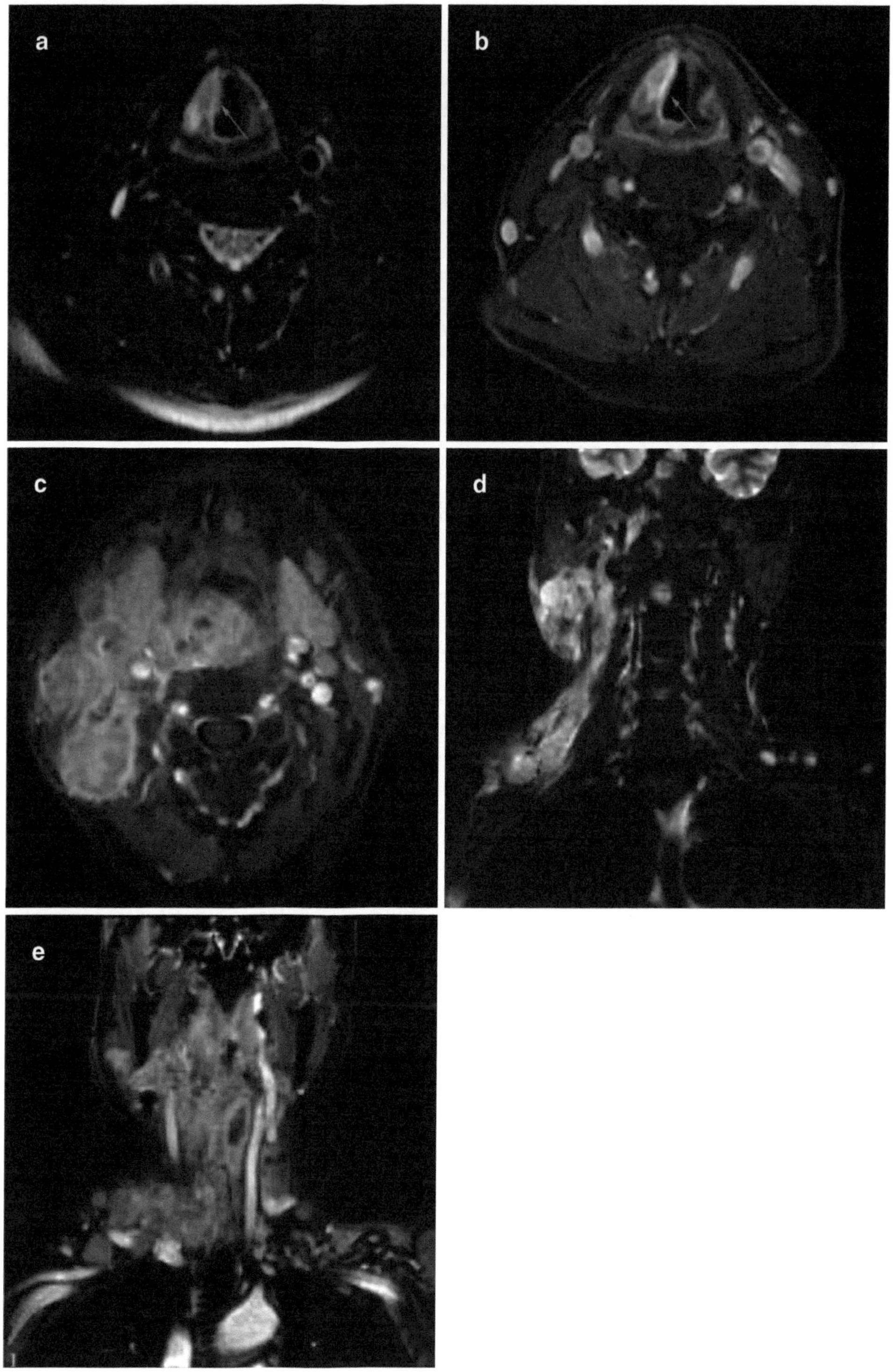


**Fig. 18.20** Axis T2 WI plain scan and axial and coronal T1WI enhanced scan images for laryngeal cancer. (**a**, **b**) Stage T1 glottic laryngeal cancer. Tumors only involve the right vocal cords, which show localized thickening and enhancement (shown by arrows). Tumors transcend the midline and thyroid cartilage (**c**–**e**). Stage T4 laryngeal cancer. Tumors involve the glottic region, supraglottic and subglottic regions; invade thyroid cartilage and extralaryngeal tissues: soft tissue of the right neck, ribbon muscles, thyroid gland and anterior intervertebral space, but not after enhancement. Homogeneous strengthening

**Treatment**

Laryngeal cancer treatment is often based on the cancer stages, the patients' constitution and requesting to living quality, etc., and it include the surgery, the radiotherapy, the chemotherapy, the biotherapy and other methods.

1. Early Lesion ($T_1$ and partial $T_2$ lesion)

To the early lesion, surgery and radiotherapy are both practicable, which have similar 5-year survival rate, 85–90%, between which the differences are the post-operation phonation quality and treatment fees. Surgery

**Table 18.2** Seventh edition AJCC larngnocancer TNM gradings in 2010

| | | |
|---|---|---|
| *Primary tumor (T)* | | |
| $T_x$ | | No evaluation on primary tumor |
| $T_0$ | | No primary tumor evidence |
| $T_{is}$ | | Carcinoma insitu (CIS) |
| Supraglottic carcinoma | $T_1$ | Tumor limits at a glottis sub-region, normal vocal cords motion |
| | $T_2$ | Tumor invade one or more adjacent glottis sub-regions, glottis region or external supraglottic region (tongue root, eipglottic vallecula, intra-piriform recess membrane), no laryngeal fixation |
| | $T_3$ | Tumor limits in larynx with vocal cords fixation and (or) invasion to any sites behind: postcriocoid region, pre-epiglottis interval, paraglottis interval and (or) thyroid cartilage intraplate |
| | $T_{4a}$ | Moderate late partial diseases<br>Tumor invade through the thyroid cartilage and (or) the outer largngeal tissues [such as trachea, cervical soft tissues (including the deep extrinsic lingual muscles), ribbon muscles, thyroid gland or esophagus] |
| | $T_{4b}$ | Very late partial disease<br>Tumor invades the prevertebral fascia, circling the cervical arteries or invading the mediastinal |
| Glottic carcinoma | $T_1$ | Tumor limits at vocal cords (may invade the anterior or posterior commissure), normal vocal cords motion |
| | $T_{1a}$ | Tumor is limited at unilateral vocal cord |
| | $T_{1b}$ | Tumor invade bilateral vocal cords |
| | $T_2$ | Tumor invade the upper and (or) lower glottic regions with (or without) limited vocal cords motion |
| | $T_3$ | Tumor limits in larynx with vocal cords fixation and (or) invasion at the paraglottic intervals and (or) thyroid cartilage intraplate |
| | $T_{4a}$ | Moderate late partial diseases<br>Tumor invades through the thyroid cartilage and (or) invades the outer laryngeal tissues [such as trachea, cervical soft tissues (including the deep extrinsic lingual muscles), ribbon muscles, thyroid gland or esophagus] |
| | $T_{4b}$ | Very late partial disease<br>Tumor invades the pre-vertebral fascia, circling the cervical arteries or invading the mediastinal |
| Infraglottic carcinoma | $T_1$ | Tumor limits at infraglottic sub-region |
| | $T_2$ | Tumor invades the vocal cords, normal or limited vocal cords motion |
| | $T_3$ | Tumor limits in the larynx, with vocal cords fixation |
| | $T_{4a}$ | Moderate late partial diseases<br>Tumor invades through the thyroid cartilage and (or) invades the outer laryngeal tissues [such as trachea, cervical soft tissues (including the deep extrinsic lingual muscles), ribbon muscles, thyroid gland or esophagus] |
| | $T_{4b}$ | Very late partial disease<br>Tumor invades the pre-vertebral fascia, circling the cervical arteries or invading the mediastinal |
| *Distinct lymph node (N)** | | |
| $N_x$ | | Region lymph nodes can't be evaluated |
| $N_0$ | | No region lymph nodes metastasis |
| $N_1$ | | Unilateral single lymph node metastasis, radius max <3 cm |
| $N_2$ | | Unilateral single lymph node metastasis, 3 cm < max radius < 6 cm or unilateral multiple lymph metastasis, max radius <6 cm; or bilateral or opposite lateral lymph nodes metastasis, no radius max however >6 cm |
| $N_{2a}$ | | Ipsilateral single lymph nodes metastasis, 3 cm < max radius < 6 cm |
| $N_{2b}$ | | Ipsilateral multiple lymph nodes metastasis, max radius < 6 cm |
| $N_{2c}$ | | Bilateral or opposite lateral lymph nodes metastasis, max radius < 6 cm |
| $N_3$ | | Metastasis lymph nodes max radius > 6 cm |
| Tips: same distinct metastasis is also distinct lymphatic metastasis | | |
| *Distinct metastasis (M)* | | |
| $M_0$ | | No distinct metastasis |
| $M_1$ | | Distinct metastasis exists |
| *Anatomy gradings/prognosis groupings* | | |
| Satge 0 | | $T_{is}N_0M_0$ |
| Stage I | | $T_1N_0M_0$ |
| Stage II | | $T_2N_0M_0$ |
| Stage III | | $T_3N_0M_0$, $T_1N_1M_0$, $T_2N_1M_0$, $T_3N_1M_0$ |
| Stage IV A | | $T_{4a}N_0M_0$, $T_{4a}N_1M_0$, $T_2N_2M_0$, $T_3N_2M_0$, $T_{4a}N_2M_0$ |
| Stage IV B | | $T_{4b}$ any $NM_0$, any $TN_3M_0$ |
| Stage V | | Any T any $NM_1$ |
| *Histology grading's (G)* | | |
| $G_x$: cannot be graded; $G_1$: highly differentiated; $G_2$: moderate differentiated; $G_3$:slightly differentiated; $G_4$: undifferentiated | | |

Cautions: the grading is only the cancer grading of the epithelium origin, without including non-epithelial tumors, lymph tissue, soft tissue, bone and the cartilage tumor

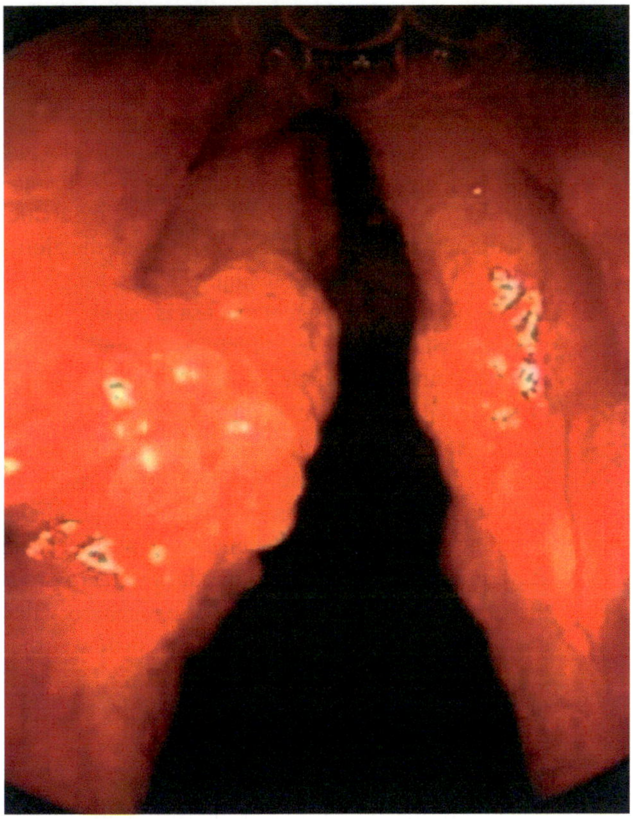

**Fig. 18.21** Bilateral vocal papilla tumor

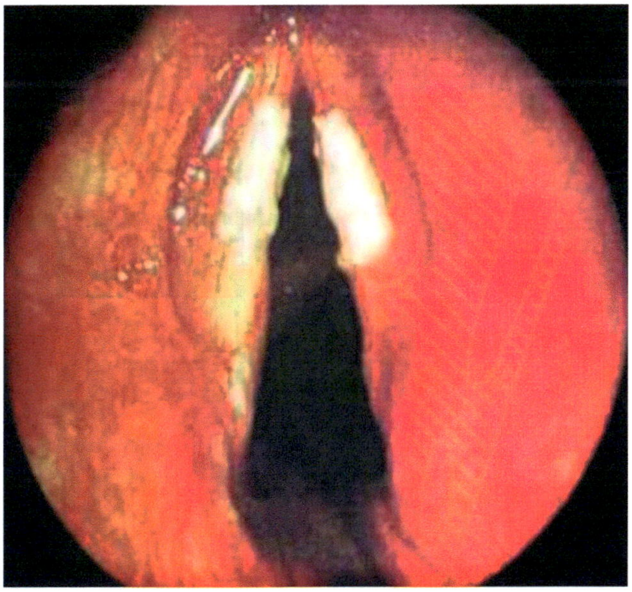

**Fig. 18.22** Vocal leukoplakia

costs less and less distinct complications. However, the voice has obvious hoarseness. Radiotherapy can preserve the original quality of voice and produce good quality, however it is difficult to eliminate the dryness of pharynx after radiotherapy, and there may be long-term complications of throat stenosis.

Laser excision under self-retaining laryngoscope is micro-invasion surgery, which causes small vulnus, short-term hospitalization and low fees, however, various degrees post operation hoarseness, which often don't influence normal communications and work can also exist. If there isn't laser surgery equipment's, open surgery can also be chosen. Simultaneous tracheal section while excising the cracking laryngosites, and removing the casing pipes after the laryngotruma heals. At the micro–wound excision or open surgery, if the excision edge is negative, radiotherapy isn't necessarily complemented after surgery.

Radiotherapy can well remain the laryngeal structure, which also means better phonation quality. However it is a long-term therapy, lasting about 2 months, and it's a bit expensive. Choosing the laser micro-wound excision or the radiotherapy should be explained to the patients about its advantages and shortcomings and then decided by the patients.

2. Middle-late Lesion ($T_3$, T4 lesion)

   To the middle-late lesion, commonly the comprehensive therapy method will be applied, generally including these as followings: (1) to the $T_3$ and the $T_4$ lesion, if the surgery could keep laryngeal function, then choose the operation and postoperative or simultaneous radio chemotherapy; if not, choose the laryngo excision surgery and postoperative radiotherapy; (2) choose simultaneous radiochemical therapy, after which examines and observe the tumor residual existing, if the residual occurs, apply the laryngeal excision, what is a pattern helpful to keep laryngeal functions, however, the repeated surgery on the postradio therapy residual or restoration may also cause more complications; (3) induction chemotherapy is also can be chosen, give 2–3 periods induction chemotherapy firstly, after which if the lesion completely remises (CR) or partially remises (PR), apply the follow-up radiotherapy or simultaneous radio chemotherapy to the patients; after which if the lesion doesn't completely remise or even partially remise, apply the surgery and the post-surgery radiotherapy.

3. Prognosis

   The overall 5-year survival rate of prognostic laryngeal cancer was 55–65%. The 5-year survival rate of surgery plus post-operative radiotherapy was about 65%, and the 5-year survival rate of concurrent radiochemotherapy was 50–60%. The 5-year survival rate of radiotherapy alone was 40–50%.

## 18.7 Laryngeal Obstruction

Laryngeal obstruction is a clinical symptom in which the larynx or surrounding tissue lesions cause the narrowing of the larynx airway and different degrees of dyspnea occur. The condition is more critical and severe, and if the treatment is not timely or inappropriate, it can lead to asphyxia.

**Etiology**

1. Inflammation

   Acute epiglottis in infants' acute laryngitis and others could evoke laryngeal stasis. Laryngeal adjacent sites' acute inflammation, such as the post laryngeal abscess, the submaxillary space infection, the inferior sub maxillary lymphatic etc.; laryngeal periostitis and other severe inflammation; leprosy, syphilis and other specific inflammation can also cause the laryngeal stasis.
2. Foreign Body in Throat: foreign body in throat can stimulate reflex laryngospasm and laryngeal edema resulting in dyspnea; Children's upper esophagus embedded foreign bodies, such as plastic caps, glass balls and other direct compression on membranous posterior wall of trachea leads to dyspnea.
3. Laryngeal Trauma: laryngeal contusion, crush injury, burn injury, laryngeal tracheal intubation injury, endoscopic damage can cause laryngeal obstruction. Laryngeal obstruction occurs in the early stage of trauma due to mucosal edema or laryngeal tissue injury, and in the later stage of trauma, laryngeal obstruction is often caused by scar adhesion or laryngeal spasm.
4. Laryngeal Edema: laryngeal inflammation, trauma, allergy, foreign body can cause laryngeal edema leads to the laryngeal obstruction. Laryngeal edema occurs mostly in supraglottic area in adults and more in subglottic area in children.
5. Tumors: laryngeal papilloma, laryngeal cancer, thyroid tumors can cause laryngeal obstruction. Hypertrophy of the tumor causes symptoms of laryngeal airway compression; it can also cause vocal cord paralysis due to secondary infection due to extensive tumor infiltration or recurrent laryngeal nerve involvement, and narrow the laryngeal airway.
6. Laryngeal Paralysis or Spasm: bilateral vocal cord paralysis cannot be extended to cause laryngeal obstruction, mostly due to thyroid surgery injury of recurrent laryngeal nerve. Tetanus infection, foreign body stimulation or electrolyte imbalance can lead to laryngeal spasm causes the laryngeal obstruction.
7. Laryngeal Deformity: congenital laryngeal webbed, thyroid cartilage deformity, laryngeal wheezing can cause laryngeal obstruction.

**Clinical Manifestations**

1. Symptoms of Hypoxia: cyanosis, cyanosis due to hypoxia, head back when inhaling, sitting and lying restlessness, dysphoria sleepless, late pulse appeared weak, fast, arrhythmia, heart failure, eventually coma and death.

   (a) Dyspnea during inspiration: Dyspnea during inspiration is a characteristic of laryngeal obstruction. The cleft glottis is the narrowest part of the larynx, formed by the slightly upward sloping edges of the vocal cords on both sides. Normally, although the inclined plane of the vocal cord is pushed by the airflow during inhalation, it is accompanied by abduction of the vocal cord, which can still make the glottis open and open, so the breathing is smooth. When lesions occur, the laryngeal mucosa is congested and swollen, which narrows the glottis. Therefore, airflow pressure on the inclined plane of the vocal cord during inhalation will make the narrowed glottis narrower and lead to breathing difficulties during inhalation (Fig. 18.23). The results showed that the inhalation movement was strengthened, the inhalation time was prolonged, the inhalation was deep and slow, but the ventilation volume did not increase. If there was no significant hypoxia, the respiratory rate did not increase. When exhaling, the airflow rushes upward to open the vocal cords, and the glottis is larger than when inhaling, so the difficulty of exhaling is not significant.

   (b) Inspiratory Laryngeal Wheezing: inspiratory inhalation of air, squeeze through the narrow glottic fissure, forming a vortex of air impact vocal cords, vocal

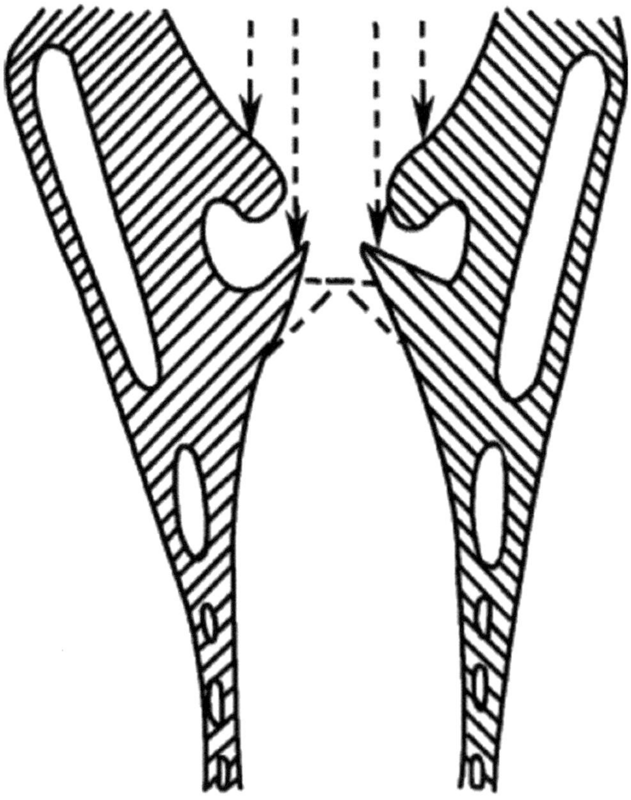

**Fig. 18.23** Dyspnea diagram at inhaling stage

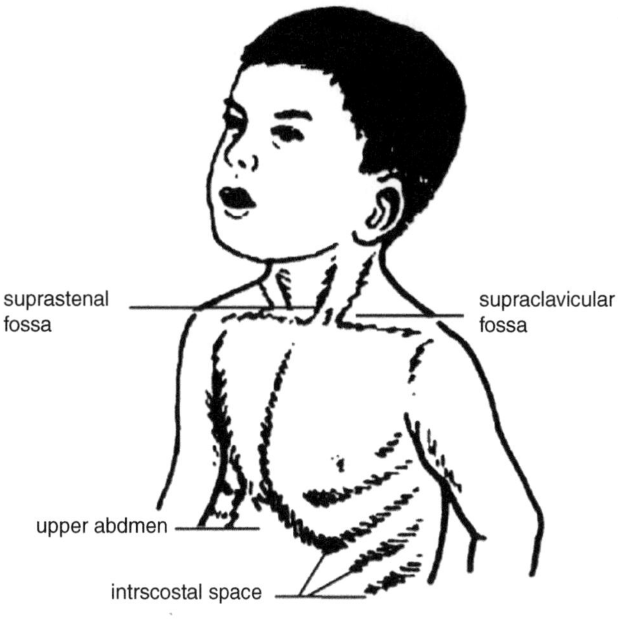


**Fig. 18.24** Sunken soft tissue

cords vibrate and send out a sharp laryngeal wheezing. Laryngeal obstruction light, throat panting sound is light; heavy, throat panting sound is loud. When exhaling, because the glottis crack is bigger, therefore, there is no this laryngeal wheezing.

(c) Soft Tissue Depression in Inspiratory Phase: it is characteristic of laryngeal obstruction. Because the air is not easy to enter the lungs through the narrow glottis, chest and abdomen auxiliary breathing muscles are compensated to strengthen movement, the chest expansion, to help absorb air, however,lung cannot expand accordingly, make the chest cavity negative pressure increases, the chest wall and its surrounding soft tissue suction, therefore, appear sternal fossa, supraclavicular, sub-clavicular fossa, sternal hilum or upper abdomen, intercostal space inspiratory depression (Fig. 18.24), called four concave sign, the degree of depression often varies with the degree of difficulty in breathing, children's muscle tone is weak, the depression signs are more obvious.

2. Hoarseness: it is a common symptom of laryngeal obstruction. If the lesion occurs in vocal cords, it often has hoarse or even lost voice. Laryngeal obstruction caused by other lesions is not obvious.

**Diagnosis**

1. The classification of laryngeal obstruction diagnosis according to the severity of the disease, laryngeal obstruction can be divided into four degrees.
   (a) Once: no symptoms when calm, crying, activity with mild inspiratory difficulties.
   (b) Second Degree: mild inspiratory dyspnea in quiet time, increased activity, however did not affect sleep and eating, hypoxia symptoms are not obvious.
   (c) Third Degree:

   Dyspnea is obvious during inspiration, laryngeal sounds are louder, and the depression of external soft tissues such as suprasternal fossa and supraclavicular fossa is obvious during inspiration. Because of lack of oxygen, it is restless, difficult to fall asleep and unwilling to eat. Patient's pulse is quickened, blood pressure is raised, heart rate is strong and powerful, that is, the compensatory function of circulatory system is good.

   (d) Fourth Degree:

   It's extremely difficult to breathe. Due to severe hypoxia and accumulation of carbon dioxide in the body, the patient is restless, cold sweating, pale or cyanotic, incontinence of urine and urine, weak pulse, irregular heart rhythm, and decreased blood pressure. If not rescued in time, they may die of asphyxia and heart failure.

2. Diagnostic Methods
   (a) According to the history, symptoms and signs, the diagnosis of laryngeal obstruction is not difficult. Once the diagnosis of laryngeal obstruction is clear. The first thing to judge is the degree of laryngeal obstruction.
   (b) As to find out the cause of laryngeal obstruction, should depend on the severity and development speed. Light and slow development, Longer course, can do indirect or fiber (electronic) laryngoscopy to identify laryngeal lesions and glottic fissure size. However, should pay attention when doing examination, because of throat anesthesia, cough reflex weakened, secretion is not easy to cough out, can make breathing difficulties significantly increased, and may induce laryngeal spasm, therefore, should be prepared for tracheotomy. Heavy and rapid development, it should be the first emergency treatment, after removing laryngeal obstruction; further examination is carried out to determine the etiology.
   (c) Medical imaging, especially MRI and CT examination, is very valuable to understand the cause of obstruction, direct obstruction caused by tumor, inflammation and foreign bodies, and vocal cord paralysis caused by mediastinal diseases, has a good diagnostic significance. General metal and animal bone high density foreign body, with CT plain scan is advisable. Tumor, inflammation and nonmetallic foreign body should be MRI. CT is appropriate for chest lesions.

**Treatment**

The treatment of laryngeal obstruction must be actively dealt with, the first problem is to solve the difficulty of breathing as soon as possible, make breathing unobstructed. Medication or surgery should be used according to the degree and cause of dyspnea.

1. Once: clear etiology, generally do not do tracheotomy, the patient's blocking symptoms can generally be controlled within 24 h after positive treatment. Caused by laryngeal inflammation, should be timely use of hormones and antibiotics, with steam inhalation or atomization inhalation, etc.; In case of retropharyngeal abscess, it is necessary to cut and discharge pus as soon as possible.
2. Second Degree: actively treat the cause of disease, closely observe the change of the disease, do a good job in the preparation of tracheotomy. If it is a foreign body, should be taken out immediately; Tracheotomy may be considered for tumors.
3. Third Degree: if it is a foreign body, it shall be taken out in time; if for acute inflammation, first try drug treatment, and ready to tracheotomy, if the observation did not improve or blocking time is longer, tracheotomy should be implemented as soon as possible. Laryngeal obstruction caused by tumor or other reasons, appropriate first tracheotomy, after waiting for breathing difficulties to ease, and then according to the cause, give other treatment.
4. Fourth degree: emergency rescue operation should be carried out immediately. Endotracheal intubation is performed under the guidance of an anesthesia laryngoscope, or an endotracheal tube is inserted to rescue breathing or a cricothyroid incision is performed. After the dyspnea is relieved, conventional tracheotomy is performed, and then the etiology is sought for further treatment.

## 18.8 Laryngotracheal Stenosis

Laryngotracheal stenosis is a kind of stenosis caused by the collapse of laryngotracheal cartilage and the proliferation of scar tissue. Congenital laryngotracheal stenosis is mainly found in children, including thyroid cartilage's soft disease, thyroid cartilage dysplasia, small laryngeal deformity, laryngeal webbed, laryngotracheal esophageal fissure, vocal cord paralysis, etc. The main causes of acquired laryngotracheal stenosis were trauma and infection.

**Etiology**

1. Congenital Factors: congenital laryngotracheal stenosis is the result of congenital laryngotracheal stenosis or complete laryngeal atresia when the laryngeal cavity is not fully recanalized or even completely disappeared during pregnancy.
2. Trauma: laryngotracheal trauma and endotracheal intubation are the main causes of acquired laryngotracheal stenosis. Laryngeal contusions, extrusion, cutting injury, firearm injury, chemical burn, long-term intubation, tracheostomy, early non-airway surgery, throat tumor radiotherapy are the risk factors of laryngeal and tracheal stenosis.
3. Infection: such as recurrent polychondritis, soft periostitis, pharyngeal scleroma, chronic inflammatory changes caused by amyloidosis of larynx and specific inflammatory infections caused by syphilis, diphtheria, etc. Wegener's granulomatosis, collagen vascular disease and nonspecific inflammation caused by scar contraction after thyroid cartilage's inflammation necrosis.
4. Other Factors: including chemical and physical damage of larynx and trachea, such as accidental inhalation of strong acid, strong alkali or radiation damage, etc.

**Typing**

1. According to the Location: divided into supraglottis, glottis, subglottic and intersecting glottis or across glottis narrow four types.
2. According to the Degree of Stenosis: currently widely used in clinical classification method is cotton classification, according to the narrow diameter classification scheme. Once: laryngotracheal obstruction <70%; second degree: the lumen obstruction is between 70% and 90%; third degree: lumen obstruction >90%, however still visible lacuna, or subglottic complete occlusion; fourth degree: totally occluded without lumen, vocal cords could not be identified.

**Clinical Manifestations**

The main manifestations were abnormal breathing, vocalization and swallowing. According to the different degree of laryngotracheal stenosis and showed different clinical symptoms, light person cannot obviously uncomfortable, some congenital laryngotracheal stenosis of children have light symptoms, even did not get diagnosis and treatment before preschool, however often misdiagnosed as asthma. For patients with tracheostomy, it was found that they could not tolerate plugging or extubation. Some patients develop eating choking cough, aspiration or even respiratory tract infection. Patients with long-term laryngotracheal stenosis may be accompanied by hoarseness and hypoxia with corresponding clinical signs (Fig. 18.25).

**Diagnosis**

According to the history, symptoms and signs, through direct laryngoscope, stroboscopic laryngoscope, electronic laryngoscope visual examination of narrow parts, combined with X- ray, CT, MRI examination can be diagnosed. The key is to determine the location, scope and degree of stenosis.

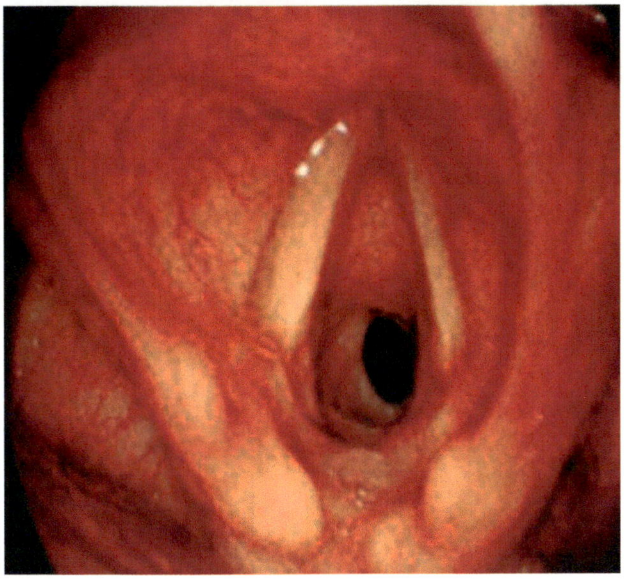

**Fig. 18.25** Laryngorepiratory tract stenosis

**Treatment**

Laryngotracheal stenosis should be focused on prevention; treatment should be based on the location, extent and scope of the lesions to choose the appropriate methods.

1. Drug Treatment: glucocorticoid, oral zinc sulfate inhibit granulation tissue growth can inhibit scar formation.
2. Surgical Treatment:
   (a) Narrow Throat
   - Thyroid Cartilage without Defect, Only Scar Hyperplasia: under the direct laryngoscope, laryngoscope scar tissue resection or laser, low temperature plasma resection, due to laser gasification, less bleeding, postoperative scar formation is less likely; the scar tissue was removed and the laryngeal expansion model was placed. Early tracheoscopic expansion of laryngotracheal stenosis.
   - Thyroid Cartilage Collapse: epiglottis laryngoplasty was used. Splitting larynx to remove narrow scar tissue, turning epiglottic cartilage over free epiglottic cartilage root, cutting periosteum at epiglottic edge with a sharp knife, respectively sewing the cut edge with the internal and external membrane of the residual thyroid cartilage to ensure that the lingual surface of epiglottic is the mucosa of laryngeal cavity, sewing the epiglottic laryngeal surface as the external periosteum of thyroid cartilage to form a bracket, reestablishing laryngeal cavity, and placing an expander; The fixation of hyoid bone flap should be paid attention to when repairing the cartilage of laryngeal and tracheal defects with hyoid bone flap with muscular pedicle.

   (b) Tracheal stenosis: tracheal defect is divided into partial defect and annular defect, local defect and extensive defect ($\geq$ 6 cm).
   - Intermittent Dilation Treatment: under direct laryngoscope, dilate with dilators or bronchoscopy 1–2 times a week until scar no longer contracts and unobstructed airway is established.
   - Continuous Expansion Treatment: titanium memory alloy stent and polyethylene tube were placed under bronchoscope for continuous expansion.
   - Thyroid Cartilage Tracheal Anastomosis: suitable for patients with subglottic stenosis within 2 cm.
   - Tracheal Reconstruction: it is difficult to perform end-to-end anastomosis for general tracheal defect exceeding 6 cm. it is advisable to resect scar under mucosa and reconstruct the defect stent with graft to achieve the goal of reconstruction of tracheal cavity.

At present, the development of tissue bioengineering has brought hope to find an ideal repair material for laryngeal and tracheal cartilage defects.

## References


1. Xia J. Medical genetics. Beijing: People's Medical Publishing House; 2004.
2. Xie J. Application of Stroboscopy at acoustic surgery. Sinoforeign Health Abstracct. 2012;9(1):421.
3. Xu W, Han D, Hou L, et al. Laryngomuscular electrogram characteristics of vocal cords dysfunction. Chin J Otorhinolaryngol Head Neck Surg. 2006;41(9):653–6.
4. Liu Y, Sun L, Li W, Ma R. Research progress of preventive nine-valent HPV vaccine [J]. Modernoncology. 2017;25(05):827–9.
5. Ligier K, Belot A, Launoy G, et al. Descriptive epidemiology of upper aerodigestive tract cancers in France:incidence over 1980-2005 and projection to 2010. Oral Oncol. 2011;47(4):302–7.

# Common Laryngeal Surgery

# 19

Yongjun Feng and Dasong Lu

## 19.1 Tracheotomy

1. Indications and Contraindications
   (a) Indications
      - Dyspnea caused by laryngeal obstruction, such as throat inflammation, trauma, tumor, foreign body, cicatricial stenosis and *recurrent laryngeal nerve paralysis,* etc. results in acute or chronic laryngeal obstruction.
      - Coma caused by various reasons, respiratory tract inflammation, trauma or operation on the chest and abdomen, decreased/incompetent clearance of tracheobronchial secretions, keep the airway unobstructed, reduce airway invalid cavity, increase the exchange of oxygen, etc.
      - Central or peripheral respiratory muscle paralysis, laryngeal spasm, etc. airway access for prolonged mechanical ventilation, tracheotomy can be done.
      - Occasionally, tracheotomy can be done to remove foreign bodies in trachea.
      - Respiratory deficiency caused by all kinds of reasons, tracheotomy can be done for auxiliary breathing.

   (b) Contraindications
      - Serious, coagulation dysfunction.
      - Unstable cardiopulmonary status (shock, extremely poor ventilatory status)
      - Without the consent of the patient or family members.
2. Preoperative Preparation
   (a) A comprehensive understanding of the etiology of the illness, grasps the initiative of the operation.
   (b) Quickly prepare and check the surgical instruments, lighting, tracheal cannula, retractor, oxygen, emergency medicine and anesthesia, intubation or bronchoscopy, etc., in order to cope with emergency rescue at any time.
   (c) According to the patient's different ages, choose suitable casing (Table 19.1).
3. Commonly Used Surgical Instruments

   Scalpel, tracheotomy knife, scissors, curved forceps, straight forceps, leather pliers, plate retractor, tooth retractor, thyroid retractor, tracheal cannula, intubation, long curved pliers, needle and thread and other emergency equipment.
4. Anaesthesia

   Generally, local infiltration anesthesia is used, Arising from the lower margin of the thyroid cartilage, to the upper margin of the sternum, equivalent to the skin incision site (Fig. 19.1). For very critical patients, tracheotomy can be done without anaesthesia; even use a simple knife for emergency operation.
5. Surgical Procedures
   (a) Posture

   Supine position is generally used: head up, neck mat high, head is extended as far as possible, and is fixed by the assistant, chin, Adam's apple and *suprasternal notch* incised three points into a straight line.

**Table 19.1** Tracheal casing size parameter table (unit: mm)

| Age | Diameter/length of outer tube of age sleeve |
|---|---|
| under 1 year old | 4/40–45 under |
| 1–2 years old | 5/50 |
| 3–6 years old | 6/60 |
| 7–11 years old | 7/65 |
| 12–17 years old | 8/70 |
| Over 18 years old | 9–10/75–80 |

Y. Feng (✉) · D. Lu
Department of Otorhinolaryngology Head and Neck Surgery, The Second Affiliated Hospital of Hainan Medical University, Haikou, China



Z. Mu, J. Fang (eds.), *Practical Otorhinolaryngology - Head and Neck Surgery*, https://doi.org/10.1007/978-981-13-7993-2_19

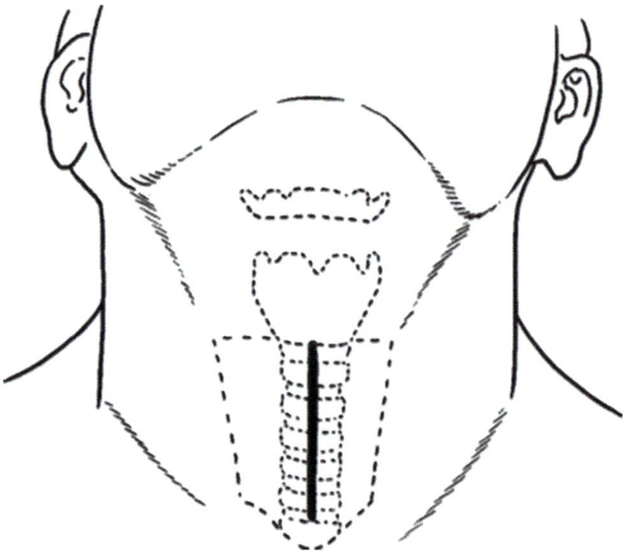

**Fig. 19.1** Anesthetic range and skin incision aperture

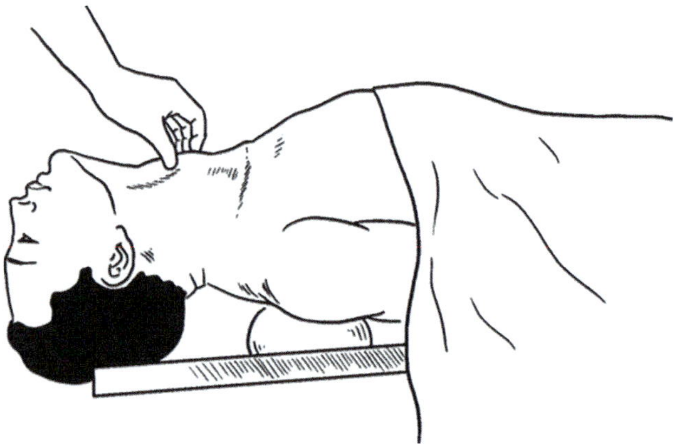

**Fig. 19.2** Common surgical position

Strictly keep on the median position, facilitate the exposure of trachea, fix limbs in case of displacement. In an emergency, the tracheal cannula or bronchoscope may be inserted before operation (Fig. 19.2).

(b) Incision

There are two kinds of incision: straight incision and transverse incision.

- Straight incision is often used in clinic, the skin and subcutaneous tissue are cut from the lower edge of the thyroid cartilage to the upper edge of the sternum. Through a straight incision—anterior median cervical incision, the trachea is exposed better, but scar is obvious after wound healing.
- The transverse incision can be cut along the front of the neck with a fine appearance (Fig. 19.3), but the trachea is poorly exposed. Notice that the incision should not be lower than the width of a finger on the sternum.

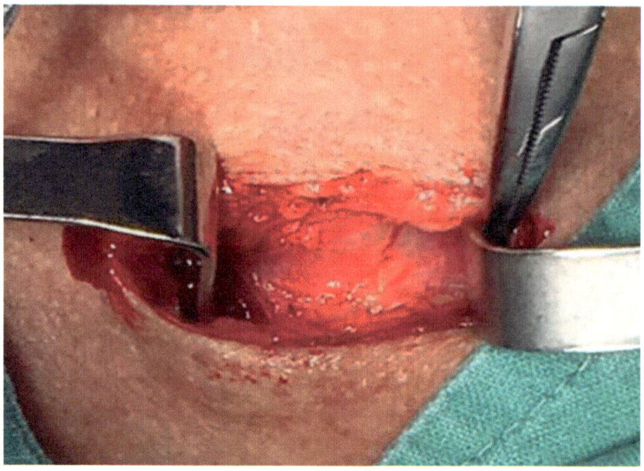

**Fig. 19.3** Transverse incision

- Low tracheotomy indication: Such as laryngectomy, upper tracheal tumor resection, open throat trauma, need to do low tracheotomy (5, 6 tracheal ring). In the suprasternal fossa transverse incision, keep away from the thyroid isthmus, no large blood vessels in the middle, less bleeding and high safety. This procedure requires more time. The surgical incision should not go beyond the upper edge of the sternum.
- Contraindication: It is not recommended for patients with short neck, acute throat obstruction or abnormal anatomy of the tracheolaryngeal structures.

(c) Exposed Cervical Fascia

Separate subcutaneous tissue and superficial fascia, revealing the white line at the junction of external laryngeal muscles on both sides. If the anterior jugular vein hinders the operation, it can be ligated and cut off. After incision of the deep cervical fascia at the white line of the neck, the sternohyoid muscle and sternothyroid muscles were separated from the midline by vascular forceps and then pulled apart with equal force from both sides. Keep the trachea in the middle of the incision, and often use the finger to touch the trachea ring, in case the trachea is pulled and displaced.

(d) Exposed Thyroid Isthmus

Keep the median along the white line, separate to the deep, pull the muscle bundles on both sides with a retractor, revealing thyroid isthmus, pay attention to balance the force on both sides of the retractor, in order to keep the surgical field in the median, and can often touch the trachea position with your fingers.

(e) Separation of The Thyroid Isthmus

After separation of the sublingual muscles, the thyroid gland can be seen covering the anterior wall of the trachea (Fig. 19.4), roughly corresponding to

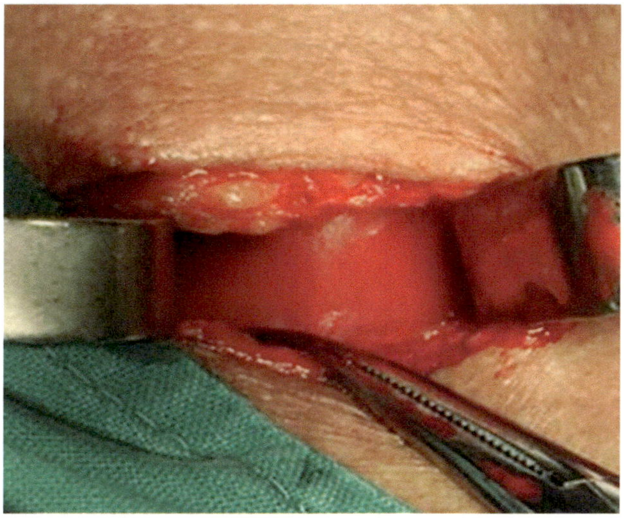

**Fig. 19.4** Thyroid isthmus exposure (transverse incision)

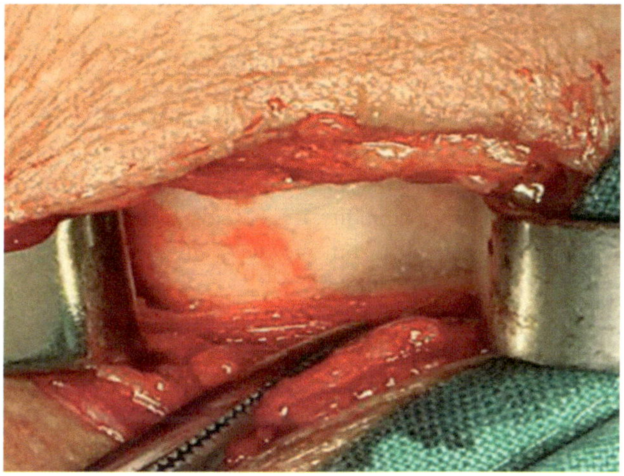

**Fig. 19.5** Tracheocricoid could be inspected after exposing thyroid gland (transverse incision)

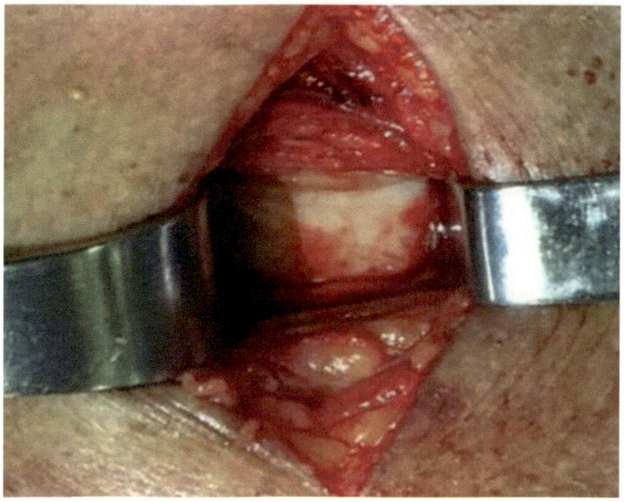

**Fig. 19.6** Tracheocricoid could be inspected after exposing thyroid gland (straight incision)

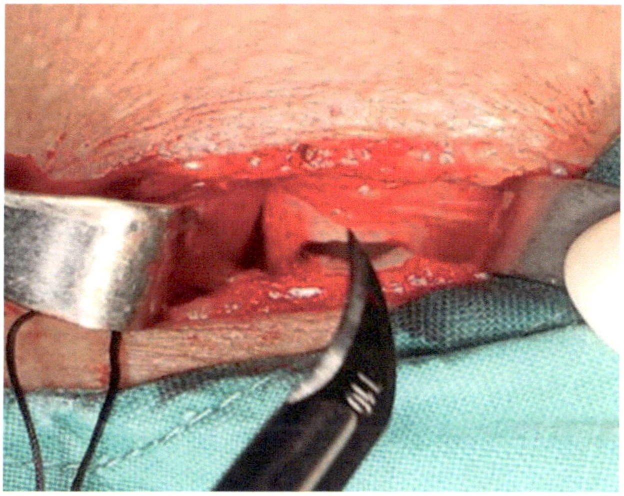

**Fig. 19.7** Tracheal fenestration

the 2nd to 4th rings of the trachea. If the thyroid isthmus is not wide, as long as it is pulled up, the anterior wall of the trachea can be clearly exposed (Fig. 19.5); If the isthmus is too wide, use vascular clamp to separate and clamp it, seam and tie at the middle after cutting the vessel, then stretch to both sides to properly expose the tracheal anterior wall (Fig. 19.6).

(f) Incision of Trachea

The anterior fascia of trachea should not be peeled off too much, and the tissues between the third and fourth trachea rings should be cut transversely in the middle of the anterior wall of trachea with a curved blade (Fig. 19.7). For long term need of the tube, appropriately remove part of the tracheal cartilage into a circular fistula. Tip into the lumen, the handle should be flat, so as not to damage the trachea rear wall.

(g) Insert The Tracheal Cannula

Open the tracheal incision with a curved vascular forceps or tracheal dilator, absorb the secretion (Fig. 19.8), fully stop bleeding, then insert the prepared cannula conveniently into the incision with the thumb against the tube core. At this time, if the secretion flows out from the tube orifice, it confirms that the cannula has been inserted into the trachea. If no secretion flows out, place a little gauze fiber on the tube orifice to see if it can flap with breathing. If it is confirmed that the cannula is not in the trachea, immediately pull out the cannula and reinsert it. If you need to perform artificial respiration or head, facial Operation and cut the trachea, the application of tracheal cannula with air bag, insert the force direction should be along the cannula bending radian,

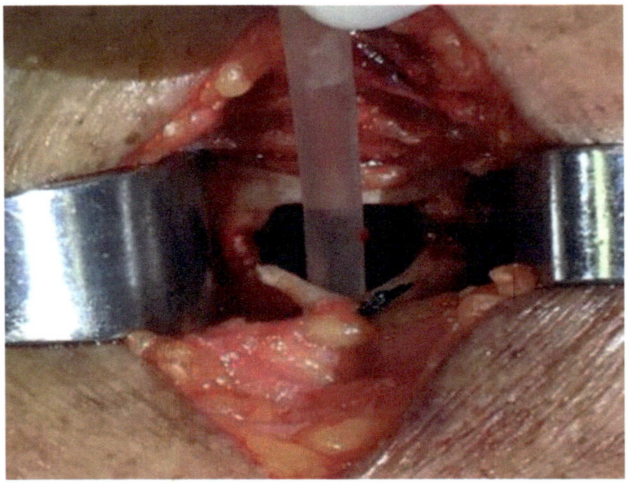

**Fig. 19.8** Sputum suction tube for removing secretions (straight incision)

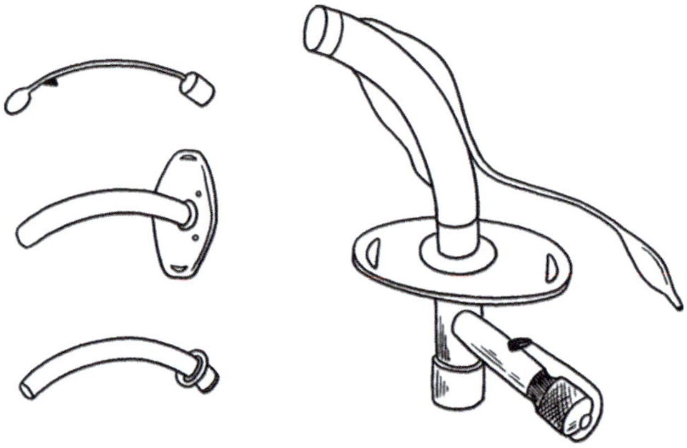

**Fig. 19.9** Common tube casing and gasbag tube casing

and pay attention not to make the tube wall to collapse, pull out the tube core after insertion, commonly used cannula is shown in Fig. 19.9.

(h) Fixing Sleeve

If the incision is too long, the upper section of the incision can be sewed with 1 or 2 Needles. The ethanol gauze which is sterilized and snipped is placed under the endotracheal tube. Insert the inner tube, tie the tiewraps with two knots, and pay attention to appropriate tightness (Fig. 19.10). Cover with a layer of warm brine gauze.

(i) Postoperative Treatment

- After tracheotomy, patients rely on cannula breathing, the original respiratory physiology changed; so they need care, in order to reduce the occurrence of complications. At the same time actively treat the primary disease.
- Close monitoring within 24 h after operation; generally take half lie or supine position. Encourage patients to turn over frequently, promote the lower respiratory tract secretion expulsion.
- The environment requires room temperatures of 20–22 °C, relative humidity of more than 80%. When oxygen inhalation, pay attention to respiratory tract humidity, it is best to cover a single layer of wet gauze at the nozzle of the tracheal cannula to increase humidity.
- After tracheotomy, patient needs specialist care, with a sputum aspirator timely clean secretions, timing dripping medicine into the cannula and cleaning cannula, in order to keep the cannula and lower respiratory tract unobstructed; and change the gauze pad in time. At the same time, check and adjust the tightness of the fixing belt every day to prevent the cannula from coming out or being too tight.
- Sputum drainage can be promoted by instilling or inhaling mucolytic drugs into the trachea.
- Keep the incision clean, prevent infection.
- If the original disease has been cured, dyspnea relieved, patient should be extubated timely. Before pulling out the pipe, try plugging the pipe first, wear the pipe for a short period of time can be a onetime plugging pipe, observe 24–48 h without dyspnea can be removed; For larger cannula, air bag cannula or wear tube for a long time, can replace the small cannula or gradually plugging pipe, until the total plugging pipe after more than 48 h without dyspnea, can pull out the pipe. After exudation, the neck incision is aligned with butterfly tape. If the wound is not easy to heal caused by the radiation treatment and other rea-

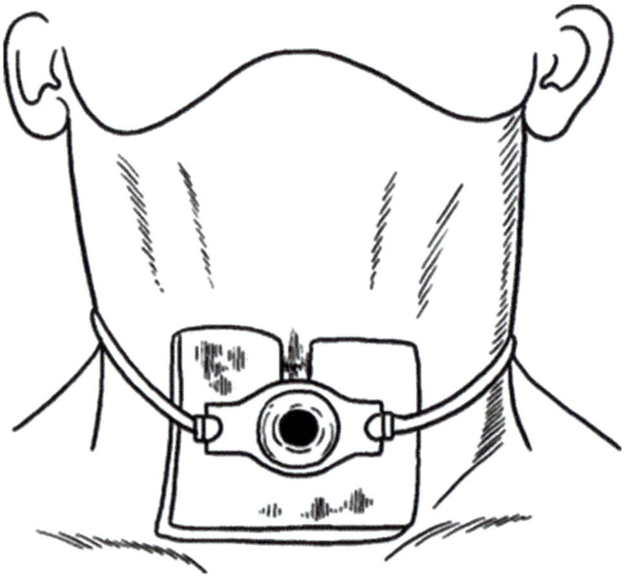

**Fig. 19.10** Fixed tube casing

sons, or fistula skin inversion, a little skin next to the fistula can be removed before suturing.

## 19.2 Tracheal Intubation

Endotracheal intubation refers to the insertion of a special endotracheal tube, through the mouth or nasal cavity into the patient's trachea, for emergency relief of upper respiratory tract obstruction. It keeps the respiratory tract unobstructed, suctions lower respiratory tract secretions and is an effective emergency method for auxiliary breathing, is also a safety measure for the implementation of anesthesia.

1. Indications
   (a) During general anesthesia, to ensure that the respiratory tract is unobstructed for example in intracranial Operation, thoracotomy, need special position such as prone position or sitting position of general anesthesia operation; Jaw, face, neck, facial features and other general anesthesia Operation; Cervical tumors compress trachea, obese patients; A person who has a marked inhibition of respiration by general anesthetics or who applies muscle relaxants.
   (b) Respiratory failure requires mechanical ventilation, cardiopulmonary resuscitation, drug poisoning and neonatal asphyxia.
   (c) Some special anesthesia, such as cooling, decompression and intravenous anesthesia, etc.
   (d) Easy to perform difficult tracheotomy.
2. Preoperative Preparations
   (a) Check the basic situation of patients before Operation, to estimate the difficulty of the operation and choose what kind of route (through the mouth or through the nose), at the same time ready to take emergency measures, such as tracheotomy bag and oxygen supply, etc.
   (b) The instrument used to prepare appropriate laryngoscope (Fig. 19.11), catheter guide wire, suction tube, dental pad, syringe, etc., It is expected that patients with intubation difficulties should prepare a fiberoptic bronchoscope. For intubation under fiberoptic bronchoscopy; Select the appropriate type of tracheal tube.
   (c) Preoperative anesthesia with 1% tetracaine or 2% lidocaine does laryngotracheal mucosal surface anesthesia, or general anesthesia. Sedative and atropine may be combined before operation. Emergency Operation is critical and may not be anesthetized.
3. Methodology

   Endotracheal intubation can be divided into orotracheal intubation and nasal endotracheal intubation according to the intubation route. According to the anesthesia method before intubation, it can be divided into general anesthesia induction tracheal intubation, semi-conscious tracheal intubation and conscious tracheal intubation. According to whether that glottis is exposed during intubation, the intubation can be divided into direct laryngoscopy intubation, fiberoptic laryngoscopy guide intubation and blind endotracheal intubation. At present, anesthesia laryngoscopes with an imaging display system can clearly display the glottis, thereby being convenient for intubation and teaching. The following is an introduction to orotracheal intubation and transnasal endotracheal intubation.

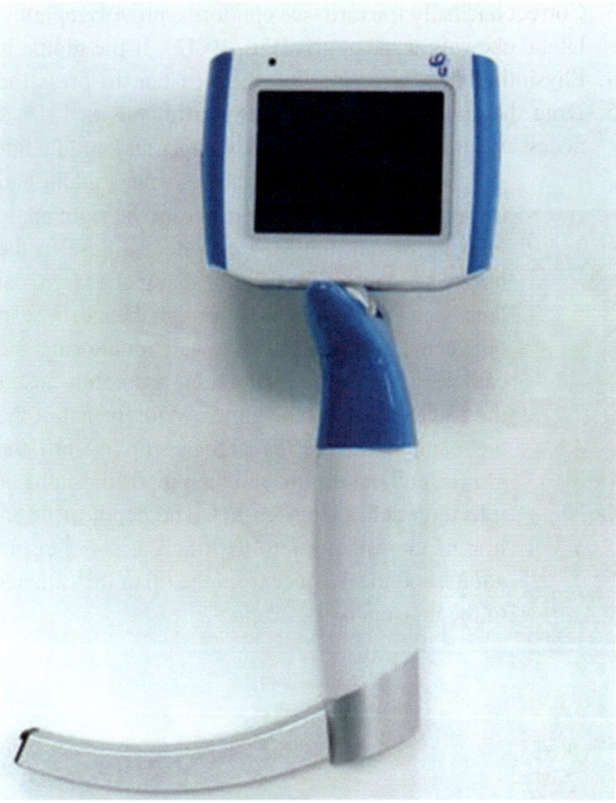

Fig. 19.11 Visibility laryngscope

   (a) After the glottis is exposed under the direct vision of laryngoscope through the orotracheal intubation, the catheter is inserted into the trachea through the oral cavity.
      - The patient take supine position, the operator tilts the patient's head back and raises the lower jaw forward with both hands to open the mouth, or with the right thumb facing the lower dentition, pointing the index finger against the upper dentition, by a rotating force to open the mouth.
      - The left hand holding laryngoscope handle to insert the laryngeal lens into the mouth from the right corner, push the tongue to the side after slowly advancing, can see the uvula. Lift the lens

vertically forward, see epiglottis, provoke epiglottis, reveal the glottis (Fig. 19.12). If the glottis is not fully exposed, ask the assistant to press the Adam's apple to assist in exposing the it.

- With the right thumb, index finger and middle finger, such as holding a pen hold the middle and upper section of the catheter, from the right angle into the mouth, until the catheter is close to the larynx and then move the tube end to the laryngeal lens, at the same time look through the narrow gap between the lens and tube wall monitoring the catheter in a forward direction, accurately insert the catheter tip into the glottis. With the aid of the die cannula, when the catheter tip is into the glottis, pull out the die and then insert the catheter into the trachea (Fig. 19.13). The depth of insertion of the catheter into the trachea is 4–5 cm in adults, and the distance from the tip of the catheter to the incisors is 18–22 cm.

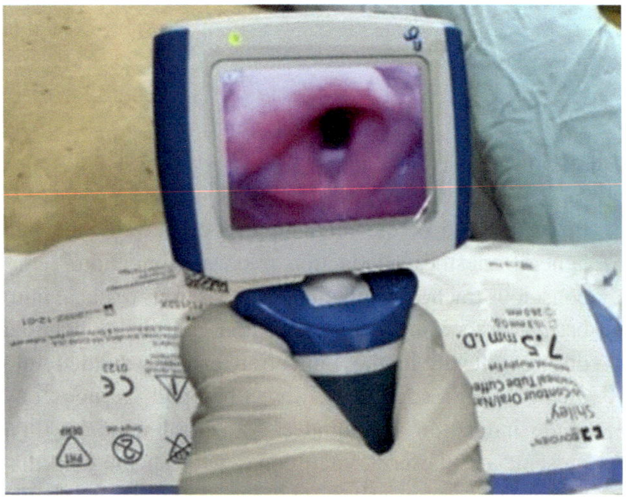

**Fig. 19.12** Raise the epiglottis and reveal the glottis

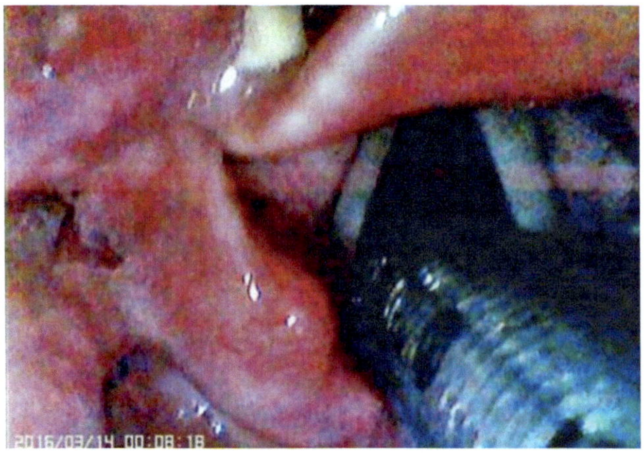

**Fig. 19.13** Insert the catheter into the trachea

- After the completion of the intubation, confirm the catheter has entered the trachea. Confirmation methods are:
  - Pressure chest, duct mouth has airflow.
  - Artificial respiration, visible bilateral thoracic symmetrical ups and downs, and can hear clear alveolar breathing.
  - If using transparent catheter, on inspiration tube wall is clear, on expiration there is an obvious visible "white fog" change.
  - If the patient has spontaneous breathing, after receiving the anesthesia machine, the respiratory sac can be seen to expand and contract with the patient's breathing.
  - End-tidal CO2 (et CO2) concentration is detected after intubation and clear alveolar breathing sound can be heard.

(b) Transnasal Endotracheal Intubation

- Nasal mucosa contraction and surface anesthesia should be done before intubation, catheter front daub a small amount of lubricant to prevent damage to the mucosa.
- Choose appropriate pipe diameter of trachea catheter, with the right hand holding the catheter, face a vertical direction from the nose and insert, along the bottom of the nose forward to the posterior nasal orifice, through the nasopharynx and oropharynx, continue to push the catheter until reaches the above position, cross the epiglottis ready to enter the glottis.
- When the glottis is opened, the catheter is rapidly pushed forward. When the catheter is into the glottis, the resistance decreases, the exhaled air flow is obvious, sometimes the patient has a cough reflex, after receiving the anesthesia machine, the respiratory sac can be seen to expand and contract with the patient's breathing, indicating that the catheter was successfully inserted into the trachea.
- If the exhaled air flow disappears after the catheter is advanced, it may be inserted into the esophagus. The catheter should be withdrawn to the nasopharynx and the tip of the catheter should be tilted upward with the head tilted back to align the glottis for insertion.
- The intubation method does not affect swallowing and instrument through the oral path into the operation, and is easy to fix, but it, may cause epistaxis in the process of operation.

4. Complications of Endotracheal Intubation

(a) If the intubation operation technology is not skilled; it may cause damage to the teeth, oral mucosa, or cause dislocation of temporomandibular joint.

(b) Endotracheal intubation under oral anesthesia can cause severe choking cough, laryngeal and bronchial spasm; Heart rate increases rapidly and blood pressure fluctuates violently, resulting in myocardial ischemia. Severe vagal reflex can lead to arrhythmia, even cardiac arrest.
(c) If the endotracheal tube diameter is too small, can cause respiratory resistance to increase; If the inner diameter of the catheter is too large, or the texture is too hard, it can easily damage the respiratory mucosa, and even cause acute laryngeal edema, or chronic granuloma, laryngeal web, and laryngeal stenosis. If the catheter is too soft, it can be easily deformed, due to compression, twisting which may lead to respiratory tract obstruction.
(d) If the catheter is inserted too deep, it can go into one side of the bronchus, causing insufficient ventilation, hypoxia or postoperative atelectasis. When the catheter is inserted too shallow, it can be accidentally removed due to the change of body position, resulting in serious accidents.

## 19.3 Rupture of Larynx

Laryngectomy, also known as thyroidectomy, the thyroid cartilage is cut from the midline, the laryngeal cavity is fully exposed, and handles the intralaryngeal lesions as appropriate.

1. Indications and Contraindications
   (a) Indications
   - In the early stage of vocal cord cancer, the tumor was confined to the anterior segment of one side of the vocal cord, 2/3 of the middle segment did not invade the anterior commissure, the posterior segment did not affect the vocal cord process, did not invade the deep tissue, vocal cord movement is normal.
   - A large benign tumor in that larynx, with a wide base or located in the subglottic region, cannot be removed completely by indirect or direct laryngoscope; Anterior commissure lesions, prone to adhesions (including laryngeal webs) require placement of an expansion mold.
   - Some exploratory operations, such as clinical manifestations of suspected malignant tumors, however, repeated biopsy is negative, or tumor rich in blood supply, biopsy has a large risk of bleeding asphyxiation.
   - The foreign body in the throat can not be taken out by the direct laryngoscope.
   - Repair of laryngeal trauma and laryngeal stenosis.

   (b) Contraindications
   - If the tumor has reached the anterior commissure or even more than the anterior commissure invading the contralateral vocal cords, conventional laryngeal dehiscence is no longer suitable, can choose the anterior commissure laryngeal dehiscence, partial laryngectomy or total laryngectomy.
   - Untreated acute inflammation of pharynx, larynx or neck.
   - Cardiopulmonary insufficiency.
2. Preoperative Preparation
   (a) Detailed examination before operation, laryngoscopy, laryngeal CT, determines the location of the tumor, vocal cord activity and subglottic area with or without invasion.
   (b) The neck skin, ready to tracheotomy bag, casing.
   (c) Check the whole body condition, preoperative 6 h fasting, forbid taking of water and preoperative half an hour injection phenobarbital and atropine.
3. Anesthesia and Posture
   (a) Anesthesia
   - General Anesthesia: endotracheal intubation is generally adopted. After the larynx is cracked, the endotracheal tube is inserted in the third to fourth ring of trachea. The air bag on the endotracheal intubation is properly inflated to block the upper segment of trachea, to avoid blood flows into the lower respiratory tract during operation, and the operation can be carried out safely.
   - Local Anesthesia: is performed with 2% lidocaine along the lower edge of the anterior median hyoid bone of the neck to the suprasternal incision for infiltration of the anesthesia, superior laryngeal nerve block anesthesia on both sides of the laryngeal mucosa. However, local anesthesia can easily cause irritative cough, bleeding, making the operation difficult. It is suitable for patients with small focus and short operation time.

   (b) Position the Patient in supine position; head back, shoulder slightly mat high, chin, Adam's apple, sternum incised three point a line, head on both sides with sandbags fixed, keep the median (Fig. 19.14).
4. Surgical Procedures
   (a) Incision: there are two kinds of incisions; vertical and horizontal. Most of them adopt longitudinal incision of the midline of the neck, similar to tracheotomy, incision of skin, subcutaneous tissue, direct to the thyroid cartilage, cricoid cartilage. The inferior hyoid muscles are separated, the thyroid isthmus is cut off, and the upper segment of trachea exposed. Lateral incision (Fig. 19.15) along the lower edge of the cricoid cartilage, cut skin layer by layer, subcutaneous

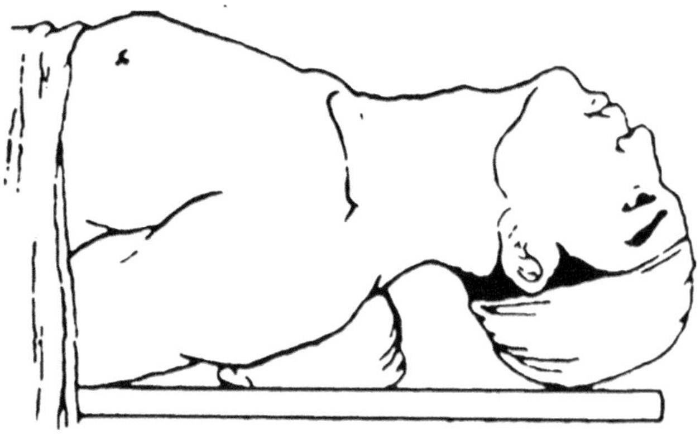

**Fig. 19.14** Common anesthetic position

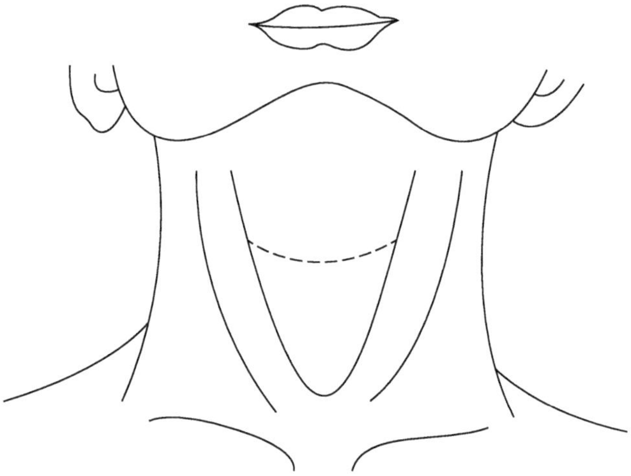

**Fig. 19.15** Transverse incision aperture

tissue can be directly cut to the thyroid cartilage, subcutaneous tissue, muscle, etc. can not be separated, because separation can affect the thyroid cartilage nutrition, resulting into cartilage infection or partial necrosis.

(b) Exposure to Thyroid Cartilage and Cricothyroid Membrane: separate the muscles under the hyoid bone, thyroid isthmus can not be cut off, if isthmus is too large, suture after cutting it off, expose the upper tracheal ring. Tracheotomy may be performed by conventional methods before or during Operation. Insert anesthesia catheter with balloon.

(c) Incision of The Cricothyroid Membrane and Thyroid Cartilage: after exposure of the cricothyroid membrane, several drops of 2% lidocaine are injected into the cricothyroid membrane, and a short transverse incision is made (Fig. 19.16). The cut on the thyroid cartilage is either made from the midline of the upper edge, or from the midline of the lower edge (Fig. 19.17), or may be sawed by an electric circular saw (Fig. 19.18).

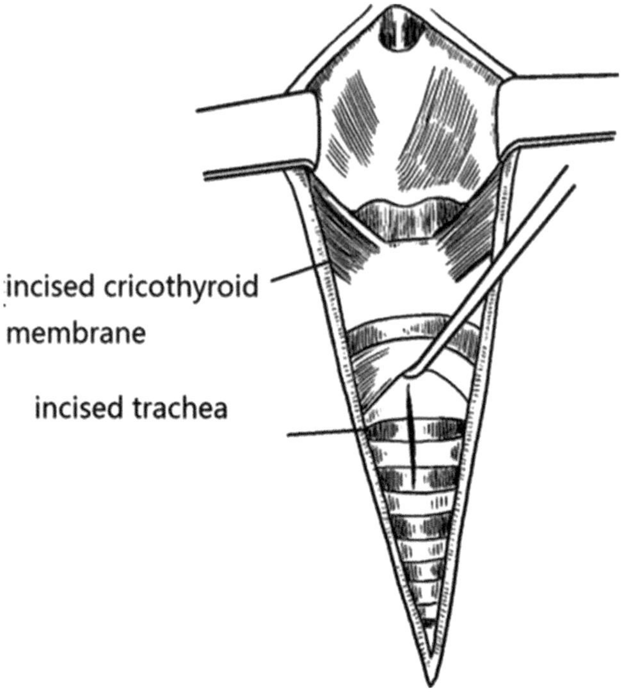


**Fig. 19.16** Tracheal incision and incised cricothyroid membrane

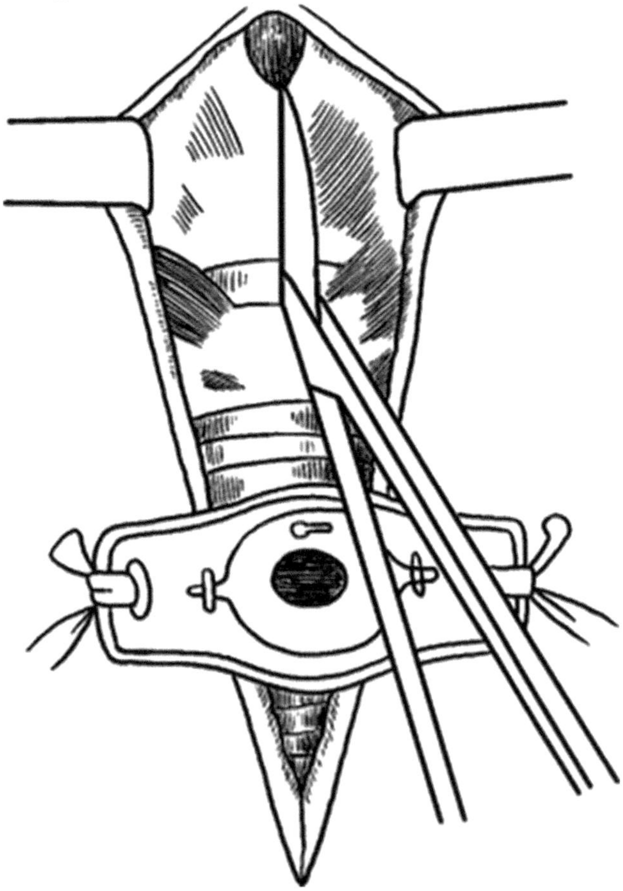

**Fig. 19.17** Cut thyroid along with midline

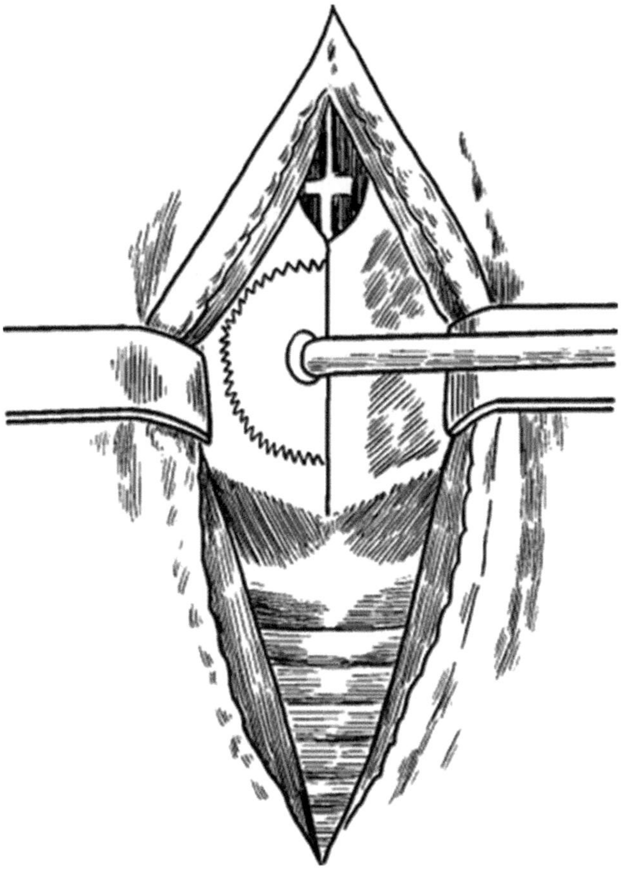

Fig. 19.18 Saw thyroid at midline with buzzsaw

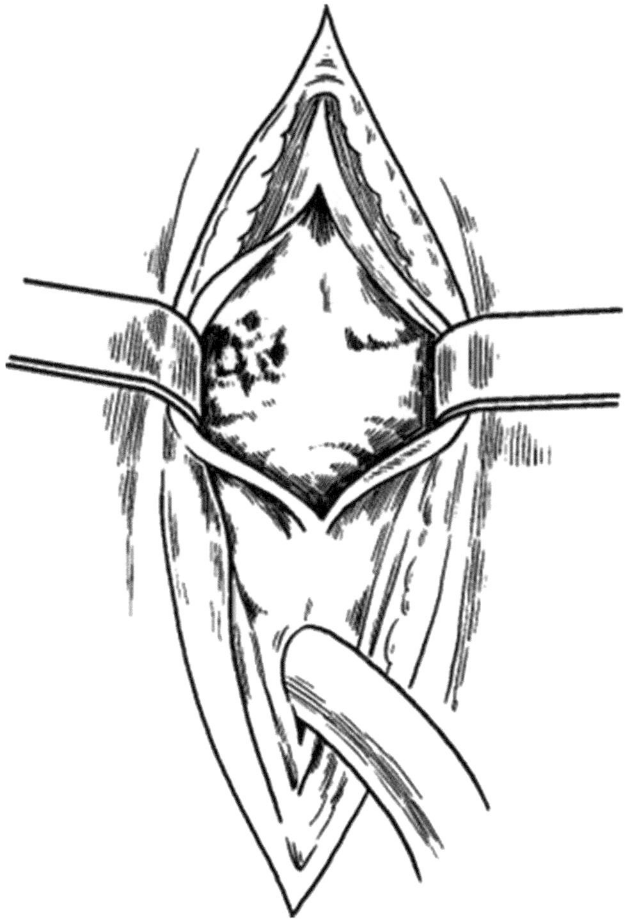

Fig. 19.19 Incise mucosa then enter laryngocavum

(d) Cut the mucosa, around the laryngeal cavity and along the midline. After entering the laryngeal cavity; explore the laryngeal lesions (Fig. 19.19).
(e) Resect The Lesion: fully expose the laryngeal cavity (Fig. 19.20), peel off along the inner wall of the thyroid cartilage, leave enough safe boundaries, and resect the tumor (Fig. 19.21).
(f) Repair The Wound: If the tumor resection area is small, can do a free mucosa traction suture. If the wound is large, can use the upper mucoperiosteal flap repair (Fig. 19.22), or in the lower mucosa do a pedicled mucosal flap transfer repair (Fig. 19.23).
(g) Suture incision carefully check the wound, and stop bleeding. Simple benign tumors with small mucosal resection do not require suturing the mucosa, if the operation needs to remove too much mucosa, can suture after being repaired with mucous membrane or muscle flap. Just suture the perichondrium (Fig. 19.24), suture the submucosal musculature of hyoid bone and subcutaneous soft tissue in layers, and finally suture the anterior cervical skin incision (Fig. 19.25).
(h) Pull out the anesthesia cannula and replace with trachea cannula

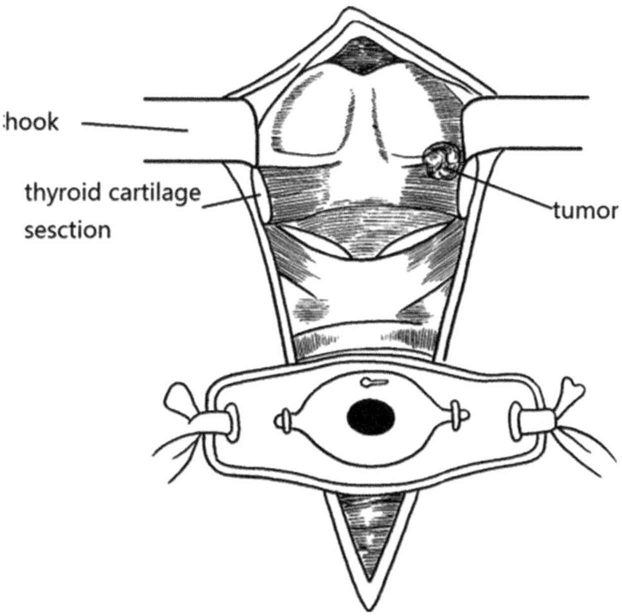


Fig. 19.20 Sufficiently expose the laryngocavum

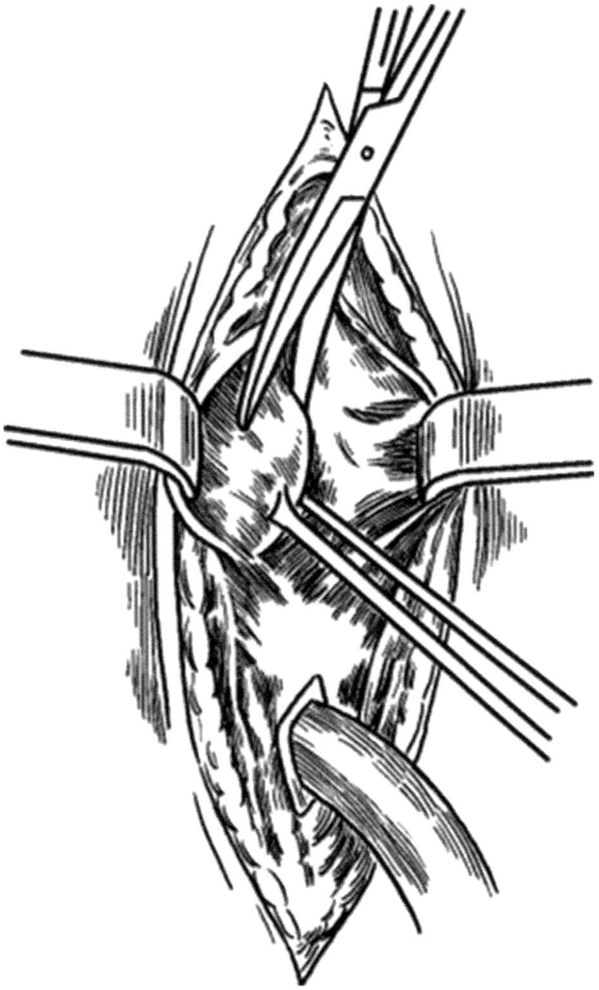

Fig. 19.21 Cut entire tumor along with safe boundary edge

5. Postoperation Disposal
   (a) Intimately investigate patients' respiratorion and hemorrhage.
   (b) Regular nurse after the tracho-incision operation and draw tubes earlily. There aren't any reports about laryngofissure without trachoincision recently.
   (c) Take liquid or semiliquid diet at second postoperation day.
   (d) Apply antibiotics for 5–7 days after operation and change medical prescriptions.
   (e) Try to obstruct the tube after 7–10 postoperation days, and if the patient can breathe freely in the following 48 h, the trachea casing pipes could be plucked.
   (f) Avoid phonating in the following 2 weeks' postoperation time.

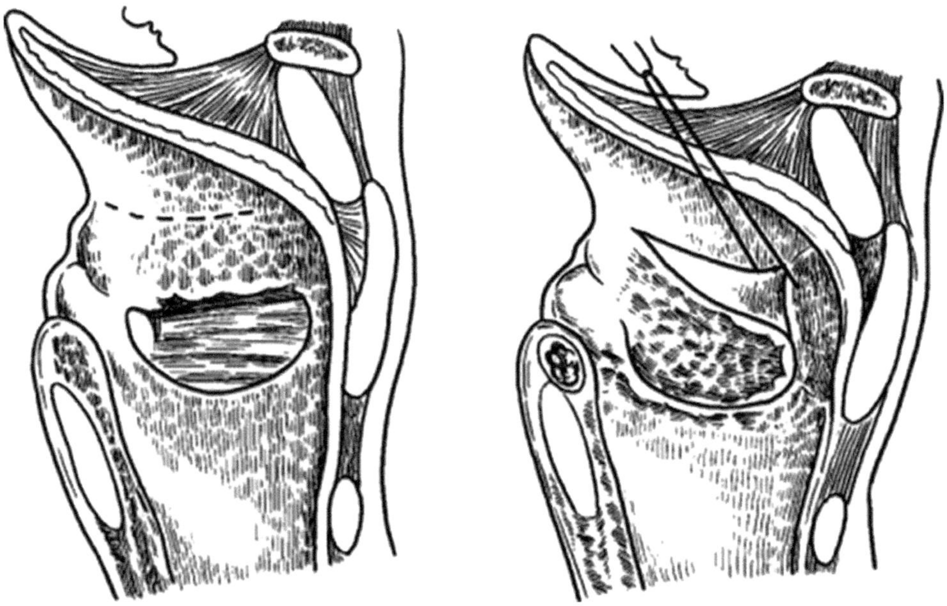

Fig. 19.22 Incise superior mucoperiost flaps, with which repair wound surface

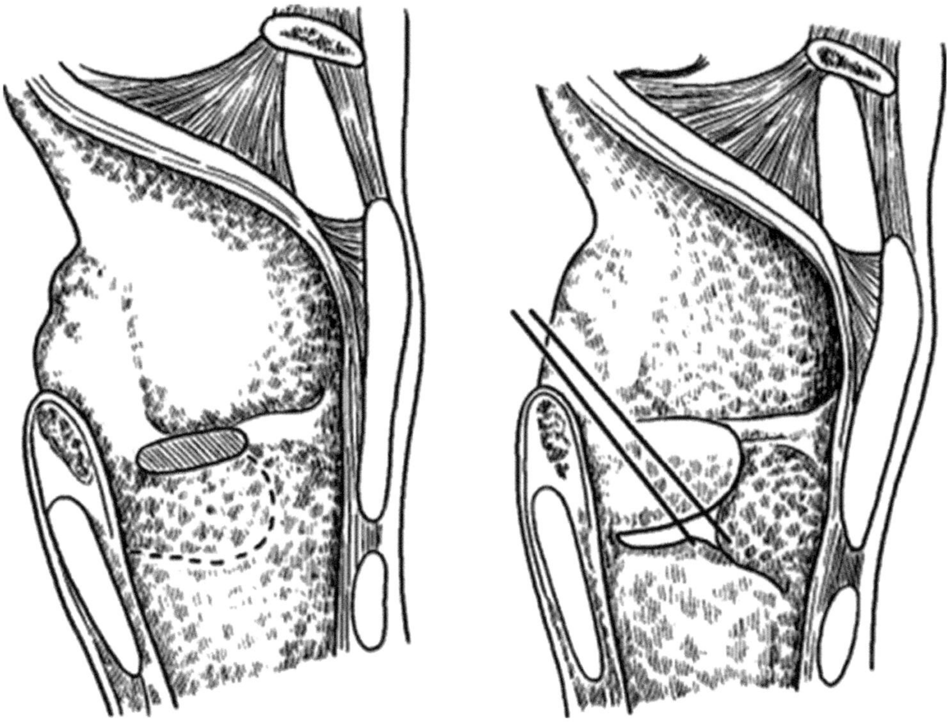

**Fig. 19.23** Incise inferior pedicle mucoflaps, metastasis and repair wound surface

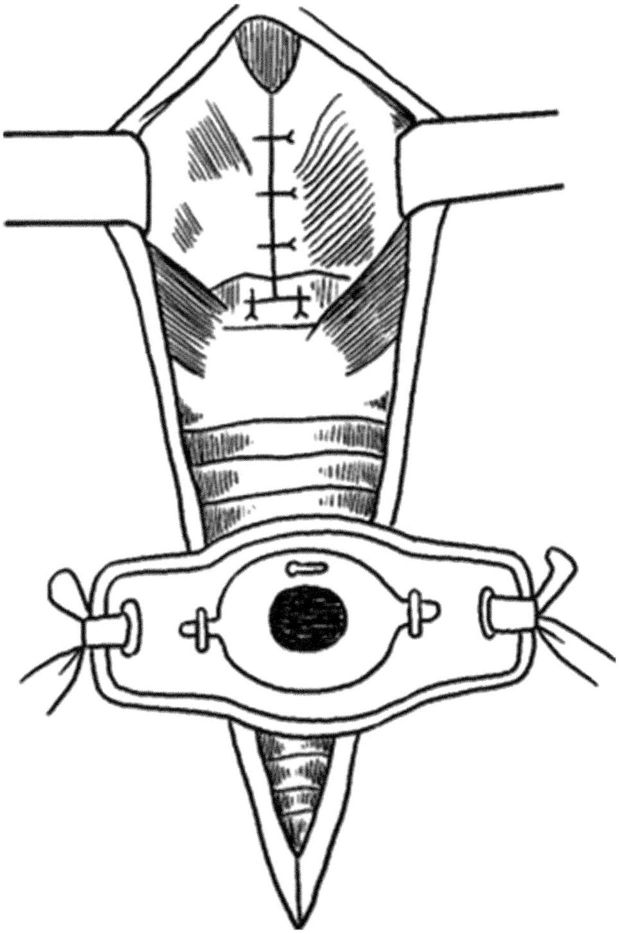

**Fig. 19.24** Suture thyrocartilage membrane

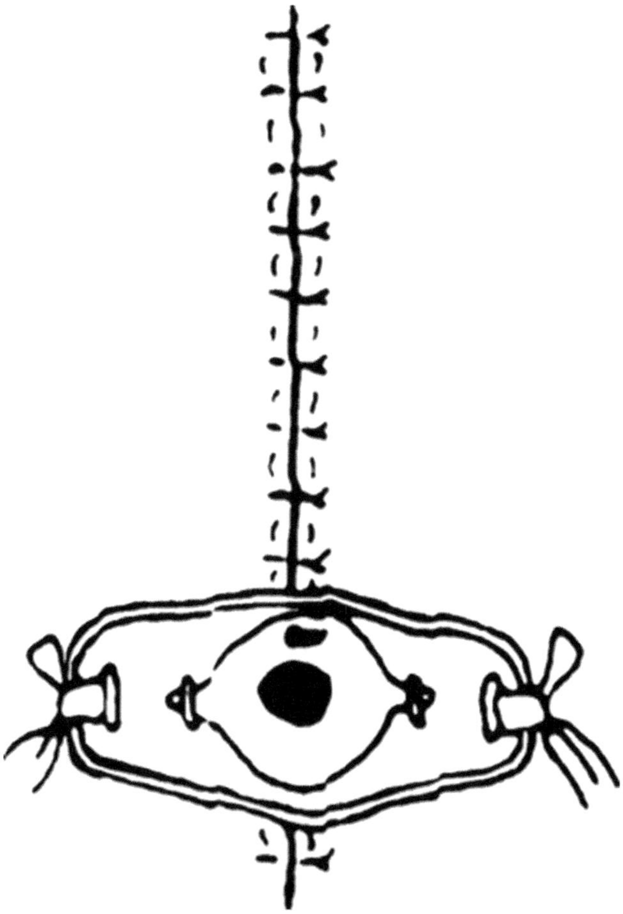

**Fig. 19.25** Suture skin incision

# Part VI

# Tracheoesophagology

The trachea constitutes the cartilage, muscle, connective tissue and mucosa and it is the joint canal between the larynx and the lung. It is not only where the air flows but also adjusts the air temperature and humidity, and it aslo help defense the alien. Esophagus is part of the alimentary tract between the larynx and the stomach and it acts on transporting. This part is for emphasizing the anatomy, physiology, examining methods and common clinic diseases diagnosis and treatment of the trachea, bronchus and esophagus.

# Applied Anatomy and Physiology of Trachea, Bronchus and Esophagus

# 20

Xiaohui Mi

The trachea, bronchus and esophagus are all located in the mediastinum. Mediastinumis generic is a term of the organs, structures and connective tissues between the right and the left mediastinum pleura. Figures 20.1 and 20.2 illustrates the relationship among the trachea, the bronchi and the esophagus clearly. Set sternal angle as bounder line, divide the mediastinum into upper mediastinum (Fig. 20.3) and inferior mediastinum. The inferior mediastinum contains three parts whose boundary is pericardium, anterior, middle and posterior parts. The trachea settles at the upper mediastinum, and the esophagus settle at the post mediastinum.

The trachea superiorly originates from the lower cricoid cartilage margin and inferiorly approaches the sternal angle plane. It is a set of tracheal cartilage that supports and remains persistently open; the esophagus is a long squamous muscular pipeline, whose upper margin attaches to the pharynx at lower sixth cervical vertebra edge and the lower margin attaches to the gastric cardia, it is over 2 times longer than trachea. The superior esophagus goes along with the slightly-left-inclined post trachea, and an esophageal stenosis is constituted at the site where the trachea separates the left-main bronchus. The clinic significance between the superior trachea and superior esophagus is; they both have a straight relationship with the pharynx. While breathing, the airway leading to the trachea opens; while taking food and swallowing, the esophagus aperture opens and the airway closes, simultaneous both of which avoid making mistakes.

X. Mi (✉)
Department of Otorhinolaryngology Head and Neck Surgery, Chinese People's Liberation Army 91458 Military Hospital, Sanya, China

## 20.1 Applied Anatomy of Trachea and Bronchus

Trachea originates upwards from the laryngeal cartilage, it ends downwards at the carina plane between the fourth and the fifth thoracic vertebral body (similar to the sternal angle) and simultaneously attaches to bronchi (Fig. 20.4). Adults' trachea are from the inferior cricocartilage edge to the carina, totally 10–12 cm long: adult male's is about 12 cm and adult female's is about 10 cm. Anterior and bilateral tracheal walls are constituted with support made with 18–22 reverse 'U' cartilage annulus and the smooth muscles form tube-like cartilage annulus space; tracheal posterior wall is membranous fibro smooth muscle, called membranous site, and it attaches to the esophagus with loose connective tissue. Infants' trachea is round-like; adults' tracheal anterior wall is arc like. The infants' post wall is flat, with a 'horse shoe like' cross section, the anterior and inferior diameter is about 1.8–2.0 cm, their transverse diameter is about 2.0–2.2 cm and the female's is slightly smaller than the male's. Bronchia's caliber, posterior to the main bronchus, gradually diminishes and even the ending bronchia's caliber is only about 0.1 cm. Based on the route, the trachea consists of the cervical segment and the thoracic segment of which the cervical segment is relatively more superficial and located upwards the sternojugular venous incisura.

1. Tracheal Structure

   From outside in, the tracheal wall contains the outer membrane, a muscle layer, cartilage, submucosa layer and a mucosa layer. The outer membrane is thin, constituting of fibrous connective tissues; the muscle layer is a smooth muscle, maintaining the elasticity of the tracheal wall; the cartilage annuli is 3–4 mm wide, occupying 2/3 tracheal cross section some of which bifurcate and some of which have a fused partial



Z. Mu, J. Fang (eds.), *Practical Otorhinolaryngology - Head and Neck Surgery*, https://doi.org/10.1007/978-981-13-7993-2_20

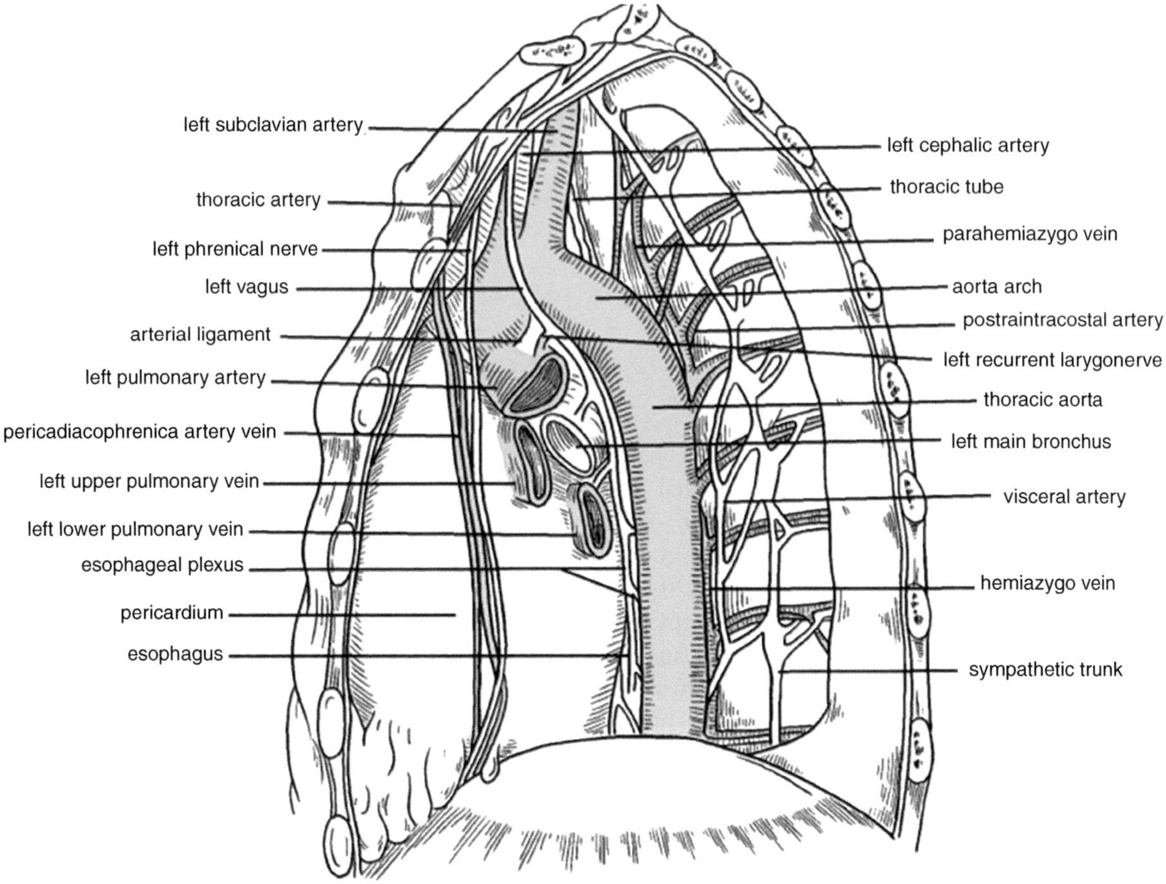


**Fig. 20.1** Mediastinum left lateral view

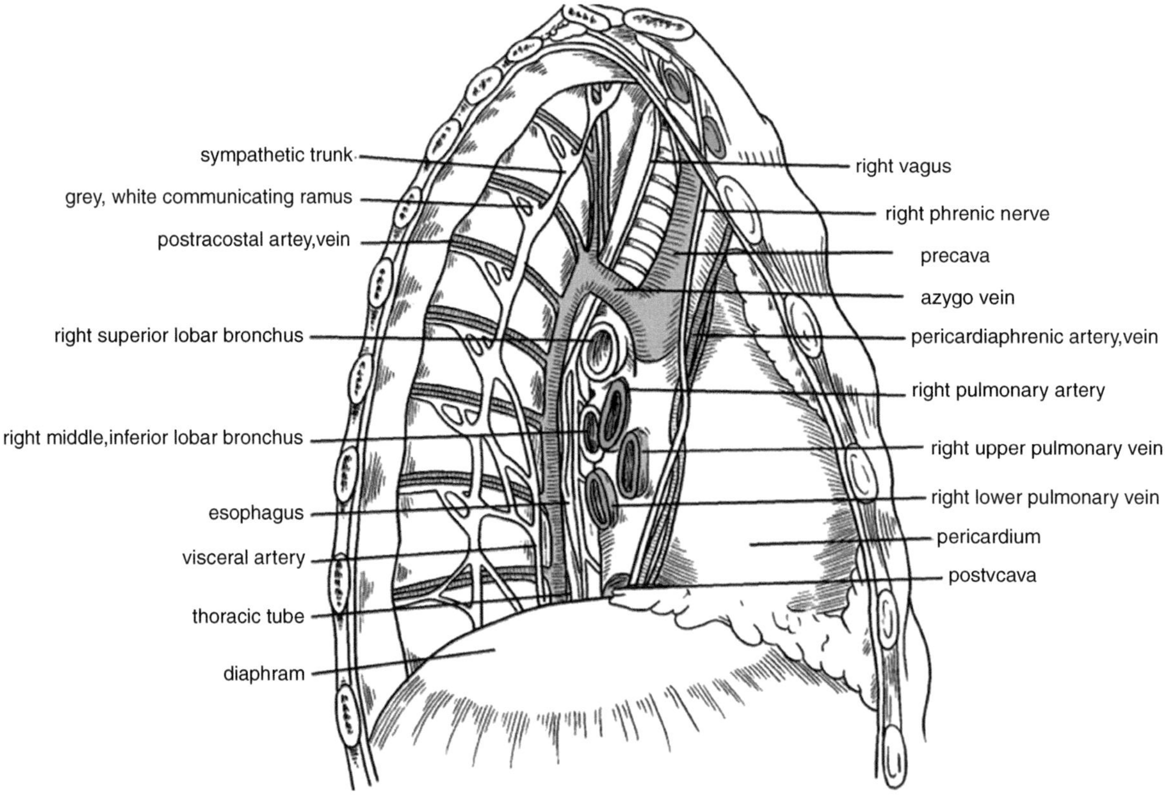


**Fig. 20.2** Mediastinum right lateral view

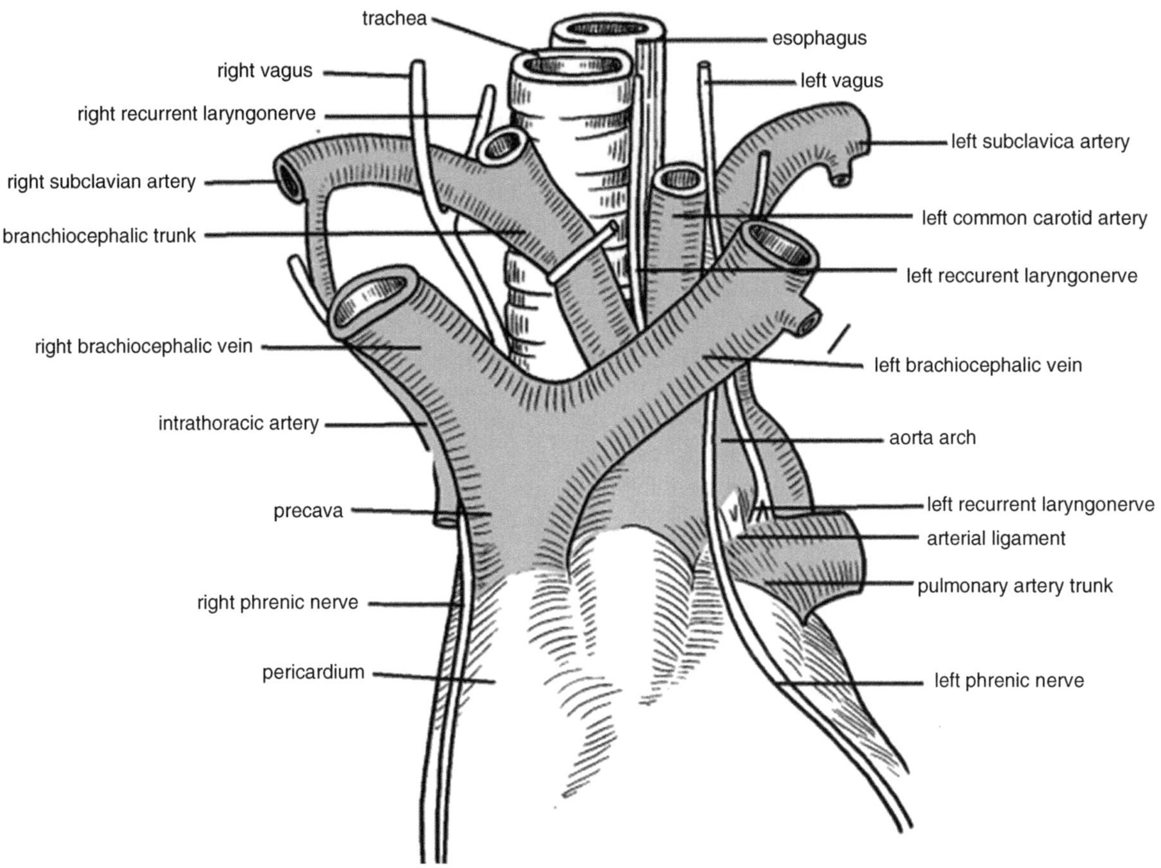


**Fig. 20.3** Upper mediastinum

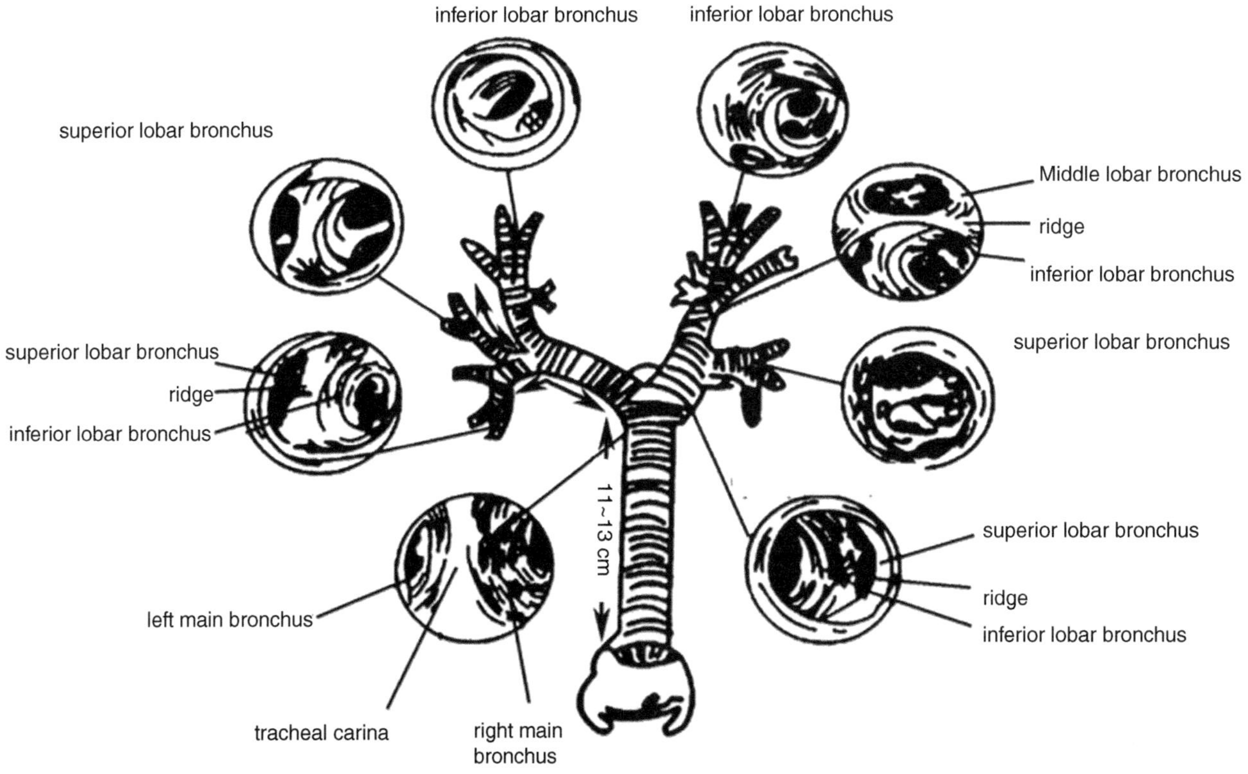


**Fig. 20.4** Bronchia aditus

annuli. At submucosal layer, abundant micro vessels, lymph nodes and nervous fibers. The mucosal layer is a columnar epithelium, cilia appears at its surface and the cilia help push forwards the secretion. The trachea could move up and down along with the cervical extension and flexion. While lowering one's head, the trachea almost enters the mediastinum and the cricoid cartilage also approaches the sub sternal incisor; while raising one's head, nearly half of the trachea is raised and a long segment trachea can be touched at the neck. Infants' tracheal elasticity is good and they have a large flexibility range. People over 45-year-old often have a post sterno vertebral process and a limited tracheal lifting exists. Because the fibrosis increases, the trachea hardens and embrittles, the excision length should be conservative while doing the tracheal resection surgeries.

2. Tracheal Blood Supply

   Its superior segment's supply is mainly from the sub thyroid arterial bronchus, commonly consisting of 2–3 bronchioles. Besides, the sub clavicular artery, the intra thoracic artery and the intercostal artery all have bronchial supply. The inferior segment's is mainly from the anterior and the middle bronchial arterial branches at sub aorta edge. All these small vessels lie at bilateral tracheal wall, anastomosing with each other and constituting longitudinal vascular chain and they seperate the transverse vessel branches to each cartilage annulus, entering the submucosa layer through cartilage to constitute a net to supply blood to the tracheal wall. Besides, at bilateral trachea, the tracheoesophageal artery separates arteries to respectively supply the trachea and the esophagus. Because the tracheal blood supply distribution is segmental, the tracheal segmental excision and anastomosis wouldn't' cause any effect on the blood supply. Whereas, a very long free range isn't suitable while excising the trachea, so the range should normally be 1–2 cm to the incisional edge and the bilateral tracheal adhered tissues shouldn't' be clamped to avoid necrosis evoked by insufficient blood supply.

3. Tracheal Lymph Supply

   Tracheal lymph supply is abundant and lymph nodes exist at anterior and bilateral trachea. Lymph nodes meet at the subcarina collects bilateral pulmonary and bronchial lymph reflux and they are the main sites where the bronchial pulmonary cancer lymphatic metastasis occurs. Therefore, clearing the subcarina lymph nodes is necessary while operating the pulmonary cancer excision surgeries. If the carina can't move up-and-down along with the respiration, it signifies that there is already an existance of a lymphatic metastasis and infiltrative fixation.

4. The tracheal carina is similar to the plane constituted by the sternal angle, the edge of the subaorta arch and the superior fifth cervicovertebral edge, and it is the connection point of the trachea and the bronchus, among which the left and the right main bronchus crossing angle is about 70–90° and subcarinal lymphatic swelling can increase the crossing angle. Gas displays radiative flow in carina and it can be evenly distributed in bilateral lungs. The carinal deformation can influence the gas diffusion. The aorta arch locates at the anterior tracheal carina hindering the pathway making it hard to expose the carina from the left cervicocavum.

## 20.2 Applied Anatomy of Esophagus

Esophagus is the narrowest region of the digestive tract, of which the anterior and the posterior are flat, its anterior edge attaches to pharynx at the inferior sixth cervical vertebral edge, downwards descending along with the anterior vertebra, passing through the superior thoracic mediastinum and posterior thoracic mediastinum, the phrenic esophageal hiatus, then entering the abdominal cavity and sustaining the stomach and the stomach cardia parallel to the 11th cervical vertebra. It's totally 25 cm long. Adults' superior 1/3 segment is skeleton muscle, middle segment is the skeleton muscle and the smooth muscle and the inferior 1/3 segment is entirely the smooth muscle. The superior 1/3 segment is dominated by the glossopharyngeal nerve, and the other 2/3 segment's motor nerves are mainly from the cervical vagus. The lowest 2–4 cm esophageal segment lies in the abdominal cavity to constitute the functional esophageal sphincter. The subesophageal sphincter is a high pressure belt, because its internal pressure is 15–40 mmHg higher than the atmospheric pressure, it is also the initial point of the stomach. While resting, the stomach initial internal pressure is only about 5 mmHg, and it can be used to test the pressure of the esophageal body and the subesophageal sphincter by the solid manometric catheter or the perfusion catheter set in the esophagus and stomach through nose. Manometry helps to assess the coordination of the esophageal contraction pressure and the multi esophageal peristalsis and the high resolution manometry has over 30 loci. The method can also be applied to examine the subesophageal sphincter's resting pressure and relaxation degrees. Multiloca manometry also contains the impedance detection. The impedance detection tests the process the food masses pass through the esophagus through detecting the electricity flow change going through the electrode, the technique is used to monitor the food masses' forward and reverse flow and detects all types of reflux including very weak acid or alkaline reflux, It could also be used for assessing the pharyngoesophageal junctional and pharyngeal muscular functional abnormality.

Esophagus is about 25 cm long, which could be divided into three parts, the cervical, the thoracic and the abdominal segment, with the plain sternocervical venus incisura and the esophageal hiatus boundaries.

1. The cervical segment: is about 5 cm long, its anterior wall approaches the loose connective tissue, adjoins with the vertebra at the posterior and bilateral cervical segments have macro vessels;
2. Thoracic Segment: is about 18–20 cm long. At the anterior, it contains the trachea, the left main bronchus and pericardium from superior downwards, and it's adjacent to the left ventricle, partitioning with the pericardium; at the left anterior lateral superior thoracic segment, the aorta arch exists, and the thoracic aorta initially originates from the inferior left anterior region, then gradually turns to the right posterior esophagus;
3. Abdominal Segment: shortest segment, about 1–2 cm long, sustaining to the stomach cardia.

## Constrictions

The esophagus has four points of constriction. When a corrosive substance, or a solid object is swallowed, it is most likely to lodge and damage one of these four points. These constrictions arise from particular structures that compress the esophagus. These constrictions are

The first stricture is at the start of the esophagus, where the laryngopharynx joins the esophagus, behind the cricoid cartilage at a 15 cm distant from the superior incisor, it is the narrowest esophageal region and also the easiest for foreign masses to incarcerate.

The second stricture is crossed on the front by the aortic arch in the superior mediastinum. The aorta compresses the esophagus and 23 cm distant from adults' superior incisor, and pulses could be partially seen under esophagoscope.

The third stricture is located where the esophagus is compressed by the left main bronchus in the posterior mediastinum and adults' is commonly located 4 cm inferior to the second stricture.

The second and the 3rd stricture are located adjacently to each other, so they are generally called the second stricture.

The fourth stricture is at the esophageal hiatus where it passes through the diaphragm in the posterior mediastinum. The adults' is commonly located about 40 cm distant from the superior incisor and they are similar to the 10th cervical vertebral plain.

These strictures are regions where foreign bodies can easily lodge, they are also tumor predilection sites, and their planar distance to the superior incisor differs at different ages (Fig. 20.5).

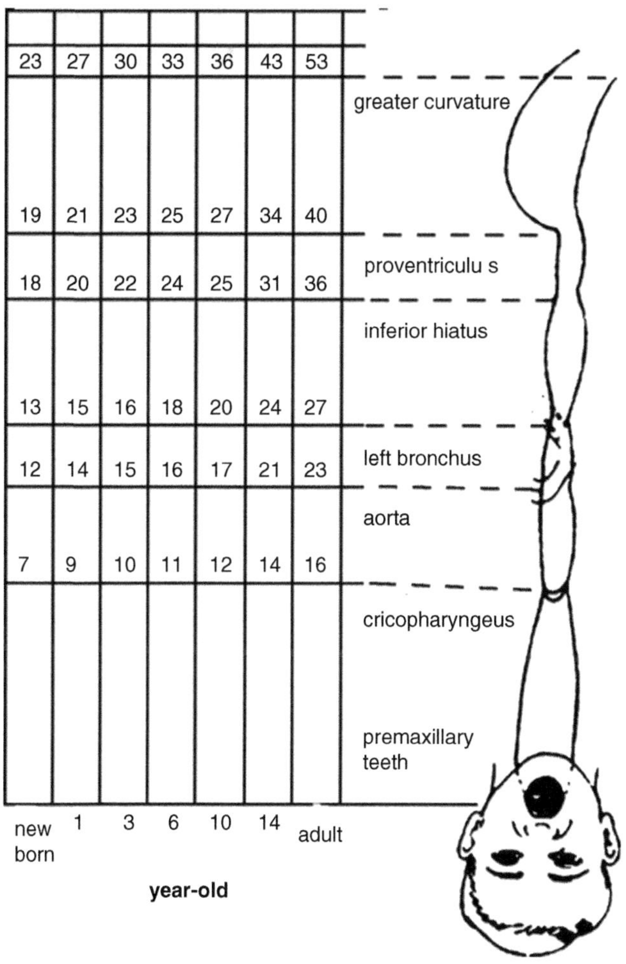


**Fig. 20.5** Each esophageal plain's distance to superior incisor (cm)

1. Esophagus Structures

   Esophagus has a typical digestive tract structure, is divided into mucosa, submucosa, muscle layer and external membrane.

   (a) Mucosal Layer: When the esophagus empties, the anterior and the posterior wall adhere to each other and 7–10 longitudinal folds constitute of the mucosal membrane; when the food passes, the muscular membrane loosens, so these folds extend and the internal cavity enlarges to help the passage of food.
   (b) Submucosal Layer: is relatively thicker, it is made up of connective tissue, inside which, has relatively large blood vessels, nerves, lymph and the esophageal glands.
   (c) Muscle Layer: It is cricoid at the internal and longitudinal at the external, it is about 2 mm thick, and the superior 1/3 muscle layer is striated, the inferior 1/3 is smooth muscle and the middle 1/3 is the mixed striated and smooth muscle. The initial esophageal cricoid myofiber is relatively thicker, which poses effect as sphincters and between which, elastic fibers exist.

(d) Outer Membrane: it is formed with loose connective tissues, it has abundant blood vessels, lymph tubes and nerves.

The whole esophageal wall is relatively thinner, only 0.3–0.6 cm thick, so puncture is easy to occur.

2. Esophagus Blood Supply

It is relatively abundant. Cervical esophageal blood supply is from the subthyroid arterial branches; superior thoracic esophageal artery is mainly supplied by the branchial artery and the descending esophageal aorta branch; the subthoracic segment is supplied by the small branch of the thoracic aorta or the intercostal artery; the abdominal segment is mainly supplied by the phrenic abdominal aorta branches. The esophageal veins contain the submucosal venous plexus and its peripheral venous plexus. The submucosal venous plexus passes through the peripheral esophageal venous plexus. The superior esophageal veins join the vena cava through the subthyroid vein and the subesophageal veins straightly join the azygos venous system.

3. Esophagus Adjacency

At the anterior esophagus, from upside down, there is the trachea, the tracheal carina, the left laryngeal recurrent nerve, the aorta arch, the left main bronchus, the right pulmonary artery, the pericardium, the left atrium and the transverse diaphragm existing.

At the posterior, there is the cervicovertebra, the thoracic vertebra and the infraesophageal space between the cervical vertebra and the esophagus, and in the space, there are the azygos vein, the semiazygos veins, the thoracic ducts and the right post intercostal artery.

At bilateral esophagus, the thoracic cavity exists, and except the right esophageal azygos venous arch, other regions all touch the pleura; under the dexter pulmonary root, the pleura extrudes to the post esophagus and constitutes the post esophageal recess. The azygos and the right vagus exist at the right lateral esophagus. The left lateral esophagus touches the pleura at the regions below the aorta arch and the seventh cervical vertebrae, but its middle region doesn't touch the pleura. And at the left lateral esophagus, from upside down, there are the left cervical aorta, the left substernal artery, the ending aorta arch segment, the thoracic aorta, the anterior thoracic duct segment and the left vagus artery.

## 20.3 Physiology of Trachea and Bronchus

1. Adjustment Protection

Tracheal mucosa is a mucinous barrier, adhering the foreign bodies in inhaled air, melting the inhaled $SO_2$, CO and other harmful gases, which are eventually coughed up. The basal cells are cone-like, located in deep epithelium, they are undifferentiated cells, which have proliferation and differentiation ability, and they could differentiate into the following two cell types.

Brush cells are columnar, whose free surface has several aligned brush-like microvilli. The brush cells' functions are unclear, which may be a certain absorption function. Basal granules can be seen at the cell top, so the brush cells may be considered as an immature ciliated cells. At some brush cells' base, a synapse constituted with the afferent nerves can be seen, so they may have stimulation proprioception function.

Neuroendocrine cells diffuse at the trachea and the intraairway tubular superior epithelium of the inferior tracheal branches, the cells are pyramidal and diffusing at the deep epithelium region. Because there are many dense core particles in cytoplasm, it is also called the small granule cell. As the immunity cellular chemical researches prove, many kinds of amines or peptides substances such as the 5-hydroxytryptamine, the bombesin, the calcitonin, the enkephalin etc; exist in the cells' secretion may join the adjusting respiratory tract blood vascular smooth muscle contraction and the glandular secretion through paracrine action or blood circulation.

2. Immunity Defense

There are relatively more elastic fibrers in proper connective tissues, so the tubular wall has a certain elasticity. The lymph tissues also exist in the proper layer, they are the same as these lymph nodes in the digestive tubular wall, having an immunity defense function. The IgA secreted by plasmocytes and the secretory piece produced at the epithelium unify to constitute the secretory IgA (SIgA), and release the SIgA into the intratubular cavum to inhibit the bacterial reproduction and the virus replication and decrease the harmful endotoxin effect.

3. Clearance and Nutrition

The submucosal layer contains the dense connective tissues, without evident boundaries between the proper layer and the outer membrane. There are also many mixed glands besides the blood vessels, the lymph tubes and the nerves in the submucosal layer. The outer layer contains the loose connective tissue, relatively thicker and mainly containing 16–20 C-like hyaline cartilage rings to form tubular wall support. Between the cartilage rings, the elastic fibers form a membranous ligament junction to keep the esophagus unobstructed and with a certain elasticity. Cartilage ring breaches open to the post tracheal wall and the ligament and a smooth muscle bundle is formed by the elastic fibersat. During coughing reflex, the smooth muscle contracts to shrink the esophagus cavum and help clear the sputum.

## 20.4 Physiology of Esophagus

Esophagus attaches to pharynx superiorly and to the cardia inferiorly, its main physical function is transmission, which is mainly achieved by its peristalsis function. After the food enters the esophagus through the mouth, the alternate esophageal relaxation and contraction display a wavelike peristalsis to pull the food into stomach. Food in esophagus can't be digested and absorbed. After the food is swallowed at pharynx and entering the esophagus, the esophageal muscles contract and relax in order, meaning the tracheal muscles above the food contracts and the tracheal muscles below the food relax, then the food is naturally pulled downwards segment by segment, finally the cardia opens, then the food enters the stomach, and whole procedure takes about 30 s. When the esophageal inflammation, stenosis and tumor occur, the esophageal peristalsis becomes irregular, then the food would stay in the esophagus and the normal esophageal aditus is closed to stop air from entering the stomach. Deglutition is a random activity in the very beginning, but after the food is chewed, it is pulled into the pharynx to touch the trigger zone and finally evoke series of complex non random reflex. The pharyngeal efferent nerve is the vagus and its afferent nerve passes through the glossopharyngeal nerve. The non random reflex includes: the glossal upwards and backwards motion to the hard palatine; the velumpalatinum muscle and the velumpharyngeal muscle combine to close the rhinopharynx; the epiglottis descends and the laryngovestibular region closes to stop the food entering the esophagus. At the moment the pharyngeal muscle contracts, the internal pressure suddenly rises up and the cricopharyngeal muscle relaxes to open. Meanwhile, what pulls the food into the esophagus from bilateral epiglottis 0.2–0.3 s after deglutition, the cricopharyngeal muscle opens, and the food approaches the cardia inside 1.5–2.5 s, which means that the food's adavancing is 10–20 cm/s. Food is pulled to the subesophageal ampulla after slow esophageal peristalsis, it stays for a short time. The subesophageal smooth muscular sphincter tension and minority of the transverse muscular fibers help the cardia to obtain the shutdown function. The cardial region is often closed, it relaxes and opens while being stimulated by then, the food enters the stomach. The deglutition motion includes three stages: oropharyngeal stage, esophageal stage and cardial stomach stage. The complex deglutition motion has several kinds of non random motion accomplished by several kinds of neural reflexes, they start from the Pommerenke regions, which distribute at the tongue root, the soft palatine and the post pharyngeal wall; when receptors at these regions touch the food, which are also the afferent impulses, it passes through the glossopharyngeal nerve, the second V cranial neural branch and the superior laryngeal nerve and approaches to the fourth ventricular floor where the swallowing motor central nerve lies. There receptors are vitally important, such as that after the oropharynx and the pharyngeal mucosa are anesthetized, the swallowing motion is influenced, and if the nerves are damaged by several kinds of diseases, the swallowing motor dysfunction will occur.

1. Oropharynx Stage

   It is from the mouth to the pharynx. It randomly starts under the effect of the cerebral cortex impulses. At the very beginning, the tongue apex rises up to touch the hard palate, then the food is pulled to the soft palate and then the pharynx under the influence of the mylohyoid muscular contraction. The glossal motion plays a very important role on deglutition motion at this stage.
2. Esophagus Stage

   It starts from the pharynx to the superior esophageal region. It can be achieved by series of rapid reflex motions. Because the food stimulates the soft palate receptors, evoking series of muscular reflexive contraction, so the soft palate rises up, the post pharyngeal wall extrudes forward and closes the rhinopharyngeal accesses; adduct the vocal cords, rise the larynx up to closely attach to the epiglottis, and close the approach between the pharynxtrachea respiration is paused; if the larynx moves forwards, the superior esophageal aditus opens, and the food is squeezed into the esophagus from the pharynx. This stage proceeds swiftly, commonly in about 0.1 s.
3. Cardia Stomach Stage

   It decends to the stomach along with the esophagus. It is achieved by the esophageal muscular contraction. The order esophageal muscular contraction is also called the peristalsis and it is a forward advancing wave-like motion. Wave inferior to the food is the diastole wave, and the wave superior to the food is the contraction wave. Therefore, the food is naturally pulled forwards. The esophageal peristalsis is a reflex motion because the food stimulates the soft palate, pharynx, esophagus and other receptors emitting afferent impulses then approaching the medullary center and finally the esophagus emits the efferent impulse and evokes the peristalsis. Between the esophagus and the stomach, though the sphincter doesn't exist in anatomy, what could be observed under the manometry is: above the esophagus and the stomach cardia junction, there is a 4–6 cm long high pressure field, whose internal pressure is commonly 0.67–1.33 kPa (5–10 mmHg) higher than that of the stomach therefore, commonly it could stop reflux of the stomach contents into the esophageal barrier, which acts similarly to the physiologic sphincter function, and it is often called the esophagus stomach sphincter. When the food passes through the esophagus, it stimulates the mechanical receptors at the superior esophageal wall and reflexively evokes the esophageal stomach sphincter diastole, then the food enters into the stomach. The gastrin is released after the food enters into the stomach, then the sphincter contraction is reinforced. Both of which may have certain effect on preventing the gastric contents from refluxing into the esophagus.

Esophagomanometry experiment confirms: at the superior about 3 cm esophageal region, the intraesophageal resting pressure is relatively higher so this region is also called the upper esophageal sphincter which is constituted with the cricopharyngeal muscle and the upper 3–4 cm esophagus. While deglutition, the upper sphincter relaxes and the pressure decreases then the esophagus returns to its resting pressure condition by immediately contracting after the food passes. The peristalsis evoked by the sphincter muscular contraction, originating from the pharynx and descending to the superior esophagus, the peristalsis wave conducts downwards the peristalsis pressure regularly crosses and approaches the whole esophagus to help in food transmission. When the superior esophageal sphincter dysfunction occurs, all the above characteristics disappear and eating difficulties occur which is often seen in cerebrovascular accident, myelitis, perineuritis, myositis, amyotrophy etc. At the inferior 3–5 cm region(esophageal hiatus), the internal esophageal cavum pressure evidently increases which is the so called high pressure region, and its pressure reduces while swallowing and restores to the normal pressure after the food passes this is all made by the lower esophageal sphincter. This sphincter has an important inside off mechanism which can stop reflux of the gastric content from the relatively higher pressure intragastric to the relatively-lower-pressure esophagus. But when its dysfunction occurs, the reflux esophagitis will happen.

Swallowing is a typical and complex reflex motion consisting series of the links occurring in order. Each link has series of motion processes and the former link's motion can evoke the latter link's motion. The deglutition afferent nerves contain the cerebral neural afferent fibers at the soft palate (the V and the IX pair cerebronerve), the postpharyngeal wall (the IX pair cerebronerve), the epiglottis (the X pair cerebronerve), the esophagus (the X pair cerebronerve) and other regions. The basic deglutition center is located in the medulla region which functions to monitor the muscular motion by the efferent nerves of the tongue, larynx and pharynx located at the V, IX and XII pair cerebronerve and whose regions monitor the esophageal efferent nerves, is the vagus.

The time cost from the beginning deglutition to the moment when the food reaches to the cardia is related to the food properties and the human position. Liquid food may cost about 3–4 s, the pasty food may cost about 5 s and the solid food is slower, costing about 6–8 s and commonly not over 15 s.

The esophageal peristalsis is the motion produced by the intraesophageal smooth muscle dominated by the vagus, its onset is from the pharynx and is accomplished by the intraesophageal reflex. This reflex could sustain its motion even after being cut off the relationship with the central nervous system, so if the vagus nerve is cut off during the experiment, the esophagus may display a complete loose condition and at the several initial days, its ataxia and abnormal reflex may occur but it would gradually restore its motion later on.

The esophageal peristalsis wave has two types: the primary type and the secondary type. The primary wave indirectly moves to the subesophageal region, it has the main power to pull the food, and a relaxation wave often appears before the contraction wave. The secondary wave has no relationship with the suboropharyngeal reflex, it mainly appears at the superior esophageal region, which is similar to the aorta region, and it is related to the intraesophageal expansion. During dog trials, the subpharyngeal or the secondary peristalsis could evoke the cardiac relaxation and if the peristalsis waves disappear before reaching the cardia, it can also open the cardia.

If the oral and the pharyngeal sensor ending nerves are stimulated, the cardiac muscular tension can be temporarily inhibited, so it stimulates the gastric mucosa, but the gastric sudden expansion can produce the reflexive cardiac muscular tension augment. The mechanically or chemically stimulated cardiac mucosa can also increase partial tension. The analysis can be rarely seen in the normal esophagus, but if there is obstruction existing, the analysis ascending from the obstructive region occurs by returning the food from the esophagus to the internal mouth.

Except the peristalsis, the esophagus still has local power, which also has the idiospasm, what may be a normal condition, but it could also be a pathologic condition, and it often occurs in local inflammation, foreign bodies, trauma and local or central neural lesion etc. Deep breath could temporarily slowly pull the food into the stomach, but the diaphragmatic sustaining contraction still can't stop the food from entering the stomach, so the diaphragm doesn't affect too much on the esophageal functions.

Under a normal condition, there is often simultaneously a little air swallowed and food, sustaining at the gastric basal region, but part of the air is often belched out after meals, which is a normal phenomenon. In esophagus, peristalsis often happens, so only a little air sustains in the esophagus. After analyzing the intragastric gas sustained in a short time after meals, the researchers found that the $CO_2$ occupies 4.2%, the $O_2$ occupies 17.1% and the $N_2$ occupies 78.8%, as we see, the air in stomach has slightly increased $CO_2$ content than the atmosphere, which could be produced by the gastric mucosa. The thoracic intraesophageal vacuum is normally about -0.5–-3.0 cm $H_2O$, and it is caused by the intrathoracic vacuum while inhaling. People may make a sound while swallowing food, which can be auscultated at thorax with a stethoscope, and it contains two types: the first sound is produced while the food rapidly enters the esophagus and it immediately occurs secondarily to the deglutition oropharyngeal stage the second sound appears after the esophageal primary peristalsis accomplishes, whose time is similar to the seventh second after the oropharyngeal stage.

There is a relative complex relationships in physiology between the gastrointestinal, the cardiac vessels and the respiratory system, and there are still not many relationships having not been mastered recently. Such as that the intraesophageal reflex could produce abnormal phenomenon in other organs by the automatic nerve systemic relationship, which is called the abnormal reflex between several vagus branches.

The esophagus sometimes presents a loosen curved condition, which is the manifestation of major irregularly local contraction and expansion, and it is also thought to be caused by each segmental muscular spasm and incoordination by Scheinmel and others. This condition often happens in middle aged males, and the painful sensation while contracting is commonly thought as a physiologic condition.

Esophageal secretion: the vagus nerve is not only related to the normal subpharyngeal and esophageal reflex action, but also dominates the esophageal secretion. The vagus contains the secretory fibers approaching to the esophageal mucosal gland. In the dog experiment, stimulating the vagus nerve can increase the secretion, which is initially sticky, then gradually change into aqueous, all this proves that the esophageal secretion is produced by domination and stimulation of the vagus nerve. The esophagus is an excretion drainage tube. Where the oral, rhinocavum's, laryngeal and tracheal secretion approach the stomach through the esophagus, then they are digested by the gastric juice in stomach and the bacteria are wiped out.

# Endoscopy of Trachea, Bronchus and Esophagus

# 21

Xiaohui Mi

## 21.1 Bronchoscopy

Bronchoscopy is a diagnosis and treatment method to examine and treat the tracheal and intrabronchial lesions through bronchoscopy. The endoscope has two types: one type is a hard metal hollow pipe which can observe every lobular bronchus; the other type is a fiberoptic bronchoscope, with a thin, soft and flexible tube body, sufficient lighting and clear images, it can be guided into several pulmonary segmental bronchi, and to diagnose the bronchial lesions, especially the early pulmonary cancer etc., the relatively harder tube is more convenient, because it causes less pain and it gains a better effect.

The bronchoscopy is a common diagnostic method for agnogenic or unknown lesion subrespiratory tract diseases, it can also be used to remove the foreign respiratory tract masses or treat the lower respiratory tract pathologic obstructions, such as the granulations, tumors, secretions, etc.

In nonurgent conditions such as severe cardiovascular diseases, recent severe hemoptysis, late stage tuberculosis, acute inflammation, cervical spondylosis etc, metal bronchoscope is unsuitable for use.

Equipments Preparation: commonly adult male use 8–9 mm diameter bronchoscope and the female use 7–8 mm diameter bronchoscope (Table 21.1).

**Table 21.1** Bronchoscope application chart

| Age (year-old) | Intradiameter (mm) | Length (mm) |
|---|---|---|
| Adult (male) | 8–9 | 400 |
| Adult (female) | 7–8 | 400 |
| 10–15 | 6–7 | 320–400 |
| 5–10 | 5–6 | 250–320 |
| 2–5 | 4–5 | 250–300 |
| 1–2 | 3.5–4 | 250 |
| <1 | 3–3.5 | 200–250 |

1. Operation Routine

   Preoperative preparation and anesthesia are same as for the straight laryngoscopy. Patients' position and assisstants' working plate are also same as for the straight laryngoscope examinations, which mainly contain two methods, including the straight intubation method and the indirect intubation method.

   (a) Indirect Intubation Method

   It suits infants. The infants' bronchoscope tube is thin and hard to expose the glottis, so after exposing the glottis with the straight laryngoscope, intubate the bronchoscope to examine and reduce the laryngeal injury chances (Fig. 21.1).

   (b) Straight Intubation Method

   The operator holds the bronchographic mirror with the right hand, and the left hand holds the scope body, of which the thumb should be at inferior scope body and the index finger should support the scope body, and enter the oral cavity along the center of the dorsum of tongue or slightly to the right, then the uvula and the epiglottis can be seen, after which, transmit the furthur scope ending to the laryngeal plain and insert it deeper to distinguish the arytenoid cartilage, then raise the epiglottis, meanwhile, the patient's head should be gradually raised to set the oral cavity, pharynx, larynx and trachea in that order then the operator's left thumb slightly raises the branchoscopic tube to expose the glottis. Inspect after

X. Mi (✉)
Department of Otorhinolaryngology Head and Neck Surgery, Chinese People's Liberation Army 91458 Military Hospital, Sanya, China



Z. Mu, J. Fang (eds.), *Practical Otorhinolaryngology - Head and Neck Surgery*, https://doi.org/10.1007/978-981-13-7993-2_21

restoring the bronchoscopic mirror handle forwards to the midcentral position, the tracheal protuberance at the bronchial cross can be seen (Fig. 21.2). While examining the right bronchus, turn the head slightly to left.

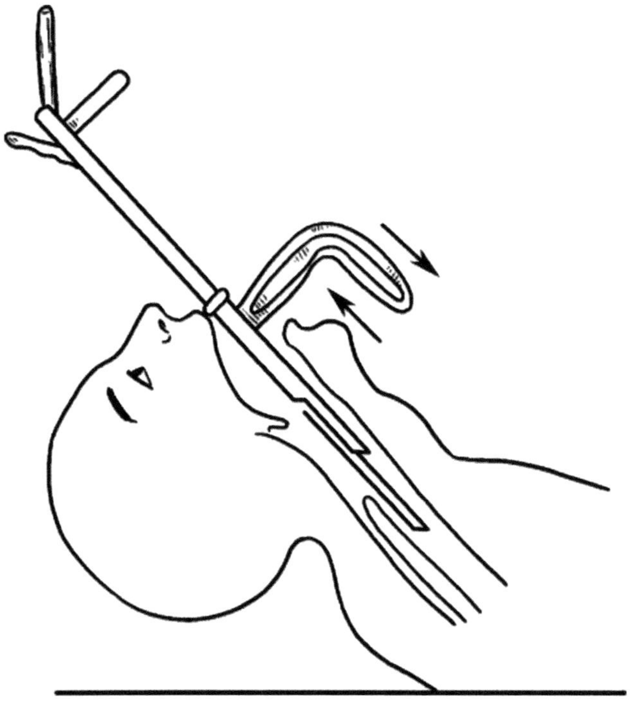

**Fig. 21.1** Insert bronchoscope by indirect method

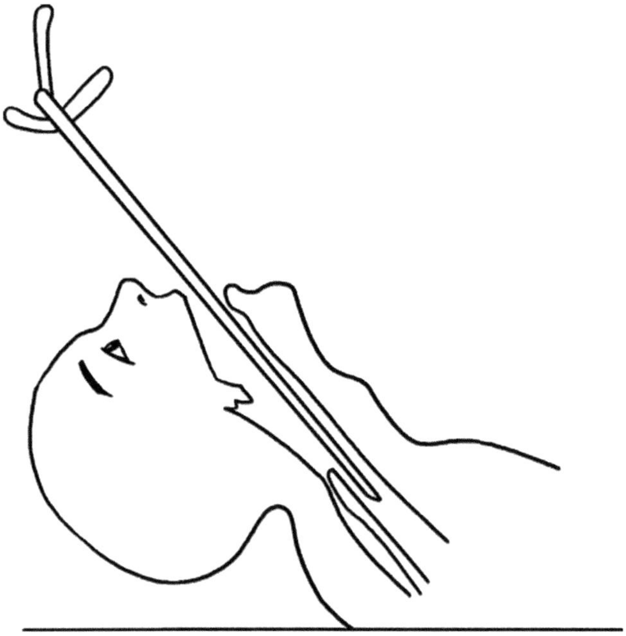

**Fig. 21.2** Insert bronchoscope by direct scope

2. Matters Needing Attention
   (a) Bronchoscopy should be kept in the middle of the trachea, should see the left and right walls before and after.
   (b) Check the bronchial health side first, and then check the affected side.
   (c) Pay attention to the mucous membrane congestion, ulcer, granulation, tumor, scar and tube wall with or without stenosis or extraluminal compression, etc.
   (d) Tracheal secretions should be fully sucked out and pay attention to the bronchial site where the secretions are coming from.
   (e) Should pay attention to the patient's general condition, such as heart rate, breathing, etc.

## 21.2 Esophagoscopy

Esophagoscopy is a method of inserting esophagoscopy into the esophagus for examination and treatment of lesions. Like bronchoscopy, esophagoscopy has two types: rigid tube and flexible tube. It is contradicted in severe cardiovascular disease, severe esophageal varices, esophageal corrosion injury in acute and critical patients.

1. Equipment Preparation

   At present, elliptical or flat circular tube are mostly used, and the selection specifications are shown in Table 21.1.

   Fiberoptic esophagoscopy, flexible, strong light intensity, wide field of vision, can observe small lesions, high diagnostic rate, less discomfort, not limited in spinal deformity, easy to operate, but it is difficult to do treatment and foreign body extraction. Clinical points for adults and children with two kinds.
2. Operating Procedures

   Operation generally takes "high and low position". Patients' head position should be the same as direct rhino-

**Table 21.1** Esophageal mirror selection table

| Age | Inside diameter (up and down diameter × left and right diameter) (mm × mm) | Length (mm) |
|---|---|---|
| Adults | (17–19) × (11–13) | 450–530 |
| Women and 5 years of age or older | 10 × 15 | 250–350 |
| Under 5 years old (foreign body in upper esophagus) | 8 × 14 | 200 |
| More than 1 years old (foreign body in the upper esophagus) | 7 × 10 | 200 |

scope. Head should be 15 cm above the table, the esophageal mirror along the right side of the mouth first inserted into the throat on the right side of the piriform recess, then the distal end of the esophageal mirror gradually moves to the midline, after arytenoid cartilage move the mirror nozzle straight to the esophagus, visible at this time the pharyngeal muscles in the rear wall uplift such as a threshold, should wait for the esophagus mouth to automatically open, or tell the patient to do the swallowing action, to see the esophageal inlet gap, conveniently slide tube end into the esophagus immediately. Because the back wall is the thinnest, forced tube insertation under improperly opened mouth should be avoided to avoid esophageal perforation. When the esophageal mirror is into the middle esophagus, the head should be gradually lowered, and slightly turned to the right so as to adapt to the direction of the esophagus the thoracic esophagus is wider than the neck section, pay attention to the esophagus and aorta at the junction of the esophagus in front of the left pulse during the examination. Examination of the lower esophagus, the patient's head is often lower than the operating table 2–5 cm. During the esophageal endoscopic examination should always keep the direction of the tube and lumen consistent, so that you can clearly see the left and right four walls in depth progress, avoid insertion on one side, to decrease the chances of esophageal wall damage. Normal esophageal mucosa is smooth, moist, soft and reddish. Should pay attention to observe mucous membrane congestion, ulcers, tumors, varicose veins, lumen stenosis, expansion, etc.

# Foreign Body of Trachea and Bronchus

# 22

Xiaohui Mi and Jianghua Wan

**Etiology**

The foreign bodies are common in children, because the children chewing and laryngeal reflex function are not perfect. Swallowing hard food without chewing, swallowing small toys or being suddenly frightened or crying with food in the mouth can easily cause choking. It is rare to observe aliens in trachea and bronchus of adults, but nothing is impossible. When adults are in coma or sleeping, they vomit or stay in bad posture, aliens, such as dentures, would fall or be inhaled into trachea or bronchus; While eating, if adults take so fast or saying at the meanwhile, things they are taking would be inhaled into trachea or bronchus as aliens; adults with bad habbits, such as remove nails with teeth and wet needle with tongue, would iatrogenicly inhale the nails or needle into trachea or bronchus.

1. The Species of Foreign Body
   It is divided into two types: endogenous and exogenous. Endogenous foreign bodies are teeth, blood, pus and secretions. There are many exogenous foreign bodies, including plant foreign bodies, animal foreign bodies and mineral foreign bodies, all from the mouth.
2. Existence Part of the Foreign Body
   According to the data, 56% of the foreign body distribution was in the total trachea, 32% in the right bronchus and 12% in the left bronchus. The right bronchial foreign body is 3 times more than the left side. The reason is:
   (a) the total tracheal protuberance is less to the left side, so the right bronchial diameter is larger.
   (b) the angle between the right bronchus and the trachea is small and straight.
   (c) when inhaling, the amount of air entering the right bronchus is more.
3. Pathophysiology
   After inhalation of a foreign body, the trachea and bronchus cause pathological changes such as inflammation, and the degree is closely related to the nature, size and the duration the foreign body stays. Plant bodies such as rice, soybean, because they contains free fatty acids, they will cause mucosal irritation, diffuse inflammation, mucosal hyperemia, swelling, increased secretions, fever and other systemic symptoms, clinically called plant bronchitis. Tissue ulceration and granulosis caused by rusting of large foreign bodies or metal foreign bodies can also obstruct the respiratory tract. Small and non irritating foreign objects such as melon seeds are less likely to block. The longer the foreign body stays, the greater the damage is. Irritant foreign bodies can be associated with pulmonary infection, causing severe complications such as pneumonia, bronchiectasis, pulmonary abscess and empyema.

**Clinical Manifestation**

The symptoms of foreign body in trachea and bronchus are related to the size, nature, location and local pathological changes of foreign bodies. It can be divided into the following 4 phases.

1. The period of foreign body inhalation: acute cough, shortness of breath. Asphyxia may occur when the foreign body is larger or stuck in the glottis.
2. Quiet period: when the foreign body is inhaled, it can stay in a certain part of the bronchus, at this time there is no symptom or only light cough. This period varies in lengths, and the nature of the foreign body and the degree of infection.
3. The period of stimulation and inflammation: due to foreign body stimulation and inflammation, or clogged bronchitis, coughing can occur, and atelectasis or emphysema may develop.

X. Mi (✉)
Department of Otorhinolaryngology Head and Neck Surgery, Chinese People's Liberation Army 91458 Military Hospital, Sanya, China

J. Wan
Department of Medical Imaging, The First Affiliated Hospital of Hainan Medical University, Haikou, China

 
Z. Mu, J. Fang (eds.), *Practical Otorhinolaryngology - Head and Neck Surgery*, https://doi.org/10.1007/978-981-13-7993-2_22

4. The period of complications: mild complications include bronchitis, pneumonia, and the severe cases have lung abscess, empyema and heart failure.

**Diagnosis**

According to the medical history, symptoms, physical examination and X ray examination, there is no difficulty in diagnosis.

1. Medical History
   History of aspiration of a foreign bodies after coughing, vomiting, shortness of breath, cyanosis and other symptoms have an important basis in the diagnosis.
2. Physical Signs
   When the smooth, hard, small foreign body is located in the positive tube, a clapping sound can be heard as the breathing moves up and down. It is more obvious when coughing. Sometimes the impact can be felt when you touch the upper part of the trachea with a finger. The foreign body in bronchus or its branches, can produce two kinds of phenomenon:
   (a) Foreign body is not completely blocking the lumen, inhale due to expand the diameter of a portion of the gas, after the foreign body and the pipe wall clearance suction to the respiratory segment, when breathing diameter has reduced and the gas can not be discharged, thus to form part of foreign body in obstructive pulmonary emphysema. In addition a prolonged "check air hissing", blocking one or a decreased breath sounds, language fibrillation is weak, on percussion was drum. In severe cases, the chest movement is limited and the heart is shifted to the healthy side when exhaling.
   (b) The foreign body has completely blocked by the cavity, the air can not be inhaled or exhaled, the air below the blocked part is absorbed, and the obstructive pulmonary atelectasis is formed. It could be found that the respiratory sound reduces, language fibrillation enhancement, and the knocking sound turbidity at the side or lobule where foreign masses clogged is heard.
3. Imaging Examination
   X-ray examination can only diagnose the foreign bodies of metal and bone tissue, but it can not directly diagnosed the translucent foreign body of plants. CT examination, especially the three dimensional multi planar reconstruction, can display the radiopaque plants or soft tissue foreign body, in addition, also need to be combined with the history of inhaling a foreign body, or indirect imaging signs to diagnose: chest X-ray shows mediastinal swing: trachea partial obstruction of bronchial pleural pressure on both sides of one side, out of balance, so that exhaling and inhaling with mediastinal swing to the both sides; if the foreign body is relatively fixed, the formation of expiratory valve, exhale tracheal narrowing, the air discharge is blocked, the formation of ipsilateral pulmonary emphysema, the ipsilateral intrapulmonary pressure is greater than the contralateral, mediastinal metastasis. If the activity of the foreign body with the suction valve down, the formation of inspiratory breath into the blocked, ipsilateral lung air content less than the healthy side, the formation of ipsilateral pulmonary atelectasis, deep breathing to the ipsilateral mediastinal mobile. However, the current chest fluoroscopy is mostly replaced by CT. The obstructive emphysema: ipsilateral lung touliangdu heighten, intrapulmonary pressure, diaphragm downward. The obstructive atelectasis, pulmonary lobe or segment foreign bodies belong there increased density, size, intrapulmonary pressure decreased diaphragmatic elevation, heart and mediastinum metastase to affected side (Fig. 22.1). Obstructive pulmonary infection: a flake fuzzy shadow

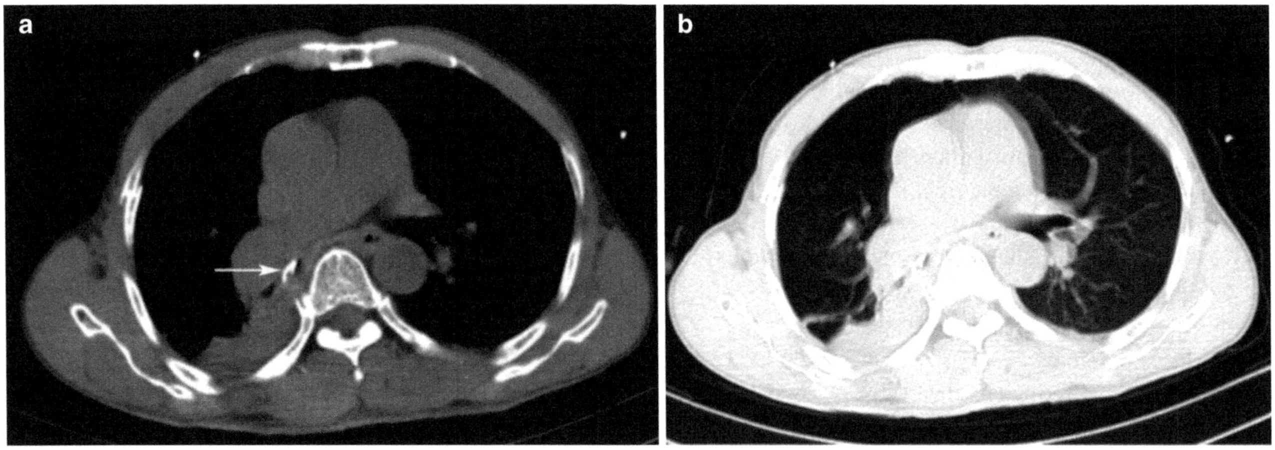


**Fig. 22.1** Thoracic axial CT plain scan displays right bronchial foreign mass. Patient is 51 year old, its thoracic pain accompanies with dyspnea for one day. (**a**) Mediastinum window displays right pulmonary midinferior lobular host intratracheal cavity high intensity foreign mass shadow (arrow). (**b**) Pulmonary window displays right pulmonary midinferior obstructive pulmonary atelectasis

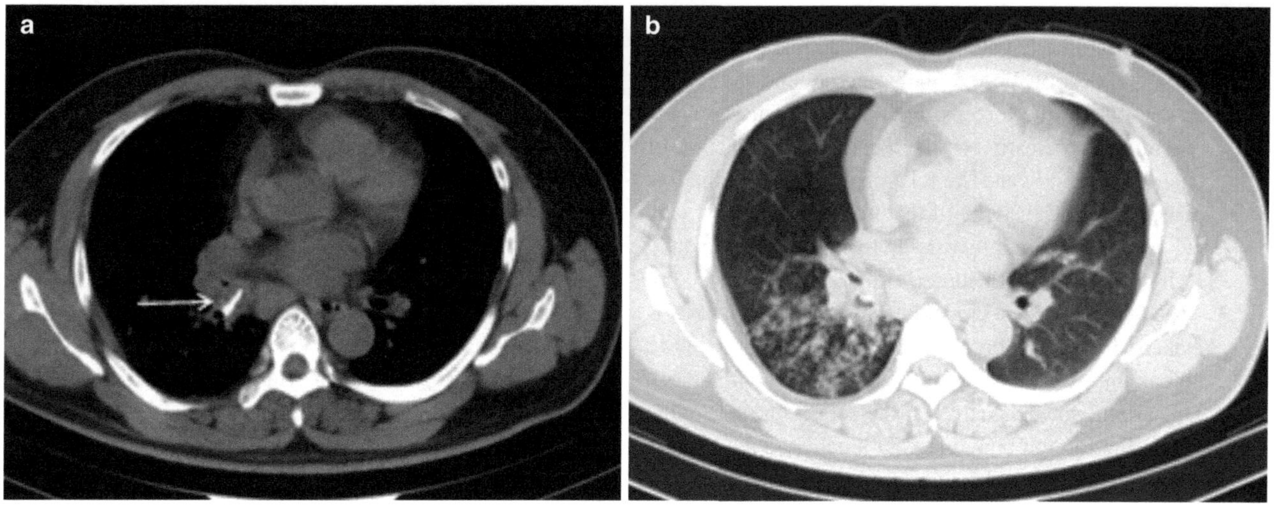


**Fig. 22.2** Thoracic axial CT plain scan displays right lateral bronchial foreign masses. (**a**) Mediastinum window displays right pulmonary inferior lobular bronchial high intensity foreign mass shadow (arrow). (**b**) Pulmonary shadow displays right pulmonary inferior lobular obstructive inflammation

(Fig. 22.2), which is characterized by uneven local density. Sometimes small foreign bodies can be found at positive and lateral faults in the chest, and CT or MR can be done to help diagnosis when necessary.

The tracheobronchoscopy is the gold standard test for the diagnosis of foreign body in the airway, if it is difficult to make a definite diagnosis if the foreign body is retained for a long time.

**Treatment**

After the diagnosis and determination of the bronchial foreign body, the hard bronchoscope (Fig. 22.3) should be selected to remove the foreign body immediately according to the clinical condition.

1. Preoperation Preparation
   The foreign body remains for more than 2–3 days. Patients with complications such as; high fever, and systemic failure should be hospitalized. First, to treat complications and correct dehydration and imbalance of water and electrolyte balance. After the whole body condition improves, repare for the operation. Patients who have not taken out of the foreign body by bronchoscopy also need to be hospitalized for anti-inflammatory, rest, and repare for the operation after trachea and bronchial mucosa swelling reduces. The time and dose of antibiotics given before and after the operation is determined according to the infection and the complications.
2. Anesthesia Method
   As a result of dyspnea, immediate rescuers and young babies can be operated without anesthesia. 1% tetracaine can be used for mucosal surface anesthesia in adults. General anesthesia can be used for those who cannot cooperate. The drugs such as atropine and promethazine should be given before operation.

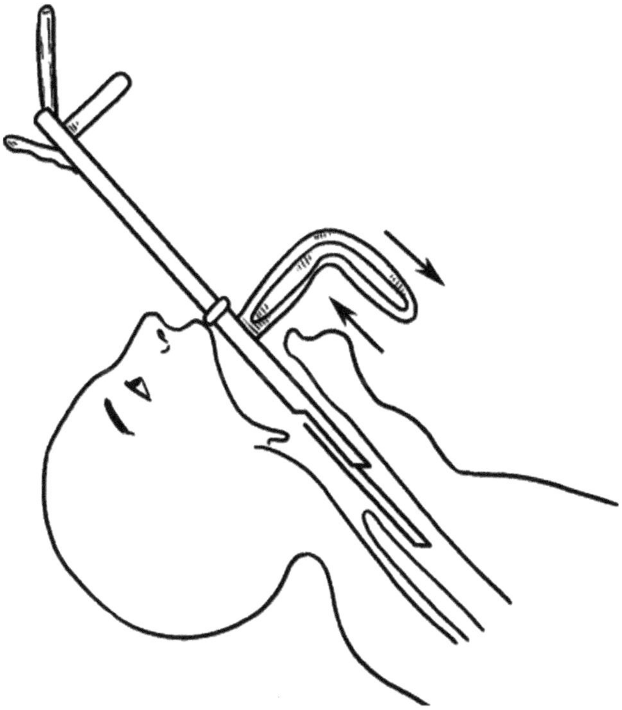

**Fig. 22.3** Tracheoscope direct laryngoscopic interposition by indirect method

3. Surgical Methods
   Different methods are used according to the nature of the foreign body, the time length, the age of the patient, and the complications.
   (a) Method of Removing Foreign Bodies under Direct Laryngoscope (with or without Lens)
      Under direct laryngoscope, open forcep beneath glottis, when patients cough, aleins would drop into the forcep.

(b) Method of Taking Foreign Body Under Bronchoscope
The foreign body with deep position must be extended into the location close to the bronchoscope and then is taken out by the forceps. First carefully suck out the secretions to clearly see the location and direction of the foreign body and the relationship between the foreign body and the wall of the bronchus. The best way to clamp the foreign body is to be studied. Usually when in the suction lumen expansion when forceps. The force should be moderate when the foreign body is taken. Too much force will cause the foreign body to break into small pieces or the foreign body will fall off. In particular, when there is an atelectasis one side of the lung, the foreign body is easily inhaled on the healthy side in the total trachea, causing severe anoxia. At this time, the bronchoscope should be sent to the healthy side and the foreign body removed. The larger foreign body can not be taken out of the bronchoscope, and the foreign body should be close to the front of the bronchoscope so that it can be taken out. With sharp spiny foreign objects such as needles and studs, the tip of the foreign body must be pinked in the bronchoscope or with a foreign body clamping tip to avoid damage to the mucous membrane. For the larger foreign bodies that can not be removed from the glottis, the tracheotomy is practicable, and the foreign body is removed from the cut opening. The use of fiberoptic bronchoscopy (Fig. 22.4) to take foreign bodies can make up for some of the shortcomings of the hard bronchoscopy (Fig. 22.5). The advantages are as follows:

- the illumination is high, the operative field is clear.
- it can be bent, and is less painful. It can be used for patients with old neck and neck weakness.
- The area not reached by rigid bronchoscope below segmental bronchus can be observed.

However, the inner diameter of the bronchoscopic attraction tube is small, which makes the respiratory tract smaller, so it is not suitable for children. Pediatric bronchoscopy is an important technique for assessing and treating children's airway diseases, saving the lives of many children inhaling foreign body (Fig. 22.6).

The indications for children's bronchoscopy include congenital larynx wheezing, larynx after intubation, hemoptysis, suspicious foreign body inhalation and refractory pneumonia.

4. Prognoses
Small foreign bodies can be naturally coughed up. If a large foreign body is not treated on time, the consequences are serious. In recent years, there are more and more hospitals that operate bronchoscopy. There are also antibiotics to prevent infection. If we can diagnose early, most of the foreign bodies can be successfully removed under bronchoscope.

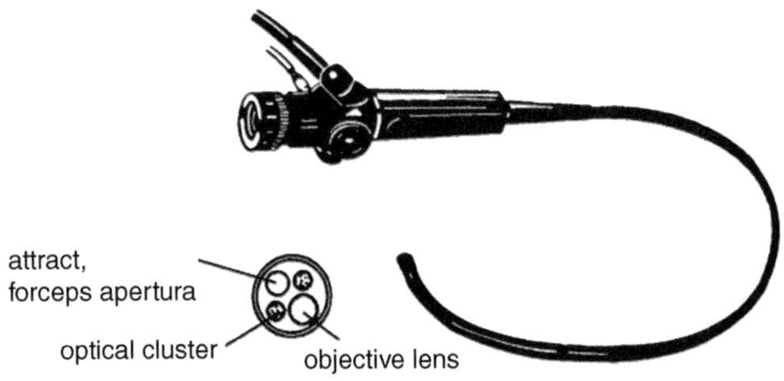


**Fig. 22.4** Fibrous bronchoscope

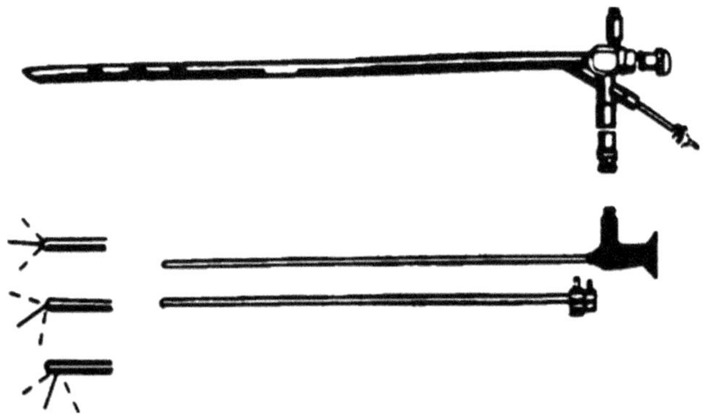

**Fig. 22.5** Rigid bronchoscope

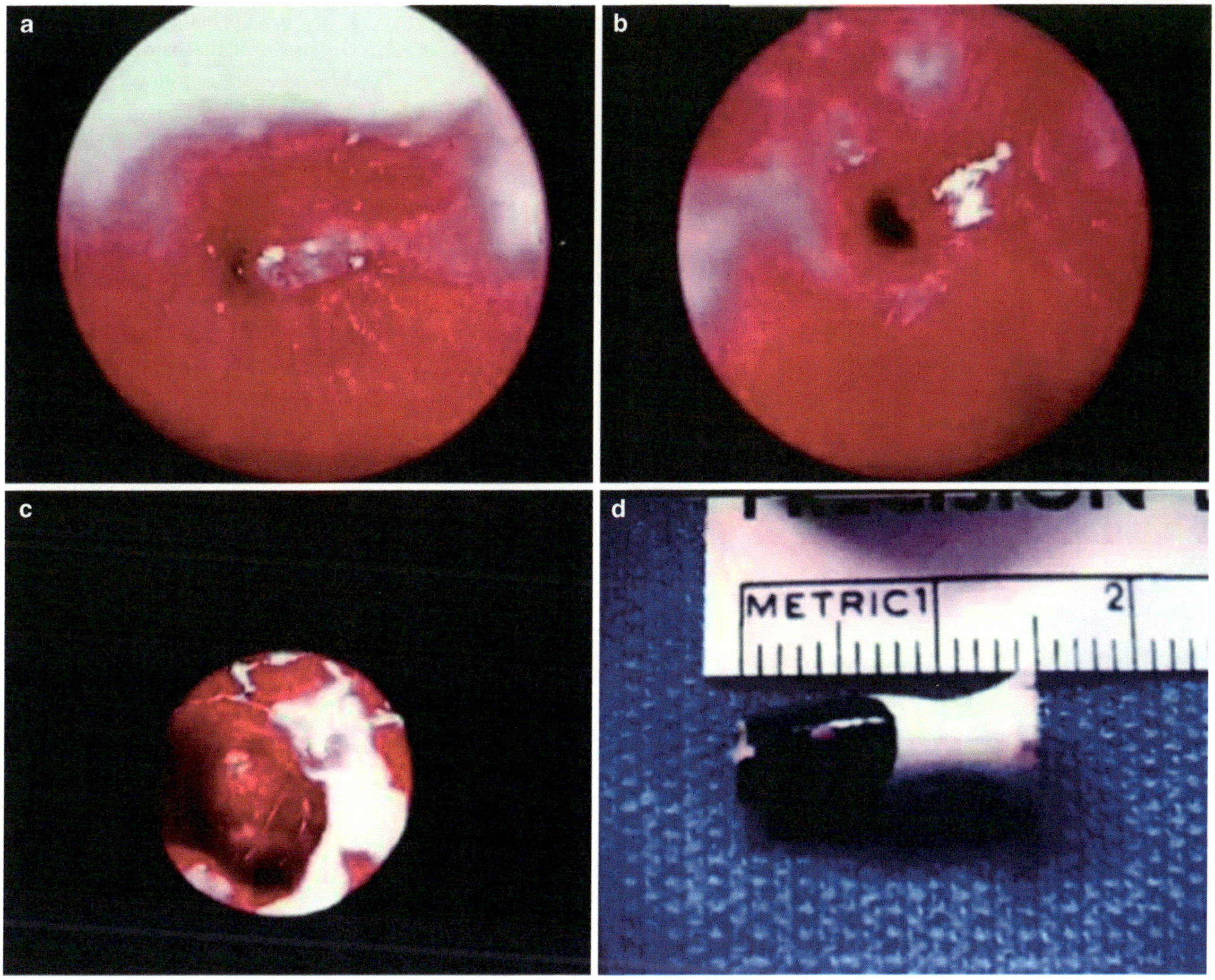


**Fig. 22.6** Apply infant bronchoscope to take wooden oldgolftee carelessly taken in 20-month-old infant trachea

# Esophageal Disease

# 23

Xiaohui Mi and Zhiqun Li

## 23.1 Foreign Body of Esophagus

The foreign body of the esophagus is a common disease of the esophagus, which is one of the emergency cases in the Department of ENT. Because the strength of pharyngeal muscle is strong enough to transmit larger irregular objects into the esophagus, the muscle strength of the upper esophagus is weak, and there are several physiological stenoses. It is easy to enter the incarceration of pharyngeal incarceration. Any object that can be terried in the esophagus can become a foreign body of the esophagus. About 70% of the foreign bodies are located at the entrance of the esophagus, followed by the aortic arch and the junction of the lower esophagus and the stomach.

**Etiology**

About half of the diseases occur in the elderly and children. At the elderly, because of teeth loss or using false teeth, they have bad chewing ability, unsensitive orosense, loose esophageal aditus and more possibility to misswallow teeth or large food; At children, almost cases are caused by mistakenly swallowing toys. At adults, almost cases are caused by mistakening swallowing the fish bones, chicken bone and others while quick or inattentive food taking. Some patients come with mistakenly swallowing false teeth while taking sticky food. Some patients are of swallowing metal needle and other things to suicide or because of mental diseases.

X. Mi (✉)
Department of Otorhinolaryngology Head and Neck Surgery, Chinese People's Liberation Army 91458 Military Hospital, Sanya, China

Z. Li
Department of Medical Imaging, The First Affiliated Hospital of Hainan Medical University, Haikou, China

**Pathology**

Most of the foreign bodies can cause edema and inflammation in the local mucosa of the esophagus. The extent and extent of the foreign bodies vary with the characteristics, the degree of contamination and the duration of the foreign body. With smooth foreign body, no irritation and no complete obstruction of the esophagus, it can stay in the esophagus for a long time and only mild swelling and inflammation of the local mucosa. The sharp foreign body easily damages the esophagus mucous membrane to spread the inflammation, and can form the esophagitis and mediastinum. A few cases broke into the trachea and formed an oesophagotracheal fistula; the serious cause of the empyema or the rupture of the aorta to the aortic arch, died of massive hemorrhage.

**Clinical Manifestations**

They are often related to property, size, shape, staying site and time, infection existing, etc.

1. Pain: a sharp foreign body piercing the wall of the esophagus causes heavier pain. According to the location of the foreign body in the esophagus, the pain can be located on both sides of the lower neck or after the sternum, and the pain is aggravated when swallowing. Sometimes the location of the patient's feeling of pain is not necessarily the location of the foreign body. Only obstruction or discomfort.
2. Dysphagia: light or early incomplete obstruction can flow into the food. The foreign body of the cervical esophagus can increase the saliva. Because of severe esophageal reflex spasm, swallowing pain and antifeedant. Inflammatory swelling of the esophagus, the large foreign body can cause complete obstruction, resulting in the saliva and fluid food can not be swallowed.



Z. Mu, J. Fang (eds.), *Practical Otorhinolaryngology - Head and Neck Surgery*, https://doi.org/10.1007/978-981-13-7993-2_23

3. Respiratory Symptoms: Large foreign body pressure trachea or retention of the saliva of the pharynx is inhaled trachea, can produce respiratory difficulties, cough and other symptoms.

**Diagnosis**

1. The history of disease: the detailed inquiry of the history and symptoms is essential for the correct diagnosis. The patient has a history of obvious foreign body, accompanied by symptoms such as dysphagia and pain, and the presence of foreign bodies should be considered.
2. Indirect Laryngoscopy: an indirect laryngoscope is used to examine the hypopharynx. If there is saliva in the pyriform recess, further examination is required.
3. Drinking Water Test: the patient's drinking water, if the facial expression of pain or dare not to swallow, there is a diagnostic significance. Pointed tips embedded in the cervical esophagus foreign body. This method should not be used in patients who are suspected of perforation of the esophagus.
4. Neck Check: in the anterior border of the sternocleidomastoid muscle to the medial compression of the esophagus when there is tingling, or moving trachea pain, this is of diagnostic significance for a stimulating foreign body.
5. Subcutaneous Emphysema: Subcutaneous emphysema may have a perforation of the esophagus.
6. X-ray Examination: Instant diagnosis of unradioparent foreign masses could be made. Barium sulphate mixed with cotton silk should be swallowed to accomplish barium hanging inspection while inspecting tiny fish bone and radioparent foreign masses. However, to patients suspected to be with esophageal perforation, barium contrast should be banned and replace with few lipiodol contrast. When the fish bone deeply stabbed in the wall, barium cotton can't hang on the foreign mass, so it can't be displayed. CT multiplane reconstruction can clearly display small fish bone and the relationship between the bone and esophagus (Figs. 23.1 and 23.2).
7. The Esophagoscopy: includes a metal esophagoscope (Fig. 23.3) and a fibrous esophagoscope (Fig. 23.4). The general situation can be clearly diagnosed by the above methods. In order to eliminate the existence of foreign body, it is necessary to do a esophagoscope examination under local anesthesia when the symptoms of the pharynx and the pain of the pharynx are negative. It was found that the foreign bodies were removed and the foreign bodies of the esophagus were excluded.
8. Complications are due to the lack of timely treatment, or due to the continued eating of foreign bodies.
   (a) Esophageal Perforation or Injury Esophagitis: sharp and hard foreign bodies, such as the hook of the denture, with piercing the esophageal wall and swallowing activity of esophageal perforation; foreign body rough and incarcerated, in addition to the direct compression injury of esophageal mucosa, food and saliva retention is conducive to the growth of bacteria, the esophageal wall infection, necrosis, ulcer etc.
   (b) Subcutaneous Emphysema or Mediastinal Emphysema: the air of the pharynx after perforation of the esophagus flows through the perforation to the subcutaneous tissue or into the cervical mediastinum to form emphysema.
   (c) Peri Esophagitis and Infection of The Cervical Space or Mediastinum Inflammation: traumatic esophagitis

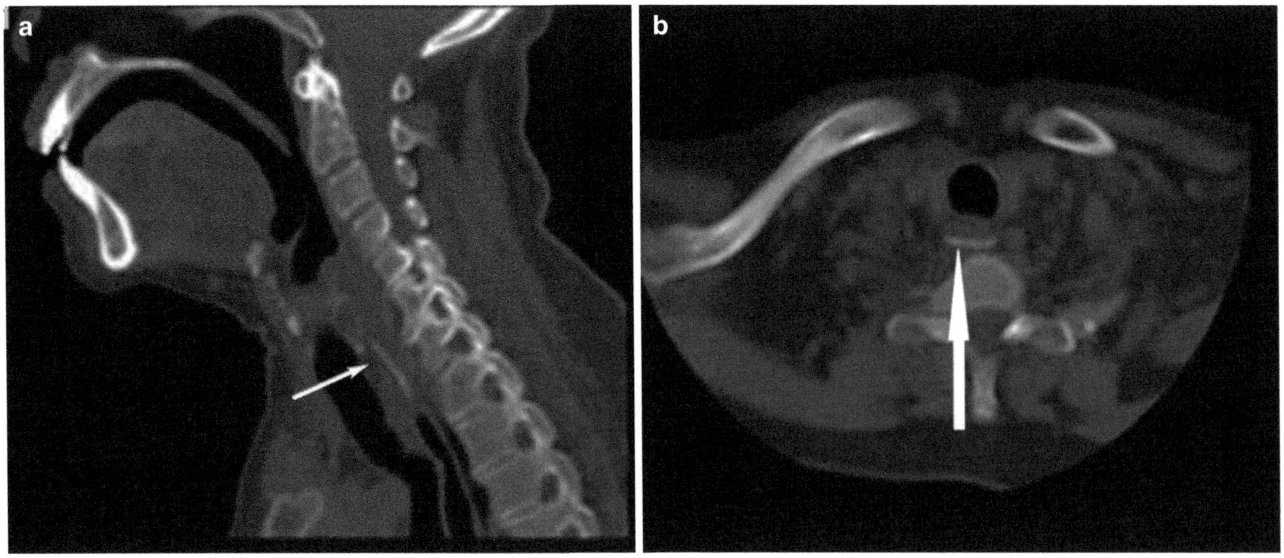


**Fig. 23.1** CT plain scan bone window. (**a**) Sagittal reconstruction, which could display esophageal upper segment linear high intensity fishbone (arrow). (**b**) Axial scan screening could display high intensity fishbone (arrow) in esophagus

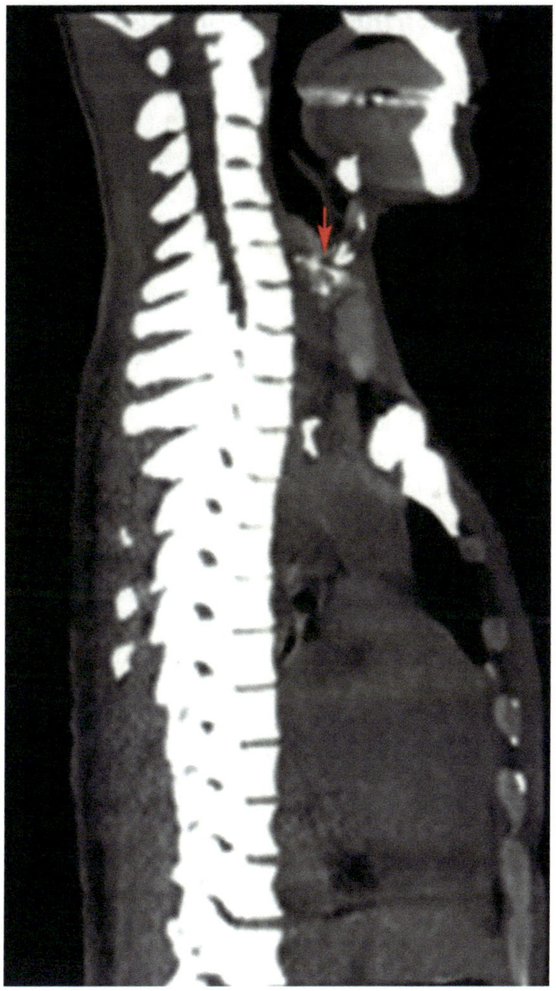

**Fig. 23.2** CT plain scan sagittal reconstruction. It could display high intensity shadow (arrow) at esophageal midupper segment thoracic aditus, which is fishbone

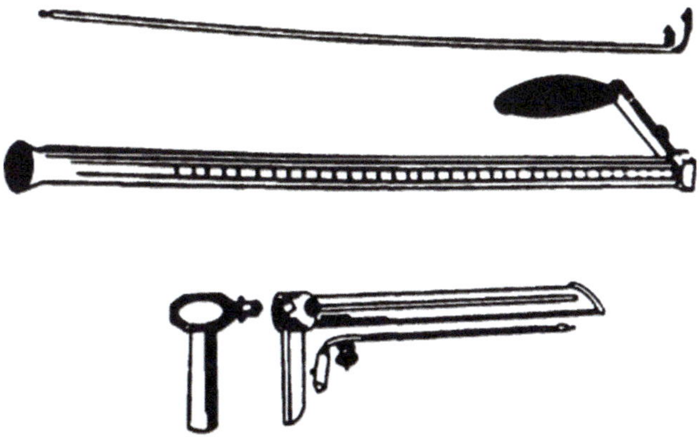

**Fig. 23.3** Metal esophagoscope

and infection can spread to the deep part, or through esophageal perforation to diffuse around the esophagus, causing esophagitis and heavy esophageal abscess. The perforation is located in the neck; the

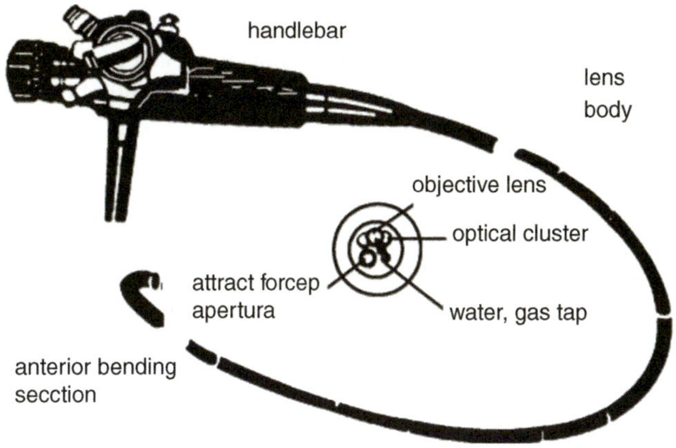


**Fig. 23.4** Fibrous esophagoscope

infection can spread to form along the neck fascial space or retropharyngeal lateral pharyngeal abscess. Thoracic esophagus perforation can occur at the mediastinum and form mediastinal abscess. Fever and other systemic symptoms would manifestate at severe condition.

(d) Rupture of Large Blood Vessels: the sharp food in the middle section of the esophagus can directly pierce the large vessels such as the esophageal wall, the aortic arch or the subclavian artery, and cause fatal bleeding. Infection can also involve blood vessels, causing rupture and bleeding. Its main manifestation is abundant hematemesis and hemafecia. Once it happens, the treatment is difficult and the death rate is high, so it should be actively saved.

(e) Tracheoesophageal Fistula: foreign body incarcerated by compression of the anterior wall of the esophagus, causing necrosis of the tube wall, and then involving the trachea and bronchus, forming tracheoesophageal fistula, which can lead to recurrent lung infection.

**Treatment**

To differentially diagnose or highly suspect esophageal foreign masses, esophagoscopy should be done as soon as possible to take it out in time.

1. Before the operation should be prepared to understand the general situation of the patient, dehydrate, if fever, should be given antibiotics and infusion and other supportive treatment. It is also necessary to understand the shape, size and inlay position of the foreign body in order to choose the suitable esophagoscope and appropriate foreign body pliers for the long and short length. 25–30 cm long esophagoscope is the best choice for foreign bodies at the upper end of the esophagus. The general foreign body can choose the crocodile mouth forceps, which depends on the shape of the foreign body in a few cases.

2. Anesthesia: Generally uses 1% tetracaine for local mucosal surface anesthesia. General anesthesia can be used for children with mental stress, foreign bodies and children. It is beneficial to remove the foreign body due to the relaxation of the esophageal muscle during general anesthesia. But should prevent the foreign body from slipping into the lower chest or stomach.
3. Surgical methods in patients with supine notation. The esophagoscope is sent down to the arytenoid cartilage along the middle line. The mucous membrane is at the radial pore, which is the entrance of the esophagus. Due to the contraction of the hypopharyngeal muscle, the entrance of the esophagus is very tight, and the esophagoscope is most difficult to pass through. It should be kept in the middle line slowly, not to use force, so as not to damage the esophagus or penetrate the pear shaped recess. When you see the food slag, barium and pus in the esophagus, it should be carefully observed, often the location of the foreign body. Take the cover carefully out or out, fully expose the foreign body, and observe the position of the foreign body and the surroundings. The sharp foreign bodies often damage the esophageal mucosa. If there is a certain distance between the foreign body and the front end of the esophagoscope, the esophagoscope can be gently sent down close to the foreign body, after that clamp the foreign body. Then the esophagoscope is removed together with the foreign body forceps.

Esophageal foreign masses taken with Foley tube has been reported by some scholars. The method is to send the Foley tube to the bottom of the foreign body first, and fill the water sac attached to the end of the tube with water, and then pull the pipe out slowly. Let the water sac carry the foreign body up to the pharynx and then take it out or spit it out. This method is suitable for large and smooth foreign objects which are inconvenient to be removed with pliers.

In recent years, the author has also used the cold light fiber esophagoscope or gastroscope to take out the foreign body of the esophagus. The advantages of the mirror are as follows: (1) The mirror is soft and thin, and the patient's pain is small and easy to accept. (2) the brightness of the cold light source is high; third, the mirror body can be bent, and the patient can also change the posture to facilitate the removal of foreign body.

However, the structure of the fibrous esophagoscope and the type and performance of the pliers are far from suitable for the operation of all foreign bodies. Therefore, metal esophagoscope is still the main means of taking out foreign bodies.

## 23.2 Erosion Injury of Esophagus

Esophageal Corrosive Injury due to esophageal damage caused by swallowing or swallowing of strong acid and alkali corrosion agent is called Esophageal Corrosive injury. In general, there are two kinds of corrosive agents: strong acid and strong alkali. Alkaline people have sodium hydroxide, lime water, ammonia water etc. Strong acids such as sulfuric acid, hydrochloric acid, nitric acid, etc.

There are two kinds of acid corrosion and alkali corrosion. The superficial damage of acid corrosion is heavy. The alkali corrosion can lead to a perforation of the esophagus or a sequelae in the deep layer. Swallowing corrosive agents, corrosion agent contact mucosa immediately hot pain is felt, at the lips, mouth, pharynx to the sternum and upper abdomen and radiate to the back of the spine on both sides, the sudden increase of saliva outflow, corrosive odor stimulation induced nausea and vomiting, vomit saliva, gastric juice and food and mixed color blood. The corrosion of laryngeal muscle membrane and vocal cords causes and hoarseness, spastic cough, dyspnea, increased heart rate. If the corrosion dose is large, the symptom of acidosis will be seen after the acid solution is absorbed, and the burn of the esophagus is heavy after the alkaline solution is absorbed. Complications such as dyspnea, pneumonia, swelling of throat and mouth, dysphagia, ulceration, necrosis and perforation of esophageal wall, esophageal and tracheal fistula, hyperthermia, shock and coma can occur later.

**Clinical Manifestation**

1. Acute Period: 1–2 Weeks
   (a) Pain: the pain occurred immediately after contact with the corrosive agent in the mouth, pharynx etc. The pain of the esophagus is often located behind the sternum.
   (b) Dysphagia is mainly related to swallowing pain, its degree depends on the severity of injury. Commonly, only liquid food could be taken, and while under severe condition, even water can't be swallowed and saliva would overflow accordingly.
   (c) Hoarseness and Dyspnea: when the corrosive invade the throat, causes mucosal edema, hoarseness and laryngeal obstruction symptoms.
2. Remission Period: 2–3 weeks after the onset of the disease. The wound gradually healed, the pain relieved, the dysphagia relieved, and the diet was gradually restored to normal.
3. Stage of Stenosis: If the lesions were lighter, and the symptoms improved 2–3 weeks after the injury, until they

recover. If the lesion involved muscle layer, the acute stage and remission is 3–4 weeks after the onset, due to connective tissue hyperplasia, followed by scar contraction of esophageal stenosis, the re emergence of dysphagia, and can be gradually increased, therefore, for the patients with esophageal corrosive injury must be observed closely.

To understand the site, range and degree of damage, the following examination can be done.

(a) Laryngeal and Pharyngeal Examination: Local mucosa hyperplasia would occur while corrosive objection contracts lips and pharynx; Pseudomembrane would be bulit after epithelium sheds; erosion change would appear when there is secondary inflammation. Indirect laryngoscopy when the larynx is involved could display mucosal edema at epiglottis, arytenoid cartilage, etc.
(b) X-ray Examination of The Esophagus: it is usually done after the remission of the acute symptoms, which helps to understand the nature, location and degree of the damaged esophagus. Barium should be avoided in those suspected of perforation of the esophagus. In order to understand the location, degree and scope of the stricture of the esophagus, the X-ray examination of the esophageal barium can also be made for the cases of narrow period. If the first examination is negative, it should be reviewed regularly in 2–3 months.
(c) Esophagoscope: it is an important method to directly observe the damage of the esophagus. The appropriate time should be selected for the first time after 2 weeks of injury, which may lead to a premature perforation.

**Treatment**

1. Emergency Treatment of Esophageal Caustic Injury in Acute Period
   (a) Local Treatment: the use of neutralizer should be used to protect the esophageal mucosa.
   (b) Tracheotomy: tracheotomy should be performed to keep the respiratory tract unobstructed when the symptoms of obstruction of the larynx are obvious.
   (c) Whole Body Treatment: to give pain relief, sedative, and anti shock treatment. Intravenous infusion or blood transfusion was given according to the condition of the disease, and electrolyte disturbance and insufficient blood volume were corrected in time.
   (d) Antibiotics and hormones: early application of antibiotics and hormones antibiotics can prevent infection; application of glucocorticoids can reduce the trauma response, anti shock, eliminate edema, inhibit the formation of fibrous tissue, preventing scar stenosis, but we should strictly control the indications and dosage, if the amount is too large, can spread the infection, and there may be complicated with esophageal perforation. Therefore, for serious burns, patients suspected of perforation of the esophagus should not be used.
   (e) Insertion of Gastric Tube: If the disease is slightly stable, can be carefully inserted into the stomach, for tube and nasal feeding, set aside a certain time, not only to maintain nutrition, but also to maintain the expansion of the cavity.
   (f) Dilatation of Esophageal Stricture: it should be found in the early stage of esophageal stricture, and it should be treated in time. The specific treatment method will be described below.
   (g) Esophagoscope: esophagoscope is an important method for direct observation of the damage in the esophagus. It should be carried out at the appropriate time, and the first examination will be carried out after 2 weeks of injury, and the possibility of causing perforation is prematurely. Fibrous esophagoscope is safer than hard esophagoscope.
2. Remission Period
   (a) The use of antibiotics and hormones according to the severity of the disease for several weeks and gradually reduced to discontinuation.
   (b) Can do X-ray examination and esophagoscope examination, and review regularly for early detection of esophageal stricture, timely treatment.
3. Memory Metal Stents
   (a) Esophageal Endoscopic Probe Dilation: It could be applied to the slighter narrowness and the limited range. There are several kinds of bungies, including the metal, the silica, etc. Under straight esophagoscopy, insert bungies at suitable sizes and increase the sizes to expand gradually. To take food more smoothly, commonly it should be expanded once per week.
   (b) Swallow Line Expansion: the most used clinically is circulation method, method is connected with the thread, and both ends of the expansion form a ring, and then pull the pull into the mouth of retrograde gastric fistula is the expansion of the sub esophageal stenosis at the back down in the stomach, can be repeated expansion, weekly 2–3 and enlarge the expander gradually, simultaneous both of which could effect on the esophagostenosis.
   (c) Titanium or Memory metal Support Dilatation.

(d) Surgery: If other treatments are not effective, surgery is necessary. According to the conditions, apply the bottleneck excision esophagus anastomosis, the esophageal replacement with colon, the free jejunal transplantated esophagus replacement, the esophago-gastric anastomosis, and the jejunostomy, etc.

## 23.3 Reflux Esophagitis

Reflux esophagitis (RE) is esophageal inflammatory lesion caused by the gastrial and the duodenal contents' reflux into the esophagus, which could be recognized as the esophago-mucosal damage under the endoscope, such as the esophageal anabrosis and (or) the esophageal ulceration. The RE could occur at any age and the morbidity increases at adults as they grow older. The morbidity is high in western countries and relatively lower in Asian area. Regional difference above may be related to the heredity and the environment factors. But at recent two decades, global morbidity tends to increase, and its high risks include advanced age, obesity, smoking of tobacco, taking of alcohol and high mental stress.

**Etiology**

The prerequisite to evoke the RE is that the gastric contents back flow into the esophagus through the lower esophageal sphincter (LES), but the esophagus can't clear the content as soon as possible itself and it causes longstanding gastric content in esophagus. What matters is the damage of the esophageal mucosa and eventually causing the reflux esophagitis are the injury factors, such as the gastric acid, the bile acid, the pepsin etc.

**Pathogenesis**

RE's pathophysiological basis is the gastroesophageal dyskinesis, including the esophageal body's motor function, the LES functions and the gastromotility disturbance. Not only the anatomy abnormality (such as the hiatus hernia) can cause these disturbance, but also some diseases (such as the diabetes), drugs (such as the smooth muscle relaxant) and food (such as the high fat food, chocolate and the coffee) can cause LES dysfunction and finally cause the RE.

**Clinical Manifestation**

Substernal burning or pain sensation is the main manifestation of RE. The manifestation mostly occur about 1 h after dinner; the semi-reclining position, the somatic proneness or strenuous exercise can evoke it as well. It would often resolves after taking antacids, but the overheating and the over acidic food could aggravate the conditions. On the hypochondriac, the burning sensation is mainly caused by the bile reflux, on which taking the antacids can't have effect. The burning severity doesn't accord with the lesion conditions. At severe esophagitis especially that occurs at the cicatrix, there might be none or slight burning sensation.

1. Gastric Esophagus Reflux
   At the time after dinner, somatic proneness or nocturnal sleep, acid containing liquid or food reflux from the stomach and the esophagus to the pharyngx or the mouth. The manifestation may occur before the substernal burning sensation or burning pain.
2. Dysphagia
   At the early stage, esophagitis could evoke the secondary esophagospasm, then the intermittent dysphagia; at the late stage, because the esophageal cicatrix may produce stenosis, the burning sensation and burning pain would gradually be alleviated and it would be replaced with permanent dysphagia, which even could cause congestion or pain at xiphoid while taking solid food.
3. Hemorrhage and Anemia
   At severe esophagitis, esophagomucosal anabrosis could occur and cause hemorrhage, which is often the chronic minimal bleeding. Longterm or abundant hemorrhage can both evoke hypoferric anemia.

**Complications**

RE not only could cause the esophageal stenosis, hemorrhage and ulceration, but also the gastric reflux could erode the pharynx, the vocal cords and the trachea to cause the chronic pharyngitis, the chronic chorditis and the trachiti, which is called the Delahunty syndrome in clinic. The gastric reflux inhaled into trachea could cause the aspiration pneumonia. Recent researches have already indicated that the gastroesophagoreflux is related to the partial repeated asthma, coughing, nocturnal respiratory arrest, angina pectoris.

**Pathologic Change**

1. Macroscopic esophagomucosal congestion, edema, which is fragile and easy to hemorrhage.
2. At acute esophagitis, mucosa epithelium defulvium occurs, producing anabrosis and superficial ulceration. At the related severer patients, the whole epithelial layer could fall off, but commonly not exceeding the mucosa layer.
3. At chronic esophagitis, mucosa fibrates after anabrosis, which may be beyond the submucosal muscle layer and involve the whole esophagowall.
4. The repeated esophagomucosal anabrosis, ulceration and fibration could cause the esophagocicatrical stenosis. Microscopic squamous epithelial basal cell hyperplasia occurs and extends to the epithelial epidermis, accompa-

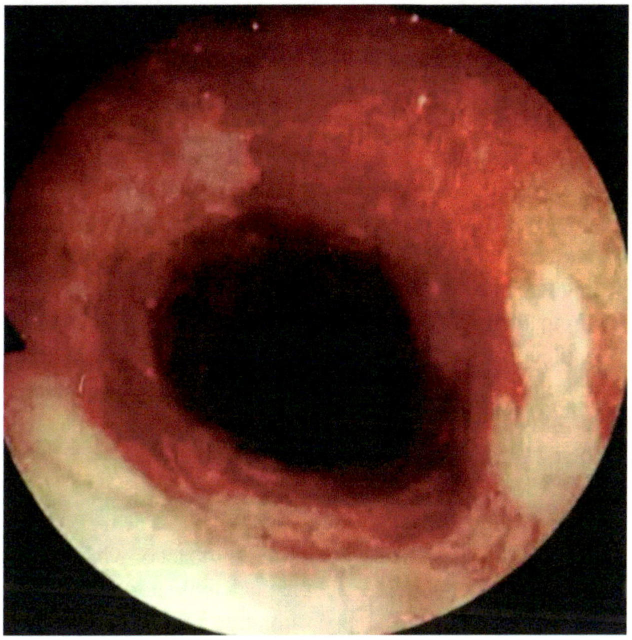

**Fig. 23.5** Barrett esophagus

nying with vascular hyperplasia and neutrophil infiltration at the lamina propria.

5. At the esophagostenosis, cicatrix formates at the submucosal or muscular layer. At the severe esophagitis, the mucosa epithelial basis is damaged and because the ulceration is too large, the squamous epithelial cells at the ulceration margin can't repair the ulceration by metaplasia, presenting as columnar metaplasia, which is called the Barrett esophagus (Fig. 23.5). Ulceration at the Barrett epithelium is called the Barrett ulceration.

**Diagnosis and Differential Diagnosis**

Reflux esophagitis diagnostic basis include: (1) Reflux manifestation; (2) Reflux esophagitis manifestation under gastroscope; (3) Objective esophageal overly-acid reflux proofs. If patients are with typical heartburn and acid reflux manifestation, RE could be primarily diagnosed. With gastroscopy and researches, the RE could be found and other esophagolesion caused by other causes could be ruled out, so the RE could be ascertained. To the patients with typical manifestations and negative endoscopy result, monitor the esophagus pH for 24 h, with which if the esophageal overly-acid reflux is verified, the diagnosis is differentiated.

Because the 24 h esophagus pH monitoring apply certain apparatus and invasion examinations, it is hard to be applied in clinic. Therefore, to the patients with suspect RE diagnosis and negative endoscopy, proton pump inhibitors(PPI) is often applied to do the experimental treatment, and if it works well, RE could be differentially diagnosed; to the patients with atypical manifestations, combine with the gastroscopy, the 24 h esophagus pH monitoring and the experimental therapy to comprehensively analyse and finally diagnose.

Through RE own manifestations and characteristics, it could be differentiated from the diseases, such as the esophagus lesion evoked by other causes (such as the fungoid esophagitis, the drug esophagitis, the esophagocancer, the esophagoachalasia, etc), the peptic ulcer and the biliary tract diseases. To those whose main manifestation is stethalgia, they should be distinguished from the cardiac stethalgia and other noncardiac chest pain evoked by other causes. So should it be distinguished from the functional diseases such as the functional heartburn, the functional chest pain and the functional dyspepsia.

**Gradings**

Based on the endoscopic esophagomucosa damage degrees, the RE could be divided into four degrees, A, B, C and D.

A. ≥1 esophagomucosa damage, whose major axis <5 mm.
B. ≥1 esophagomucosa damage, whose major axis >5 mm and without confluent lesion.
C. With mucosal damage and fusion but ≤75% pericricoid esophagus.
D. With mucosal damage and fusion and ≥75% pericricoid esophagus.

**Treatment**

RE therapy aims at curing the esophagitis, rapidly alleviating symptoms, reducing relapse and improving life quality.

1. Common Therapy

   Lifestyle changes is basis of the RE therapy, which include less take in and 80%full each dinner. Raise the bed headboard by 15–20 cm to reduce the clinostatism or the nocturnal reflux, avoid taking food before bed and it is inadvisable to immediately lie in bed after day time meal. Such daily measurements could reduce reflux: cigarettes cessation; temperance; decrease abdominal pressure; avoid tying a tight belt; the obese should lose weight; avoid taking in the high fat food, chocolate, coffee, excitable food, etc. Avoid using reducing gastroesophagokinetic drugs, such as the anticholinergic drugs, the tricyclic antidepressant, the dopamine receptor agonist, the calcium antagonists, the theophylline, the β2-adrenergic receptor agonist, etc.

2. Drug Therapy

   (a) Antacid Therapy

   RE is a motility disorder radically, and stopping the gastrocontents reflux is the treatment crux. So far, antireflux prokinetics drugs' efficacy isn't good enough, but the PPI could rapidly alleviate the symptoms and cure the RE, so the anti-acid therapy is the main method to treat the RE recently. Regular usage of H2-receptor antagonist (H2RA) could evidently inhibit the empty-stomach and the nocturnal gastro-acid secretion and alleviate majority of patients' symptoms, but it has low coalescence to over-C-degree RE. This kind of drugs inhibit weakly on the posprandial acid secretion and it has rapid resistance reaction, so it could only be applied to the A/B degree esophagitis patients. Extra-strong antacid drugs PPI could generate outstanding and lasting antacid effect, rapidly alleviate symptoms and it has high esophagitis healing rate, so it could be applied to all the RE. Common drugs include the omeprazole (OME 40 mg/day), the rabeprazole (20 mg/day), the lansoprazole (40 mg/day) etc. The RE therapy need 2 time PPI dosage than the peptic ulcer treatment, and the RE therapy course is about 8–12 weeks. The esophagitis's healing rate at eighth PPI-therapy week is about 90% and after 8-week treatment, gastroscope reexamination is necessary for mastering the esophagitis's healing conditions; if the esophagitis isn't completely cured, the course should be prolonged to 12 weeks.

(b) Prokinetics

It could make certain effect, but its efficacy is bad while being singly used and its adverse reaction limits its application as well.

(c) Others

Antacid drugs could neutralize the gastric acid, which commonly apply the basic salt and its compound agents which contain aluminum, magnesium, bismuth, etc. Both above could help release the symptoms and the hydrotalcite could absorb the bile to protect the esophageal mucosa and it is helpful to restore the esophagitis.

(d) Maintenance Treatment

PPI could almost cure all kinds of the esophagitis, but the recurrence rate is about 80% after the sixth withdrawal month. To the RE, remaining treatment is vital. PPI remaining therapeutic effects is better than the H2RA and the prokinetics, but the remaining therapeutic dosage isn't unified, and the PPI is always under regular dose. There is on-demand medicine taken, which means that the patients take medicines when the symptoms occur till the symptoms are under control, and it is also a good choice. To reduce the medicine dosage and save the costs, apply the relative-rapider-on setting PPI.

3. Endoscopy Therapy

Several patients recur after withdrawing treatment, so they need long-term medication. Endoscopy therapy could be made inspirable efficacy, but the long-time efficacy and the complications still need the followup, which include the methods following: radio-frequency energy input method, injection method and folding method; its indication is the patients who need largedosage remaining treatment; its contraindications include the C or D degree esophagitis, the Barrett esophagus, the >2 cm hiatus hernia, the esophagus body dysperistalsis etc.

4. Prevention

(a) Cigarette Cessation and Temperance

Because there is nicotine in tobacco, which could decrease the lower esophageal sphincter (LES) pressure, set it in a loosen condition and aggravate the reflux; liquor mainly contains the alcohol, which could not only stimulate the gastroacid secretion, but also it could relax the LES, which is one cause of the gastroesophageal reflux.

(b) Taking small but more meals and low-fat diet could reduce the reflux symptoms after taking food. Adversely, high fat diet could promote the small intestine mucosa by relieving the cholecystokinin (CCK) and it could evoke the gastrointestinal contents reflux.

(c) Inadvisable to take too much at supper and avoid lying immediately after meals.

(d) The obese patient should lose weight. The obese has high abdominal pressure, which could evoke the gastroreflux and especially lying could evoke a more severe condition, so losing weight could help improve the reflux symptoms.

(e) Keep a delightful mood and do suitable physical exercise.

(f) Raising the bed head-board by 10–15 cm while sleeping is helpful to reduce the nocturnal reflux.

(g) Decrease the activities which could increase the intra-abdominal pressure, such as overly-bowing, wearing the tight clothes, tying tight belts, etc.

(h) Take medicines only under doctors' guide and avoid taking chaos drugs to produce side effects.

# Part VII

# Head and Neck Surgery

Cervocranial site involves the motion, speech, respiratory, the deglutition and other important physical functions, so the cervocranial diseases measurement is bit complex and tedious with consideration of all functions above. Cautiously researching the diseases' characteristics has an important meanings on improving the survival incidence and the patients' living quality. Therefore, this part would expound the cranial base and the cervical pathology and anatomy angle, based on which emphatically states the common cervocranial diseases and their diagnosis and therapy.

# Applied Anatomy of Head and Neck

# 24

Jugao Fang and Jiajun Huang

## 24.1 Applied Anatomy of Skull Base

Cranial base is initially developed at the early embryo. It firstly appears as the anterior notochord cartilage, then it grows to the bilateral and the anterior to constitute the rudimental cartilage cranial base; then several gasified centers appear in the cartilage, gradually extend and interconnect to constitute the cranial base bone. The cranial base is cartilaginous osteogenesis and the other cranial part is intramembranous ossification, which is firstly differentiated into the fibrous membrane from the mesenchyme, secondly one or multiple gasified centers appear in the post-membrane and then they unify into the cranium.

Cranial base is a complex area. Above the irregular cranial base bone, there are the brainstem and other important structures; below it, there is the mouth, the ear, the nose, the nasal sinus, the pharyngocavum and other bacteria-containing structures; and several life-related blood vessels and cranial nerves have their accesses in this area. The cranial base bone has 7 bones, consisting of 3 unpaired bones (sphenoid bone, ethmoid bone and occipital bone) and 2 pairs of bones(frontal bones and temporal bone) (Fig. 24.1). The skull base isn't only the base of the cranial cavum, but it is also the roof of the eye orbit, the rhinocavum, the sphenoid sinus, the ethmoid sinus, the rhinopharynx and the infratemporal fossa; from top to bottom, the internal skull basal boundary is the post-small-sphenoid-wing edge and the temporal crest, based on which the skull base is divided into 3 cranial fossa, including the anterior, the middle and the posterior cranial fossa, which are corresponding to the anterior, the middle and the posterior skull base (Fig. 24.2). At recent years, to help make accurate operational approaches, cross partition at the inferior skull base surface from the anatomy and the clinical aspects has been made, but there's not a unified standard.

The cranial basal diseases are not rare, but they don't have a unified standard: based on the their anatomical sites, which means dividing the lateral cranial basal surface into the midline area and the lateral area and partitioning the medial cranial basal surface into the anterior, the middle and the inferior cranial fossa; based on the pathologic classification methods, they could be divided into 4 types: the tumor, the trauma, the inflammation and the congenital diseases.

## 24.2 Applied Anatomy of Neck

Neck is located between the head and the chest, it connects the skull, the truncus and the upper extremity. The cervical appearance is closely-related to gender, age and bodily form: female's and infants' necks have relative-thicker subcutaneous fat and relative-round outline. The cervical support is the cervical spine, the anterior spine is the respiratory tract and the cervical alimentary canal, there are diagonal macro vessels and nerves ending at the cervical root at bilateral upper respiratory-alimentary canal and the cervical pleura and the pulmonary apex appear at the cervical root. Loose connective tissues stuff up the cervical structures and constitute several anadesma and fascial space closely-related to clinical diagnosis and treatment. The cervical motility range is relative-bigger and the length and all organs' location change while moving the neck. During head hypsokinesis, the anterior neck lengthens, the cervical trachea approaches to skin; while rotating head, the larynx, the trachea and the blood vessels shift to the rovolved side and the esophagus shift to the opposite side. Mastering these characteristics mean much to all cervical organs' operations.

**Electronic Supplementary Material** The online version of this chapter (https://doi.org/10.1007/978-981-13-7993-2_24) contains supplementary material, which is available to authorized users.

J. Fang (✉)
Department of Otorhinolaryngology Head and Neck Surgery, Beijing Tongren Hospital, Capital Medical University, Beijing, China

J. Huang
Department of Otorhinolaryngology Head and Neck Surgery, The First Affiliated Hospital of Hainan Medical University, Haikou, China



Z. Mu, J. Fang (eds.), *Practical Otorhinolaryngology - Head and Neck Surgery*, https://doi.org/10.1007/978-981-13-7993-2_24

**Fig. 24.1** Inferior aspect of the cranial base anatomy diagram

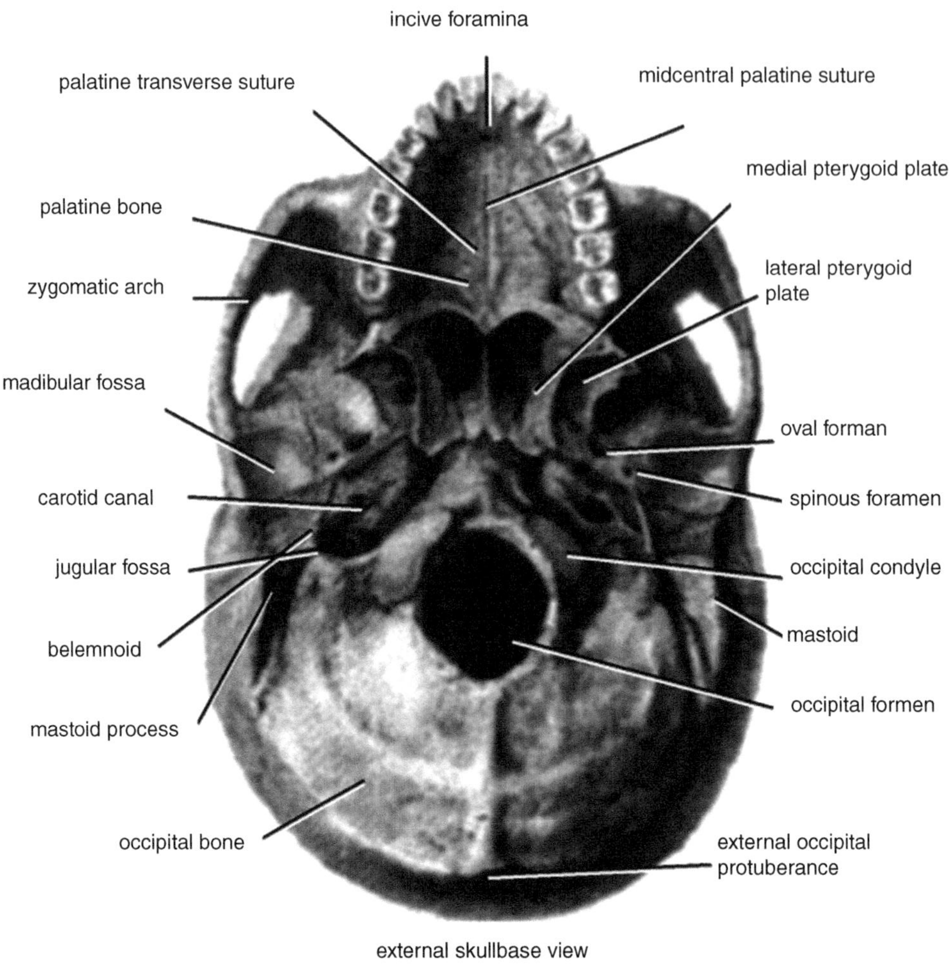


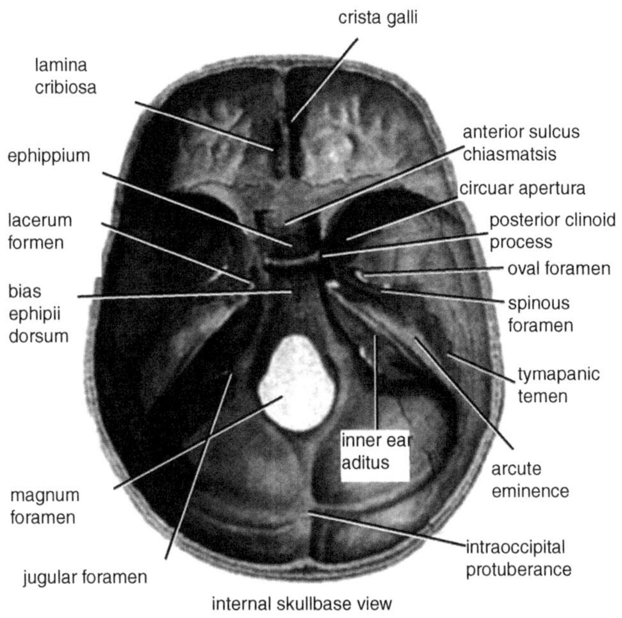


**Fig. 24.2** Superior aspect of the cranial base anatomy diagram

There are abundant lymph nodes at cervical region, whose quantity are about 380 and occupying 1/3 of the total lymph nodes. It is divided into zone 1–6, mainly lining peripheral to the macro-vessels. Therefore, when the cervical tumor extends along with the lymph tubes, certain meta-basis rules exist and the corresponding ranges' lymph nodes' clearance should be done, basing on the specific characteristics, while doing the cervical malignant tumor surgeries.

1. Important Cervical Surface Signs
   (a) Thyroid Cartilage Incisura

   It is also known as male's Adam's apple, which is the top of the site where the bilateral thyroid cartilage join each other and also the mid cervical most upheaval sign; the female's Adam's apple can also be touched, but unobvious like the male's. It can also be set as the surface sign of the emergency tracheotomy and other surgeries.

   (b) Cricoid Cartilage Arch

   It is 2–3 cm below the Adam's apple and its inferior margin is the boundary sign between the larynx and the trachea. It is a hard bony structure at inferior thyroid cartilage, slightly upheavaled than trachea. At acute laryngopharyngitis, it could be used to ascertain the cricothyroid membranous location and it is an important sign of doing the cricothyroid laryngotomy.

(c) Sternocleidomastoid

It originates from mastoid and ends at the upper sternum incisura and the inner clavicular segment; it is an important sign of the cervical partitions. Its deep area contains the cervicovascular vagina constituted with the carotid artery, the jugular vein, the vagus, etc., and the sheath is encircled by several lymph nodes.

2. Cervical Zones

Cervical zone could be partitioned into the anterior and the posterior zones by antero-trapezius edge: the sites at the anterior is called the anterolateral cervical zone or the proper cervical zone, which is also the neck in narrow sense; the part posterior to the trapezius is called the post-neck or the napex. To help elaborate accurately in clinic, the neck could be partitioned into several triangle zones according to the important muscular signs. The neck could be partitioned into the anterocervical triangle and the postcervical triangle: the anterocervical triangle contains the inferior submandibular triangle, the submental triangle, the carotid triangle and the deltoid; the postcervical triangle contains the supraclavicular triangle and the occipital triangle.

(a) Inferior Submaxillary Triangle

It lies among the anteroventral digastric muscle, the post-ventral digastric muscle and the inferior submaxillary edge.

(b) Submental Triangle

It lies among bilateral digastric muscle and the hyoid bone.

(c) Carotid Triangle

It lies among the antero-sternocleidomastoid edge, the postventral digastric muscle and the anteroventral omohyoid muscle.

(d) Muscotriangle

It lies among the anterosternocleidomastoid edge, the centro-anterocervical midline and the supventral omohyoid.

(e) Supclavicular Triangle

It lies among the poststernocleidomastoid edge, the subventral omohyoid bone and the clavicle.

(f) Occipital Triangle

It lies among the poststernocleidomastoid edge, the sub-ventral omohyoid and the trapezius.

3. Cervical Blood Vessels

(a) Common Carotid Artery

Left common carotid artery (CCA) originates from the aorta arch and the right originates from the brachiocephalic trunk. The flat hyoid large angle site could be partitioned into the external (ECA) and the internal carotid artery (ICA). The outward lateral CCA is the internal jugular vein, between which there is vagus existing and the vagus is the main content of the cervicocarotid sheath. The extremity of the CCA inflates, which is called the carotid sinus and it has the baroceptor; the carotid body, chemoreceptor, is at the post-CCA bifurcation.

(b) ICA

After separating from the CCA, it firstly ascends at the postECA, it secondarily turns to the internal ECA, vertically approaching upwards the skull base and entering the carotid canals through the foramen lacerum, then the mid-cranial fossa through the cavernous sinus. It mainly distributes at brain and optic organs. The ICA has no branches in neck.

(c) Carotid Body and Carotid Sinus

Carotid bodies lie at the posterior sites of the bifurcation of the ICA and the ECA and they connect to the artery wall by the connective tissues. They are chemoreceptor, sensing blood $CO_2$ concentration change and reflexively adjusting the respiratory movement. The carotid sinus is the inflation part of the ICA origination and there are specific sensory nerve endings in the carotid sinus, which is a kind of the baroceptor: when the arterial blood pressure rises, which also means the carotid sinus extension, stimulating the baroceptor, providing nervous impulse from the central nerve, reducing heartbeat by central reflex and extending the terminal blood vessels, finally the blood pressure is reduced.

(d) ECA

After seperating from the CCA, it firstly lies at the internal ICA, secondarily turns to the outward lateral, asscends across the post-ventral digastric muscle and the deep stylohyoid area and descendingly separates into two terminal branches at the cervico-submaxillary plane, the superficial temporal artery and the maxillary artery. The ECA issues such branches from bottom to top: sup-thyroid artery, lingual artery, facial artery, superficial temporal artery and the maxillary artery.

(e) Jugular Vein

- Superficial Jugular Vein
  - Anterior Jugular Vein

    It is joined by the mental and submaxillary veins. It descends along with bilateral anterior cervical mid line and finally joins the external jugular vein. The veins don't have valves.
  - External Jugular Vein

    It lies at the superficial sternocleidomastoid and it is joined adjacent to the submaxillary angle with the postsubmaxillary vein and the post-auricular vein. Eventually it would join the subclavian vein or the subintracervicovein at the anterior scalene muscle.

- Internal Jugular Vein

  It locates in the cervicoarterial sheath, along with the CCA, and the vagus and it is the sustaining of the intracranial sigmoid sinus. It descends downwards to the superior thoracic aperture from the skull base, and its ending combines and the subclavicular vein join each other, constituting the brachiocephalic veins. It is also the main approach of the cervicocranial venous circulation reflux.

4. Cervical Nerve

(a) Cervical Plexus

It is constituted by the preramus of the 1st–4th cervical nerve and it locates among the deep sternocleidomastoid area and the superficial layer of the midiscalenus and the omohyoid muscle. The superficial cervicoplexus branch is also the cutaneous nerve and its deep branch could be divided into two groups, the anterior group and the posterior group, between which the phrenic nerve, which is mainly issued by the anterior vertical nerve branch, locating at the deep prevertebral fascia layer and vertically descending into the thoracic cavity across the superficial anterior scalene, is the most important branch of the anterior branch.

(b) Brachial Plexus

It is constituted by the anterior 5th–8th cervical nerve and the first thoracic nerve and it would go through the scalene muscular space to form the three trunks, which consist the superior, the middle and the inferior trunk and each trunk contains the anterior and the posterior trunk. The anterior branch of the superior and the middle trunk constitute the outer lateral cord, the anterior post trunk branch constitutes the internal lateral cord, and the posterior branches of the three trunks merge into the posterior cord. These three cords enter the axilla at the central clavicle and encircle the axillary arteries at the interior, the external and the posterior. The brachial plexus mainly branches into the Bell's nerve, the thoracic spinal nerve, the anterior thoracic nerve, the musculocutaneous nerve and the median nerve, and they distribute at the skin of the thorax, the shoulder, the neck and the upper limb. The branchial plexus is relatively centralized above the clavicular midpoint and its position is shallow, so the midpoint is often set as the site doing the branchial-plexus conduction-block anesthesia.

(c) Phrenic Nerve

After being issued from the branchial plexus muscular branch, phrenic nerve descends to the internal sub-anterior trapezius along with anterior outer-lateral sub-anterior trapezius, then it enters the thoracic cavum between the subclavicular arteries and veins. The phrenic nerve damage mainly manifest as the diaphragm paralysis and the reduced or disappeared abdominal respiration; when the phrenic nerve is irritated, hiccup may occur.

(d) Vagus

It locates in the cervical sheath and the posterior site between the CCA and the internal jugular vein. Its main branches are the superior laryngonerve and the recurrent laryngonerve.

The internal suplaryngonerve branch goes along with the suplaryngoartery, entering the pharynx through the thyroid hyoid membrane and distributing at the supglottic laryngomucosa, and it masters feeling; the external suplaryngonerve branch descends along with the outer-lateral supthyroid blood vessel, then it turns to the internal lateral of the supblood-vessel, going through the infraconstrictor at sites 0.5–2.0 cm distant to the sup-internal site of the location where the upper thyroid artery enters the supthyroid apex and entering and dominating the cricothyroid muscle. The outer suplaryngonerve branch is closely related to the supthyroid artery, so attention should be paid to the nerve damage while doing the thyroidectomy.

Bilateral recurrent laryngonerve differs at directions, of which the left side ascends encircling the aorta and the right side ascends encircling the subclavicular artery. Bilateral nerves both go in the tracheoesophagogroove at neck, all terminal branches all enter the larynx through the postcricothyroid joint and dominate the intralaryngomuscle except the cricothyroid muscle.

(e) Accessory Nerve

It is constituted by medulla oblongata and spinal cord. The medulla oblongata root forms the internal accessory nerve branch after leaving the cranium through the jugular foramen and joins the vagus, dominating the laryngopharyngostriated muscle. The spinal cord root constitutes the external accessory nerve branch after leaving the cranium and the branch goes by or passing through the sternocleidomastoid and issues the sternocleidomastoid muscle branches along the way, downwards approaching the junction of the middle and the inferior 1/3 anterior trapezius edge and entering the trapezius. The accessory nerve is the motor nerve of the sternocleidomastoid muscle and the trapezius muscle, if it is cut off, the shrugging and the upper extremity lifting function would be influenced.

(f) Hypoglossal Nerve

It is issued from the hypoglossal nucleus, leaving the cranium through the hypoglossal nerve tube. At the outer lateral vagus and between the internal jugular vein and the internal carotid artery, vagus descends, then goes forward after passing through between the internal and the external carotid artery, entering the submandibular interval through the deep post ventral digastric area, forward ascending from the deep inferior submaxiallary gland area, distributing at the tongue and matering all the intra-glossal muscle and partial external glossal muscle. When either lateral hypoglossal nerve is injured, the lingual apex deflect to the affected side while lolling and the atrophy may occur at the affected lingualis.

5. Cervical Muscle
   (a) Sternocleidomastoid (SCM)

   It is at outer lateral neck, each at one side. Its origination has two endings, and they respectively originate from the manubrium and the internal 1/3 clavicle, diagonally ascending and ending at the outer lateral mastoid and supnuchal occipital bone. The SCM is dominated by the accessory nerve and the anterior branches of the second and the 3th cervical nerves. The SCM is thewy and it is an important muscular sign at cervical surgeries. The carotid artery, the internal jugular vein and the vagus all locate at the deep SCM region.

   (b) Hyoid Muscular Cogroup

   It locates between the submaxillary bone, skull base and the hyoid bone and it includes four muscle masses.

   - Digastric Muscle

     The digastric muscle lies at the submandibular bone and it has the anterior ventral part and the postventral part, the anterior ventral part originates from the submaxillary digastric fossa, obliquely posteriorly-descending; the post ventral part originates from the temporal mastoid incisura, obliquely anterior-descending and both the two parts join each other, constituting the intermediate bond, then being fixed at the basihyoid.

   - Mylohyoid muscle

     It locates at the deep anterior ventral digastric muscle, originating from the intralateral submaxillary bone and obliquely descending till the midline and the hyoid bone.

   - Geniohyoid

     It locates at the deep mylohyoid muscle, originating from the mental spine and ending at the hyoid bone.

   - Stylohyoid

     It originates from the belemnoid and ends at the hyoid bone.

   (c) Infrahyoid Muscles

   The infrahyoid muscles locate at bilateral midcentral subhyoid, consisting 4 pairs of muscles.

   - Sternohyoid Muscles

     They originate from the post manubrium and ends at the inferior hyoid edge.

   - Sternothyroid Muscles

     They locate at the deep sternohyoid muscle, originating from the post manubrium and ending at the oblique thyroid cartilage line.

   - Thyrohyoid Muscles

     They originate from the oblique thyroid cartilage line and end at the inferior edge of the basihyoid, the large post hyoid angle edge and downlinking the sternothyroid muscle.

   - Omohyoid Muscles

     They could be divided into three parts, including superior venter, the inferior venter and the intermediate bond. The inferior venter originates from the scapula edge, ascending forward till the deep inferior sternocleidomastoid segment and ending at the intermediate bond; the superior venter originates from the intermediate bond, slightly vertically ascending and ending at the infrahyoid edge.

   (d) Deep Cervical Muscles (DCM)

   - Internal DCM

     They contain the longus capitis muscles and the longus collum mucles, locating at the anterior cervicospine, and they are commonly called the prevertebral muscles.

   - External DCM

     They contain the anterior, the middle and the posterior trapezius, all of which originate from transverse cervicovertebral processes and end at the ribs. The space between the anterior and the middle trapezius and the first rib is called the trapezius space, through which the branchial plexus and the subclavicular arteries pass. At the superficial trapezius, the phrenic nerves pass; at the crossing angle the anteriorinferior anterior trapezius and the ribs join each other, the subclavicular vein goes through.

6. Cervical Lymph Nodes

   They contain five groups: submental lymph nodes, submandibular lymph nodes, anterior cervical lymph nodes, superficial cervical lymph nodes and deep cervical lymph nodes.

   (a) Submental Lymph Nodes

   They locate in the submental triangle, containing 2–3 lymph nodes and which is mainly the combination of the mental, the lingual apex's, the mandibular incisor's and other lymph nodes, and their efferent tube eventually immit into the submandibular lymph nodes.

   (b) Submandibular Lymph Nodes

   It locates at the submandibular triangle zone, consisting 4–6 lymph nodes and which is the combination of the facial, the gingival, the anterior lingual, the submental lymphatics' lymph etc., and they eventually mainly-immit into the superior deep cervical lymph nodes.

(c) Anterior Cervical Lymph Nodes

They contain two groups: deep and shallow layer. The shallow distribute along with the shallow anterior cervical vein and the deep locate anteriorly to the larynx, the cricothyroid membrane and the trachea, collecting the lymph from the larynx, the trachea, thyroid gland, etc. All their efferent tubes immit into the deep subcervical lymph nodes.

(d) Shallow Cervical Lymph Nodes

They locate at shallow sternocleidomastoid, linging along with the external jugular vein and collecting the facial, the retroauricular, the parotid lymph etc., and they eventually immit into the deep supcervical lymph nodes.

(e) Deep Cervical Lymph Nodes

They line along with the internal jugular vein and they could be divided into the superior and the inferior deep cervical lymph nodes, bondering with the junction of the omohyoid muscle and the intrajugular vein.

- Deep Supcervical Lymph Nodes

  They are the lymph nodes between the site above the omohyoid muscular intermediate bond and the intrajugular vein. They collect the lymphatic circulation reflux from the rhinolarynx, the palatine tonsil, the tongue, the submental site and the submandibular site, and they finally immit into deep subcervical lymph nodes.

- Deep Subcervical Lymph Nodes

  They are the lymph nodes between the site below the omohyoid muscular intermediate bond and the intrajugular vein, able to extend to the subclavicular artery, the peripheral brachial plexus and transverse cervical artery, of which the former two is commonly called the supclavicular lymph nodes. The deep subcervical lymph nodes mainly collect the cervicocranial lymph nodes, they also collect partial thoracic and epigastric lymph vessel. Their efferent tubes leftly immit into the thoracic ducts and rightly the right lymphatic trunk or straightly the intrajugular vein. The thoracic and the abdominal malignant tumor cell retrograde at cervical trunk through the thoracic duct and metastasize to the supclavicular lymph nodes, commonly the abdominal and the left thoracic organs' malignant tumors metastasize to the left subclavicular lymph nodes and the right thoracic organs' malignant tumors metastasize to the right subclavicular lymph nodes.

Based on the cervical lymph nodes' metastasis rules and the requestion of the cervical dissection, the American Otorhinolaryngopharyngocervicocranial surgery funds institutes (AOSFI) have divided the cervical lymph nodes into 6 zones at 1991:

- Zone I (Level I): Submental and submandibular lymph nodes, containing two subregions, A and B;
- Zone II (Level II): Intrajugular venous lymph nodes cogroup, containing two subregions, A and B;
- Zone III (Level III): Intrajugular venous lymph node midgroup;
- Zone IV (Level IV): Intrajugular venous lymph node subgroup;
- Zone V (Level V): Postcervical triangle lymph nodes, containing two subregions, A and B;
- Zone VI (Level VI): Precervical lymph nodes.

# Common Cervical Diseases

# 25

Jugao Fang, Zhonglin Mu, Jihong Huang
and Yongjun Feng

## 25.1 Thyroglossal Cyst

It is a common cervicocongenital disease and it is related to the embryonic thyrolingual tube dysplasia, which include the undegenerated or uncompletely degenerated thyrolingual tube.

**Etiology**
During the embryonic development, a tubule initiately linked the original base, called the thyrolingual tube, grows during the process, the origional thyroid base downwards shift from the lingual base to the neck. At the sixth week embryo, the thyrolingual tube degenerates and completely disappear at the eighth week, retenting a superior lingual foramen cecum; If the thyrolingual tube is undegenerated or uncompletely degenerated, the thyrolingual tube cyst or fistula occurs. The left and right hyoid bones fuse at the midcentral line during the thyrolingual tube degeneration, so the undegenerated tube may locate at the ventro or the dorso-hyoid bone side or in the lingual bone but the cyst locates in the deep precervial ribbon muscles.

**Clinical Manifestation**
Cysts are different in size; no symptoms at most of times and unnoticable; always be found occasionally or at physical examinations. Cysts are round with clear boundary, no adhesion to the peripheral tissues and skin, no pressing pain, soft texture, cystic sensation and movability along with deglutition motion, some of which can be palpated a cable-like mass in the superior. While accompanying with infections, the cysts grow rapidly and the partial pain and the pressing pain occur.

**Diagnosis**
Cysts locate at the midcentral preneck and ocassionally deviating to a side, but it can be diagnosed along with deglutition up-down motions. To the complete fistula, inject the methylene blue (MB) from the external fistula to observe the MB overflow from the lingual foramen cecum and finally ascertain the diagnosis. B-ultrasound examination can help diagnose the cysts. Nuclide imaging displays a non-isotope imaging, no specific manifestation on MRI but cystic lesion could be recognized at the mid-central preneck (Fig. 25.1).

**Differentiate Diagnosis**
The thyrolingual tube cyst should be differentiated from the diseases following:

1. Dermoid Cyst
   It is congenital, locating at the centra-middle anterior neck; the cyst adheres to the skin and it can't move up and down along with the deglutition. At the ultrasound imaging, the dermoid cyst's contents echo is higher than the thyrolingual tube cyst.
2. Submental Lymphnoditis
   There could be adjacent tissues' inflammation, such as the periodontal, the submaxil, the lower lip, etc. The lumps have relative hard texture and pressing pain and they don't move up and down along with the deglutition.
3. Ectopic Thyroid Gland
   Majority of them locate at the lingual root, and minority of them at the mid-central anterior larynx would be misdi-

J. Fang (✉)
Department of Otorhinolaryngology Head and Neck Surgery,
Beijing Tongren Hospital, Capital Medical University,
Beijing, China
e-mail: fangjg@trhos.com

Z. Mu · J. Huang
Department of Otorhinolaryngology Head and Neck Surgery,
The First Affiliated Hospital of Hainan Medical University,
Haikou, China

Y. Feng
Department of Otorhinolaryngology Head and Neck Surgery,
The Second Affiliated Hospital of Hainan Medical University,
Haikou, China



Z. Mu, J. Fang (eds.), *Practical Otorhinolaryngology - Head and Neck Surgery*, https://doi.org/10.1007/978-981-13-7993-2_25

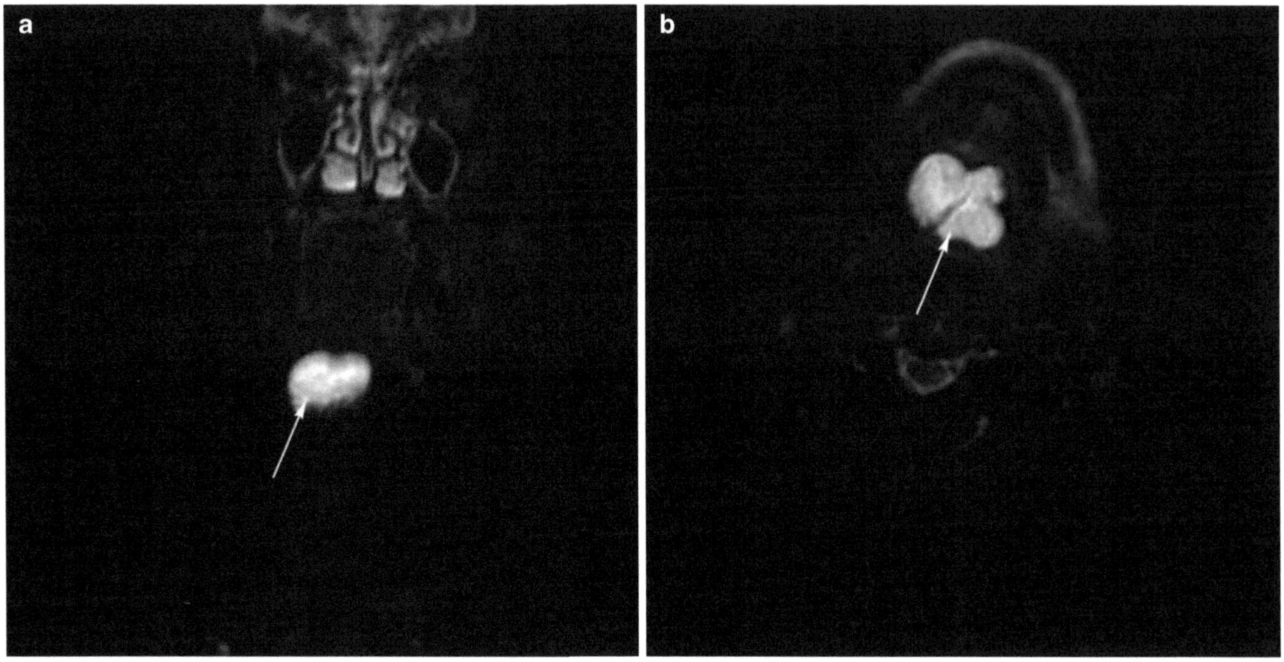


**Fig. 25.1** MRI T2WI displays the thyrolingual tube cyst. The coronary (**a**) and the axial (**b**) imagings display lobulated mid-central high signals between the tongue root and the thyroid gland (arrow)

agnosed as the thyrolingual tube cyst. B-mode ultrasound and radionuclide 131I examination could help differentiate diagnosis. Whether the thyroid tissues exist at the normal precervical sites or not merits special attention.

4. Pyramidal Thyroid Tumor or Cyst

   Pyramidal thyroid lobe could lie between the subcrico-cartilage thyroid isthmus and the hyoid bone. The tumor and the cyst may occur at the pyramidal lobe, especially the cyst is hard to be differentiated from the thyrolingual cyst. At the ultrasound imaging, there are thyroid tissues surrounding the pyramidal lobular cyst.

**Treatment**

Except the inflammation stage, once the diagnosis is ascertained, surgery should be opted as soon as possible. Before the excision surgery, the normal thyroid tissues; existing should be ascertained by the ultrasound, the nuclide scanning or the CT and the MRI examination. Infants should take operation after 4 years old. No choices could be better than taking systemic anesthesia during surgeries. Transversely excise parallel to the hyoid bone at the hyoid plane or the most upheaved cyst and its two ends should be slightly beyond the cyst range; longitudinally excise the cervical albline and stretch the subhyoid muscular flaps towards left and right to expose the cyst. If adhesion exists, electrotome, secateur or vessel forceps could be used to do the anatomy dissection; and stretching the lesion tissue shouldn't be over-exerted. Under the cyst, the superficial thyroid cartilage separate from top to bottom and straightly approach the subhyoid edge. After seperating the middle hyoid up and down adhered muscle and the hyothyroid membrane, absciss together the middle small hyoid angle basihyoid bone with the periosteum. Clamp the midbasihyoid bone with forceps and stretch outwards, then continue seperating the fistula striking the lingual foramen cecum orientation, and while almost approaching the submucosal lingual foramen cecum, ligate and excise. Sturate straticulately, but if the operative space is relatively larger, vacuum drainage setting is suitable.

## 25.2 Cleft Cyst and Fistula of Branchus

Branchial cleft fistula is developed by the communication of the branchial pouch and the branchial groove or disappear branchial groove. The branchial cleft cyst is developed by the unfused brachial groove and its closed external aperture, often existing together with the fistula. The branchial cleft fistula contains four types (Table 25.1):

**Table 25.1** The four types of branchial cleft fistula

| Fistula canal type | External fistula orificial location | Internal fistula orificial location |
|---|---|---|
| First | The cervical lateral skin at the post-submandibular angle and at the plane above the hyoid bone | External auricular cancal cartilage or anterior or posterior auricle, tympanum or eustachian tube |
| Second | Junction at mid-inferior-1/3 anterior sternocleidomastoid edge | Superior tonsillar fossa |
| Third | Substernocleidomastoid | Ending at piriform recess |
| Fourth | Same as second fistula cancal | Superior esophagus |

### Etiology

At common consideration, fistula canal is developed because of the incomplete closure of either the branchial cleft or the pharyngodiverticulum or both of them and the cyst is caused by the remaining epithelium cells during embryonic development. As recent researches say, the branchial cleft cyst or abnormality is related to dominant autosomal heredity.

### Clinical Manifestation

Branchial cleft cyst often manifests no symptoms, but a cervical lateral painless lump may be occasionally found, and the lump is without unified size, round or oval, none-adhered to skin, movable, without cystic sensation, and it could enlarge rapidly with partial pressing pain while secondary infection. The cyst upheaves toward the pharyngolateral, evoking the pharyngeal pain, dysphagia etc. At the branchial fistula canal, it mainly manifests the external fistula orificial intermittent or persisting secretion spillover, some patients may have smelly odour in their mouth and repeated onsetting of the perifistula orificial swelling pain and the purulent secretion spillover may occur during secondary infection (Fig. 25.2).

### Differential Diagnosis

1. Otitis Externa or Otitis Media

   When the first branchial fistula's secondary infection occurs, because its inner mouth is communicated with the inner part of the external auditory canal, the canal infection can be easily misdiagnosed as pus otitis externa or otitis externamedia. At this time, the pus from the external auditory canal can be absorbed. The pus can be observed from the fistula of external auditory canal, and the upper neck may touch the cyst or observe the external opening. When the upper neck or cyst is compressed, the pus overflow from the external auditory canal can help to diagnose.
2. Parotid Pleomorphic Adenoma (Mixed Tumor)

   The first branchial cleft fistula or cyst can be located in parenchyma of the parotid gland, and can be misdiagnosed as pleomorphic adenoma of the parotid gland. In particular, the pleomorphic adenoma of the parotid gland originated from the posterior mandible. The tumor is mostly solid and cystic. But the symptoms such as red and pain are not common, and the diagnosis needs postoperative pathology.
3. Neck Cold Abscess

   Branchial cleft cyst should be identified with cold abscess. Can do tuberculin test; take the chest X-ray film to know whether the patient has tuberculosis infection. Fine needle puncture and acid bacilli smear examination could be used before operation. After the operation, the *Mycobacterium tuberculosis* could be cultured and the diagnosis further clarified.
4. Cystic Lymphangioma of the Neck (Cystic Water Tumor)

   Cystic lymphangioma is caused by abnormal lymphangiogenesis in the embryonic stage, and also a cystic tumor with slow growth of the neck. Most of the disease is in infantile period. There is no infection in general. The test of translucent test was positive. The puncture can suck out the green water like liquid, and a large number of lymphocytes can be seen under the microscope. The wall of the capsule consists of fibrous tissue and endothelial cells, containing lymphocytes and lymph nodes. The above features can assist in the diagnosis.

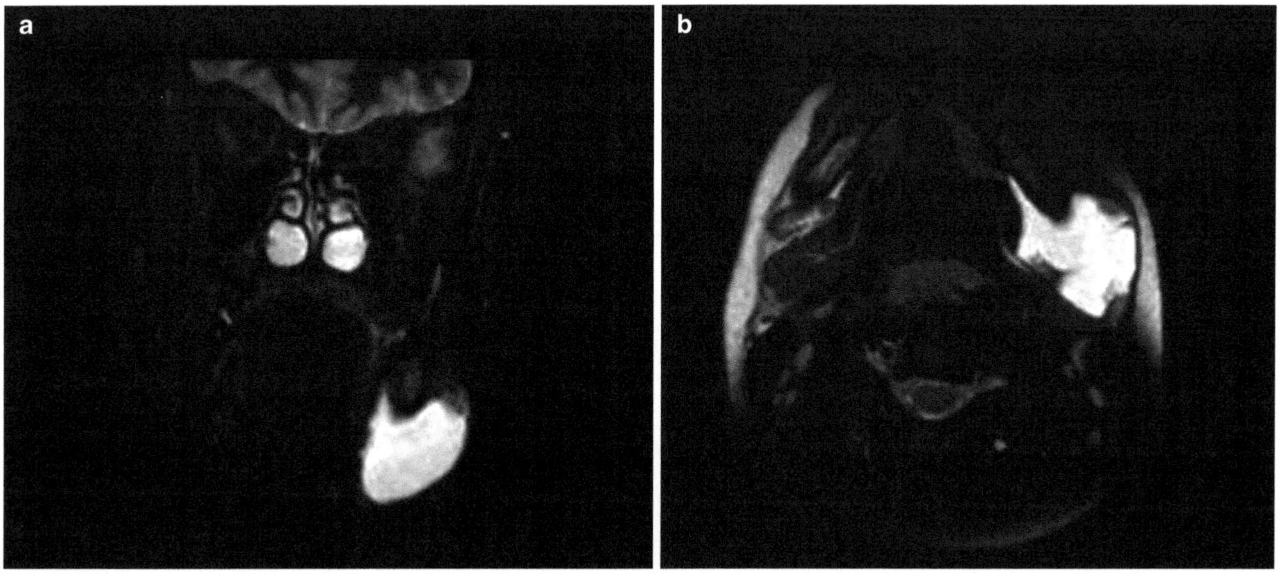


**Fig. 25.2** Branchial cleft cyst MRI $T_2$WI. Coronary (**a**) and axial (**b**) MRI display the lobular irregular high signals at postinferior left cervical submaxillary bone, which is branchial cleft cyst's manifestation

5. Larynx Gas Cyst

Third branchial fistula through the thyroid hyoid membrane, its associated cyst is easily misdiagnosed as laryngeal gas cyst. The characteristics of laryngeal cyst are: as Valsalva action, deep breathing, severe cough, crying or swallowing, the pressure can be reduced. The above characteristics can be distinguished from branchial cleft cyst.

**Treatment**

The cyst and the fistula were completely removed. In particular, fistulae are thinner or branched, and should be more vigilant for fistula and postoperative recurrence. If secondary infection occurs, the first is control of the infection, and then operation.

The first branchial fistula often wears parotid parenchyma and has multiple branches. During facial resection, facial nerve anatomy and protection, partial parotidectomy and fistula anatomy and protection should be done. Otherwise, it is easy to relapse.

The second branchial fistula often occurs in both sides, and should be distinguished.

The third branchial fistula is the most common cervical branchial fistula, often prone to infection, the infection after surgery, in the anatomy of the thyroid and parathyroid protection, recurrent laryngeal nerve and the external laryngeal nerve after the lateral thyroid and carotid sheath, soft tissue above clavicle to piriform fossa was excised. Similarly to that of cervical lymph node dissection, and excision method.

## 25.3 Acute and Chronic Cervical Lymphadenitis

**Etiology**

Cervical lymphadenitis secondary to dental and oral infection is the most common, can also be derived from facial skin damage, furuncle, carbuncle. The majority in children are caused by upper respiratory tract infection and tonsillitis. Cervical lymphadenitis caused by pyogenic bacteria, such as staphylococci and Streptococcus, is called purulent lymphadenitis; the tuberculous lymphadenitis is infected by *Mycobacterium tuberculosis*.

**Clinical Manifestations**

May come from odontogenic lesions, and most of them in infants are secondary to upper respiratory tract infection. Most of the clinical symptoms are rapid. A swelling and tenderness of a single lymph node in the early stage. After involving multiple lymph nodes, can also results in adhesion, skin redness, spreading or perforation of lymph node capsule formation cellulitis. There are different systemic reactions with the condition of the virulence of the cell and the patient's body resistance, especially in children.

**Diagnosis**

Cervical lymph node enlargement, tenderness, lymphatic drainage area of internal organs have acute inflammation; the body may have chills, fever and other symptoms. Neutrophils increased in leucocyte count. The cervical ultrasonography is helpful to understand the location, size and number of lymph nodes and the relationship with the surrounding tissues. This disease should be identified with cervical lymph node tuberculosis, malignant lymphoma and metastatic malignant tumor (Fig. 25.3). Lymph node puncture or biopsy should be done when necessary.

**Treatment**

Treating primary lesions includes anti infection, strengthening nutrition, enhancing the body's resistance, etc.

Children may have a single lymphadenitis. Lymphadenopathy, swelling and swelling of the surface of the neck. Selection of antibiotics for staphylococci is often effective, but some children continue to develop until they are involved in lymph node necrosis and abscess formation. At this point, local incision and drainage should be performed.

A group of lymph nodes in the corresponding drainage lymphatic chain are caused by the common head and neck infection in the clinic. The lymphadenopathy in the region was characterized by swelling and tenderness, which resulted in a reduction in the activity of the neck. The muscle tissue around the affected lymph nodes can be spasmodic and tetanus. At this time, the primary infection should be treated in order to effectively control lymphadenitis.

In adults, if the lymph nodes are not treated after 1 week of antiinflammatory treatment and no symptoms of inflammation such as fever and pain, we should pay attention to the possibility of metastasis of malignant tumors in the external head and neck.

## 25.4 Tumor of Carotid Body

The origin of carotid body tumor in the carotid body is a chemical sensor in the dorsal carotid bifurcation receptors belonging to the tumor, paraganglioma, mostly benign lesions, few (10~15%) for low grade. Near the tumor easily infringe the vagus, sublingual nerve can cause vocal cord movement disorder, skew.

**Etiology**

It is unknown and may be associated with chronic anoxia. Recent studies have shown that some of them are autosomal dominant hereditary diseases, with familial and autosomal recessive inheritance.

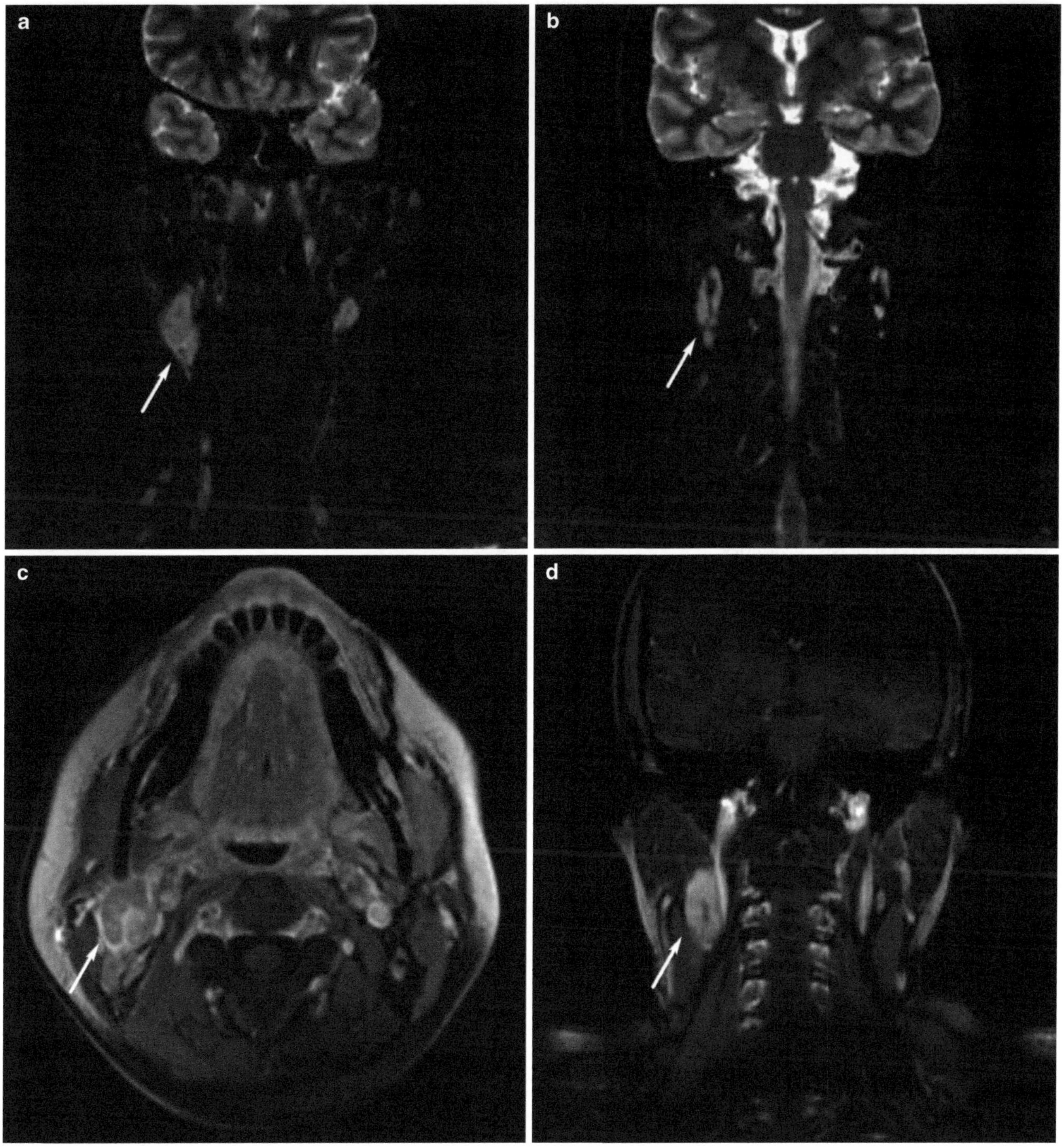


**Fig. 25.3** MRI, $T_2WI$, coronal and axial and coronal $T_1WI$ enhanced images show chronic inflammation of lymph nodes. (**a**) Showed enlargement of the right neck lymph nodes, with a slight high signal (arrow). (**b**) Showed that the border of the skin and medulla (arrow) (**c**, **d**) was enhanced with irregular ring enhancement (arrow)

**Clinical Manifestations**

This disease is mostly seen between the age of 30 ~ 50, and there is no significant gender difference. It can change the neck lymph node in zone II and III, and the distant metastases are common bone metastases, followed by lung and liver.

1. Neck Mass: it can happen in any part of the neck with a lump. Most of the masses are located in the front and lower of the mandibular angle, usually unilateral, round, smooth and toughened (Fig. 25.4). On the surface of the tumor, the carotid artery pulsation can be palpated on the

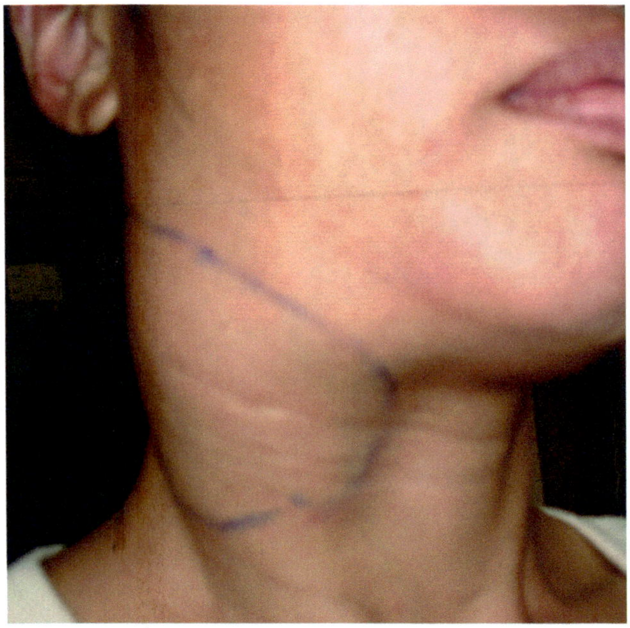

**Fig. 25.4** Right cervical masses external view

superficial side, and the internal and external carotid arteries are pushed to the sides by the mass. Sometimes on the tumor itself, can also palpate the pulsation.

2. Carotid Sinus Syndrome: dizziness or faintness in a low head or an oppressive mass.
3. Nerve compression symptoms such as sympathetic nerve compression, can cause Horner syndrome; vagus nerve compression, can present with hoarseness, irritating cough, choking water, etc. Hypoglossal nerve involvement can have dysphagia, disfluency, ipsilateral tongue bias.

**Diagnosis**

The mass is located in the triangle of the carotid artery. It is round, with a tough texture and clear boundary. It can move around and move up and down. The masses can be palpabled and sometimes have vascular murmur. B ultrasonography and DSA examination are of great value in the diagnosis of this disease. Ultrasound visible at the carotid bifurcation mass will be separated from the internal and external carotid artery, the distance widened. DSA showed that the tumor was located behind the carotid artery, and the bifurcation of the common carotid artery was pushed forward. The bifurcation of the carotid artery widened. The internal and external carotid arteries showed "high feet cup sign". The tumor was rich in blood vessels (Fig. 25.5). Enhanced MRI showed enhancement the clear boundary of the tumor located in the carotid artery bifurcation. Tumor signal, magnetic resonance image shows the carotid triangle area significantly enhanced clear boundary, neck vascular sheath wrapped around vessels

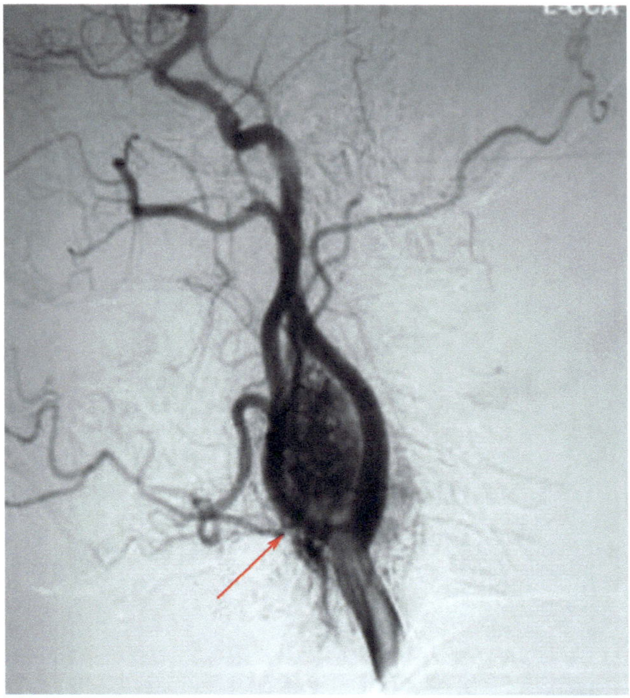

**Fig. 25.5** DSA manifestation of left carotid artery aneurysm. According to the bifurcation of the common carotid artery group of vascular tumors, internal carotid and external carotid artery separately, showed a typical "goblet" sign (arrow)

(Fig. 25.6). The internal carotid artery and external carotid artery (Fig. 25.7) were found in the carotid body tumor by enhanced CT.

According to the degree of tumor wrapped in internal carotid artery, Shambling of carotid body tumor were divided into three types: type I is not only around the tumor or artery of not more than 1/3 weeks, type II is the tumor around the artery more than 2/3 weeks but not all week, type III is completely wrapped around the tumor artery, the artery may change fine (Fig. 25.8).

**Treatment**

Surgical treatment of carotid body tumor is usually performed. The smaller the tumor, the easier the operation is to be excised and the less the complications. The internal carotid artery should be preserved as much as possible in the operation. If it is not easy to retain, it should be rebuilt to minimize the probability of intracranial complications. Generally, type I and type II are easier to retain the internal carotid artery, and type III retention of blood vessels is difficult. All patients should be examined by DSA before operation, to observe the blood supply of the tumor and the blood vessels of the brain, and to measure the internal carotid artery reflux pressure. If the reflux pressure is >70 mmHg, it is safer to block the artery during operation. The reflux pressure is

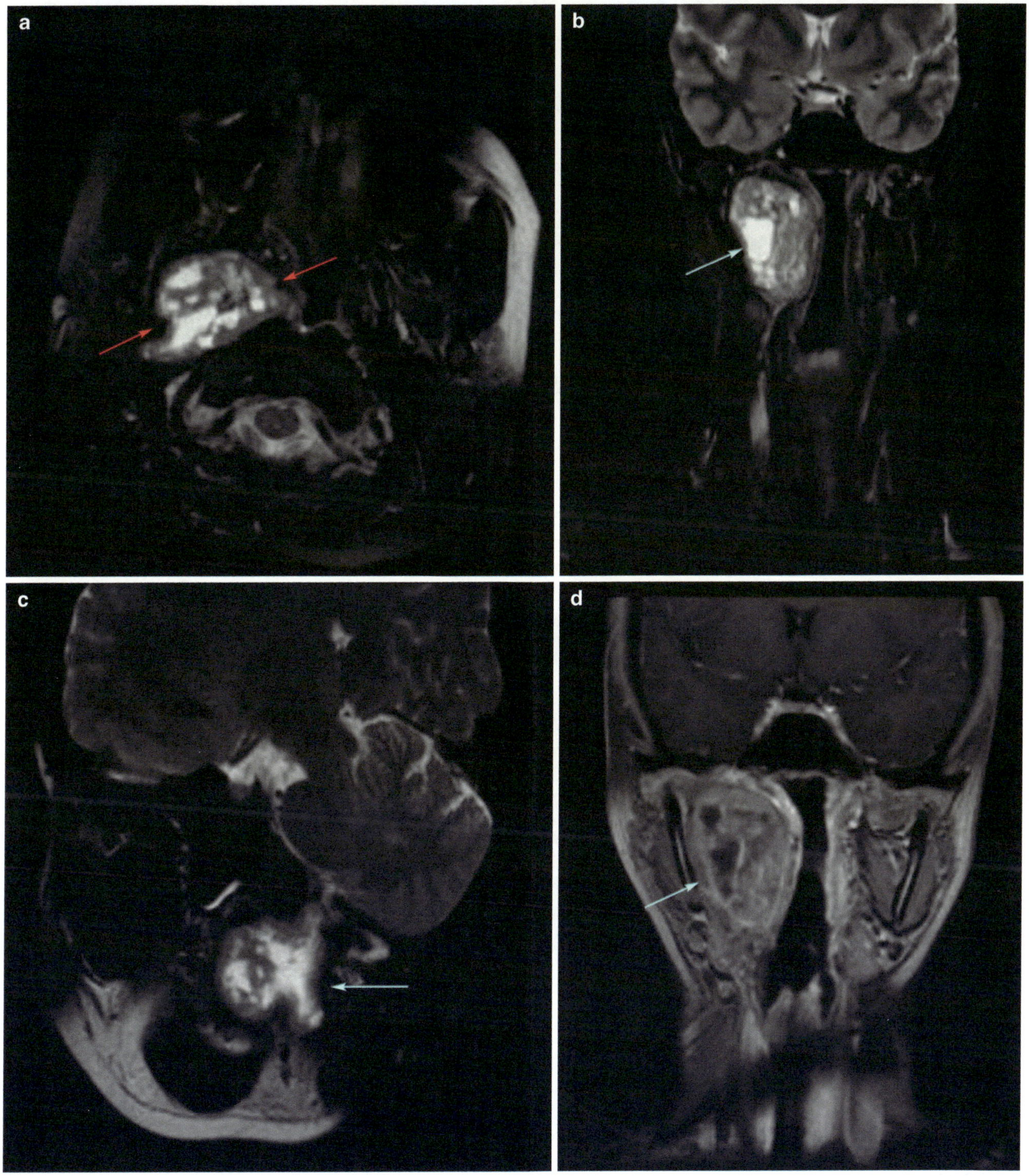


**Fig. 25.6** MRI plain scan and enhancement showed right carotid body tumor. (**a**) $T_2$WI axis showed a mixed $T_2$ signal tumor in the right carotid artery, which showed irregular ellipse. The inside and outside of the rounded flow vessel (red arrow) showed, respectively, as the internal and external bifurcated vessels of the carotid artery, which was a characteristic change. (**b**) $T_2$WI showed coronal compression of the lateral wall of the pharynx (arrow). (**c**) $T_2$WI. Sagittal display of the anterior and posterior relationship of the tumor (arrow). (**d**) T1WI coronal enhancement showed abundant blood supply (arrow)

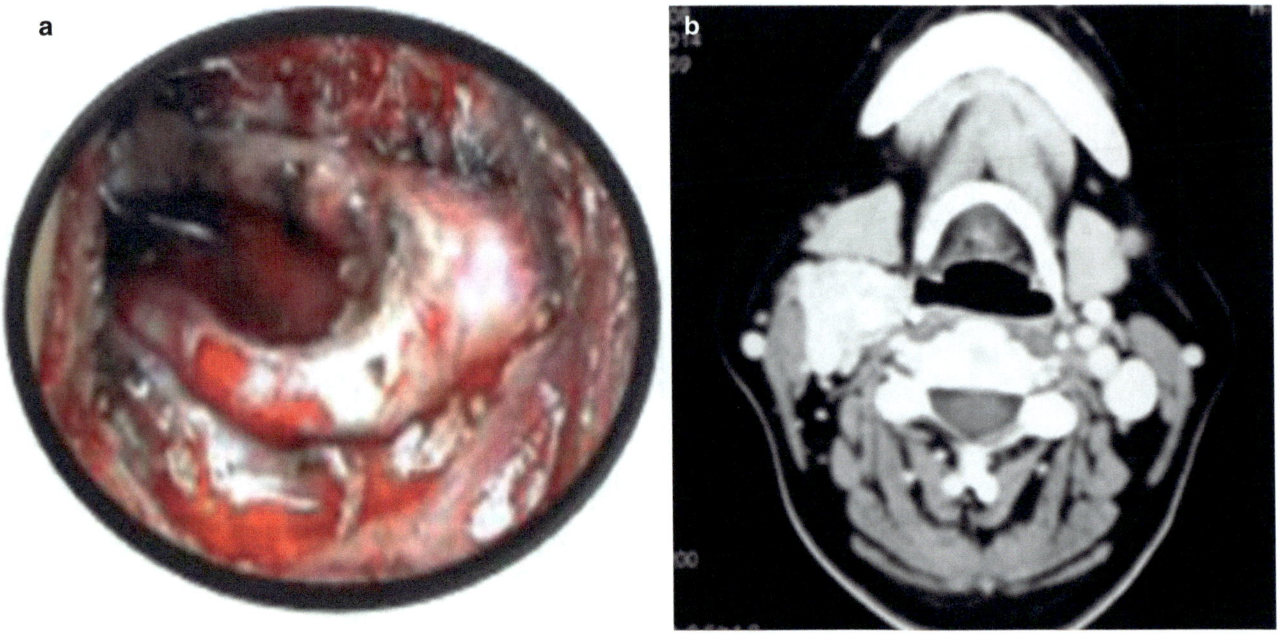

**Fig. 25.7** (**a**) Intraoperative graphy (**b**) enhanced CT displays carotid arterial tumor circling internal carotid (short arrow), external carotid (long arrow)

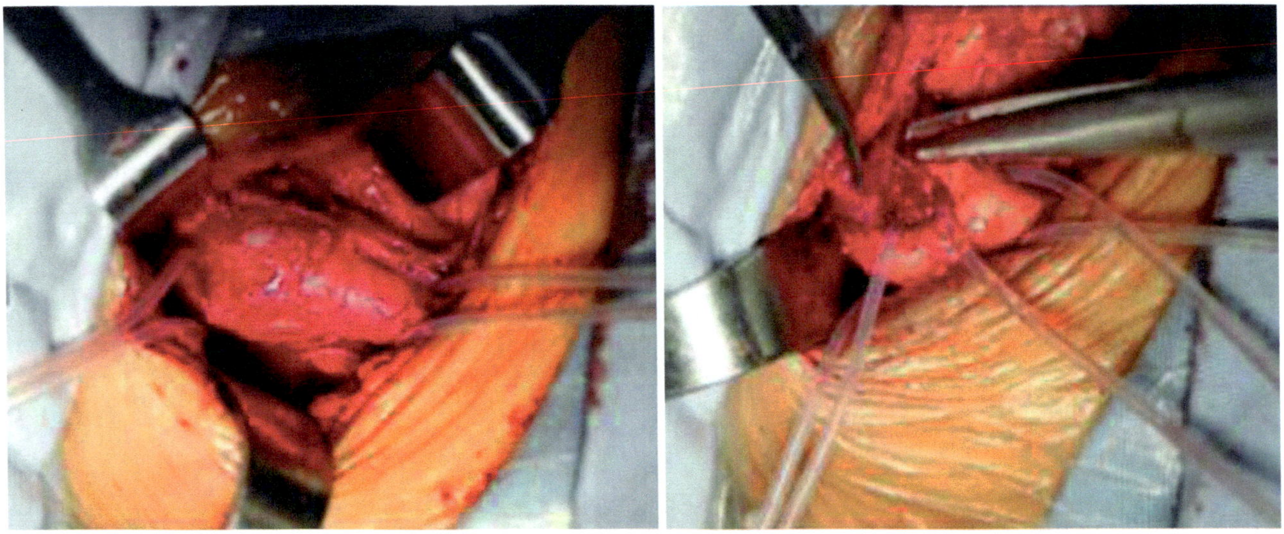

**Fig. 25.8** Carotid body tumorectomy

relatively safe from 50 to 70 mmHg, and the risk of stroke after blocking the artery is larger than 50 mmHg. During operation, we should remove lymph nodes around the tumor and send it to frozen disease inspection. A few malignant carotid body tumors do not show obvious malignant characteristics. The methods of operation are divided into several kinds.

1. Preservation of the artery under the adventitia tumor resection: because the tumor originates from the carotid body connected with the outer carotid artery, it has very rich blood supply, and is closely adjacent to the carotid artery, veins and nerves, and the operation is difficult (Fig. 25.8). It is suitable for type I and type II tumors.
2. The tumor is removed together with the carotid artery. The first stage of vascular reconstruction is type III and larger tumor. If the carotid artery is adhered or wrapped around the carotid artery, the lump and part of the carotid artery should be removed together. Then the artery can be reconstructed. The artificial blood vessel or great saphenous vein can be used (Fig. 25.9). Attentions should be paid to the protection of the vagus and hypoglossal nerves during the operation.

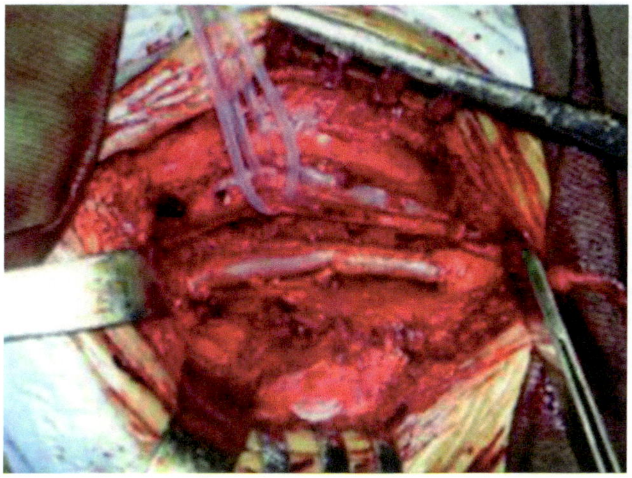

**Fig. 25.9** Carotid body tumor resection and internal saphenous vein reconstruction

## 25.5 Tumor of Nerve Sheath

**Etiology**

It originated from Schwann cells of nerve sheath tumor, can occur in the glossopharyngeal, vagus, side, diaphragm, cervical sympathetic, cervical plexus, brachial plexus nerve, vagus, higher incidence of cervical sympathetic and glossopharyngeal nerve. The tumor has a centrifugal distribution along the peripheral nerve, which can have cystic and degenerative changes. The typical pathological features were Antoni A and Antoni B.

**Clinical Manifestation**

This disease is common in a 30~40 year old male with a longer course of disease.

1. Neck Mass: any part of the neck can occur. Tumors originating in the vagus or sympathetic nerves, sometimes from the parapharyngeal space into the lateral wall of the pharynx, are called parapharyngeal neurilemmoma. The edge of the tumor is clear, the surface is smooth, the surface of the skin or the mucous membrane of the pharynx are normal, and it is active and has nothing to do with the swallowing movement (Fig. 25.10).
2. Symptoms of Nerve Function: according to the location of the tumor, the corresponding symptoms of nerve function can be caused. The hypoglossal nerve compression, can present with ipsilateral tongue muscle atrophy; phrenic nerve involvement, ipsilateral diaphragmatic elevention; brachial plexus compression, muscle atrophy, tapping mass, radiation to hand electric shock; sympathetic nerve involvement, can produce Horner (Horner) syndrome, namely, ptosis of upper eyelid miosis, enophthalmos, ipsilateral facial flushing, sweating less; vagus nerve involvement can produce hoarseness, choking cough, etc.

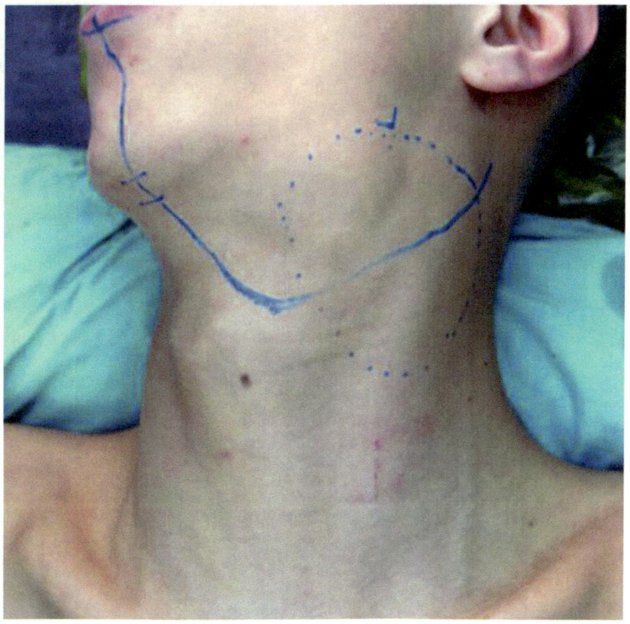

**Fig. 25.10** Left nerve sheath tumor's external cervical view. Visible left submandibular carotid trigono

3. Transposition of The Carotid Artery: the main lesion of the cervical sympathetic or vagus nerve, which can squeeze the anterior internal displacement of the carotid artery. At this point, the pulsating artery can be palpated on the surface of the tumor.

**Diagnosis**

There was a solitary painless mass in the neck, with slow growth, round or oval shape, well-defined boundary, good left and right movement, limited upper and lower activities, and no symptoms associated with nerve compression. The diagnosis of B, CT, MRI and DSA can be further diagnosed (Fig. 25.11). But neurilemmoma in carotid triangle is sometimes difficult to identify with carotid body tumor, the former located in the common carotid artery and internal carotid artery external carotid artery posterior, often goes forward, in the surface of the mass was palpable pulses, open the artery, palpable mass in the lower, which is located in the carotid artery bifurcation mass, superficial palpable carotid artery pulsatile compression transfer, carotid artery proximal, mass can be reduced. DSA is of great significance in the identification of two kinds of tumors.

**Treatment**

Once the disease is diagnosed, it should be excised in time; otherwise the enlargement of the tumor can result in oppression and destruction. Most tumors can be excised through the neck, and the higher position can be removed through the

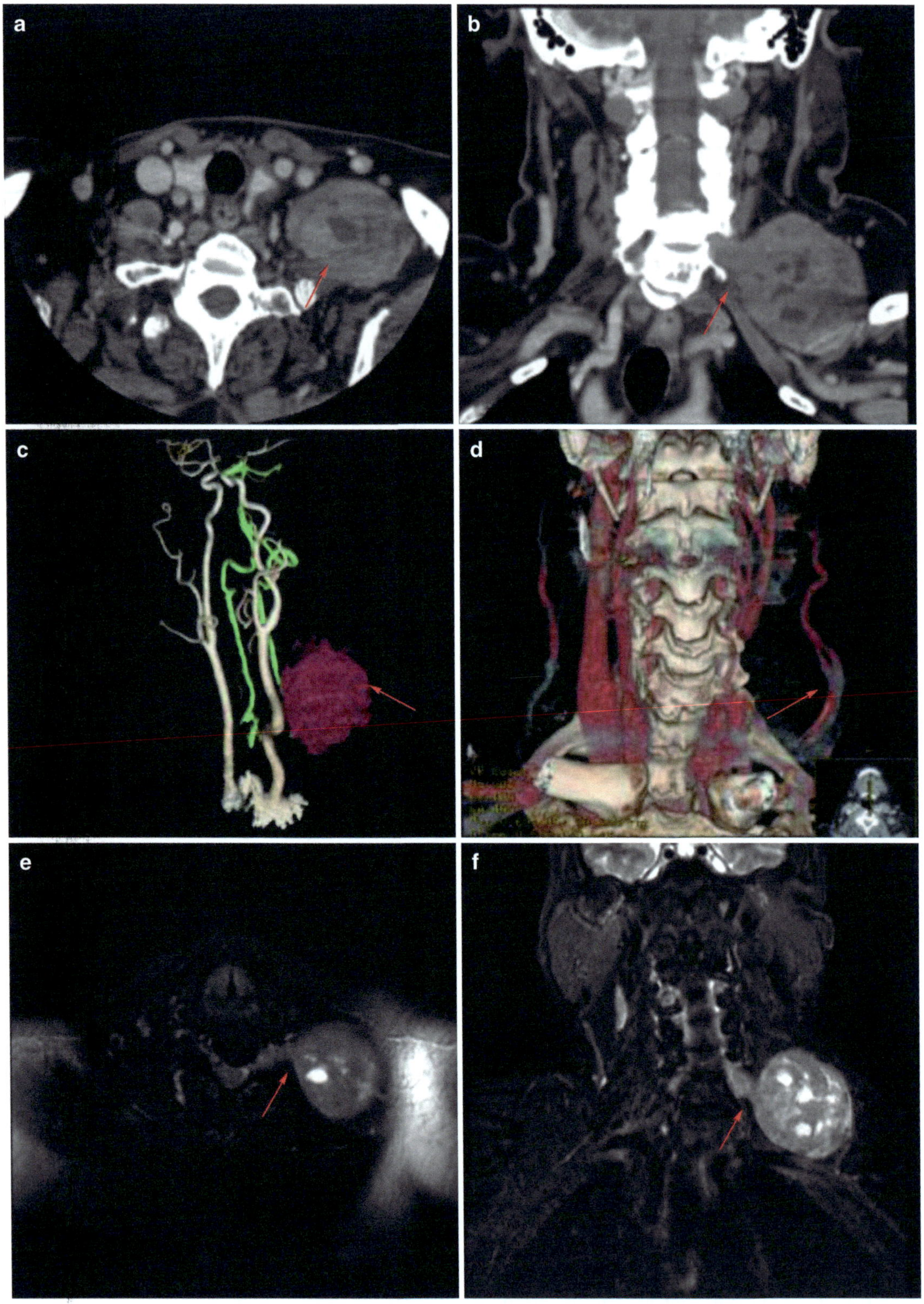


**Fig. 25.11** Cervical CT and MRI graphy displays left neurogenous tumor. (**a**, **b**) CT enhanced axial and coronary reconstruction imaging: left carotid space mass, heterogeneous enhancement, carotid moves forward, and vertebral canal and tumor are related to each other (arrow). (**c**, **d**) CT angiography says that the tumor does not locate in the carotid bifurcation, which is suggesting that it is not carotid body tumor, and on the other hand, the external jugular vein arc moves under compression (arrow). (**e**, **f**) MRI axial and coronary $T_2$WI, visible within the tumor hyperintense cystic, and it is connected with the left pedicle (arrow), which is characteristic of neurogenic tumors

posterior and parotid approach. For high parapharyngeal neurilemmoma, transoral endoscopy or endoscopic assisted resection can also be used. The operation should be stripped of the tumor on the basis of the preservation of the nerve trunk as much as possible. During operation, the nerve fiber bundles are tightly wrapped around the tumor. At the same time, the superficial tissue should be cut along the direction of the nerve along the tumor surface, and then the tumor surface can be separated by layer. The tumor will be blunt. Sometimes the nerve is preserved, but the nerve function is often damaged after the operation.

## 25.6 Trauma of Closed Trachea

**Etiology**

When blunt force is directly from the front to the neck, the trachea is extruded on the hard spine, which cause tracheal cartilage ring disruption and posterior soft tissue can tear. Even the trachea is separated from the cricoid cartilage, and the damage is more serious. When the blunt force strikes the neck from the side, the trachea can metastasis to the contralateral side with light damage, often without fracture and dislocation, and only causes the injury of the trachea mucous membrane. Tracheal rupture can be caused by elevated endotracheal pressure, tracheal intubation anaesthesia, and high pressure of air bag.

**Clinical Manifestation**

The symptoms of closed trauma of the trachea often accompanied by the contusion of the larynx.

1. Pain in the wound of the trachea: the pain increases when swallowing or head rotation can radiate to the same ear.
2. Cough and Hemoptysis: Tracheal wall injuries after blood flow into the trachea, caused by paroxysmal irritating cough, cough with phlegm and blood bubbles, if the damage is to the blood vessels, then it can cause bleeding.
3. Dyspnea: tracheal mucous membrane damage swelling, cartilage injury, or concurrent mediastinal emphysema, pneumothorax, etc., can cause difficulty in breathing and more progressive. If the tracheal cricoid dislocation occurs, it can cause severe dyspnea and even death of asphyxia.
4. Subcutaneous Emphysema: gas enters subcutaneous tissue through the broken wall of the trachea and produces emphysema, which is an important sign for the injury of the trachea. Emphysema can be localized. It can be progressive, that is, it will expand rapidly and even involve in the whole body in a short time. Severe cases are often accompanied by mediastinal emphysema and pneumothorax.
5. Laryngeal contusion or hoarseness associated with recurrent laryngeal nerve injury, severe cases can produce hoarseness, aphonia.

**Diagnosis**

After neck contusion or thoracic crush injury, cough foamy bloody phlegm, dyspnea, high suspicion of tracheal contusion, X-ray examination should be carried out immediately. CT scan can show the damage of tracheal cartilage ring. If the patient's condition is allowed, the bronchoscopy can also be carried out to determine the location and degree of the injury.

**Treatment**

The principle is to keep the airway open, repair the injury of the trachea and prevent the stenosis of the trachea.

1. Conservative Treatment: A mild injury without dyspnea, closes observation of the respiratory situation, and gives antibiotics and hormone treatment.
2. Early Tracheotomy trachea injury without dyspnea, if CT showed tracheal cartilage ring fracture or tracheal deformation, then the patient can have difficulty breathing after a few hours, tracheotomy should be done as early as possible.
3. Repair Injury: according to the extent and location of the injury, different surgical methods are taken. Less damage to the tracheal mucosa, without suture; long mucosal laceration, sutured; and the displacement of fracture of trachea should be reset, suture the perichondrium, and do routine tracheal incision, or implantation of T tube; if the tracheal cartilage is comminuted or tracheal injury completely broken off, to the upper and lower trachea retreat, this can free the damage in the upper and lower ends of the trachea, tracheal anastomosis; injury of the thoracic trachea, to relieve dyspnea (such as low tracheotomy or insertion of the bronchoscope) under the premise of thoracic tracheal repair.

## 25.7 Trauma of Open Blood Vessels and Nerves

**Etiology**

Because of the anatomical relationship, vascular injury is often accompanied by nerve damage. Open vascular injury is caused by direct injury of the neck. In addition to direct injury of the nerve, the hematoma formed by vascular injury can oppress the nerve. According to the degree of injury, vascular injury can be divided into three types: (1) traumatic artery spasm; (2) the injury of vessel wall is mainly intimal or medial injuries and the outer membrane is still intact; (3) partial or complete rupture of a blood vessel.

**Clinical Manifestation**

1. Bleeding: there can be massive hemorrhage or hematoma in the damaged area, and if serious in a patient, can cause hemorrhagic shock. A small wound with small blood ves-

sels outside the wound can cause a large number of internal bleeding, but the external bleeding is very small, and this situation is easily ignored. The blood pressure and the pulse status of the patients should be closely observed, and the internal bleeding should be paid attention to.

2. Neurological Symptoms: often accompanied by vagal and hypoglossal, glossopharyngeal, facial nerve injury, hoarseness, cough, facial paralysis, tongue deviation etc.
3. Cerebral Ischemia: carotid artery injury can cause cerebral ischemia of the injured side, manifested as coma, hemiplegia, aphasia, etc.
4. Dyspnea: the injury of the carotid artery is often accompanied by the trauma of the larynx and trachea, which causes dyspnea. In addition, the hematoma formed after the injury of the carotid artery can also oppress the larynx and trachea, and aggravate the difficulty of breathing.
5. Air Embolism: after internal jugular vein injury, when the inhaled air enters the vein through the damaged vein due to the negative pressure of the thoracic cavity, causing air embolism, it causes damage to important organs such as brain, liver and kidney.
6. Injuries of The Other Organs of The Neck: the more commonly affected organs are: the larynx, the trachea, the esophagus and the thyroid gland.
7. Artery hematoma caused by injury of artery pseudoaneurysm in the second days after the injury, its characteristic is obvious and can hear the pulse, systolic murmur often spread along the artery, often accompanied by headache and disease side radioactivity. The internal carotid artery hematoma has the edema, congestion, venous dilatation and decrease of visual acuity in the diseased side of the optic disc. The symptoms of mobile and venous hematoma appear earlier, and the murmur is often heard within hours after injury, and the murmur is more obvious. Not only along the blood vessels, but also far away from the wound site, it can also hear murmur and palpate the persistent tremor locally.

**Diagnosis**

There is a history of open trauma in the neck. There is local bleeding or hematoma formation, obvious hematoma beating, and systolic murmur can be heard, accompanied by cerebral ischemia, nerve compression and systemic bleeding symptoms. Cervical vascular and nerve injuries should be considered. In the diagnosis, cervical B-ultrasound, CT and DSA is helpful (Fig. 25.12). If necessary, neck wound exploration should be done in order to understand the location and extent of damage. But it must be done on the premise that the blood is fully prepared.

**Treatment**

1. The Treatment of Cervical Artery Injury: it is effective for innominate small artery injury, local pressurization and tamponade. For the neck artery injury, first, we must stop bleeding when we can with first aid. To send the patient quickly in the supine position, head to the injured side, the sternocleidomastoid muscle in the chest with the thumb on the edge of a palpable pulsatile carotid artery, and there will be pressure to the cricoid cartilage plane sixth cervical vertebra transverse process, and into the

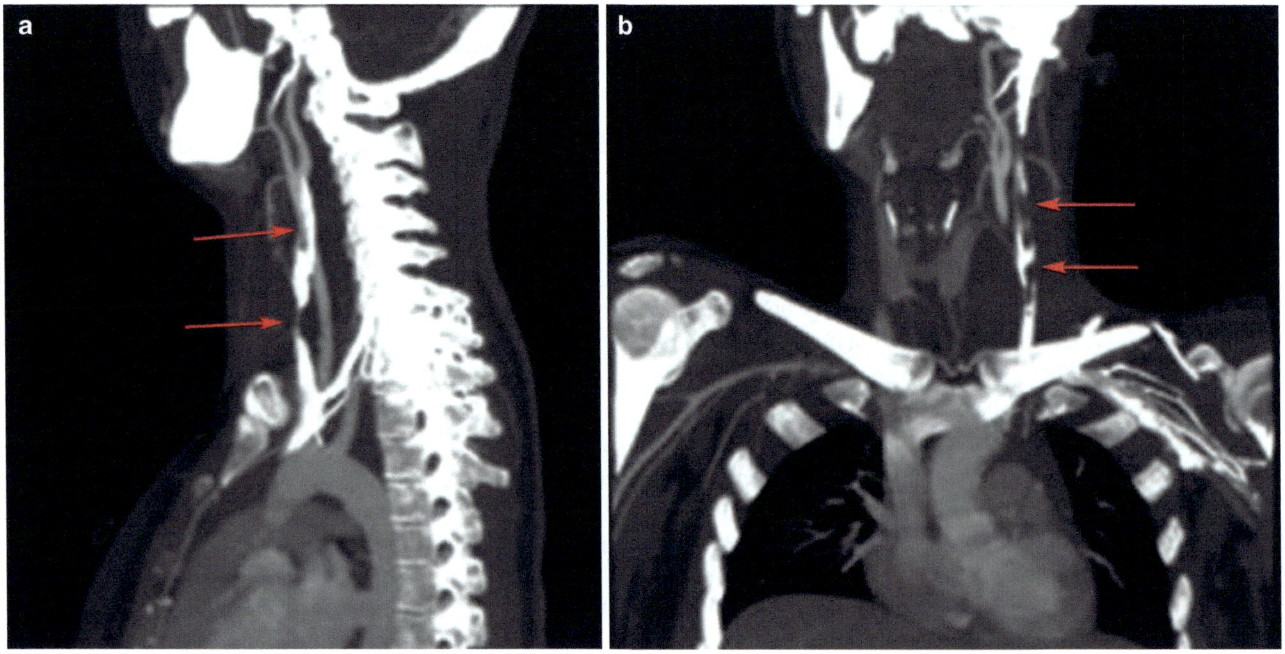


**Fig. 25.12** Thrombosis occurred 6 h after left internal jugular veous puncture. (**a**) CT sagittal MIP reconstruction (**b**) CT coronary site MIP reconstruction

wound dressing, bleeding local oppression, in order to achieve the purpose of reducing bleeding. At the same time, we should be active in anti shock treatment, and the blood volume is supplemented quickly. If blood is not available in time, we can use the vasoconstrictor temporarily to boost the blood pressure, which helps maintain the cerebral perfusion pressure and maintain the coronary blood flow, but it can never replace the supplementary blood volume. After the shock is corrected, it should be debrided in time and look for the bleeding point carefully. In finding the bleeding point, it can often be caused by severe tissue congestion, poor visual field, or serious tissue damage and the broken ends of the blood vessels are reduced to the soft tissue and are not easy to find. For large blood vessel bleeding, look carefully along its path, clamp and ligate the bleeder. Attention should be paid to keeping the respiratory tract unobstructed while dealing with bleeding.

2. The Treatment of Cervical Vascular Rupture: cervical artery injury, common carotid artery and internal carotid artery injury should be repaired in time, so as to avoid serious complications such as cerebral ischemia, necrosis and cerebral softening. The repair methods include end anastomosis, side repair, or vascular transplantation. In addition, the trauma of the common carotid artery can also be performed by the internal carotid artery and the external carotid artery anastomosis, to debride and repair the arteries as early as possible. If the rupture is difficult to repair, the great saphenous vein can be used for revascularization. The injury of external carotid artery, vertebral artery and external jugular vein needs simple ligation. However, the rupture of vertebral artery is often not easy to ligate. Because it sometimes needs to use the bone-biting forceps to remove the transverse process of cervical vertebrae in the cervical transverse foramen, so that it can be ligated. The injury of the external carotid artery and its branches can be ligated. When ligating, the original mouth is enlarged or the incision of the anterior margin of the papillomastoid muscle is not <5 cm. For the injury of the vein of the neck, it can be ligated when treated. It should be noted that the formation of the embolus should be prevented when the internal jugular vein is handled. It is most effective to use tamponade and pressure hemostasis during first aid. When debridement is done, we should find the ruptured vascular stump to ligate.
3. Surgical Exploration of Vascular Injury of the Neck: the injuries of the large vessels in the neck are mostly open and easy to diagnose. Bleeding from the veins and arterioles usually oppresses the hemostasis. If the pressure can't stop the bleeding, it may be the big artery bleeding. Hemorrhagic shock after cervical trauma is mostly seen in larger vascular injuries. However, some neck vascular injuries are not easy to observe because of small wound, bleeding at the time of consultation, or wound dressing. If there is a large vascular injury, when removing operative conditions of debridement and hemostasis, it is not easy to remove gauze and remove blood clots from wound. When patients have the following conditions, Surgical exploration should be done.
   (a) Active bleeding in the wound, the blood pressure continued to decrease, accompanied by a history of bleeding of the wound.
   (b) There are active bleeding in the mouth, and the oral mucosa is normal.
   (c) Thickening of the neck and subcutaneous congestion.
   (d) Pressure and displacement of the trachea.
   (e) The pulsation of the superficial temporal artery and the facial artery disappeared.

# 26 Common Skull Base Disease

Jugao Fang and Zhonglin Mu

## 26.1 Fracture of Skull Base

Skull fracture is a common clinical craniocerebral injury disease, its incidence accounted for 22.9% with skull fracture, skull fracture joint. The clinical classification of skull base fractures can be divided into anterior skull base fracture, middle skull base fracture, posterior skull base fracture and occipital condyle fracture according to the location of skull base fracture.

**Etiology**

1. By Extending to Skull Fracture.
2. The violence on the surface of the base of the skull.
3. The crush and violence of the head caused the general bending and deformation of the skull.
4. In an individual case, the buttocks are located at the top of the head or falling from the height in the vertical direction. It is divided into the anterior cranial fossa fracture, the middle cranial fossa fracture and the posterior fossa fracture according to its anatomical location. The fracture of the skull base is usually closed, and the fracture itself does not need special treatment. It is mainly aimed at the serious complication of the skull and skull base and the prevention of infection. The general prognosis is better.

**Clinical Manifestation**

1. Anterior skull base fracture: many times after the injury for several hours, there is subconjunctival hemorrhage and delayed blepharal subcutaneous congestion, which is purple blue. Commonly known as "panda eye", it is important for diagnosis. The fracture involves the ethmoid roof or plate, with cerebrospinal rhinorrhea and (or) pneumocephalus, unilateral or bilateral olfactory disorder; hemorrhage of orbital with exophthalmos, affected optic nerve or the optic canal fracture, can produce different degree of visual impairment.
2. Skull fracture of skull base fracture often involving the sella and parasellar petrous bone, with II~VIII of the symptoms of cerebral nerve injury, mainly manifested as dizziness, hemotympanum, hearing impairment, peripheral facial paralysis, pharyngeal congestion swelling, cerebrospinal fluid rhinorrhea and mouth, (or) otorrhea and fracture; intracavernous internal carotid artery, can cause carotid cavernous fistula, vascular pulsatile cranial tinnitus and ipsilateral exophthalmos and conjunctival congestion and edema, traumatic carotid artery pseudoaneurysm or traumatic internal carotid artery thrombosis features severe internal carotid artery rupture in the hole or the internal carotid artery tube rupture can be fatal, massive epistaxis. A small number of concurrent diabetes insipidus are associated with the sellar fracture of the hypothalamus or hypophyseal stalk.
3. After the skull fracture: after fracture of the skull base mainly occipital, mastoid or subcutaneous ecchymosis, muscle swelling, tenderness, delayed subcutaneous ecchymosis of mastoid region (Battle syndrome) and pharyngeal mucosa congestion and edema. The fracture line through the transverse sulcus may be associated with supratentorial and infratentorial epidural hematoma straddling transverse sinus sulcus or micro hematoma. The foramen magnum ring fracture, with craniocervical joint dislocation and fracture (or), cranial nerves (IX, X, XI and XII nerve) injury symptoms (such as hoarseness, dysphagia, etc.) and cerebellar and brainstem symptoms.

J. Fang (✉)
Department of Otorhinolaryngology Head and Neck Surgery, Beijing Tongren Hospital, Capital Medical University, Beijing, China

Z. Mu
Department of Otorhinolaryngology Head and Neck Surgery, The First Affiliated Hospital of Hainan Medical University, Haikou, China



Z. Mu, J. Fang (eds.), *Practical Otorhinolaryngology - Head and Neck Surgery*, https://doi.org/10.1007/978-981-13-7993-2_26

4. Fractures of the occipital condyle: occipital condyle fracture is traumatic neck pain and limitation of activity, spasmodic torticollis, hours after injury appeared Napex swelling and ecchymosis, can also cause low spinal cord injury, incomplete or complete paraplegia, vertebral artery ischemia symptoms and signs. In those with the level of the inferior lingual canal and the jugular hole, the traction, pressure and avulsion of the cerebral nerve were found, with the symptoms and signs of cerebral nerve paralysis.

**Diagnosis**

1. Clinical Signs
   (a) Fracture of The Anterior Cranial Fossa: periorbital subcutaneous and subconjunctival congestion of the eyeball, showing the "Panda" eye sign. Nasal bleeding with cerebrospinal fluid rhinorrhea. It can be combined with the symptoms of contusion of the olfactory nerve, optic nerve, pituitary, thalamus and frontal lobe.
   (b) Mid-cranial Fossa Fracture
   The external ear canal bleeds and combines with cerebrospinal otorrhea, always accompanying with manifestations like injuries at the auditory, the facial, the trigeminal, the abducent nerves and the temporal lobe. Minority of the patients may combine with the intracarotid cavenous fistula (ICCF) or the trumatic aneurism.
   (c) Post-cranial Fossa Fracture
   Sub-mastoid-thelium congestion, swelling, pressing pain and occasional post laryngeal wall swelling, congestion or cerebrospinorrhea are all its manifestations. Sometimes, it combines with injuries at the glossopharyngonerve, the labyrinth, the accessory nerve, the subglossonerve and the cerebellum, the brainstem.
2. Cranial base CT section imaging (Fig. 26.1), on whose three dimensional imaging straight fracture signs and secondary hemorrhage especially manifested clearly.

**Treatment**

Most of the skull base injury doesn't need any specific management, and its treatment is mainly against complications and sequelae evoked by fracture. The major treatment principle is infection-prevention and management of the complications and the timely management of sequelae.

1. Precranial Base Fracture
   (a) Conservation Treatment
   - Set with semi-fowler's position and free the cerebrospino-rhinorrhea from flowing or being swallowing, then the manifestations may disappear within 2 weeks spontaneously, during which, if there isn't any rhinocavum active bleedings, avoid the rhinocavum plugging.
   - Pay attention to the otorhinolaryngeal and oral clearance and nursing, avoid violently blowing nose and set a rhinogastric tube.
   - Infection-provention
   Choose and apply antibiotics that could pass through the blood brain barrier (BBB).
   (b) Surgery
   To the patients with uncurable cerebrospino-rhinorrhea over 4 weeks or repeated evoked meningitis and abundant discharge, apply cerebrospino-rhinorrhaphy. It may be under endorhinoscope and apply preoperative magnetic resonance hydrography (MRHG) to help determine the location.
2. Mid-Cranial Base Fracture
   (a) To those who accompany with crebrospino-rhinorrhea, clear and sterilize the outer rhinocancal skin, cover with sterilized absorbent cottons or gauzes and change timely; set with semi-fowler position, head tends to the affected side to promote its self-healings, and if the weeping lasts over 4 weeks, surgery should be considered.
   (b) To those who accompany with cavernous arteriovenous fistula, apply Meta test at the early stage, which means pressing affected-side cephalic artery at sixth cervicovertebral transverse process, 4~6 times/day and 15~30 min/time, and it could affect on part of the related smaller fistula aperture; but to those who suffers from midcranial base fracture for a long time, whose condition aggravates or who have tardive arteriovenous fistula, surgery should be applied as early as possible. Operation method could be the interventional therapy, which means to implant the covered stent through catheter in intracervical artery to interdict the communication between the arteries and the veins.
   (c) To those who have severe post-trumatic epistaxis, apply the first-aid management to avoid shock or asphyxia death; or apply the endotracheal intubation surgery, keep the respiration free, rapidly replenish the blood loss, stanch with the anterior nostril packing surgery, if all above don't make any sense, apply the choana packing surgery or simultaneous anterior and inferior nostril packing operation, and if necessary, apply the urgent digital subtraction angiography (DSA) examination to determine the hemorrhagic spots, then apply the vascular thrombosis surgery or implant the covered stent. Open surgery management is also viable if necessary.

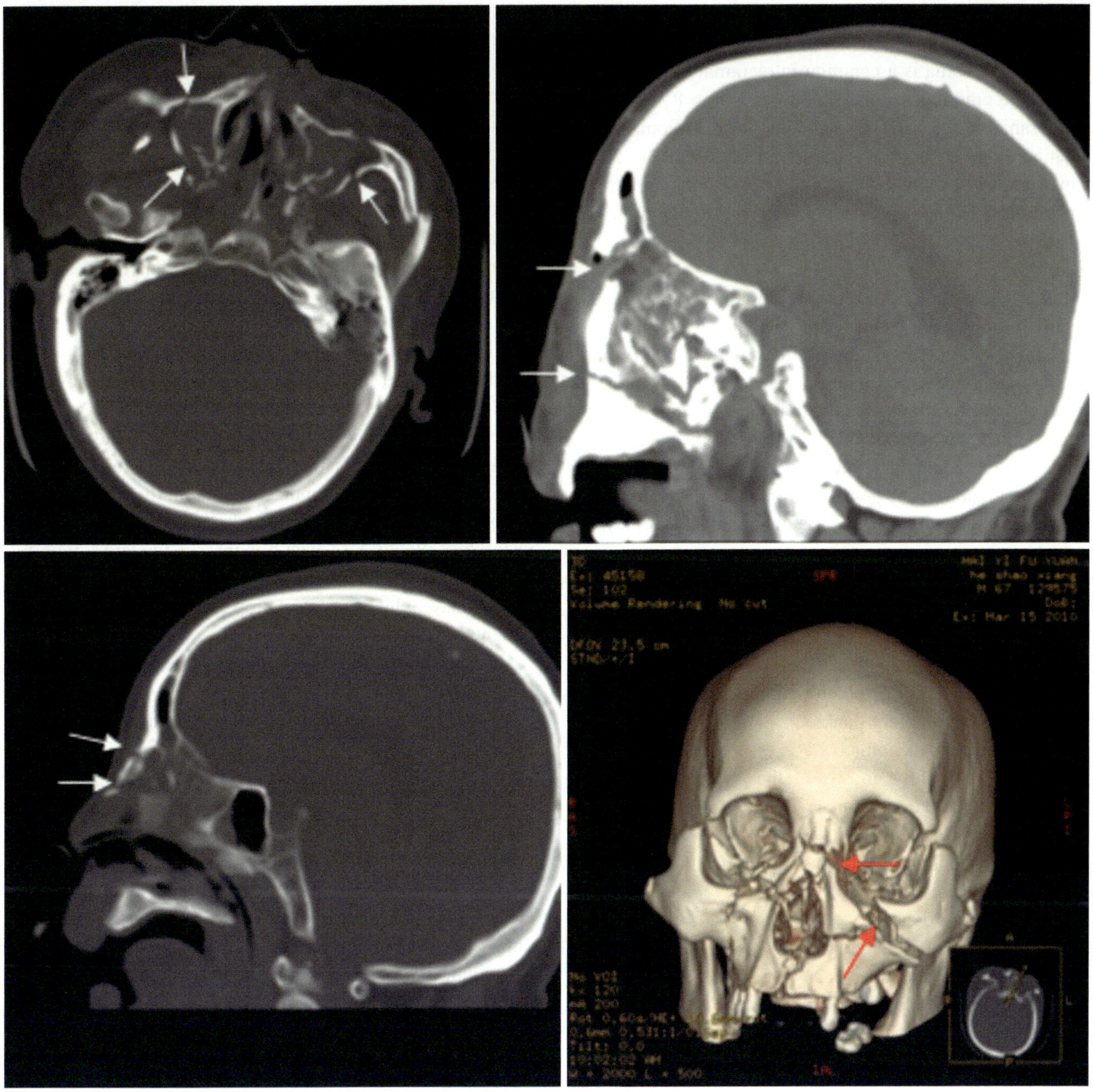

**Fig. 26.1** Bilateral maxilla, multiple precranial base fractures axial CT scan, sagittal and three dimensional rebuildment imaging. Bilateral maxillofacial bones, multiple precranial base fractures and aboard rhinosinus congestion display

3. Postcranial Base Fracture

   At the acute stage, the management should be mainly against the foramen magnum's and the upper cervical vertebral fracture or dislocation, such as the respiratory dysfunction and (or) the pressed cervicoverterbra, those with which should be applied the tracheotomy, the skull traction, and if necessary, the assisting respiratory or the artificial respiration, the cranial fossa and the cervical vertebral lamina decompression surgery could be applied.

4. Occipital Condyle Fracture

   Its treatment is decided by influence fracture makes to the occipitocervical stability. But to those who accompany with unsteady occipitoneck, converse treatment should be applied at very early, if inefficient, apply the Halo support fixation or the occipitocervical fission surgery at later period.

## 26.2 Pituitary Adenoma

Pituitary adenoma is a common intracranial tumor, belonging to the epidural neoplasm and occupying 8~10% of the intracranial tumor and only secondary to the glioma and the meningioma. It favorably occurs in adults at 30~50 age range, mostly originates from the anterior lobe and 25% of the pituitary adenoma doesn't have secretion function.

**Etiology**

Pituitary adenoma is the most commonly-seen adenoma, whose etiology isn't clear. But recently, by combing the immunity cell chemicostraining, the micro structure observation under electromicroscope, the endocrine hormone, the clinical manifestations etc., the hormone existing classification is made, which includes: (1) prolactin adenoma; (2) somatotropin adenoma; (3) corticotropin adenoma; (4) thyrotropin adenoma; (5) gonadotropin adenoma; (6) multisecretory cytoadenoma (mixed functional adenoma); (7) non-secretory cytoadenoma.

Hormone type (or types) the pituitary adenoma secrets have certain relavance to the cytostraining characteristics:

1. Prolactin Adenoma:
   It is acidophily or chromophobia, scattered, originating at lateral pituitary flank;
2. Somatotropin Adenoma:
   It is acidophily, mostly at the lateral anterior lobe, originating at lateral pituitary flank;
3. Corticotropin Adenoma:
   It is basophily, mostly distributing at the pre-internal lateral anterior lobe;
4. Thyrotropin Adenoma:
   It is basophily, distributing at the internal and external anterior lobe (mid 1/3);
5. Gonadotropin Adenoma:
   It includes the follicle-stimulating hormone and the luteinizing hormone adenoma, chromophobia or acidophily, distributing at outer lateral anterior lobe (mid 1/3);
6. Multi-secretory Cytoadenoma (mixed functional adenoma):
   It may be one type of cell secreting two or over two types of hormones, or multiple types of cells secret two or over two types of hormones;
7. Non-secretory Cytoadenoma
   It is chromophobia.

Adenomas' size varies much, which may be micro-adenoma (diameter $\leq$ 1.0 cm), macro-adenoma (diameter > 1.0 cm) and giant-adenoma (diameter > 3.0 cm). Pituitary adenoma is intracranial extra-meningeal tumor, most of which is benign, dilatancy—growed and often packed with fibrous capsule or pseudocapsule, which is often substantial and on 1/4 of which, necrosis, cystic change, hemorrhage or other degenerative change can occur, what can damage or perforate the diaphragma sellae and then approach the suprasellar cistern to grow up and press the optic nerve, the optic chiasma and its adjacent structures. Minority of the pituitary adenoma grows invasively, invades the peripheral constructions, such as the cavernous sinus and the embedded intracarotid artery and presses and invades the cranial nerves. The prolactin and the somatotropin adenoma both develops from the pituitary flank and could easily invade the parasellae dura mater and the cavernous sinus.

**Clinic Manifestation**

Headache, visual impairment and pituitary deficiency is the most commonly seen clinical manifestations in pituatary tumor. Bitemporal vision loss is the main pituitary visual impairment characteristics. Macro-pituitary tumor presses the optic chiasma at suboptic chiasma, firstly seeing the sup-temporal vision loss and secondarily the whole temporal vision loss. Vision loss even blindness is the late symptoms. Tumors that grow laterally trending could cause the extra-muscopalsy, which manifestation is also rare. Minority of patients suffer the stubborn headache.

**Diagnosis**

According to the history, different types' adenomas' clinical manifestations and physical signs, combining with endocrine examination and imaging examinations, commonly diagnosis could be ascertained. But to the early microadenoma cases, whose clinical manifestations isn't evident, endocrine examination isn't typical and imaging displays little, it is hard to make diagnosis. Pay attention to differentiate from the other sella lesion, such as the craniopharyngioma, the meningioma, the ectopic pineal gland, the chordoma, the optic nerve or the optic chiasm glioma, the epidermoids cyst, the trigeminal neurinoma, the empty sella syndrome, the hypophyseal cyst, the Rathke punch cyst, the intracranial aneurysm, the communicating encephalohydrop, etc. Enhanced sellar MRI is a related sensitive method, which differentiates from other tumors at microtumor discovery (Fig. 26.2), the unvisionable normal pituitary.

**Treatment**

Surgery is the first choice. To whose tumor locates under sella, excise through rhinocavum sphenoid sinus under rhinoscope; to the tumor those who are related-bigger and breaks the diaphragma sellae, accompanying with vision field disorder and multiple pressed nerve structures, excise through the subfrontal approach with craniotomy. If surgeries can't totally excise the tumor or patients can't hold surgeries because of the age and the physical conditions, radiotherapy can be applied; to the prolactinoma, postopeative bromocriptine can be used, so are other drugs, including somatostatin (SS), cyproheptadine, long-acting human growth hormone, etc.

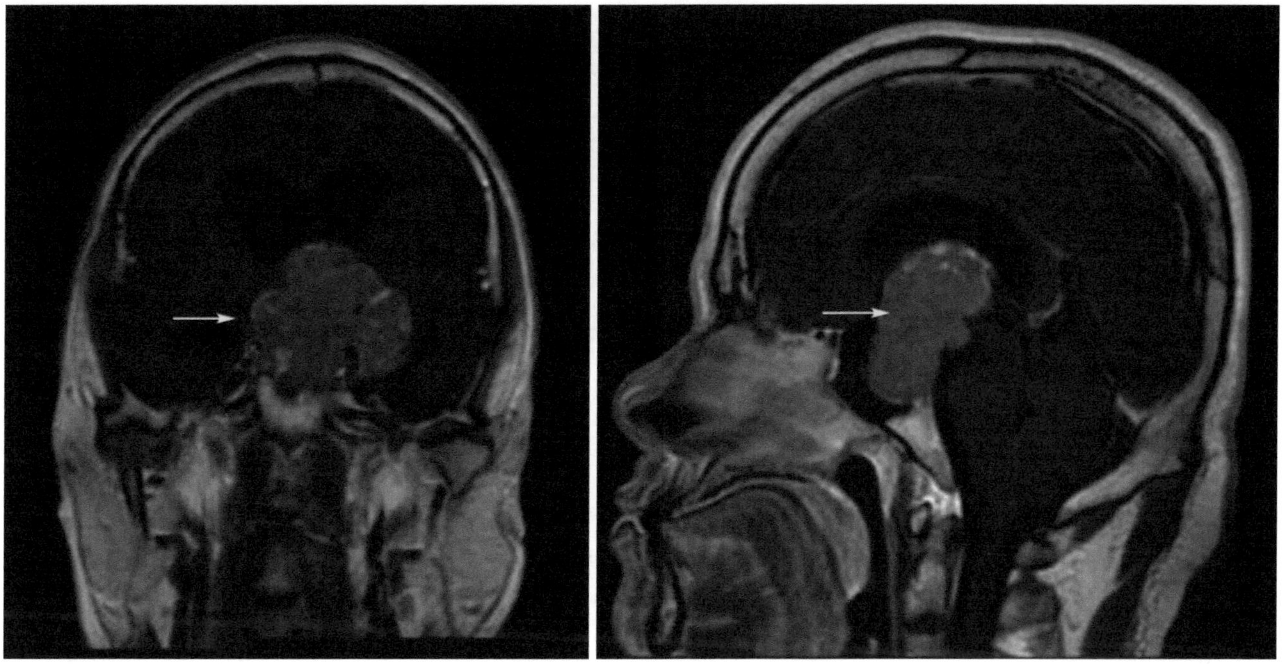

**Fig. 26.2** Enhanced coronary and sagittal MRI display pituitary adenoma. Evidently enlarged pituitary, leaves-like lumps and obvious with enhancement after enhancing, circling intra-cervical arteries (arrow)

## 26.3 Chordoma

**Pathogenesis**

It is a tumor orgionating from the residual notochord and mostly seen during 30~50 years old. Its obvious characteristic is fewer occuring at dosal spine with residual notochord and related bigger nucleus pulposus and mainly happening at the sacral district, secondary at the craniobase and less at the neck, the waist and the thorax spine. Intracranial chordoma mainly locates at the mid-clivus-line and less at the mid-cranial fossa. Through it is embryonic; it is rarely seen in infants. Clivus chordoma mainly manifestates the headache, the visual impairment, the rhinobyon and the cervicache, and may concomitant with the cerebral palsy.

**Clinical Manifestation**

Headache is the most commonly-seen manifestation, occupying about 70% and mostly is the entire head aching or extending to the occipitalia or the neck, persisting dull-pain, nonobvious change during 1 day; if intracranial pressure increases the condition agravates. The persisting chordoma cephalalgia is related to the cranial basal infiltration.

Along with the tumor location and the invasion trends direction change, the chordoma clinic manifestation and physical signs vary.

1. Saddle Chordoma

   Pituitary deficiency mainly manifestates the asynodia, the amenorrhea, the grow stout, etc.; pressed optic nerve can also produce primary optic nerve atrophy, vision loss, bitemporal hemianopia etc.
2. Parasellar Chordoma

   It mainly manifestates the uni or bilateral III, IV and VI pair's cranial nerve paralysis, more of which is the involved abducent nerve.
3. Clivus Chordoma

   It mainly manifestates the pressed cranial stem condition, also called dysbasia or pyramidal signs, and the VI and the VII pairs cranial nerve disturbance, whose mainly characteristics is bilateral abducent nerve damage. Additionally, it can cause cranial basal communicating hydrocephalus; if the tumor invades the cererbellumpons angle, the audition disturbance, the tinnitus and the dizziness could occur. The chordoma who develops from the rhinopharyngowall nearby always protrudes into the rhinopharynx or invades one or multiple pranasal sinuses to evoke the rhinobyon, headache, purulent or bloody rhinorrhea, dysphagia, tinnitus and other similar rhinopharyngo cancer symptoms. and these rhinopharyngeal symptoms always occur before that the nerves get involved, so the lumps could be found at rhinopharyngeal examination by 13~ 33%.

**Diagnosis**

According to the diseases history, the clinical manifestations and the physical signs, combing with the imaging examinations, commonly the differentiated diagnosis can be made (Fig. 26.3). To the patients with chordoma that protrudes into the rhinopharynx, biopsy should be applied as earlier as possible to ascertain the diagnosis.

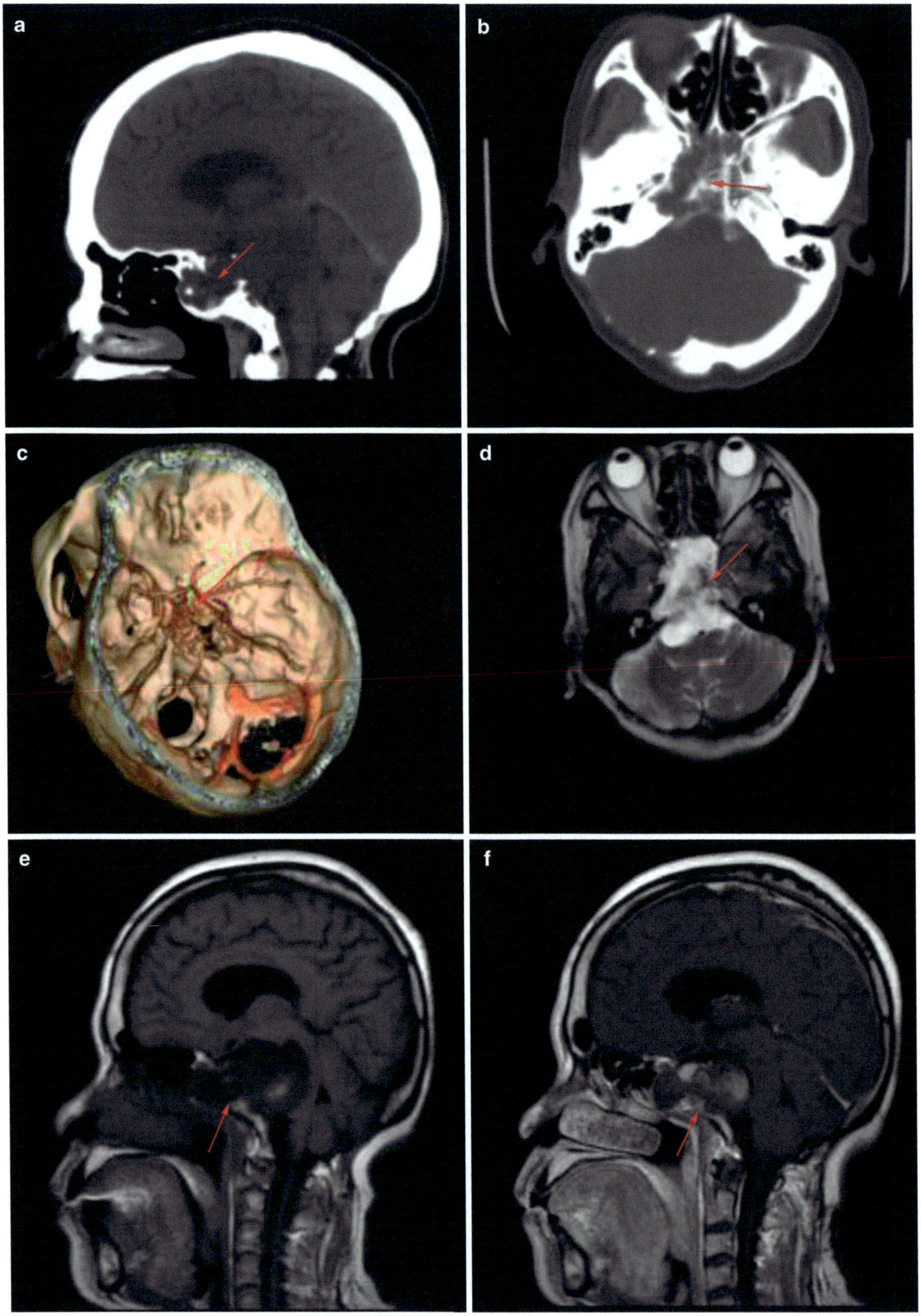


**Fig. 26.3** Cranial base CT and MRI display cranial basa chordoma. (**a**–**c**) CT plane-sagittal scan, plane axial scan and tri-dimension rebuildment imaging, which display the clivus sclerotin damage (arrow) and sellar soft tissue swellings especially the internal punctiform calcification (arrow); (**d**–**f**) axial MRI T2WI, sagittal plane T1WI and enhancement. Sellar swellings manifestate better than CT; brainstem is pressed and slightly enhanced after enhancement. They are from the relapsed post-clivus-chordoma-surgery patients

**Differential Diagnosis**
Take caution on differentiating from rhinopharyngeal cancer, meningioma, acoustic neuroma, the pituitary adenoma and the cranophrayngotubuloma.

**Treatment**
Commonly surgery excision is first choice and the postoperative persistance could be expelled by radiotherapy but with bad efficacy. The surgery approach should be chosen according to the main tumor location: to tumors at the rhinopharynx or in the sphenoid bone, apply through the nose approach to expel it under rhinal endoscope; to clivus tumor, apply the cervicoclivus entrance approach and to other tumors at suprasellar sphenoid region, and apply the tumorectomy after opening the skull through the subtemporary.

## 26.4 Meningioma

**Pathogenesis**
It is the specific tumors originating from the retina, which is also considered as tumor grown from the arachnoidea. Meningioma is always related to the supsagittal sinus, the cavernous tumor and the sphenoid apex venous sinus and it often appears at the tissues with arachnoid cells existing, so the craniobasal meningioma develops more at the sphenoid ridge. Pacchionian bodies is little at infants, They can be recognized by the naked eye 18 months after birth and grow bigger as time goes by. The tumor could locate at the cranial base, the eye orbit, the rhinosinus, etc. The tumors at intracranial sites are commonly called the intrameningioma, those outside the cranium are called the ectopic meningioma. The meningioma always has abundant blood supply.

**Clinical Manifestation**
Mostly, meningioma is benign, with slow growth, related-long-term course and several year history. Clinical manifestations is produced under a certain size and they vary a lot according to the tumor existing sites.

Its main symptoms are headache, dizziness, epilepsy and epilepsy is seen more in the elder as initial symptom. At the late stage, the intracranial hypertension symptoms and physical signs occur, for instance, headache, emesis, papilloedema; when the tumor invades the peripheral tissues, symptoms, such as the exophthalmos, the visual field diminution, the vision diminution, the dysosmia, the dysacusis, the limb movement disorder, etc., could appear. The patients with tumor developing at the rhinocavum rhinosisnus, the rhinal obstruction, the facial risement or the eyeball dislocation could occur.

**Diagnosis**
According to the history, the clinical manifestations and the physical signs, combining with the imaging examinations, could generally ascertain diagnosis. Enhanced MRI scan could display that the tumor is from the meninx and the enhanced scan causes evenly enhanced imaging and the dural tail signs, which is its characteristic manifestations (Fig. 26.4). Generally, it should be differentiated from other occupation lesion, such as the carotid-spheroid tumor, the schwannoma, the angioma, etc.

**Treatment**
1. Surgery

   Surgery is the most efficient treatment methods to completely remove the tumor, and if the tumor relapses, apply another operation excision. To those whose tumor is at precraniobasal intracranium, apply operation under rhinoendoscope through the rhinocavum.
2. Radiotherapy

   To those meningioma can't be remove entirely, its hard to accept another operation if the tumor relapses, who's unable to accept operation excision, or other specific meningioma, radiotherapy could be applied, which includes the $\gamma$ knife, x knife, intracellular radiotherapy, etc.
3. Other Treatments

   Glucocorticoid, gene therapy and other methods could treat meningioma, but they're without certain efficiency and they need further investigations.

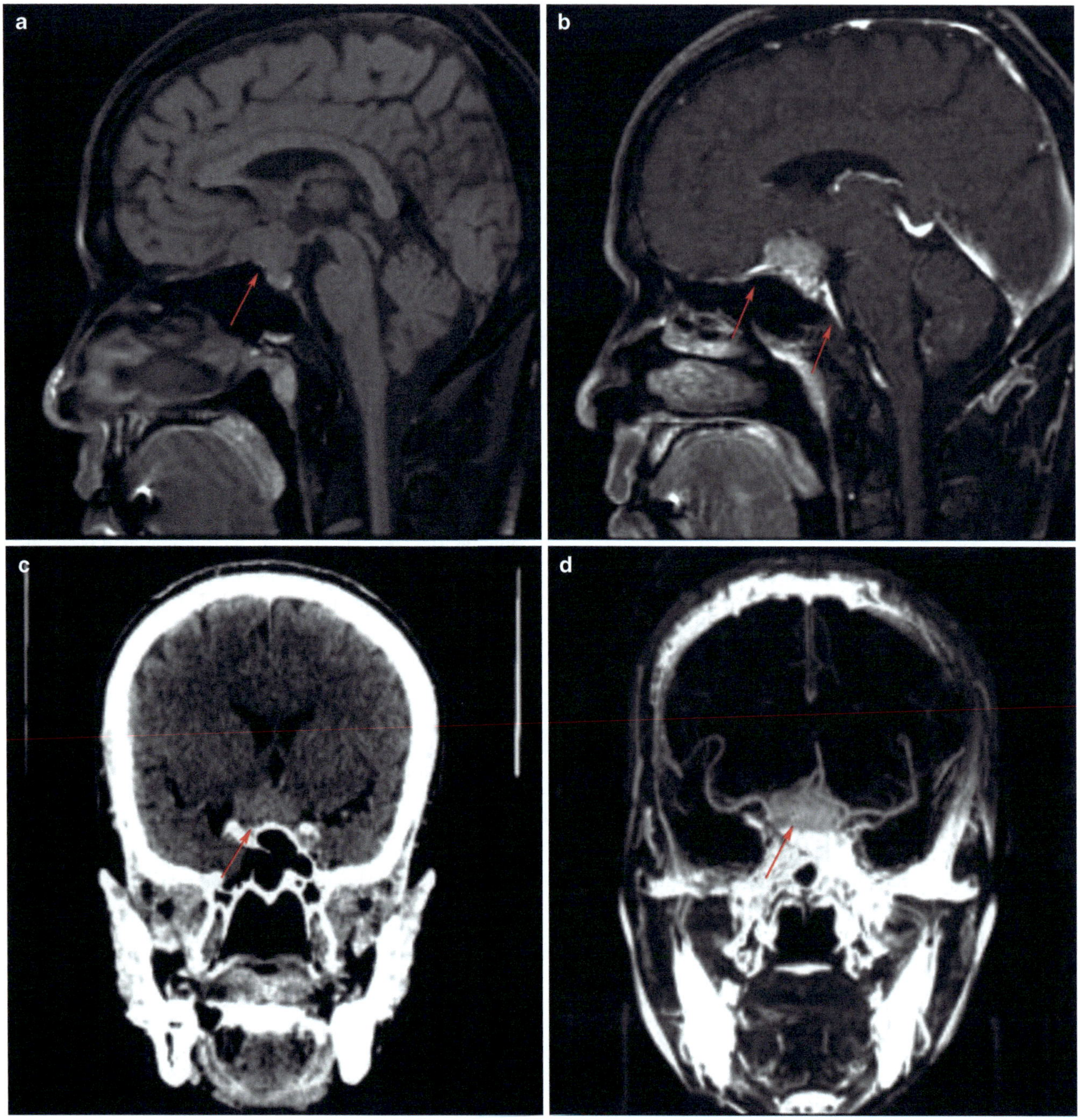


**Fig. 26.4** MRI and CT display sellar meningioma. (**a**, **b**) Sagittal MRI T1 plan scan and enhancement, displaying the suppituitary equateT1 lump, tensely-adhered meninx growth, obviously enhanced after enhancement and dural tail signs, normal pituitary gland and normal sphenoid sinus; (**c**, **d**) another patient's coronary CT rebuildment plane scan and enhanced CTA, displaying the supsellar slightly high density lump; distinguisabless relationship with pituitary gland, but be obviously enhanced after enhancement and display the relationship with cranial basal arteries

# Part VIII

# Special Otorhinolaryngopharyngology Head and Neck Surgery Disease

In the clinic, diseases include the common diseases and the special diseases. Researching the diagnosis and the therapy of the specific diseases can not only help improve the medical personnels' theories and practical level but also have important significance to improve the diseases' curative ratio and remit the patients' pain. Therefore, this part will focus on discussing the diagnosis and the therapy of the otorhinopharyngocervicocranial foreign mass, tuberculosis, syphilis, AIDS, leprosy, etc.

# Foreign Body of Otorhinolaryngopharyngology Head and Neck

27

Xiaohui Mi and Rong Tu

## 27.1 Foreign Body of Ear

**Etiology**

1. Children like to put foreign bodies into their ears when playing.
2. For most adults it is usually as a result of small objects or insects invasions by ear picking or trauma.
3. The species of animal (Fig. 27.1a), botanical (such as cereals, legumes, pits) and abiotic (Fig. 27.1b).

**Clinical Manifestation**

It varies according to the size and location of the foreign body. Small, non-obstructive, non-irritating foreign bodies can be retained for a long time without any obvious symptoms. Larger foreign bodies or plant foreign bodies sw swell in the presence of dampness, obstruct the external auditory canal, affect hearing and cause tinnitus, etc. Individual external auditory canal foreign body can cause external auditory canal inflammation and earache. When the foreign body approaches the tympanic membrane, it can compress the tympanic membrane and cause tinnitus and vertigo. Active insects can cause intolerable discomfort when they crawl and scratch. Touching the tympanic membrane can cause pain, tinnitus and even damage the tympanic membrane. On examination, foreign bodies of different sizes were found in different locations of the external auditory canal.

X. Mi (✉)
Department of Otorhinolaryngology Head and Neck Surgery, Chinese People's Liberation Army 91458 Military Hospital, Sanya, China

R. Tu
Department of Medical Imaging, The First Affiliated Hospital of Hainan Medical University, Haikou, China

**Physical Examination**

1. During examination, pay attention to the border between the external ear canal's lower wall and the inferior tympanic membrane edge where small foreign body could also be concealed.
2. Secondary infection may cause the outer ear canal congestion and swelling. Self-ear picking may cause the skin damage even tympocavum rupture.

**Diagnosis**

1. Disease History

   Pay attention to the fact that children often have no typical medical history. Children with foreign bodies are not easy found, they often cry because of pain, or often scratch the mouth of the external auditory canal with their hands. In adults, a foreign body often enters the external auditory canal. Obstruction of the external auditory canal can cause hearing loss.
2. Otoscopy

   Otolaroscopy revealed that foreign bodies remained in the external auditory canal. If the foreign body is too small and the residence time is too long, therefore inflammation of middle ear and external auditory canal should be examined carefully. Larger foreign bodies or insects can cause severe otalgia and noise
3. Reflex cough or dizziness may occasionally occur due to long-term stimulation of the external auditory canal by foreign bodies. Granulomatosis can conceal foreign bodies. The foreign body can be found only after the granulation is carefully removed.
4. Assisting Examinations

   Auxiliary endoscopy and imaging are helpful for diagnosis. If the foreign body is too deep or too long, the physical examination can not detect it, or it is difficult to remove it. Calcium-containing foreign bodies



Z. Mu, J. Fang (eds.), *Practical Otorhinolaryngology - Head and Neck Surgery*, https://doi.org/10.1007/978-981-13-7993-2_27

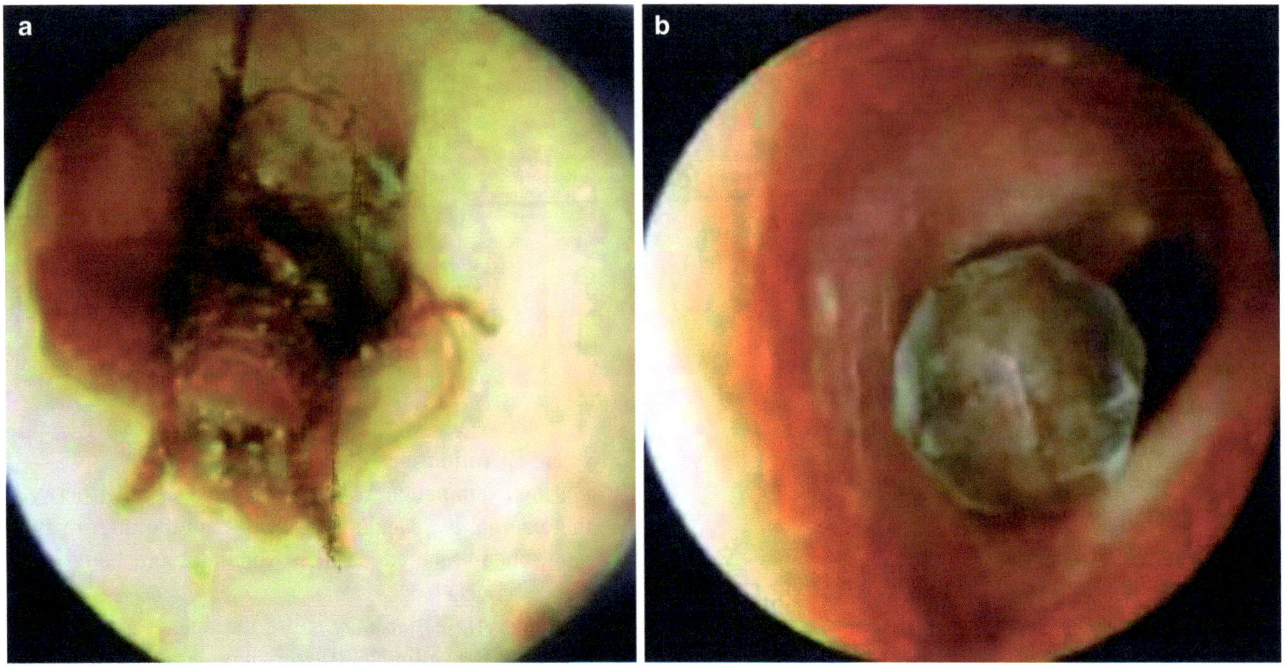


**Fig. 27.1** Ear foreign body. (**a**) animal; (**b**) abiotic foreign body

can be examined by CT, soft tissue foreign bodies can be examined by MR to understand the location of foreign bodies and the formation of granuloma around them.

**Treatment**

Timely diagnosis and treatment, early removal, according to the type, size, and location of foreign bodies, has different methods of removal.

1. Small Mass

   Fetch with cerumen hook or douche with water
2. For smooth, hard foreign bodies, such as beads, beans, etc., do not use tweezers, forceps to take, in order to prevent foreign bodies into the depth or damage the tympanic membrane. A right angle cerumen hook can be used to cross the gap between the external auditory canal and the upper part of the foreign body to hook the foreign body out (Fig. 27.2).
3. Living Insects

   For living insects, they can be anesthetized or killed by dropping oil or ethanol or ether into the ear, and then washed out or removed after about 5 min.
4. Vegetalitas Foreign Bodies (Dry Beans. etc)

   Dry legumes and other plant foreign bodies; do not wash with water, so as not to be embedded in the external auditory canal after bubbling. For inflated plant foreign bodies, ear drops with 95% ethanol solution can be used to dehydrate and shrink them before removal.

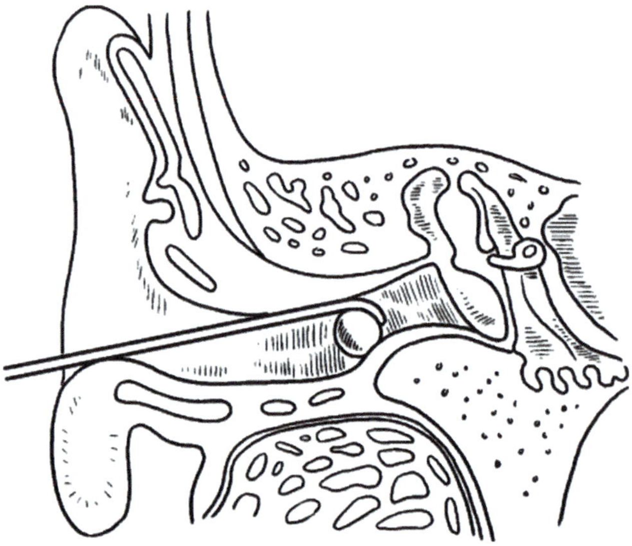

**Fig. 27.2** Extraotocanal foreign masses fetchment

5. Children often choose to remove foreign bodies under general anesthesia because they cannot cooperate. Adults can choose local anesthesia or topical anesthesia.
6. When the foreign body is removed, if the external auditory canal is damaged and bleeding occurs, gauze can be used to compress hemostasis. After removal the next day, antibiotic ointment or antibiotic eardrops can be applied to ear-drops.
7. When the foreign body in the middle ear is too large or too tight or has both, it must be removed through an incision in the ear or behind the ear under local anesthesia or

general anesthesia. If necessary, part of the posterior wall of the external auditory canal can be chiseled to facilitate the removal of the foreign body.

8. Those complicated with external auditory canal inflammation should be given anti-inflammatory treatment first, and then take out the foreign body after the inflammation subsides, or actively treat external auditory canal inflammation after taking out the foreign body.

## 27.2 Foreign Body of Nose and Paranasal Sinus

Nasal foreign bodies can be divided into two categories: endogenous and exogenous. The former includes dead bone, clot, rhinolith, crust, etc. The latter can be divided into biological and abiotic. In biology, Botany is the most common, while animal nature is relatively rare. There are many kinds of abiotic alien species, so the disease is more complicated.

**Etiology**

Children stuff small objects into the nasal cavity because of ignorance or inadvertence; or food enters the nasal cavity through the nasopharynx when eating carelessly or vomiting; foreign bodies are left in the nose because of trauma, bullet injury or explosive injury; small insects accidentally enter the nose because of camping in the wild; iatrogenic foreign bodies remain in the nose; psychiatric patients stuff foreign bodies by themselves, etc. There are three common types of foreign bodies:

1. Biologics

   Biology such as small insects, ants, leeches, etc. enters the nasal cavity, crawl and commotion, can cause pain and hemorrhage.

2. Vegetalitas

   Plant foreign bodies such as soybeans, peanuts, maize, melon seeds and fruit nuclei can cause nasal obstruction and runny nose. If they stay for a long time, foreign bodies will swell in the presence of water, and the symptoms will be aggravated.

3. Inanimation

   Non biological tissue, rubber, glass ball, chalk, buttons, foam, sand, warhead, shrapnel and other nasal retention, obstruction of the nasal cavity, can cause nasal congestion, runny nose, and even local swelling, congestion, ulceration.

**Clinical Manifestation**

1. Early Clinical Manifestations

   Early clinical manifestations of early patients can be manifested as nasal obstruction (mostly unilateral), sleep breathing, and accompanied by epistaxis, purulent discharge, headache and so on. For example, children who are afraid of or unable to express insect crawling sensation consciously will have nose rubbing and rubbing. The nasal foreign body caused by trauma can leave a wound on the face. During nasal examination, congestion, edema and secretion of nasal mucosa can be found. A shallow foreign body can be seen.

2. Late Clinical Manifestations and Complications

   Late clinical manifestations and complications, such as deep location of foreign bodies and long retention time, can cause local nasal mucosal ulcer, and then cause systemic symptoms such as fever and anemia. The symptoms of sinusitis can be caused by the obstruction of the nasal cavity for a long time and the obstruction of sinus drainage. Foreign bodies stay for a long time; inflammatory secretions evaporate, concentrate and decompose into a variety of inorganic salts gradually deposited on the surface of foreign bodies, taking this as the core to form rhinolith, which can be found by local examination.

**Diagnosis**

1. Due to the long-term presence of foreign bodies in the nasal cavity, nasal mucosa inflammation swelling, local ulceration, manifestations of one side of the nasal obstruction, bleeding or mucopurulent runny nose and odor, sometimes accompanied by runny blood, animal foreign bodies, itching or peristalsis in the nose, may be accompanied by nasal pain. Because the history of childhood patients is unclear, the diagnosis cannot be determined solely by the history of foreign body implantation. All children with unilateral nasal obstruction, bleeding or stink should consider the possibility of foreign bodies.

2. Rhinal Examination

   The foreign body in nasal examination is usually located in the front of inferior turbinate and nasal septum, and it is easy to find by nasal endoscopy. If the time is long, the nasal cavity on the affected side has a large number of purulent secretions or purulent secretions, nasal mucosa is red, erosion, bleeding or granulation growth cannot see foreign bodies, it is difficult to examine, and easy to misdiagnose. It must be cleaned and examined carefully. If the foreign body stays for a long time, the foreign body will be calm in calcium salt, rough in touch, and can form rhinolith centered on the foreign body. The foreign body of leech in nasal cavity often attaches to the mucosa at the top of nasal cavity, which is difficult to find. However, if there are symptoms such as repeated epistaxis, itching and foreign body crawling in the nose, the brown leech can be easily seen only after the mucosa has been fully converged.

3. Imaging Examination

   If the foreign body is too deep or too long for imaging examination, physical examination cannot be detected, or

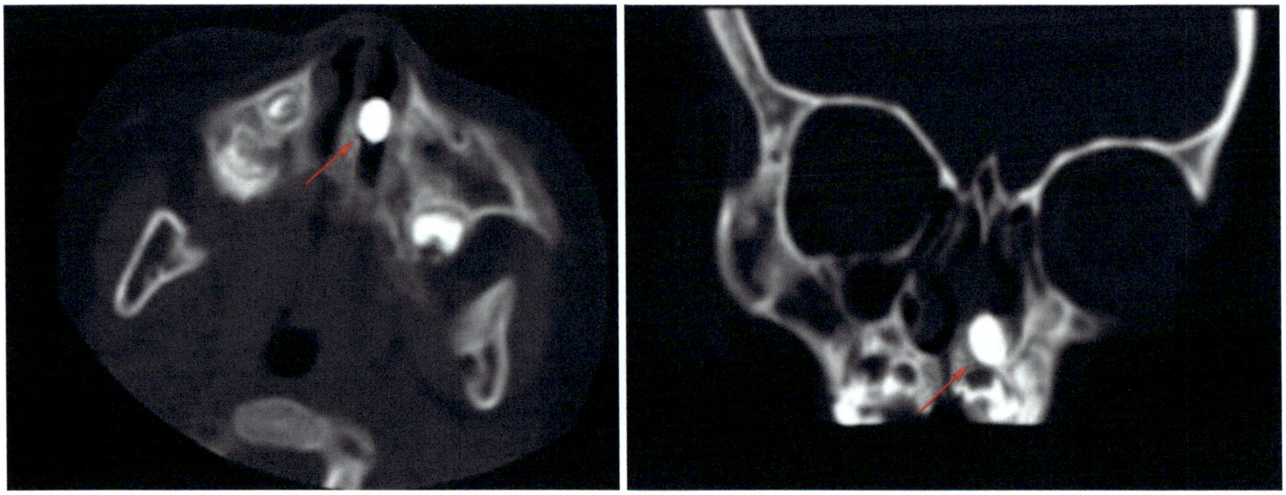

**Fig. 27.3** Plain CT scans of the nasal cavity (coronal and axial bone windows). An elliptical high density foreign body (arrow) is seen in the left nasal cavity

it is difficult to remove it. Calcium-containing foreign bodies can be examined by CT, soft tissue foreign bodies can be examined by MR to understand the location of foreign bodies and the formation of granuloma in surrounding tissues (Figs. 27.3 and 27.4).

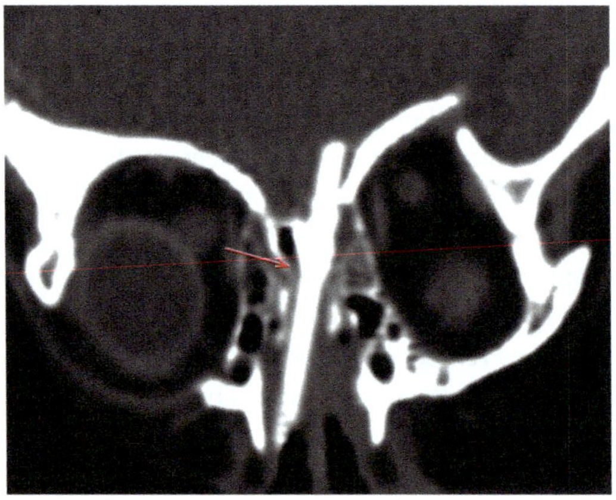

**Fig. 27.4** CT manifestations of the foreign body (chopsticks) in the skull base of the nasal cavity

**Treatment**

1. Inquire About the History of the Disease
   (a) The nature of the foreign body: inflammation of plant stimulation is large, easy to secondary infection, when necessary to give antibiotic treatment; animal can be the first to use tetracaine anesthesia; corrosive objects such as alkaline batteries after removal of available 25% vitamin C solution washing and antibiotic therapy. Small magnets can suck metal materials out.
   (b) The Duration of Foreign Body Residence: shorter time, less stimulation on nasal mucosa, and observation after routine removal. For a long time, mucosal inflammatory reaction is heavy and needs antibiotic treatment.
   (c) The Shape, Size and Blunt Condition of The Foreign Body: the round material should be hung around the outer ring with the front ring as the instrument, and the hook should not be tweezers (Fig. 27.5). the flat long tweezers can clip foreign body. Cotton paper, small residence time is not long but the contralateral nostril oppression blow out. Sharp wire and blade should be checked in with CT to avoid blind removal of bleeding and adjacent tissue damage.
2. Examination: normal ephedrine and tetracaine before the examination of nasal mucosa and surface anesthesia to reduce pain and expand the field of vision. General for-

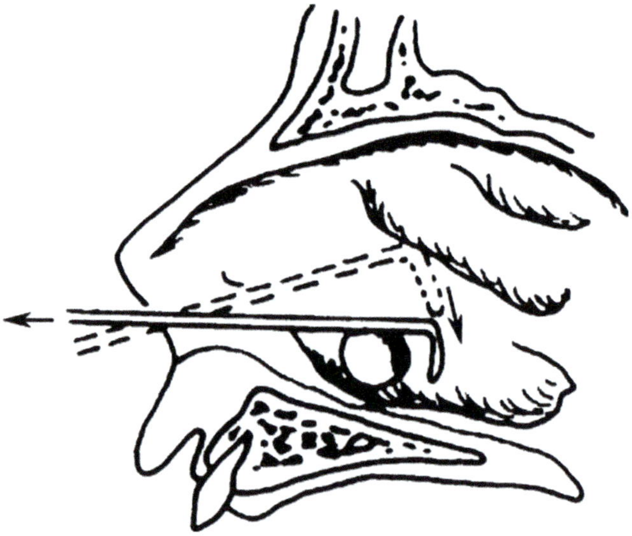

**Fig. 27.5** Removal of the foreign body in the nasal cavity

eign body to nasal mucosa irritation after nasal secretion can be sucked out. Children with poor coordination need help from family members. When the foreign body is taken, the head low or the supine head can be used to avoid the iatrogenic tracheal foreign body caused by the foreign body falling into the trachea.

3. Traumatic Nasal Foreign Body
   (a) A Assess the Condition of Injury: if there are other important parts of the injury, the nasal cavity can be disposed of according to the principle of first fast and then slow. When we lose blood, we should measure blood pressure and pulse, check blood type, open venous passages, improve plasma osmotic pressure, and avoid blood transfusion.
   (b) Evaluate the Foreign Body of The Nasal Cavity: check the situation of the face and nasal cavity, see if there is an open wound, and see the location of the nose bleeding. The location was performed with nasal endoscopy and CT examination.
   (c) Determine the time, approach and method of operation according to the above conditions.

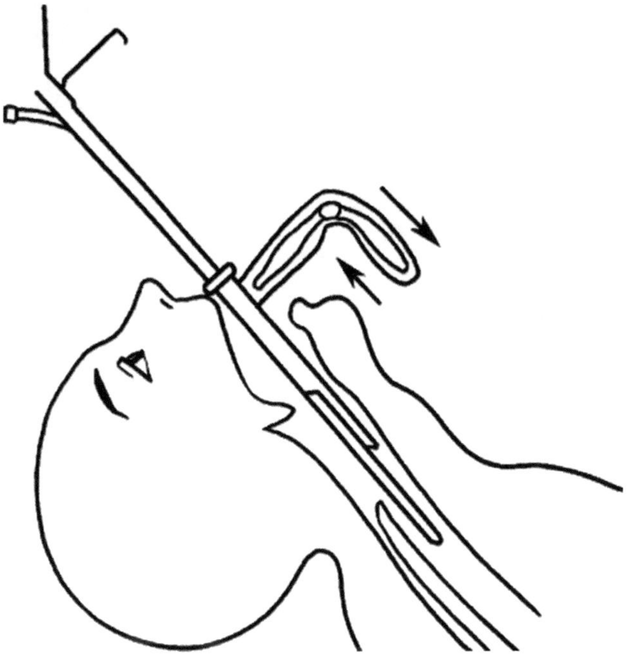

**Fig. 27.6** Direct laryngoscopic larygoforeign bodies drawing by indirect method

## 27.3 Foreign Body of Pharynx

The foreign body of the pharynx is most common in all kinds of foreign bodies in the otolaryngology. It is generally easy to diagnose and deal with.

There are many kinds of foreign bodies, including minerals, chemicals, animals, plants etc. The common causes are the following.

1. Swallowed accidentally pharyngeal fishbone, bone, stone etc. The foreign body is easy to tie in the oropharynx or hypopharyngeal mucosa, foreign body easy larger left in the hypopharynx.
2. Children play, coins, paper clips, small nails, and small toys, such as the cap into the mouth, accidentally swallowed.
3. Abnormality of the mind, sleep, coma, drunken or anaesthesia are easily deglutition.
4. Patients attempted suicide and intentionally swallowed a large sharp foreign body, such as a small fruit knife, a small scissors, and a key. Foreign body can stay in the pharynx to become the pharynx foreign body, such as the pharynx into the esophagus, can cause the foreign body of the esophagus.
5. Elderly denture loose into the hypopharynx.
6. The foreign body of the pharynx could be given to the pharynx mucosa with 1% tetracaine, and the foreign body removed under the indirect laryngoscope. The direct laryngoscope takes the supine position of the foreign body in the pharynx of the pharynx (Fig. 27.6).

**Clinical Manifestation**

1. Patients complain of pharyngache (mostly tingling, pain, odynophagia, relatively fixed position) or dysphagia, speech pain, increased saliva, punctured mucosa is sometimes associated with bleeding, visible pseudomembrane formation, concurrent infection more pain, more foreign bodies can cause swallowing and breathing difficulties of pharynx and larynx, nasopharynx foreign body less, for a long time there will be odor. The foreign bodies retained in the epiglottis and the pyriform recess not taken out in time to cause the fatal complications of the larynx edema.
2. Long course or foreign body injury can occur epiglottitis, abscess of epiglottis and lateral pharyngeal wall abscess and hemorrhage, and very few cases, foreign body from wall to the neck subcutaneous, pharyngeal thyroid, even from parapharyngeal space through the skin, piercing the carotid artery leading to fatal bleeding.

**Diagnosis**

1. Medical History: a conscious or cooperative therapist can often understand the nature of the foreign body.
2. Physical Examination: through oral oropharynx examination, indirect laryngoscopy and electronic (laryngoscopy) examination, foreign bodies and other indirect signs may be found, such as piriform recess, saliva retention and mucosal abrasion.
3. Imaging Examination: if the foreign body is too deep and too long, the physical examination cannot be detected, or it is difficult to take out. The calcium containing foreign

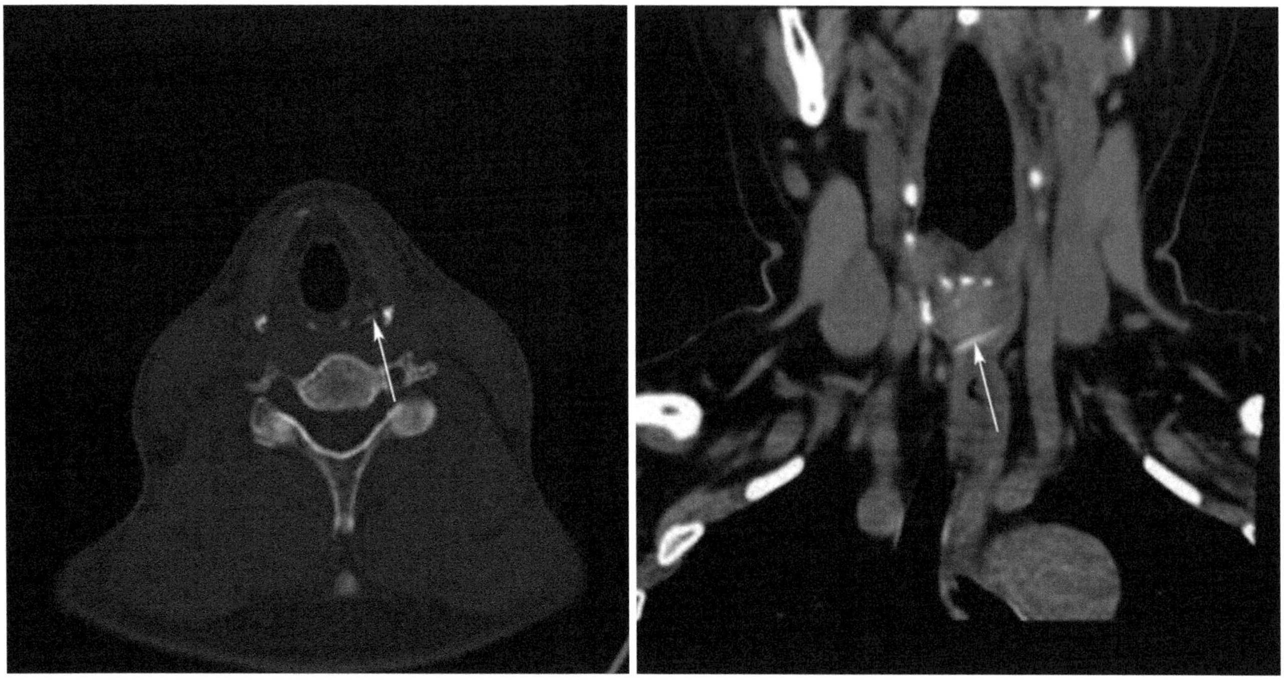

**Fig. 27.7** CT scan of the left pharynx fish-bone foreign body (axial plus coronal reconstruction)

bodies can be examined by CT (Fig. 27.7). The foreign body of the soft tissue can be examined by MR to understand the position of the foreign body and the formation of the granuloma around the tissue.

On the level of oropharynx and esophageal entrance (approximately flat C6 vertebral body), a long strip of high density shadow was seen in the soft tissue of the left posterior pharyngeal wall traveling laterally.

(The arrow shows a fish spine), about 1.7 cm long, with slightly thicker esophageal wall and no gas density in the surrounding fat space.

**Treatment**

1. Find a foreign body forceps or forceps with tweezers; remove foreign body forceps before and after the opening of transverse, longitudinal left and right opening use foreign body forceps. The openings of the pliers should be closed when they enter, and open when they are close to the foreign body. It is true that after a foreign object is caught, the foreign body is brought out with a proper force. Try to avoid long time exploration of the foreign body forceps in the pharynx. Avoid injury and mucous membrane.
2. For the hypertrophy of the tongue, the short neck, nausea, and obvious discomfort, the foreign body can be removed under the surface anesthesia by the electronic (fiber) laryngoscope or the hard tube laryngoscope.
3. Longer duration of foreign body in the laryngopharynx causes epiglottitis, laryngitis; edema, inflammation, atomization, and oxygen inhalation.
4. Pharyngeal foreign body occurs in retropharyngeal abscess or parapharyngeal abscess, incision and drainage from oropharyngeal or lateral neck abscess.

In addition, because the foreign body is stucked, the pharyngeal mucosa can be swallowed down, though the patient will also have a sense of foreign body. If there is no repeated detection of the foreign body through the above methods, it can be observed that the general pain and foreign body sensation will disappear gradually after 24 h.

## 27.4 Foreign Body of Larynx

The foreign body of the larynx is rare, and the foreign body mostly stays in the pharynx, followed by the trachea or the bronchus, and only a few stays in the laryngeal cavity.

**Etiology**

There are many causes of the throat, peanuts, beans and other nuts accounted for more than half of the fish bone, stone and bone (Fig. 27.8); and rice is also common. This kind of foreign body is mistaken in the larynx when children are suddenly laughing, crying, and frightening etc. Nail, needle, coins and other metal objects, cap, small toys, balloon debris and other plastic products also very common, children with these objects, if suddenly fell down, crying and laughing, but also easy to be aspirated into the throat. The foreign body is inhale in the glottic region and causes the foreign body in the larynx.

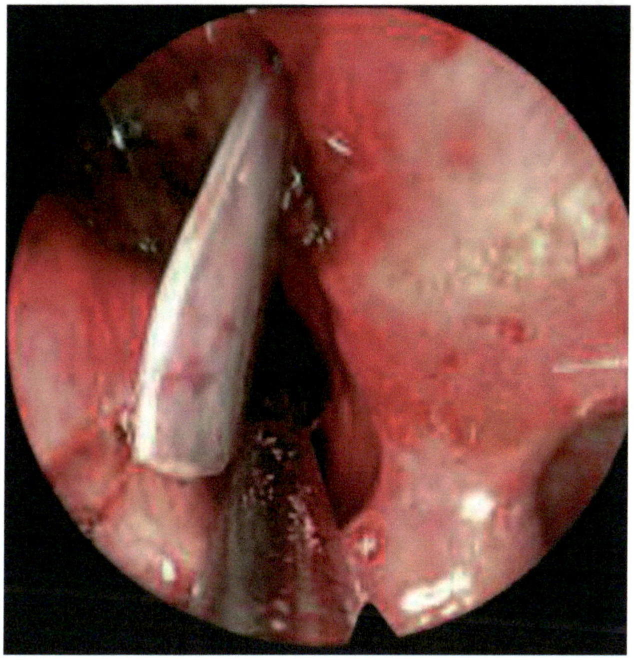

**Fig. 27.8** Laryngeal osteocomma

**Clinical Manifestation**

1. The history of foreign objects was choked.
2. Laryngeal mucosa is sensitive, so severe cough would be caused if foreign bodies drop into laryngeal cavity irritantly, which is called cough reflex, by which most of foreign bodies could be discharged.
3. Foreign bodies with difficulty breathing and wheezing stay in the laryngeal cavity, causing complete obstruction or laryngospasm, inspiratory dyspnea, wheezing, and even laryngeal obstruction and asphyxia.
4. Larynx pain, the feel of the existence in the laryngeal cavity for a period of time, induces severe cough which can be relieved, also the appearances of laryngeal pain, and the discomfort causes by the foreign body.
5. Sounds hoarse.
6. The dysphagia is difficult to swallow, even saliva spillover caused by pain; some foreign bodies stop at the entrance of the throat to the entrance to the dysphagia.
7. Laryngeal abscess, laryngeal stenosis cannot be removed by foreign body, infections caused by laryngeal abscess caused by pain, hoarseness, dyspnea, dysphagia aggravated symptoms of systemic poisoning, even sympathetic and oppression of Horner syndrome. When the foreign body is not taken out in time, it can cause excessive hyperplasia of the granulation tissue and fibrous tissue in the larynx, forming scar and causing the stricture of the larynx.

**Diagnosis**

According to the history of foreign body inhalation; laryngoscopy was used to find foreign bodies.

Imaging examination: if the foreign body is too deep and too long, the physical examination cannot be detected, or it is difficult to take out. Calcium containing foreign bodies can be checked by CT. Soft tissue foreign bodies can be used for MR examination to understand the location of foreign bodies and the formation of granuloma around their tissues. More diagnoses can be made and the location, shape and incarceration of foreign bodies can be identified, so as to provide References for the removal of foreign bodies.

**Treatment**

1. The foreign body should be removed by direct laryngoscope as early as possible. The trachea and foreign body forceps should be prepared before the operation, so that the intraoperative foreign body should be used when the trachea is falling into the trachea. If breathing is difficult, emergency tracheostomy should be performed first. After breathing difficulty is relieved, foreign body can be removed under direct laryngoscope, and foreign body can be removed upward from tracheotomy.
2. Laryngeal foreign body is highly dangerous. We should strengthen education and do not allow children to play with nails, pins and needles etc., and do not cry, or play whiles eating. Children should avoid taking food those contains lots of fishbones or other bones or bone fragments to protect children from inhaling them into respiratory tract accidently.

# Tuberculosis of Otorhinolaryngopharyngology Head and Neck

28

Xiaohui Mi and Jianghua Wan

## 28.1 Tuberculosis of Ear

Tuberculosis of external ear is extremely rare. In recent years, tubercular otitis media and mastoiditis have been reported. Middle ear tuberculosis is secondary to tuberculosis of nasopharynx and tuberculosis of cervical lymph nodes.

**Clinical Manifestations**

The onset of this disease is occult, most of which are painless ear leaks and thinner secretions. In the early stage, there is obvious hearing impairment. First, there is conductive deafness, such as the mixed deafness when the lesions invaded the inner ear. There is typical change of the tympanic membrane with multiple perforations, but because of the rapid fusion of perforation, it is generally seen as a single large perforation in the tension part and the edge can reach the drum groove. If there is no purulent infection, the tympanic mucous membrane is mostly pale white, and the proliferating granulation is visible. Facial paralysis and vertigo can occur when facial nerve canal and bone labyrinth are destroyed. The lateral osseous wall of the mastoid is destroyed and breaks through the ear, forming a posterior ear fistula. The CT of the temporal bone shows destruction of the tympanic cavity and mastoid bone, and there is a soft tissue shadow, and bone necrosis is common. Intracranial lesions can be accompanied by complications such as tuberculous meningitis.

**Diagnosis**

Diagnosis of chronic otitis media, such as recurrent otorrhea, hearing loss, and chest X-ray shows pulmonary tuberculosis. The final diagnosis depends on pathological examination, and it should be identified from suppurative otitis media and ear tumor. Pathological examination can differentiate.

**Treatment**

Early systemic use of anti tuberculosis drugs combined with mastoid radical mastoidectomy to remove the focus is the principle treatment of this disease. If there is a dead bone formation, a posterior ear fistula, a local drainage or a facial paralysis, a radical mastoid operation should be performed as long as the patient's general condition is good. If tympanoplasty is made, it should be carried out at second phase.

## 28.2 Tuberculosis of Nose

**Etiology**

Tuberculosis of the nasal cavity is rare. Most of the secondary tuberculosis focuses on other sites. The lesion is well distributed in the anterior nasal septum, and the base of the nasal cavity, the lateral wall and the nasal vestibule may also be invaded. The lesions are shades of ulcer, with uneven edges, wound coated pseudomembrane or crusts, underneath, are the pale soft callous or granulation. In severe cases there is nasal septum perforation, saddle nose, nasal and facial fistula.

**Clinical Manifestation**

1. Nasal Pain.
2. Nasal Congestion: turbinate swelling (abscess), exudation, or granuloma of the nasal cavity.
3. Nasal Bleeding: the formation of nasal mucosa ulcers which bleed on touching.
4. Malformation: the tip of the nose collapses and a scar is formed.

X. Mi (✉)
Department of Otorhinolaryngology Head and Neck Surgery, Chinese People's Liberation Army 91458 Military Hospital, Sanya, China

J. Wan
Department of Medical Imaging, The First Affiliated Hospital of Hainan Medical University, Haikou, China



Z. Mu, J. Fang (eds.), *Practical Otorhinolaryngology - Head and Neck Surgery*, https://doi.org/10.1007/978-981-13-7993-2_28

**Diagnosis**

Chronic nasal ulcers, erosions and history of tuberculosis. The possibility of nasal tuberculosis should be considered, and the diagnosis is based on biopsy.

It should be identified from nasal sclerosis, nasal leprosy, nasal syphilis and nasal tumor.

**Treatment**

In addition to the treatment of systemic tuberculosis, remove the crusts or any local ulcer etc. and give, rifampicin or 0.5% streptomycin nosal drops or, 30% three chloro acetic acid.

## 28.3 Tuberculosis of Pharynx

**Etiology**

Pharyngeal tuberculosis is secondary to the mucous membrane of tubercle bacillus infected with sputum, which is caused by ascending infection of laryngeal tuberculosis. It can also be caused by blood transmission. The incidence is mostly in young adults, more in males than females. Miliary tuberculosis of pharynx, good hair at the soft palate, palatal or pharyngeal etc. Chronic ulcer type tuberculosis of pharynx occurs in the palatal or pharyngeal wall.

**Clinical Manifestations**

It can be divided into two types; acute miliary and chronic ulcerative, miliary pharyngeal tuberculosis often secondary to active or miliary tuberculosis.

1. Acute miliary tuberculosis of pharynx, is often secondary to active or miliary tuberculosis, patients present with obvious symptoms of systemic poisoning, severe pharyngache, particularly when swallowing, and often radiation to the ear. The visible pharyngeal mucosa is pale, soft palate, palatal or pharyngeal have scattered miliary nodules, which is rapidly develops into an irregularly edged, shallow ulcer edge, with an exudate on the surface.
2. Chronic Ulcerative Tuberculosis of Pharynx: in palatal or pharyngeal mucosa, shows pale edematous ulcerative lesions ranging from one or more with slow development, ulcers with deep development, can cause soft palate perforation, palatal or uvula defect, scar after healing of nasopharyngeal tuberculosis can cause atresia. There were no special symptoms of palatine tonsil and pharyngeal tonsil tuberculosis, and most of them were found in pathological examination after surgical excision.

**Diagnosis**

History of pulmonary tuberculosis and chest X-ray examination, we can find the combined tuberculosis, but it is not a necessary condition. MR scan of the nasopharynx shows lesions, mainly manifested as thickening of the mucous membrane, granulation tissue and lymph node enlargement (Fig. 28.1). But the final diagnosis should be confirmed by the biopsy of the neck lymph node or the pharynx. It should be identified from pharynx syphilis and pharynx leprosy, nasopharyngeal tuberculosis should be identified from nasopharyngeal carcinoma and the pathological examination should be confirmed.

**Treatment**

With systemic anti-tuberculosis treatment, for those with severe local pain, 0.5~ 1% tetracaine can be used to spray throat to relieve pain temporarily, and the surface of ulcer can be coated with 30% three-chloroacetic acid or 20% silver nitrate. Surgical treatment can be considered in patients with scar contracture or atresia.

## 28.4 Tuberculosis of Larynx

Secondary laryngeal tuberculosis is the most common otolaryngology tuberculosis, primary laryngeal tuberculosis is rare, but in recent years there is a growing trend.

**Etiology**

This disease is secondary to sputum positive infiltrating tuberculosis or miliary tuberculosis. Its often accompanied by pharyngeal tuberculosis or gastrointestinal tuberculosis. It occurs in the posterior part of the larynx, such as the interarytenoid area, arytenoid cartilage, vocal cord, ventricular band, epiglottis etc. It can be transmitted through contact, blood circulation or lymphatic transmission. Contact infection is carrier's sputum directly attached to laryngeal mucosa or mucosal wrinkles, and it is more susceptible to infection when the mucous membrane is damaged. It is more in young men at the age of 20~30. However, with the increase in the incidence of tuberculosis in the elderly, there is an increased onsetof laryngeal tuberculosis in the middle aged and old aged. Laryngeal TB according to pathological changes can be divided into three types.

1. Infiltrating Type: localized congestion and edema of mucous membrane, infiltration of lymphocytes under the mucous membrane, forming nodules.
2. Ulcerative Type: caseous necrosis occurred in the center of tubercular nodules, forming tuberculous ulcers, often accompanied by secondary infection. It is characterized by an irregular lurking edge around the ulcer. The progress of the disease can invade the laryngeal perichondrium and cause soft periostitis.
3. Hyperplastic: Advanced infiltration of fibrous tissue, when the condition is better, it can be cicatricial and some of the lesions form a tuberculoma.

The early symptoms are a burning sensation and dryness in the larynx.

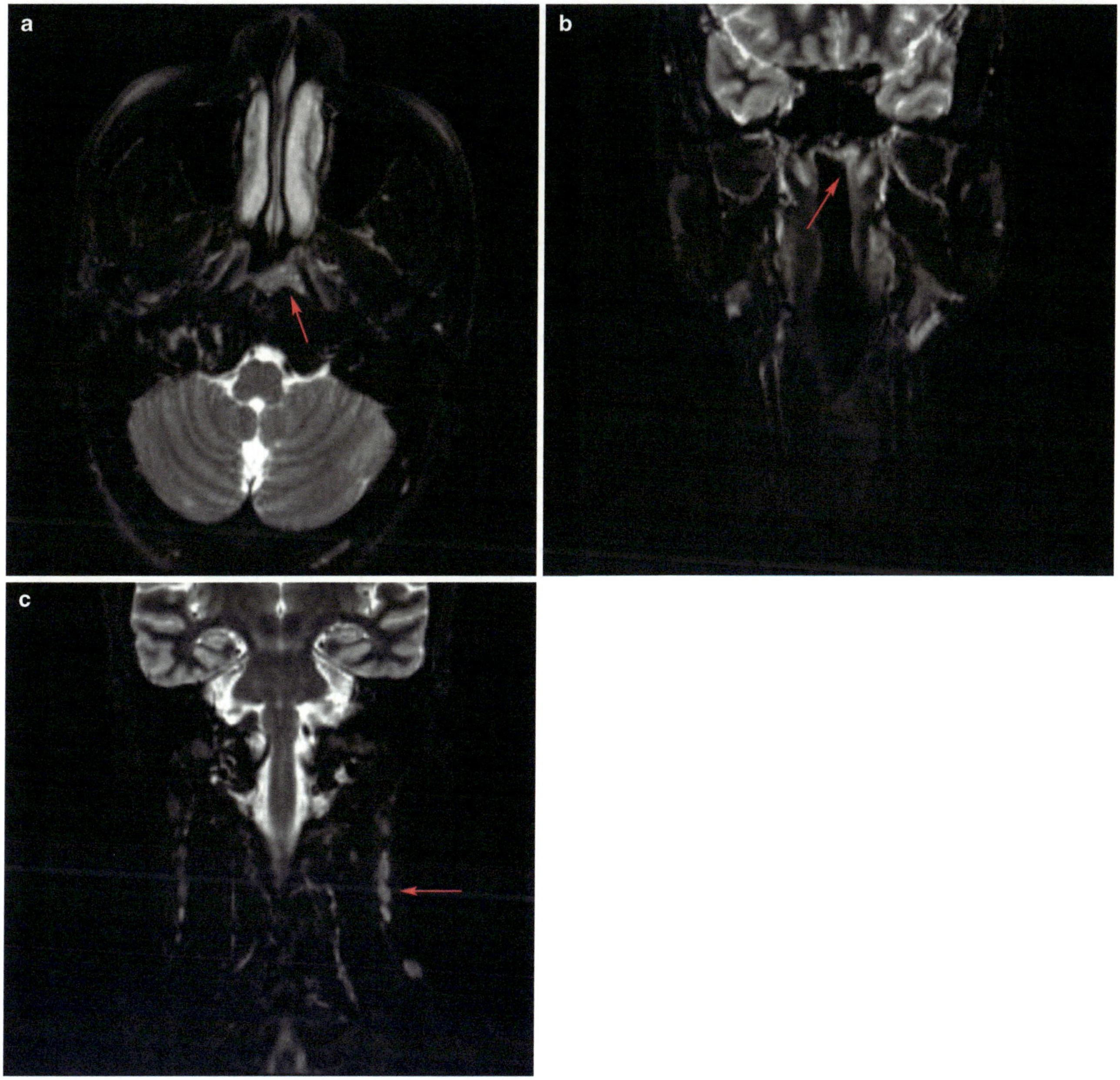


**Fig. 28.1** plain scan of nasopharynx (axial T2WI and coronal STIR) showed tuberculosis on the left side of the nasopharynx, MR. (**a**, **b**) in the left posterior pharyngeal wall and the top wall thickening of mucosa (arrow) (**c**) on the left side of the neck lymph node increased slightly, increased (arrow) is very difficult to distinguish from nasopharyngeal carcinoma, and the diagnosis is nasopharyngeal tuberculosis

1. As main symptom, hoarseness begins with a low and weak voice, then the voice would disappear gradually.
2. Pain in The Larynx: aggravated when swallowing or pronouncing, especially in the cartilage membrane.
3. Dyspnea: when the lesion is extensive, it can be difficult to breathe because of granulosis and tissue edema.

**Diagnosis**

Diagnosis can still rely on pathological examination of the pathological tissues. Chest radiography shows pulmonary tuberculosis in suspected cases. But we should be careful that a few patients have no positive lung and MR scan shows calcified or old lesions in the larynx of many cases. The main manifestations are the thickening of mucous membrane, the formation of granulation tissue and the enlargement of lymph nodes. But the final diagnosis requires a biopsy of the neck lymph node or the larynx. Bacteriological examination includes sputum smear test, acid fast bacilli and bacterial culture. The former is simple and convenient, but negative results cannot be negated by diagnosis. The latter takes too long.

**Treatment**

1. General treatment is enough rest, adequate nutrition, symptomatic treatment.
2. Reasonable early anti tuberculosis treatment is the principle, joint, regular pattern and full use of drugs; the choice of drug is isoniazid (INH), Rifampcin (REP) and pyrazinamide (PZA), etc.
3. Patients with local treatment of laryngeal TB should avoid taking excitant food. When there is severe laryngeal pain, 1% of superior Procaine could be applied to block nerve of larynx and spray 1% of tetracacine on throat before having food; When there is sever dyspnea, tracheotomy should be applied in time.

## 28.5 Tuberculosis of Cervical Lymph Node

**Etiology**

Eighty percent tuberculosis of the neck lymph node is found in children and adolescents. *Mycobacterium tuberculosis* is mostly manifested by oral (dental caries), tonsil or nasopharynx primary infection. There is no invasion site of clinical tuberculosis lesions in general, it will occur when there is immunosuppression, the bacteria is spread through the lymphatic or intrathoracic tuberculosis lesions involving the mediastinum, paratracheal lymph nodes, to cervical lymph nodes, only a handful of a blood infection.

**Clinical Manifestations**

Some patients have symptoms of tuberculosis poisoning such as fatigue, low grade fever, night sweats, lack of appetite, and emaciation. The superficial or deep lymph nodes of one or both sides of the neck are enlarged, usually located below the mandible and the anterior and posterior margin of the sternocleidomastoid muscle. At the early stage, the enlarged lymph nodes are separated from each other. They can move without pain. Afterwards, the enlarged lymph nodes adhereto each other, forming beadedtenderness. If secondary infection and tenderness are obvious, the enlarged lymph nodes often have adhesion with skin and surrounding tissues, and the mobility is poor. Later, enlargement of lymph nodes can cause caseous necrosis, forming cold abscesses, the local skin is shiny and purple, touching wave motion, abscesses and ulcers, forming uneasy healing ulcers or fistulas, and spills outside the fistula. Some patients show symptoms of pulmonary tuberculosis and laryngeal tuberculosis, such as coughing, hemoptysis, and laryngia.

**Diagnosis**

Multiple or enlarged bead-like lymph nodes on one or both sides of the neck, adhewithering to the skin and surrounding tissues, or rupture of the skin, forming a fistula which is not able to heal. It is generally diagnosed. Chest X-ray or CT scan and neck CT or MRI examination, preferably plain scan with enhancement, can clearly show the imaging features of enlarged lymph nodes and its central necrosis. MRI has better effect. Combined with the history of pulmonary tuberculosis, it can be diagnosed (Fig. 28.2). Indirect laryngoscopy

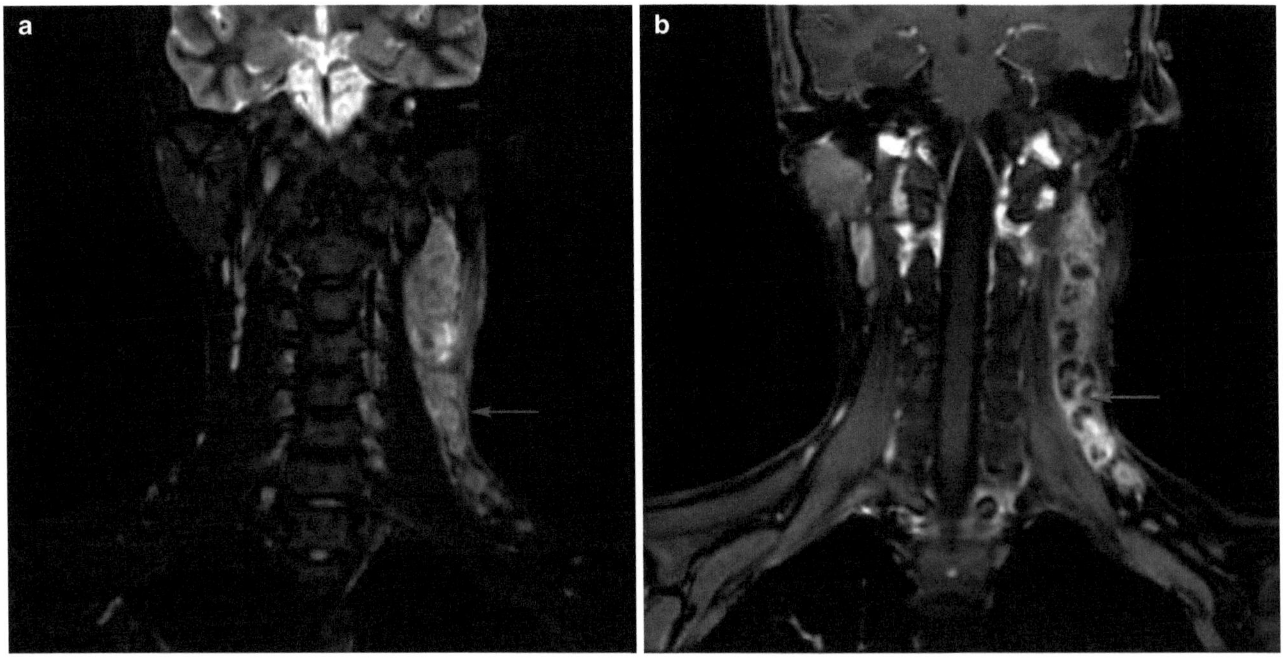


**Fig. 28.2** cervical MRI imaging displays left cervical lymphatic tuberculosis. (**a**) MRI coronal (STIR) plain scan shows that the left lymph nodes appear bead-like, $T_2$ signal increased, and (**b**) MRI coronal enhanced Scan shows irregular ring enhancement, suggesting necrosis of the center, and imaging findings of MRI feature

and posterior rhinoscopy can sometimes show laryngeal tuberculosis and tuberculosis of nasopharynx. The test of tuberculin, tuberculosis antibody and erythrocyte sedimentation rate are helpful in the diagnosis. This disease should be identified from chronic lymphadenitis of the neck, primary and metastatic malignant tumors of the neck.

**Treatment**

1. The general treatment includes proper nutrition.
2. Anti tuberculosis drugs commonly used are streptomycin, isoniazid, rifampicin and pyrazinamide.
   (a) Local treatment of abscess or fistula, through local aspiration, washing, and injection of anti tuberculosis drugs.
   (b) Immunotherapy: use of transfer factor, levamisole, immune ribonucleic acid, dead BCG skin scratch, and intramuscular injection of BCG polysaccharide nucleic acid.
3. Surgical excision is not general advocated treatment method, surgical excision would only be applied when there are a few large solitary lymph nodes.

# 29 Other Special Diseases and Treatment

Xiaohui Mi and Jianghua Wan

## 29.1 Syphilis of Otorhinolaryngopharynx

**Etiology**

Syphilis is a systemic infectious disease caused by Treponema pallidum, which can involve multiple or single organs. Syphilis can be divided into congenital and acquired syphilis. Congenital syphilis is transmitted through mother to child. Acquired syphilis is transmitted mainly through sexual pathways, blood transfusion and breastfeeding. Damaged skin and mucous membrane can also be infected by body fluids and saliva with pathogens.

Treponema pallidum can intrude skin or mucous membrane of the human body, which can invade multiple organs and become complex. The disease is asymptomatic for many years but later causes various various symptoms. The early invasion of the skin and mucous membrane is manifested by an ulceration. In the late stage, the heart, central nervous system, viscera, and bones can be invaded. There is no internal and external toxin in Treponema pallidum, and the pathogenesis is still not clear. The strength of the immune system determines the outcome of the infection. The organism can produce humoral immunity and delayed allergy to the pathogen, and local granulomatosis is formed. There are two basic diseases of syphilis: (1) focal occlusive arteritis and perivascular inflammation; (2) syphilis granuloma. The progression of invading pathogens can be divided into three stages: first stage: hard chancre period, second stage: syphilis rash and third stage: syphilis tumor stage.

X. Mi (✉)
Department of Otorhinolaryngology Head and Neck Surgery, Chinese People's Liberation Army 91458 Military Hospital, Sanya, China

J. Wan
Department of Medical Imaging, The First Affiliated Hospital of Hainan Medical University, Haikou, China

**Clinical Manifestations**

Syphilis has a certain specificity in Otolaryngology, and it is sometimes easy to diagnose with the epidemiological characteristics of the patients. However, some patients begin to appear only in general inflammation, which is difficult for clinical diagnosis.

1. Ears Syphilis: early congenital syphilis patients are mostly in the first 1~2 years of birth, and late congenital syphilis often occurs at the age of 8~10 years. The patient has deafness and vertigo. Hutchinson triad is called labyrinthine, interstitial keratitis and serrated teeth in patients with congenital syphilis. If the bone is broken into the labyrinthine fistula or annular ligament to soften the stapes loose, it appears normal and the middle ear fistula test is positive, known as Herbert syndrome. Labyrinthine and facial paralysis can also occur in patients with acquired syphilis. The symptoms of acquired inner ear syphilis and late congenital inner ear syphilis are basically the same, and facial nerve paralysis and labyrinthine can occur.
2. Nasal Syphilis is divided into congenital and postnatal nature. The syphilis may infringe on the nose at all stages, which is seen in the three stages. Primary syphilis is rare. Second stage syphilis often involves nasal septum and anterior inferior turbinate. The local mucosa is red, swollen and erosive. It can form white mucous patches. It is called syphilitic rhinitis, which is highly infectious. The characteristics of early congenital syphilis are similar to that of this period, and can be found at 1~3 months after birth. Secretion block make the children crying uneasy, breathing and suckling are difficult. Late congenital syphilis and acquired syphilis are manifested in three stages, and the nasal septum is mainly damaged which causes the nasal shape to change. At the age of 3 to puberty, the Hutchinson triple sign is often accompanied by the collapse of the nose. Patients with syphilis tumor invasion of nasal septum and the hard palate bone have a perforated nasal septum and hard palate, a saddle nose and even nasal damage.


Z. Mu, J. Fang (eds.), *Practical Otorhinolaryngology - Head and Neck Surgery*, https://doi.org/10.1007/978-981-13-7993-2_29

3. Pharynx Syphilis: the pharynx lymphoid tissue is rich, and the syphilis may occur in the pharynx at various stages. Pharynx syphilis is rare, and is usually on one side tonsil chancre, ipsilateral cervical lymph node hardens second stage syphilis of pharynx in about 2 months after the emergence of scarlet fever and rash manifested by pharyngitis, throat congestion, swollen tonsils, oral and pharyngeal mucosa often appears with gray round or oval infiltrating.

   Third stage is often accompanied by generalized lymphadenopathy and diffuse rash. The third stage of syphilis of the pharynx occurs years after the initial infection, syphilis lesions by tumor infiltration, softening, ulceration, and finally the formation of scar contracture, can appear. There is perforation of the hard palate pharyngeal tissue, adhesion, stenosis or atresia deformity.
4. Laryngeal Syphilis
   (a) A period of Laryngeal Syphilis: is extremely rare. It can appear as an epiglottis chancre.
   (b) Second Stage Laryngeal Syphilis: Is similar to catarrhal laryngitis, there is laryngeal mucosa diffuse hyperemia. In addition, the mucous plaque can occur in the vocal cords and the dipper area, which is often accompanied by systemic rash and pharynx mucous plaque.
   (c) Third stage laryngeal syphilis: first or second stage syphilis is slightly more common, the common symptoms vary, change of voice to a light, or hoarseness, cough and a mild pharyngache (this is different from the laryngeal tuberculosis), dysphagia (epiglottis, tongue and lateral pharyngeal wall involvement). There are four common types: (1) gumma, mostly located in epiglottis, is a dip-like epiglottis, dark red or purple red arytenoid cartilage, involving the vocal cord or ventricular zone (2) The ulcer formation, the gum swells after the formation of an ulcer covered with yellow rotting tissue, the surrounding tissue is hyperemic There is soft periostitis and necrosis, the ulcer develops in depth, caused by laryngeal cartilage necrosis deformity. If the thyroid cartilage or cricoid cartilage is necrotic, then laryngeal stenosis will occur. The scar and adhesion, due to ulcers and perichondritis after healing, fibrous tissue hyperplasia evolved between the epiglottis and tongue, adhesion between or on both sides of the vocal cords, can also occur in arytenoid cartilage causing a deformity.

**Diagnosis**

1. There is a history of an unprotected sexual contact with a syphilis partner.
2. The clinical symptoms and signs conform to the characteristics of mucous syphilis.
3. Histopathological examination reveals histologic evidence of mucous syphilis.
4. Serological screening tests for syphilis and positive test for syphilis specific diagnosis are positive.

**Treatment**

1. Treatment: penicillin is the first choice for syphilis. Erythromycin can be used in patients allergic to penicillin.
2. Symptomatic treatment with saline, boric acid, hydrogen peroxide solution, Furacilin Solution to clean the wound, and keep it clean; for the repair of the scar deformity, a plastic Operation is feasible.

Otolaryngology syphilis has its specific manifestations. However, it is difficult to diagnose patients with general inflammation and deny the history of epidemiology. Therefore, serious medical examination and medical history collection are very important for the diagnosis.

## 29.2 AIDS Manifestation at Otorhinolaryngopharyngology Head and Neck

40~70% of AIDS patients have otolaryngology head and neck lesions. The neck of AIDS patients is mainly manifested as cervical lymph node enlargement, which is one of the early symptoms. Due to HIV infection, follicular hyperplasia is often seen, and cervical lymph node enlargement is common, especially in the posterior cervical trigone area. Kaposi's sarcoma can also occur in the skin of the head and neck. When it invades the lymph nodes of the neck, they increase rapidly, a on Hodgkin's lymphoma and mycobacterial infection should also be considered when there are neck masses. A fine needle aspiration is helpful for the diagnosis and differential diagnosis. Squamous cell carcinoma in the head and neck is also more common in AIDS patients. The virus infection can cause parotid enlargement.

**Etiology**

HIV is a virus in the family lentivirus. It is a single strand RNA virus, which has a lifetime in the host. When HIV invades the human body, it can adsorb on the surface of CD4+T cells, enter the cells through the cell membrane and integrate into the DNA of CD4+T cells, resulting in the decrease of CD4+T cell number, the CD4+T lymphocyte dysfunction and cause an abnormal immune activation. The inhibitory/cytotoxic lymphocytes (CD8+T lymphocytes) in HIV infected patients show normal or increasing number of functions, which may contribute to further immunodeficiency and lead to CD4+T/CD8+T < 1. HIV can also infect non lymphocyte, such as macrophages, small neuroglia cells, various endothelial and epithelial cells. HIV can adhere to the surface of dendritic cells in the lymph nodes but does not invade the cells. HIV infection results in the number of functional of T cells, B cells, natural killer cells, monocytes and macrophages, which are characterized by opportunistic infections, malignancies, neurological dysfunction and other syndromes.

**Clinical Manifestations**

There are a variety of general manifestations of HIV infection, but it is often non-specific. It is easy to be misdiagnosed. Some patients have HIV infection before physical examination or preoperative examination. In general, infected people usually have infection and new organisms in the otolaryngology. These symptoms and signs can occur in one site or in multiple sites. In addition, the degree of immunosuppression in patients can affect the severity of the infection, the probability of occurrence, and the response of the infection to a new biological treatment.

1. Ear Manifestations: the ear manifestations of AIDS patients show multiple hemorrhagic card Posey's sarcoma, Pneumocystis carinii infection, otitis media, hearing impairment etc. Multiple hemorrhagic Posey's sarcoma can occur in the auricle and external auditory canal, showing red purple patches or nodules slightly higher to skin surface, with different sizes, unequally from several millimeters to several centimeters. The outer otic pneumocystis carinii infection manifestates the multilocular cyst, and the protozoon could be found on the biopsy. The pneumocystis serous otitis media often occurs in adults, and HIV can be detected from the tympanic effusion. Among the infants, acute otitis media caused by the fungi, protozoan, virus or myobacteria can be observed from the pus culture. The HIV easily invades the central nervous system or auditory nerve, commonly leading to a sensory neural hearing loss at an early stage.
2. Rhinal and Rhinosinuses' Manifestation

   The AIDS patient's nose and rhinosinus mainly manifest all kinds of symptoms and signs evoked by the amebic protozoa, cytomegalovirus, herpes virus, cryptococcal infection etc. The amebic protozoa infection could cause the rhinal and rhinosinus mucosa to swell and cause a pus snot or the epistaxis to the rhinobyon and other symptoms. The cytomegalovirus infection can cause suppurated rhinitis, the granules and the erythema existing at the rhinomucosa, and the cytomegalovirus inclusion body and the squamous metaplasia at the intravascular endothelial cells can be seen at rhinomucosal biopsy. The herpes virus infection can cause a herpetic ulcer, expanding from the rhinovestibule to the rhinoseptum and the adjacent rhinoala and facial segment. The cryptococcal infection can cause the whole group rhinosinusitis. Besides, the lymphoma and Kaposis sarcoma can also occur.
3. Lingual and Laryngeal Manifestation

   The AIDS patients' oral and pharyngeal manifestations are mainly monilial infection, villous mucosal leukoderma, single herpes, amygdalitis, and Kaposi's sarcoma, etc.
4. Laryngeal Manifestation

   The AIDS patients' laryngeal manifestations are mainly the Kaposi's sarcoma and the monilial infection, that finally leads to hoarseness, laryngostridor and laryngostasis.
5. Cervicocranial Manifestation

   The AIDS patients cervical manifestation is based on early symptoms. It mainly manifests as cervicolymphatic swelling, Kaposis sarcoma, non-hodgkin lymphoma, mycobacteria infection and other infections, squamous cell carcinoma, parotid swellings etc. The cervical lymphatic swelling is commonly seen and is HIV evoked. Follicular hyperplasia is usually seen at the supracervical triangle region. The Kaposis sarcoma can occur on the cervicocranial skin, and when it invades the cervical lymph nodes, they will rapidly enlarge. The cervicocranial squamous-cell carcinoma is also oftenly seen. The virus infection and other infection can cause the parotid to swell, and it is also tagged as the AIDS omen.

**Diagnosis**

Based on the disease history, clinic manifestation and lab examination results, diagnosis could be made.

1. History Detail Enquiry

   Especially in the homosexuality, promiscious sexual behavior, intravenous drug-taking, blood transfusion and other histories should be taken.
2. Infection-Possibility Manifestation

   Such as to the pneumocystic carnii pneumonia and the Kaposi's sarcoma patient, this is an important diagnosis. Long-term and low-grade fever, diarrhea, emaciation and systemic lymphatic swelling combined with oral, pharyngeal and other regions' monilial infection, this is all similar to the AIDS premonitory symptoms and they should be paid attention to cautiously.
3. Immunity-Deficiency-Metrics CD4+T Cells Reduction

   The Center for Disease Control and Prevention (CDC) revised-diagnosis-gist noticed in 1991 that the CD4+T < $200/mm^3$ could be diagnosed as the AIDS. Besides; there should be CD4+T/CD8+T < 1.
4. HIV Lab Diagnosis

   It include virus isolation culture, antigen detection, antibody detection, virus nucleic acid detection, etc.

When the primary screening test result is positive, recheck to avoid false positive results and if latter result is positive, ascertain an HIV infection existence. HIV antibody can be commonly detected 2 months after the time of infection.

**Treatment**

1. Anti-HIV-virus drug
2. Immunoregulation drug
3. Prevention and treatment of opportunistic infections.
4. Traditional Chinese Medicine treatment

AIDS otorhinopharyngocervicocranial manifestations vary, but they lack specificity, so it's not hard to misdiagnose. The AIDS incidence is higher, and the medical personnel should enhance the vigilance to the AIDS and improve its cognition.

## 29.3 Leprosy of Otorhinolaryngopharyngology

**Etiology**

Leprosy is a chronic inflammatory disease evoked by the mycobacterium leprae. The pathogenic bacteria's detection rate is related to the leprosy types. Relatively more mycobacterium leprae can be found in the lepra lepromatosa patients' mucosa, skin and lymph nodes; but the tuberculoid leprosy's pathogenic bacteria isn't easy to detect and it mainly damages the skin, mucosa and the peripheral nerves. The rhinoleprosy is the most favored type, and the nose is also the earliest invaded region. Leprosy is mainly acquired through touching and after being infected, the incubation period is very long and the lesion develops slowly.

**Clinical Manifestation**

Except the systemic manifestations, its otorhinopharyngolaryngeal manifestations are as follows.

1. Otic Leprosy

   It mainly occurs at the auricle, especially the ear lobule. Its main manifestations are the local infiltration, nodular formation, ulceration, cicatrix, and the skin folds and tissue defects etc. The great auricular nerve bulges and there is pain on palpation. These are the diagnosis valuable symptoms. The facial nerve spasm and (or) paralysis is caused by the stimulation from the lesion invasion.
2. Rhinal Leprosy

   Rhinal leprosy is the most common one in the otorhinopharyngolaryngeal leprosy, and nose is one of the leprous earliest invaded regions. It is nearly all lepra lepromatosa. The early lesion invades the rhinovestibular hair follicle, which causes loss of the rhinothrix, there is an ulcer formation and the rhinocavum submucosal nobular infiltration, then the nubular diabrosis could cause the refractory ulcer or cicatrical synechia; at the late stage, the mucosal gland bodies shrink, the dry rhinocavum incrustates and presents a change similar to the atrophic rhinitis. In severe patients, their rhinoseptum cartilage perforates, the rhinocolumella damages, the rhinal apex collapses and abutts to the upper lip, so it is easy to differentiate it from the saddle nose caused by the atrophic rhinitis and syphilis. In rhinoleprosy secretion, abundant of the mycobacterium leprae often exist, so this disease has high infectivity.
3. Pharyngeal Leprosy

   It is mostly caused by the desposingly extending rhinal lepra lepromatosa. Except presenting the acute edema at the early stage, the pharyngomucosa commonly manifest as dryness, escharosis, infiltrated nubule and ulceration; if necrosis exists, the open rhinolalia symptom and eating reflux symptom may occurs.
4. Laryngeal Leprosy

   It is mainly secondary to the rhinal and the pharyngeal leprosy, favorably occurring at the epiglottis root and its anterior commissure, secondarily at the arytenoid epiglottis folds and the ventricular cords. It manifests the nobular infiltration and ulceration, and finally cicatrizates. On examination, there is epiglottis congestion or paleness, incrassation, crinked deformity, and even damage can occur. Hoarseness, stridor and slight dyspnea can occur.

   Leprosy commonly incubates for a long time and develops slowly. But under some conditions, like climate change, infection, emotional change and others, the acute or subacute symptoms suddenly occur, which is also called the leprosy reaction. The reaction contains two types: the type I and the type II. The type I is the cellular immunity allergic reaction, manifesting as skin redness and swelling, local pyrexia, nerve trunk lesion sudden augmentation and obvious pain, but no systemic symptoms. The type II is the immunity complex allergic reaction, consisting the systemic symptoms, such as fever, headache and systemic lymphatic swelling, joint gall, existance of a skin erythema, pain and acute iris conjunctivitis, acute orchitis, etc.

**Diagnosis**

Primary diagnosis can be made based on the leprosy contraction history and the typical damage manifestations at the skin, the mucosal and the peripheral nerves, and the diagnosis could be ascertained if the mycobacterium leprae is found on examination from the secretions got from the lesion or the biopsy. The upper respiratory tract leprosy lesion should be differentiated from tuberculosis and the syphilis.

**Treatment**

Systemic anti-leprosy treatment is the main method, accompanied with each otorhinopharyngolaryngeal regional symptomatic therapy.

1. Systemic Treatment

   Main leprosy bacillus's therapeutic drugs include the dapsone, the rifampicin, protionamide, clofazimine etc., and the recent proposition is the alternative-three drugs combination.
2. Symptomatic Treatment

   It is mainly used to dispose the leprosous reaction, from preventing and avoiding the aggravated abnormality. Its main therapeutic drugs include glucocorticoid, thalidomide (thalidomide), etc. If there is relatively more severe neurodynia, procaine could help the local sealing.
3. Local Treatment

   Clearing the rhinocavum crusta prevents the secondary infection. Lubricate the rhinocavum with the liquid paraffin, peppermint oil etc., or relieve the symptoms by daubing the rhinocavum with the Aureomycin or the erythromycin ointment. The local ulcerations can be cauterized with the 30% trichoroacetic acid (TCS).

## 29.4 Diphtheria of Otorhinolaryngopharyngology

**Etiology**

Diphtheria is a kind of acute respiratory tract inflammation caused by the corynebacterium diphteriae. Its main lesion includes the pharyngeal and the laryngeal mucosal congestional swelling, necrosis and exudation, which develops its specific hard-deciduous incanus pseudo-membrane and the systemic poisoning symptoms evoked by the diptheria exotoxin. The air droplets or the bacterial-contaminated towels, table ware, toys, books and newspapers and other methods, mainly transmit it. Diphtheritis commonly occurs in autumn, winter and spring, and is mainly in infants younger than 10-year-old, of which the 2~5-year-old incidences are the highest. Because of improved living conditions and widely arranged prophylactic vaccination, the diphtheric incidence has evidently decreased, and is rarely seen at recent time.

**Clinical Manifestation**

1. Pharyngeal Diphtheritis

   It is the most common type of the diphtheritis, with 80% incidence. In clinic, it is divided into three types: the limited type, the dispersal type and the poisoning type.

   (a) The Limited Type

   This type onset is slow, its systemic manifestations are fever, weakness, inappetence etc. Its local symptoms are mild, with slight pharyngeal pain. On the tonsil, the incanus pseudomembrane can be seen, and the pseudomembrane surpasses the palatoglossal arch, covering the soft palatine and the uvula or the postpharyngeal wall. The pseudomembrane adheres closely to the tissues, indelible, and if forcibly peeled, bleeding will occur. With the pseudomembranous smear or culture, the corynebacterium diphtheriae will be seen.

   (b) The Dispersal Type

   Its lesion often surpasses the tonsil, involves the palatina arch, soft palatine, uvula or the postpharyngeal wall, rhinopharynx or the larynx. The pseudomembrane is lamellar. The systemic symptoms are relatively evident, including slight or moderate fever, accompanied by weakness, the inappetence, nausea, emesis, headache and cervical lymphadenectasis.

   (c) The Poisoning Type

   This type onsets acutely, the pseudomembrane expands rapidly, and the systemic poisoning symptoms soon occur, such as high fever, fidget, polypnea, pallor, lips' cyanosis, cold limbs, fine-speedy pulse, low blood pressure, arrhythmia, etc. The pharyngomucosa, tonsil, uvula and palatina arch obviously swell. There is cervical lymph nodes tumefication, soft tissues edema, even neck augments like a 'bovine neck', and severe complications can occur, such as the myocarditis, leading to heart failure, cardiogenc shock (CGS), etc.
2. Laryngeal Diphtheritis

   It occurs in 20% diphtheritis cases, it is also caused by the pharyngo-diphtheritis despondingly extending to the larynx, and occasionally it originates from the larynx. It onsets is slow, its tussiculation sounds like barking and there is hoarseness. When the laryngeal tumidness or the pseudomembrane obstructs the glottis, it causes inhaled dyspnea and laryngeal stridor, the three-concave sign and cyanosis can occur if the obstruction becomes more severe, even the patients will die from suffocation if the obstructions aren't relieved. The laryngeal lesion extends downwards to the trachea and the bronchus to evoke lower respiratory tract obstruction.
3. Rhinodiphtheritis

   It is rarely seen, and it includes the primary type and the secondary type. Its rhinal symptoms are similar to the common rhinitis, manifestating as the rhinobyon and a running nose (often stained with blood). At examinations, the rhinovestibular and the upper lip skin versenkbar and erosion can be seen, and it is found that the rhinocavum mucosal surface is covered with the incanus pseudomembrane, especially seen at the rhinoseptum, and if the pseudomembrane is removed, there will be bleeding at the ulceration.

4. Ear Diphtheritis

   It is rarely seen. It is often secondary to the rhinal and the pharyngeal diphtheritis. Nearly none of this type is primary. This type often occurs in 1~6-year-old infant. Its symptoms are similar to the common suppurative otiti media, with severe otalgia, and smelly hemorrhagic pus or the polluted pseudomembrane-like discharge after the tympanic tresis occurs.

**Diagnosis**

According to the disease history, the symptoms and the physical signs, combined with the bacterial examinations, the diagnosis is often not hard. But one time of the negative bacterial result can't exclude the diagnosis, so the bacterial examination should be repeated several times to ascertain the diagnosis at early stage. The bacterial examination methods include; the secretion smear scope, the immunity fluoroscopy and the bacterium culture, and if necessary, the Schick test and the immunochromatographic method should assist diagnosis.

**Treatment**

1. Common Treatment

   Rigorous isolation, 2~4 weeks bed rest (the severe patients should take 4~6 weeks). Pay attention to the oral and the rhinal clearance. Supply enough nutrition. Tracheotomy should be done as early as possible if laryngeal obstruction exists.
2. Etiology Treatment

   The diphtheria antitoxin should be used at the early stage, combined with intravenous sensitive antibiotics drips, whose first choice is penicillin.
3. Complications Treatment

   Pay a close attention to the cardial conditions, if heart damage exists, ask the cardiovascular physicians to assist in the treatment.

## 29.5 Rhinoscleroma

It is a chronic process, inflammatory granulomatous lesion; was first reported in 1870 by Habra. At the International Otorhinopharyngolaryngeal Conference convoked in 1932, it is named as the 'rhino scleroma'. It is a sporadic disease. It has been reported around the world, in China it is mostly in Shandong province, occupying 46% of the total rhinoscleroma cases.

**Etiology**

It usually originates from the nose, and extends to the nasal sinus, soft palatine, hard palatine, pharynx, larynx, trachea, bronchus, rhino lacrimal canals and the middle ear. Besides, this disease can sporadically supervene or secondarily occur at several respiratory regions, so it is also called the respiratory track scleroma.

**Clinical Manifestation**

1. Catarrhal Period

   At this stage, it manifests as the local mucosal desiccation, atrophy, escharosis and hemorrhage. Its primary symptom is the rhinobyon, and if it invades other regions, the manifestation will be the corresponding regional catarrheal symptoms. The patients can restore to normal after treatment. This period could last for several months even several years.
2. Scleroma Stage

   This stage mainly manifestates as rhinal obstruction, external rhinal deformation and nobular lumps exist in the rhinocavum, with a cartilage-like texture, often lying at the rhinovestibule, prenaris, anterior rhino-septum segment, upper lip and other regions, whose surface lightens and aubergine. and if there is secondary infection purulent scab festers could presents at the lump surface and can be smelly or not. This period could last several years or longer a time.
3. Scar Stage

   Because the cicatrix contracts, symptoms, such as closed rhinolalia, hoarseness or dyspnea and others, and physical signs such as the anterior rhinal stenosis, atresia, the nasal alae ingression, uvula disappearance, laryngopharyngostenosis, etc., can occur.

**Diagnosis**

1. Long term, progressive development
2. It always locates at the anterior rhinocavum with hard texture and mostly without ulceration. Outer nose transformation may occur.
3. Without partial pain.
4. Plenty of plasmocyte infiltration with lymph cells and froth cells may manifest on the biopsy under the microscope. Ascertain diagnosis with the Mikulicz cells and the Russel globules appearance and sometimes repeated biopsies are also necessary (Fig. 29.1).
5. Germiculture

   Rhinoscleroma bacillus is positive.
6. Serology Examination

   Complementary fixation butter has high reliability. Apply the early cases more than other stages'.

**Treatment**

1. Antibiotics Treatment

   Commonly, intramuscular 1 g/day streptomycin injection totals 60~120 g, or intramuscular kanamycin or cefazobenzidazole injection.

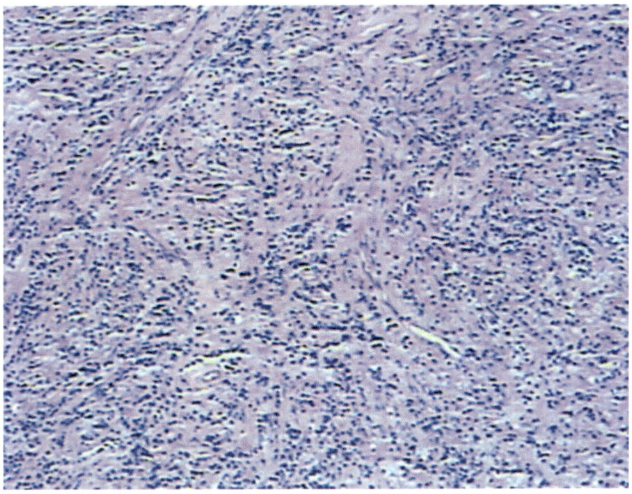

**Fig. 29.1** Rhinoscleroma pathogenesis slice (HE × 10)

2. Radiotherapy

   It could remit the disease progression; total radial quantity is 40~70 Gy.

3. Operation

   Based on the conditions, scar malformation excision Operation can be applied. The scleroma excision Operation can not be applied, or it would evoke severe scar contraction. Do a tracheotomy in case of dyspnea.

# Appendix A: Preoperative Auditory-Speech Development Assessment and Postoperative Restoration Evaluation at Cochlear Implant

| Material name | Contents | Form | Examination system | Applied population |
|---|---|---|---|---|
| Hearing disorder infants audition evaluation gists and methods | Enviromental sound, tone, inital conconant, vowel, disyllable recognition | Closed or open cards | Computer-guiding audition-speech evulation system | Over 2-year-old |
| Hearing disorder infants language skills assessment gists and methods | Speech pronunciation, grammatical competence, sawy, expression ability, communication ability | Speech articulation test, long imitation sentences, computer-guiding audition-speech assessment system | Listen to read images, images description, language function assessment questionnaire | 1~6-year-old |
| Madarin Early Speech Perception Test (MESPT) | Speech sound detection, syllable paradigm, disyllable, initial conconant, vowel, tone perception | Close cards | MAPP software | 2~3-year-old |
| Madarin pediatric speech intelligibility test (MPSIT) | Phrase recognition | Close cards | MAPP software | 3-year-old |
| Madarin Audio-Picture of Infants Distinguishment (MAPID) | Numbers, disyllable and tones (uncer silence and noise) | Close (touch screen images) | MAPPID-N software | 3~9-year-old |
| Lexical Neighbourship Test-Madarin (LNT-M) | Syllable, disyllable recognition | Open | LNT-M software | 4~6-year-old |
| Madarin beta Kids' Brief-sentence Test (MBKBT) | Infants phrases recognition (under silence or noise) | | Fly-love madarin speech test platform | Over 4.5-year-old |
| Madarin Speech Test Materials (MSTMs) | Syllable, disyllable, sentence | | MSTMs software | Adults |
| HOPE speech test materials (HOPE-STMs) | Syllable, disyllable, phrases under silence and noise (audio pattern, vision pattern, audio-vision pattern) | | Fly-love madarin speech test platform | Adults |
| Madarin Hearing In Noise Test (MHINT) | Sentence in noise | | HINT pro software adults version | Adults |
| Madarin Hearing IN Noise Test-Chilren version (M-HINT-C) | Long sentence in silence and noise | | HINT pro software infants version | 6~14-year-old |
| Beta Kids' Brief-sentence Standard-Chinese In Noise Test (BKB-SINT) | Infants phrase in noise | | Fly-love madarin speech test platform | School-children and adults |
| Tone In Noise Test (TINT) | Tone in noise | Close | HINT software | School-children and adults |

Tips: test according to introductions



Z. Mu, J. Fang (eds.), *Practical Otorhinolaryngology - Head and Neck Surgery*, https://doi.org/10.1007/978-981-13-7993-2

# Appendix B: Informed Consent of Cochlear Implant

Name ______ gender ______ age ______ scase no. ______ Preoperation diagnosis ______

I know my relatives/children apply articochlea implantation surgery, which may help it restore auditory ability, but i also master that the surgery may cause risks, such as:

1. Intra-operative risk
   - 1.1 Possible anesthesia risk
   - 1.2 Possible cardiovascular risk and cranial-vascular risk
   - 1.3 Possible intra-operative huge blood transfusion
   - 1.4 Possible temporary or permanent facial paralysis caused by facial nerve damage
   - 1.5 Possible postoperative gustation change caused by tympanic nerve damage
   - 1.6 Possible tympanic membrane puncture and external audio canal puncture
   - 1.7 Possible sigmoid sinus and dura mater damage
   - 1.8 Possible perilymphorrhea and cerebrospinorrhea
   - 1.9 Possible removal and shifting of otosteon, chorda tympanic nerve and other middle ear structures
   - 1.10 Possible incomplete active-electrode implantation or partial electrode damage caused by electrode implantation obstruction
   - 1.11 Possible occurrence of the infeasible electrode implantation caused by internal ear deformity or severe ossification
   - 1.12 Possible operation suspension or first-aid measures caused by sundry factors

2. Postoperative risks
   - 2.1. Possible flap hemorrhage, subcutaneous hematoma, intracranial hematoma
   - 2.2. Possible partial (incision, middle ear, internal ear) infection, flap necrosis, intracranial infection
   - 2.3. Possible postoperative incision cicatrix and post-otic subcutaneous swelling of implanted device
   - 2.4. Possible electrode transposition or prolapse
   - 2.5. Possible skiving reapportion because incrassate flaps effect device usage
   - 2.6. Possible remnant hearing loss or deafness
   - 2.7. Possible tinnitus, vertigo and equilibrium disorder
   - 2.8. Possible facial muscular spasm and other non auditory stimuli during electrical stimulation
   - 2.9. Possible skin allergies caused by wearing devices in vitro or allergies to implant units in vivo

3. other risks
   - 3.1. Possible inconsistent pre-operative expectancy value and post-operative effect
   - 3.2. Possible device failure, requesting operative withdrawing or change
   - 3.3. Possible un-adaptability to new voice, even request to withdraw implanted devices
   - 3.4. Patients can't accept medical treatment, which produce inducing electricity and these treatments include: electrosurgery, diathermy, neuro-stimulation, electroconvulsive therapy and ionizing radiotherapy. Reoperation to withdraw magnet in vivo temporarily during taking MRI.
   - 3.5. Sundry risks increased by other diseases conditions.
   - 3.6. Other unknown risks and accidents.

Patients' family members' (parents) signature______relationship with patients____physician signature_____

____(year)___(month)___(day)



Z. Mu, J. Fang (eds.), *Practical Otorhinolaryngology - Head and Neck Surgery*, https://doi.org/10.1007/978-981-13-7993-2

GPSR Compliance

*The European Union's (EU) General Product Safety Regulation (GPSR) is a set of rules that requires consumer products to be safe and our obligations to ensure this.*

*If you have any concerns about our products, you can contact us on ProductSafety@springernature.com*

In case Publisher is established outside the EU, the EU authorized representative is:

Springer Nature Customer Service Center GmbH
Europaplatz 3
69115 Heidelberg, Germany

**Batch number: 10731661**

Printed by Printforce, the Netherlands